The Paperless Medical Office
Using Harris CareTracker

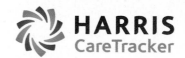

The Paperless Medical Office
Using Harris CareTracker

Virginia Busey Ferrari
Michelle E. Heller

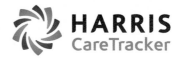

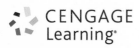

Australia • Brazil • Mexico • Singapore • United Kingdom • United States

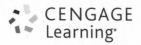

The Paperless Medical Office:
Using Harris CareTracker
Virginia Busey Ferrari, Michelle E. Heller

General Manager: Dawn Gerrain

Product Director: Matthew Seeley

Product Team Manager: Stephen Smith

Senior Director, Development: Marah Bellegarde

Product Development Manager: Juliet Steiner

Content Developer: Lauren Whalen

Product Assistant: Mark Turner

Marketing Director: Michele McTighe

Marketing Manager: Jessica Cipperly

Senior Production Director: Wendy Troeger

Production Manager: Andrew Crouth

Content Project Manager: Thomas Heffernan

Senior Art Director: Jack Pendleton

Cover image(s): iStock.com/traffic_analyzer

For product information and technology assistance, contact us at
Cengage Learning Customer & Sales Support, 1-800-354-9706
For permission to use material from this text or product,
submit all requests online at **www.cengage.com/permissions.**
Further permissions questions can be e-mailed to
permissionrequest@cengage.com

Library of Congress Control Number: 2014931294

ISBN-13: 978-1-133-27895-5

Cengage Learning
200 First Stamford Place, 4th Floor
Stamford, CT 06902
USA

Cengage Learning is a leading provider of customized learning solutions with office locations around the globe, including Singapore, the United Kingdom, Australia, Mexico, Brazil, and Japan. Locate your local office at:
www.cengage.com/global

Cengage Learning products are represented in Canada by Nelson Education, Ltd.

To learn more about Cengage Learning, visit **www.cengage.com**
Purchase any of our products at your local college store or at our preferred online store **www.cengagebrain.com**

Notice to the Reader
Publisher does not warrant or guarantee any of the products described herein or perform any independent analysis in connection with any of the product information contained herein. Publisher does not assume, and expressly disclaims, any obligation to obtain and include information other than that provided to it by the manufacturer. The reader is expressly warned to consider and adopt all safety precautions that might be indicated by the activities described herein and to avoid all potential hazards. By following the instructions contained herein, the reader willingly assumes all risks in connection with such instructions. The publisher makes no representations or warranties of any kind, including but not limited to, the warranties of fitness for particular purpose or merchantability, nor are any such representations implied with respect to the material set forth herein, and the publisher takes no responsibility with respect to such material. The publisher shall not be liable for any special, consequential, or exemplary damages resulting, in whole or part, from the readers' use of, or reliance upon, this material.

Printed in the United States of America
6 7 19 18 17 16

Contents

List of Activities   ix
How to Use the Book   xi
Preface   xv
System Requirements for Harris CareTracker   xxiii

CHAPTER 1

Introduction to the Paperless Medical Office   1

Paper Records vs. Paperless Records   4
   Sustainability   4
   Government Health Initiatives   5
   Converting the Practice   7
Introduction of CEHRS™ Exam Outline   7
   The EHR Specialist—Administrative and Practice Management   9
Administrative Workflows in Harris CareTracker   10
Practice Management   12
   Front Office   12
   Billing   12
   Administrative   14
Classification Systems   15
Coding Systems   16
   International Classification of Diseases (ICD)   17
   Current Procedural Terminology (CPT®)   23
   Healthcare Common Procedural Coding System (HCPCS)   24
Electronic Medical Records   26
   Core Functions of the EMR/EHR   27
   Advantages of Electronic Medical/Health Records   28

   Duties of an EHR Specialist   29
   Pitfalls of the Electronic Health Record   30
Clinical Workflows in Harris CareTracker   31
Common Acronyms and Terminology   33
CEHRS™ Clinical Components   36
   Computer Physician Order Entry   36
   Medical Terminology   37
   Coding Fundamentals   41

CHAPTER 2

Introduction to Harris CareTracker PM and EMR   45

Log in to Harris CareTracker   46
Help System   51
   Using the Harris CareTracker PM and EMR Help Window   51
   Contents   52
   Search   52
   Training   53
   Support   56
   Glossary   57
   Print   57
   Forward and Back   58
Main Menu and Navigation   58
   Home Overview   58
   Dashboard Overview   59
Administration Features and Functions   65
   Practice– Daily Administration   66
   Practice – System Administration   71
   Clinical– Daily Administration   82

Clinical–System Administration   84
Clinical Import/Export   86
Setup   86
Message Center   99
Accessing the Messages Application   99
Message Center Templates   100
ToDo Application   100
Mail   103
Queue   107
Fax Capabilities of Harris CareTracker   108

CHAPTER 3
Patient Demographics and Registration   113

Name Bar   114
Demographics   118
Patient Search   118
Patient Alerts   120
Name   122
Photos   123
Addresses   123
Phones   124
Chart Number   125
Date of Birth   125
Social Security Number   125
Gender (Sex)   125
Notes   126
VIP Flag   127
Responsible Party   129
Insurance Plan(s)   129
Employers   129
Search for a Patient   130
Register New Patients   135
Scan/Attach Insurance Card(s)   146
Print Patient Demographics Report   148
Edit Patient Information   149
Eligibility Checks   151

CHAPTER 4
Appointment Scheduling   157

Book Appointments   159
Booking an Appointment Using Find   166
Forcing an Appointment   169
Reschedule Appointments   171
Cancel Appointments   175
Appointment Conflicts   178
Non-Patient Appointments   180
Add Patient to the Wait List   183
Mini-Menu   185

Daily Schedule   187
Month Application   187
Calendar Display   188
Family   191
Advanced   192
Recalls   193
History   195
TeleVox®   196
Check in Patients   201
Create a Batch   203
Setting Operator Preferences   204
Accept a Payment   211
Journals   216

CHAPTER 5
Preliminary Duties in the EMR   225

Electronic Medical Records   226
Meaningful Use   226
Background of Meaningful Use   226
Tools within Harris CareTracker to Assist Providers with Meaningful Use   229
Activating Care Management   233
Navigating the Medical Record Module   235
Patient Detail Bar   236
Viewing Encounter Information   239
Patient Medical History Pane   241
Clinical Toolbar   243
Chart Summary   245
Maintenance Functions That Affect Harris CareTracker EMR   247
Room Maintenance   247
Custom Resources   250
Favorite Lab Maintenance   251
Manage Immunization Lots   254

CHAPTER 6
Patient Work-Up   263

Setting Operator Preferences in the Batch Application   264
Overview of the Clinical Today Module   265
Appointments   265
Tasks Menu   267
Retrieving and Updating the Patient's Electronic Medical Record   274
Updating the Patient's Medication List   275
Updating the Patient's Allergy Information   280
Updating the Patient's Immunization Status   283
Accessing the History Application   284

Recording Patient's Vital Signs and Chief Complaint 291
Viewing Flow Sheets 296
Pediatric Growth Chart 298
Accessing the Patient Care Management Application 302
Creating Progress Notes 306
Progress Note Templates 306

CHAPTER 7
Completing the Visit 315

Completing Requisitions for Diagnostic Orders 316
Enter New Lab Orders 319
Creating and Printing Prescriptions 330
Create Prescriptions 332
Print Prescriptions 339
Accessing the Immunization Application 346
Add Immunizations 347
Print Immunization Records 352
View the Activity Log of an Immunization 353
Pulling Up and Recording Patient Education 354
Advanced Features for Patient Education 356
Creating Clinical Letters 357
Access the Correspondence Application 359
Add Patient Correspondence 360
Work with Patient Correspondence 363
Activate and Deactivate Correspondence 363
Print the Correspondence Log 364
Creating Referrals 366
Access the Referrals and Authorizations Application 367
Create Outgoing Referrals 367
Create Incoming Referrals 371
Completing a Visit for Billing Purposes 376
Completing a Visit 376
Open Encounters 382
Unsigned Notes 387

CHAPTER 8
Other Clinical Documentation 397

The Progress Notes Application 398
Access and View Progress Notes 399
Filter Progress Note Templates 404
Manage Progress Note Templates 406
Access and Record Results 414
Entering Results Manually 416
Viewing Results 420

Recording Messages 427
Message Center Templates 427
ToDos 428
Mail 432
Recall Letters 443
Add Recalls 444
Update Recall Details 447
Running an Immunization Lot Number Report 448
Immunization Export 448
Immunization Lot Number Report 449

CHAPTER 9
Billing 455

Create a Batch 457
Setting Operator Preferences 457
Manually Enter a Charge 461
Edit an Unposted Charge 471
Journals 475
Generate Claims 478
Electronic Submission of Claims 478
Paper Claim Batches 481
Electronic Remittance 488
Post Payments and Adjustments 489
Insurance Payment Reconciliation and Follow-Up 497
Matching Unmatched Transactions 498
Print Insurance EOBs 499
Denials 502
Credit Balances 509
Unapplied Payments 513
Billing Statements 516
Verify Payments 517
View or Edit Batch Deposits 523

CHAPTER 10
ClaimsManager and Collections 529

ClaimsManager 530
EncoderPro 531
Claims Worklist Overview 532
Claim Summary Fields and Features 535
Work the Claims Worklist 536
Work Crossover Claims 544
Work Unpaid Claims 545
Electronically Checking Claim Status 546
Working Unpaid/Inactive Claims 550
Generate Patient Statements 554
Reprinting Statements 558

Patient Collections   560
  Financial Classes   560
Collection Status   563
  New Status   564
  Open Collection Status   564
  Review Status   564
  Collections Actual Status   564
  Collections Pending Status   565
  Collections Pending – NS Status   565
  Hold Status   565
  Transfer Private Pay Balances   565
  Moving Patients to Collections   566
Collection Actions   567
Collection Letters   573
  Adding a Form Letter to Quick Picks   578
Generate Collection Letters   579

CHAPTER 11
Applied Learning for the Paperless Medical Office   587

Case Study 11-1: Julia Hernandez   587
  Step 1: Register a New Patient and Schedule an Appointment   587
  Step 2: Enter Payment, Check In Patient, and Complete Patient Registration   588
  Step 3: Patient Work-Up   588
  Step 4: Complete the Visit   592
  Step 5: Capture the Visit and Sign the Note   592
  Step 6: Other Clinical Documentation   593
  Step 7: Verify Charges   593
  Step 8: Process Remittance (EOB) and Transfer to Private Pay   593
  Step 9: Work Claims and Generate Patient Statement   593
Case Study 11-2: Delores Simpson   594
  Step 1: Search the Database and Schedule an Appointment   594
  Step 2: Check In Patient   594
  Step 3: Patient Work-Up   594
  Step 4: Complete the Visit   596
  Step 5: Capture the Visit and Sign the Note   596
  Step 6: Verify Charges   597
  Step 7: Process Remittance (EOB) and Transfer to Private Pay   597
  Step 8: Work Claims and Generate Patient Statement   597

Case Study 11-3: Adam Zotto   597
  Step 1: Search the Database and Schedule an Appointment   597
  Step 2: Enter Payment and Check In Patient   598
  Step 3: Patient Work-Up   598
  Step 4: Complete the Visit   601
  Step 5: Capture the Visit and Sign the Note   602
  Step 6: Other Clinical Documentation   602
  Step 7: Verify Charges   603
  Step 8: Process Remittance (EOB) and Transfer to Private Pay   603
  Step 9: Work Claims and Generate Patient Statement   603
Case Study 11-4: Barbara Watson   603
  Step 1: Search the Database and Schedule an Appointment   603
  Step 2: Enter Payment and Check In Patient   604
  Step 3: Patient Work-Up   604
  Step 4: Complete the Visit   606
  Step 5: Capture the Visit and Sign the Note   606
  Step 6: Verify Charges   606
  Step 7: Process Remittance (EOB) and Transfer to Private Pay   606
  Step 8: Work Claims and Generate Patient Statement   607
Case Study 11-5: Craig X. Smith   607
  Step 1: Search the Database and Schedule an Appointment   607
  Step 2: Enter Payment and Check In Patient   607
  Step 3: Patient Work-Up   607
  Step 4: Capture the Visit and Sign the Note   609
  Step 5: Verify Charges   609
  Step 6: Process Remittance (EOB) and Transfer to Private Pay   609
  Step 7: Work Claims and Generate Patient Statement   609
Case Study 11-6: Transfer to Collections   609
Case Study 11-7: Operator Activity Log   610
Case Study 11-8: View the VIP Log   610
Case Study 11-9: Close the Fiscal Periods and Fiscal Years   610

Appendix A   611
Appendix B   663
Glossary   679
Index   684

List of Activities

Activity 2-1: Clear Your Cache   47

Activity 2-2: Log in to Harris CareTracker PM and EMR   48

Activity 2-3: Recorded Training—General Navigation and Help   54

Activity 2-4: Snipit (S) Fiscal Period   55

Activity 2-5: Operator Audit Log   67

Activity 2-6: Open a New Fiscal Year   71

Activity 2-7: Open a Fiscal Period   73

Activity 2-8: Change Your Password   75

Activity 2-9: To Add an Operator   77

Activity 2-10: Add a Favorite Lab   83

Activity 2-11: Add Patient Visit Summary Items   85

Activity 2-12: Search for Then Add a New Location   89

Activity 2-13: Add Item(s) to a Quick Pick List   91

Activity 2-14: Add a Cancel/Reschedule Reason   94

Activity 2-15: Add a Chief Complaint   95

Activity 2-16: Add a Custom Resource   96

Activity 2-17: Add a Room   98

Activity 2-18: Create a ToDo   100

Activity 2-19: Create a New Mail Message   104

Activity 3-1: Searching for a Patient by Name *(currently in the database)*   130

Activity 3-2: Searching for a Patient by ID Number   132

Activity 3-3: Searching for a Patient by Chart Number   133

Activity 3-4: Searching for a Patient by Social Security Number (SSN)   135

Activity 3-5: Register a New Patient   137

Activity 3-6: Print the Patient Demographics Summary   148

Activity 3-7: Editing Patient Information   150

Activity 3-8: View and Perform Eligibility Check—Electronic Eligibility Checks   152

Activity 4-1: Book an Appointment   163

Activity 4-2: Book an Appointment Using the Find Button   166

Activity 4-3: Book an Appointment Using the Force Button   169

Activity 4-4: Reschedule Appointments   171

Activity 4-5: Reschedule Appointments Using the Find Button   173

Activity 4-6: Cancel Appointments   176

Activity 4-7: Booking a Non-Patient Appointment with No Patient in Context   180

Activity 4-8: Add Patient to the Wait List from the Mini-Menu   185

Activity 4-9: View Appointment Totals for a Month   187

Activity 4-10: Generate a Calendar   188

Activity 4-11: Linking Existing Patients as Family Members   191

Activity 4-12: Entering an Appointment Recall   194

Activity 4-13: Remove a Patient from the Call List   198

Activity 4-14: Check in Patient from the Mini-Menu   202

Activity 4-15: Setting Operator Preferences   205

Activity 4-16: Create a Batch   208

Activity 4-17: Accept/Enter a Payment   212

Activity 4-18: Print Patient Receipts   216

Activity 4-19: Run a Journal   218

Activity 4-20: Post a Batch   220

Activity 5-1: Viewing the Meaningful Use Dashboard   231

Activity 5-2: Activating Care Management Items   233

Activity 5-3: Viewing a Summary of Patient Information   237

Activity 5-4: Viewing the Encounters Application, Active Medications, Allergies, and Problems   239

Activity 5-5: Viewing Patient Alerts in the Patient's Medical Record   240

Activity 5-6: Accessing a Patient Chart Summary Using the Name Bar   246

Activity 5-7: Adding a Room   247

Activity 5-8: Editing a Room   249

Activity 5-9: Adding Custom Resources   250

Activity 5-10: Adding Favorite Labs   252

Activity 5-11: Remove a Favorite Lab   254

Activity 5-12: Adding an Immunization Lot   255

Activity 5-13: Modify an Immunization Lot   257

Activity 6-1: Setting Operator Preferences in Your Batch Application   264

Activity 6-2: Viewing Appointments   266

Activity 6-3: Transferring a Patient   266

Activity 6-4: Viewing Tasks   268

Activity 6-5: Viewing Rx Renewals   273

Activity 6-6: Bringing Up the Patient's Chart   275

Activity 6-7: Adding a Medication to a Patient's Chart   276

Activity 6-8: Adding an Allergy to a Patient's Chart   281

Activity 6-9: Entering Past Immunizations in a Patient's Chart   283

Activity 6-10: Entering a Patient's Medical History   286

Activity 6-11: Recording a Patient's Vital Signs   291

Activity 6-12: Viewing a Flow Sheet   296

Activity 6-13: Creating a Growth Chart   299

Activity 6-14: Accessing and Updating Patient Care Management Items   303

Activity 6-15: Accessing and Updating the Progress Notes Application   307

Activity 7-1: Access the Orders Application   317

Activity 7-2: Add a New Lab Order   320

Activity 7-3: Add a Medication as a Function of Managing the List of Favorites   334

Activity 7-4: Reprint a Prescription   339

Activity 7-5: Search for a Pharmacy   341

Activity 7-6: Access the Immunizations Application   346

Activity 7-7: Add a New Immunization   348

Activity 7-8: Print Immunization Records   352

Activity 7-9: View the Activity Log of an Immunization   353

Activity 7-10: Access and Search for Patient Education   355

Activity 7-11: Create Clinical Letters   357

Activity 7-12: Add a Patient Correspondence   360

Activity 7-13: View and Print Correspondence Attachments   363

Activity 7-14: Set an Item as Inactive or Active   364

Activity 7-15: Print the Correspondence Log   364

Activity 7-16: Create an Outgoing Referral   368

Activity 7-17: Add Your Providers to the Quick Picks List   371

Activity 7-18: Create an Incoming Referral   372

Activity 7-19: Capture a Visit   377

Activity 7-20: Resolve an Open Encounter   385

Activity 7-21: Sign a Note   390

Activity 8-1: Access the Progress Notes Application   399

Activity 8-2: Access Progress Notes from the Clinical Toolbar   402

Activity 8-3: Access the Progress Note from the Encounter Dialog Box   403

Activity 8-4: Filter the List of Notes   404

Activity 8-5: Edit a Progress Note   407

Activity 8-6: Delete a Progress Note   408

Activity 8-7: Add an Addendum to a Progress Note   410

Activity 8-8: Sign a Progress Note   411

Activity 8-9: Unsign a Progress Note   412

Activity 8-10: Print the Progress Note   413

Activity 8-11: Enter Results Manually   416

Activity 8-12: Create Customized Result Views   421

Activity 8-13: Filter the Patient's Result List   422

Activity 8-14: Graph Patient Results   424

Activity 8-15: Print a Single Result   425

Activity 8-16: Access the Messages Application   427

Activity 8-17: Create a ToDo   428

Activity 8-18: Create Mail Message   433

Activity 8-19: View Mail Messages   437

Activity 8-20: Move a Mail Message   438

Activity 8-21: Reply to a Mail Message   440

Activity 8-22: Forward a Mail Message   441

Activity 8-23: Delete a Mail Message   442

Activity 8-24: Add Recalls   444

Activity 8-25: Update Recall Details   447

Activity 8-26: Run an Immunization Lot Number Report   449

Activity 9-1: Create a Batch for Billing and Charges   457

Activity 9-2: Posting a Patient Payment   461

Activity 9-3: Manually Enter a Charge for a Patient   462

Activity 9-4: Reversing a Charge   471

Activity 9-5: Run a Journal   475

Activity 9-6: Post a Batch   477

Activity 9-7: Workflow for Electronic Submission of Claims   478

Activity 9-8: Apply Settings to Print Paper Claims   481

Activity 9-9: Generate a Paper Claim   483

Activity 9-10: Process a Remittance   494

Activity 9-11: Enter a Denial and Remittance   504

Activity 9-12: Work Credit Balances   511

Activity 10-1: Work the Claims Worklist   540

Activity 10-2: Search Crossover Claims   545

Activity 10-3: Individually Check Claim Status Electronically   546

Activity 10-4: Work Unpaid/Inactive Claims   550

Activity 10-5: Generate Patient Statements   555

Activity 10-6: View and Reprint a Patient Statement Using the Financial Module   558

Activity 10-7: Transfer a Balance   566

Activity 10-8: Create a Custom Collection Letter   573

Activity 10-9: Add a Form Letter to Quick Picks   578

Activity 10-10: Generate Collection Letters   580

How to Use the Book

Chapter Openers

Key Terms

accounts receivable
(A/R)
cache
clearinghouse
event type
fee schedule
Knowledge Base
macros

open order
override
recall
resources
revenue codes
roles
task classes
template

Key Terms identify important vocabulary for the chapter. Each term appears in boldface color the first time it is used in the chapter and also appears in the glossary with a definition.

The **Learning Objectives** state chapter goals and outcomes.

Learning Objectives

1. Log in to Harris CareTracker to begin your training

2. Use the Help system to become familiar with key features of Harris CareTracker PM and EMR and to access step-by-step instructions on using each aspect of the system to quickly and successfully complete required tasks.

3. Demonstrate knowledge of the Main Menu, Navigation, Home, and Dashboard overview.

4. Discuss Administration features and functions for Practice Management and Electronic Medical Records.

5. Demonstrate understanding and use of the

Certification Connection

1. Perform basic keyboarding skills (e.g., Microsoft Word®, Excel®, etc.).

2. Manage patient flow (e.g., front office, back office, administrative tasks).

3. Access the Internet to obtain patient- and practice-related information and transmit patient data for external use (e.g., insurance, pharmacies, other providers), complying with HIPAA and office protocol regarding security.

4. Operate office machines and devices such as scanners, fax machine, signature pads, and cameras integrated with EHR software.

5. Define clinical vocabularies in a health information management (HIM) system and related patient safety standards regarding abbreviations.

6. Coordinate office workflows regarding patient flow such as scheduling, patient registration and verification, patient referrals, and more.

7. Participate in end-user training of EHR software; provide training to others.

8. Adhere to federal, state, and local laws relating to exchange of information.

9. Identify the impact of HIPAA for the medical assistant and apply security standards related to the confidentiality and release of protected health information (PHI); de-identify PHI.

10. Develop and execute a plan for data recovery in case of downtime or a catastrophic event.

The **Certification Connection** feature highlights sample competencies that are covered in each chapter for a generic EHR certification exam.

The **Sustainability icon** appears throughout the book to highlight chapter material that addresses the responsible use of resources. Each "print prompt" throughout the text is accompanied by the Sustainability icon to encourage electronic submission of activities.

PM SP⬤TLIGHT

If *Chief Complaints* have not been set up for your groups, this list is disabled. If the chief complaint is linked to a progress note template, Harris CareTracker PM and EMR will automatically apply the associated progress note template and select the chief complaint that is linked to the appointment. If the complaint is entered manually, this text will be pulled into the CC/HPI text box in certain templates.

Spotlight boxes highlight important material included throughout the text. It is critical that users of EHR software are familiar with this information. There are different types of spotlight boxes included in the text, depending on the information being presented. These types include Administrative Spotlight, PM Spotlight, Clinical Spotlight, and Legal Spotlight.

Critical Thinking boxes help you think about and deal with issues you may face on the job.

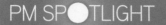

Critical Thinking

List times when it may be necessary to delete or edit a family member from a patient's record and why. Explain what the consequences might be for not deleting or editing the record and how you reached your conclusion.

⚠ Alert

You will need to schedule appointments for Activities 4-1 through 4-8 approximately one week in the future because certain features will not work on "past dates"; that is, you cannot reschedule an appointment on a day that has already passed. Scheduling patient appointments approximately one to two weeks in the future should give you enough time to complete all of the activities in this chapter. Avoid booking too far in advance because that would affect future patient visit and billing activities. For example, if today's date is May 15, it would be best to book your appointments sometime between May 22 and May 29.

Alert boxes present critical information to know when completing activities in Harris CareTracker PM and EMR.

Tip boxes provide helpful hints for using Harris CareTracker PM and EMR.

📦 Tip Box

Do not use any symbols when entering appointment notes or patient complaints. Using symbols will cause an error when you try to print encounter forms.

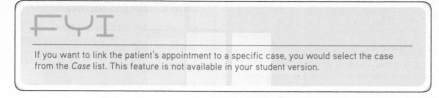

If you want to link the patient's appointment to a specific case, you would select the case from the *Case* list. This feature is not available in your student version.

FYI boxes provide details on functions of Harris CareTracker PM and EMR that are available in real-world settings but are not available in your student version of Harris CareTracker.

Exam Tip boxes highlight information relevant to EHR certification exams.

CEHRS™ Exam Tip

What are the benefits of NHA certification?

• Many employers prefer and often require employees to obtain certification
• Demonstrates commitment to a chosen profession
• Enables recipients to work anywhere in the country because it is a national certification
• Gives a competitive edge during the job search
• Improves earnings potential, career opportunities, a higher pay scale, job security, and advancement options

ACTIVITY 4-12: Entering an Appointment Recall

1. Pull patient James Smith into context.
2. Click the *Scheduling* module and then click the *Recall* tab.
3. Click *New Recall*. Harris CareTracker PM displays the *Add Patient Recall* box (Figure 44-4).
4. Select the time frame for the recall from the *Time Frame* list (select "1 Year"). When Days, Weeks, Months, or Years is selected, you must also enter a numeric value to correspond to the selected time unit.
5. Select the type of appointment from the *Appointment Type* list. (Select "Lab.")
6. Select the provider from the *Provider* list. (Amir Raman)
7. Select the location from the *Location* list. (Napa Valley Family Associates)
8. If the recall appointment needs to be linked to a case, select the appropriate case from the *Case* list (not applicable here).
9. (Optional) Select an alert type from the *EMR Alert Status* list. (Select "Soft Alert.")
10. (Optional) Enter a note about the recall in the *Recall Notes* field. (Free text note: "Annual CPE Labs")

Step-by-Step Activities, included throughout the text, give instruction on how to complete front and back office functions in Harris CareTracker PM and EMR. They feature detailed information on steps to be performed as well as full color screenshots that illustrate key steps.

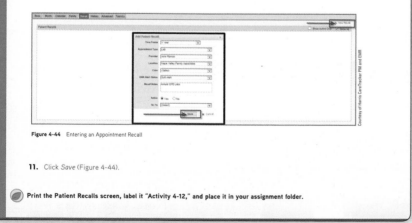

Figure 4-44 Entering an Appointment Recall

11. Click *Save* (Figure 4-44).

Print the Patient Recalls screen, label it "Activity 4-12," and place it in your assignment folder.

SUMMARY

This chapter wraps up the patient scheduling module of front office/practice management responsibilities in Harris CareTracker that are required before the clinical application of the EHR can be used. Mastering the various methods of scheduling, rescheduling, and canceling appointments lays the foundation for the patient visit and billing activities.

Other duties associated with managing the appointment schedule include appointment reminders (*TeleVox®*) and the effect on the practice and patients; scheduling non-patient appointments, which are vital to prevent appointment conflicts with a provider's schedule; and creating a wait list. There are many reasons an appointment would need to be canceled or rescheduled and this happens frequently in today's busy medical practice. You are now familiar with the steps to complete the scheduling process in Harris CareTracker PM and EMR, and the importance of creating and maintaining an effective wait list within the program, which helps to fill open time slots with other patients waiting to see the provider and in turn increases revenue to the practice.

Creating a batch is the initial function that establishes defaults and assigns a name to a batch (group) of financial transactions you enter into the system. A new batch must be created to enter financial transactions. You have completed activities that include setting operator batch preferences, accepting a payment, generating a patient receipt, running a journal, and posting the batch. These front office activities related to the batch links the patient visit to the financial module, which is covered in Chapters 9 and 10. You will continue to refer to batch activities throughout this book and when completing many future activities.

The **Chapter Summaries** provide an overview and summation of the main learning outcomes within the chapter.

Check Your Knowledge

Select the best response.

_____ 1. Booking non-patient appointments must be done directly from the:

      a. Dashboard   c. Schedule
      b. Administration module   d. None of the above

_____ 2. How do you access the mini-menu?

      a. Left-click on patient's name
      b. Click on the *Dashboard Schedule*
      c. In the batch setup
      d. None of the above

_____ 3. How long does the mini-menu schedule display on the screen?

      a. As long as you are operating in the *Schedule* module
      b. 8 minutes
      c. As long as the patient is in context
      d. 8 seconds

The **Check Your Knowledge** multiple-choice quizzes at the end of each chapter solidify your understanding of the material presented.

mini-case studies

Case Study 5-1

Repeat Activity 5-6 (Accessing a Patient Chart Summary Using the *Name Bar*). Instead of bringing up Caroline Sweeney's chart, bring up Brad Training's chart. Change the view of the chart summary by changing it to *Chronological* view.

Print the screen with Brad Training's chronological chart view, label it "Case Study 5-1," and place it in your assignment folder.

Case Study 5-2

Repeat Activity 5-7 (Adding a Room), but add the following two new rooms: X-Ray and Laboratory.

Print a copy of the screens that illustrate you added the rooms. Label the *X-Ray* screenshot "Case Study 5-2A" and the *Laboratory* screenshot "Case Study 5-2B." Place each one in your assignment folder.

The **Mini-Case Studies** provide additional opportunity for students to test their ability to complete key chapter activities without the benefit of step-by-step instructions. **Note:** Case studies MUST be completed in every chapter since future chapter activities build upon them.

Preface

Electronic technology is the major means through which workers communicate in today's health care environment. *The Paperless Medical Office: Using Harris Care-Tracker PM and EMR* is an electronic health record (EHR) solution that integrates instructional theory with a state-of-the-art practice management (PM) and electronic medical record (EMR) software.

Harris CareTracker PM and EMR is one of the most advanced web-based PMs and EHRs in the industry. The product is certified through the Certification Commission for Health Information Technology (CCHIT®) and is used by thousands of providers throughout the country. The Harris CareTracker product provides state-of-the-art features and user-friendly software and is compliant with governmental mandates.

The PM side of Harris CareTracker is a sophisticated practice management system that automates time-consuming administrative tasks such as eligibility checks, scheduling, reminders, patient visit documentation, and claims submission. Its features include:

- Interactive dashboards that prioritize work lists automatically
- A rules-based, front-end clinical editing tool that scrubs outgoing claims prior to submission
- An online code lookup software that boosts coding accuracy

The EMR side of Harris CareTracker monitors and measures all clinical data and prioritizes anything that needs attention. Some of the features of Harris Care-Tracker EMR include:

- Automatic refill requests
- Chart management
- Lab management

- Medication history
- Prescription (Rx) writing
- Report management

Purpose of the Text

The Paperless Medical Office: Using Harris CareTracker PM and EMR was written to fill a void in today's EHR training market. There are many EHR training solutions available but this text integrates advanced content on EHR concepts and meaningful use guidelines with 30–40 hours of step-by-step training activities that simulate typical workflows in ambulatory health organizations. This text takes students through critical information on integrating EHR software into the medical practice, and then offers step-by-step guidance on how those principles can be applied using the Harris CareTracker PM and EMR software.

Chapter 1 serves as an introduction to the EHR, including its benefits and core functions. Chapters 2 through 11 contain step-by-step front and back office activities for the students to complete. At the end of each activity, students are asked to print a screenshot or report that captures the work they have completed. Students are encouraged to keep this documentation in an "assignments" folder to be turned in to their instructor.

Features

The *Help* system within the Harris CareTracker software includes a plethora of educational materials and training tutorials that provide tips for using Harris CareTracker PM and EMR. In addition to text materials, the Harris CareTracker *Help* system provides training videos that walk users through each function within the system. Because this product is a live program, updated training materials containing the most recent information for meaningful use, ICD-10, and HIPAA are available.

The 30–40 hours of hands-on, step-by-step training activities include critical thinking components. The students not only learn how to use the different functions of the Harris CareTracker software but also how to change settings in the software to meet meaningful use goals and to satisfy individual preferences. The *Clinical Today* module within Harris CareTracker PM and EMR assists students in learning how to manage daily, weekly, and monthly tasks, promoting organization and time management.

Unique features of the text also include:

- Full color screenshots throughout the text that illustrate the step-by-step activities and allow students to check their work
- End-of-chapter Check Your Knowledge quizzes that test the students' retention of information
- Feature boxes such as Critical Thinking questions; PM, Clinical, and Legal Spotlights; Harris CareTracker PM and EMR Tips

- Guidance on how Harris CareTracker PM and EMR could map to an EHR certification exam
- Mapping to the latest CAAHEP and ABHES Medical Assisting Standards

Disclaimer

Due to the evolving nature and continuous upgrades of real-world EMRs such as this one, as you log in and work in your student version of Harris CareTracker there may be a slightly different look to your live screen from the screenshots provided in the text.

Keep in mind that you will be asked to work in "current dates" when completing activities, so your appointment and encounter dates will not match those used in the textbook screenshots.

When prompted, follow the instructions given in the text to complete the activites.

Organization of the Text

The Paperless Medical Office is organized to match the daily flow of an office. Chapters 1 and 2 address theoretical EHR concepts that are essential to foundational learning. Beginning with Chapter 3, Patient Demographics and Registration, and continuing throughout the text, students follow the logical sequence of what occurs from the time the patient registers and schedules an appointment through to processing the insurance claim form generated from the patient's visit.

The following breakdown summarizes what is included in each chapter:

Chapter 1: Introduction to the Paperless Medical Office
- This chapter discusses the process of converting paper health records to electronic health records and illustrates what occurs in an electronic health network. Students are provided with a list of common acronyms and terms associated with EHR and PM technology. A variety of common coding and classifications systems are presented in this chapter and students are introduced to the CEHRS™ exam.

Chapter 2: Introduction to Harris CareTracker PM and EMR
- Students will learn how to log in to Harris CareTracker in this chapter and use the *Help* system. Basic navigation functions of the Main Menu, Home, and Dashboard are presented here as well as the discussion of administrative features available within Harris CareTracker PM. Students will gain a firm understanding of using an electronic messaging system and will demonstrate their knowledge by performing messaging activities.

Chapter 3: Patient Demographics and Registration
- In this chapter, students will learn the fundamentals of entering patient demographics, registering new patients, and viewing and performing eligibility checks.

Chapter 4: Appointment Scheduling

- Scheduling is the central theme of this chapter. Students will learn how to book, reschedule, and cancel appointments; add patients to the wait list; and perform activities managing the daily schedule. Users will also learn how to check in patients, create a batch, accept payments, print patient receipts, run a journal, and post the batch.

Chapter 5: Preliminary Duties in the EMR

- This chapter is where the EMR side of Harris CareTracker is introduced. Students will learn the significance of meaningful use and receive training in how to activate the care management registries. In this chapter, users will perform basic maintenance functions such as adding a room, adding a custom resource, adding a favorite lab, and managing immunizations. Learning how to navigate through the medical record is a large focus of the chapter.

Chapter 6: Patient Work-Up

- In this chapter, students will learn the major applications of the *Clinical Today* module—the clinical or EMR side of Harris CareTracker. Students will perform basic check-in duties, and track patients throughout the visit. Learning how to read the tasks menu and complete those tasks is a central focus in this chapter. Tasks may include items such as prescription renewals, electronic ToDos, outstanding lab reports or lab reports waiting for a response, and managing open encounters. This chapter emphasizes the importance of time management. In addition to these items, students will learn how to record vital signs and chief complaints, view and create flow sheets, create and print growth charts, update the patient on preventive testing and health maintenance items, and create progress notes.

Chapter 7: Completing the Visit

- This chapter focuses on what occurs following the patient's examination. Students will learn how to use computerized provider order entry (CPOE) for medication, laboratory, and radiology orders. Users will also learn how to access the correspondence application, create outgoing and incoming referrals, and complete the visit by capturing ICD and CPT® codes required for billing services.

Chapter 8: Other Clinical Documentation

- In this chapter, users will learn how to edit progress notes, add addendums, sign progress notes, and enter results into the patient's medical record. Students will learn how to view, customize, graph, and print patient results and record messages. Additionally, users will create and update patient recall letters, use the clinical export feature, and run an immunization report.

Chapter 9: Billing

- Students switch back to administrative tasks in this chapter. Once the visit is completed the financial activities begin. Creating a batch for financial activities, manually entering charges, and editing an unposted charge are just a few of the activities in this chapter. Users will also learn how to generate electronic and paper claims and perform activities related to electronic remittance.

Chapter 10: ClaimsManager and Collections

- In this chapter users will learn how to use the *ClaimsManager* feature in Harris CareTracker and will check the status of unpaid or inactive claims. Generating patient statements and collection letters are also introduced in this chapter.

Chapter 11: Applied Learning for the Paperless Medical Office

- This chapter is the finale of the text. It includes several case studies that test the users' comprehension of the material presented throughout the text without providing step-by-step instructions. Students will build both competence and confidence from performing activities in this chapter.

Student Supplements

CourseMate

CourseMate helps you make the grade with several components: (1) an interactive eBook with highlighting, note-taking, and search capabilities; (2) interactive learning tools, including quizzes, flashcards, videos, games, and presentations; and (3) Engagement Tracker, a first-of-its-kind tool that monitors student engagement in the course. Go to www.cengagebrain.com to access these resources and look for this icon ⸙CourseMate, which denotes a resource available within CourseMate.

Billers and Coders Workbook

The Paperless Medical Office for Billers and Coders workbook provides hands-on practice that is focused on billing and coding activities within Harris CareTracker PM and EMR. This workbook contains 8–10 hours of activities with screenshots and step-by-step instructions.

Instructor Supplements

Instructor's Manual

The customizable Instructor's Manual can be found on the Instructor Companion Site. Features include:

- Curriculum guide and lesson plans
- Answer keys to all Mini-Case Studies and Applied Learning case studies
- Answers to Critical Thinking boxes and Check Your Knowledge quizzes in the text

Instructor Companion Site (Access at www.cengage.com/login)

The Instructor Companion Site offers extra content to instructors. Log on to www.cengage.com/login to get these resources and more:

- A Cognero Test Bank with more than 300 questions and answers organized by chapter
- Instructor slides created in PowerPoint for each chapter, which cover key concepts presented in the text
- Complete, customizable Instructor's Manual files
- Mapping to Snipit (S) recorded training videos found in the Harris CareTracker *Help* system

About the Authors

Virginia Ferrari is a former adjunct faculty member at Solano Community College in the Career Technical Education/Business division, where she taught medical front office, medical coding, and small business courses. In addition, she has been a contributing author for other Cengage Learning textbooks, including the Seventh and Eighth Editions of *Medical Assisting: Administrative and Clinical Competencies* and the Second Edition of *Clinical Medical Assisting: A Professional, Field Smart Approach to the Workplace*. Prior to joining Solano Community College, Virginia served as the manager of extended services for one of the fastest-growing physicians networks in the San Francisco Bay area. In addition to overseeing the conversion and implementation of electronic medical records, she served on the Best Practice Committee, Customer Satisfaction Committee, Pilot Project for Risk Adjust Coding, and Team Up for Health, a national collaborative for Diabetes Self-Management Education. Virginia holds dual bachelor degrees in sociology and family and consumer studies from Central Washington University and a master's degree in health administration from the University of Phoenix. Virginia also holds certification from the National Healthcareer Association as a Certified Electronic Health Record Specialist (CEHRS) and is a member of the AAMA Editorial Advisory Committee.

Currently a faculty member at Columbus State Community College, Michelle Heller has worked in health care and health care education for the past 30 years. She has received a variety of "Outstanding Teacher" awards from institutions in which she has taught and from the Ohio Council of Private Career Schools and Colleges. A frequent presenter and the author of multiple textbooks, Michelle has served as both director of education and director of the Medical Assisting Program for the Ohio Institute of Health Careers. She also serves on the ABHES Medical Assisting programmatic accreditation committee.

Acknowledgments

To Guy, my husband and best friend, who has believed in me from the day we met nearly 40 years ago. Thank you for your inspiration and unwavering support of me on our life's journey and in my pursuit of these generous opportunities. Thank you for sharing me with all my personal and professional commitments, for keeping me focused, and offering encouragement when I needed it most.

To the entire team at Cengage Learning, and especially Lauren Whalen, thank you for the opportunity to write and share my passion for learning, leadership, and excellence. Your continued support, guidance, attention to detail, and utmost professionalism (always going above and beyond) to see this project through has been invaluable.

Special thanks to my colleague and co-author, Michelle Heller. I couldn't have done it without you. It's truly been a great pleasure to work with you on this project and I'm honored to call you a dear friend and mentor. I look forward to collaborating on many projects in the future.

—Virginia Busey Ferrari

I would like to thank my best friend and husband, Kevin, for his continued support throughout the project! Babe, you had some difficult health challenges this past year, but you fought hard and never gave up! I am so proud of you!

To my co-author and friend, Virginia Ferrari, thank you for picking up the slack and lightening my load when life threw out some obstacles. It was a pleasure getting to know you throughout this project! Your passion for quality and attention to detail are two of the assets that make you such a wonderful author! I look forward to working with you on future projects, but even more importantly, I look forward to a lifelong friendship!

A special thanks to the Cengage team, especially Lauren Whalen, our project manager. I have watched you develop from an editorial assistant into an amazing editor! You have such a keen eye for details. I will miss working with you but know that you are going on to bigger and better things. Thanks for going above and beyond to get this project to fruition!

—Michelle Heller

SYSTEM REQUIREMENTS FOR HARRIS CARETRACKER

Minimum Requirements

- Intel core or Xeon processor
- Operating System: Windows 7, Windows 8, Windows 10, iPad IOS6
- Windows 7: 8 GB
- Microsoft Internet Explorer 9, 10, or 11.
- Please note that the Windows 8 and Windows 10 OS will not support IE 9. IE 9 can be used with Windows 7.
- Acrobat Reader
- Adobe Flash
- Java
- 1024 × 768 resolution

Third-Party Software

Third-party software (such as Yahoo! and Google toolbars, or Norton and McAfee, etc.) does not follow the rules setup in Internet options; therefore it tends to block Harris CareTracker functionality with respect to Pop-ups. If this does happen, then you need to add training.caretracker.com, rapidrelease.caretracker.com, and optum.webex.com to the allowed or safe sites lists of those programs. Follow the instructions in the next section, Internet Settings (Add as Safe Site).

Internet Settings (Add as Trusted Site)

1. Open Internet Explorer browser window.
2. On the menu bar, click Tools and then select Internet Options from the menu. Internet Explorer displays the Internet Options dialog box.
3. Click the Security tab and then click Trusted Sites.

4. Click Sites. Internet Explorer displays the Trusted Sites dialog box.
5. In the Add this website to the zone box, type: training.caretracker.com
6. Click Add. Internet Explorer adds the address to trusted sites.
7. Repeat Steps 5 and 6 for rapidrelease.caretracker.com and optum.webex.com
8. Deselect the Require server verification (https:) for all sites in this zone checkbox.
9. Click Close to close the Trusted Sites box.
10. Click OK on the Internet Options box to save your changes.

Bandwidth Recommendations

If there are multiple workstations utilizing Harris CareTracker, then each will require a minimum of 300kb of bandwidth per active workstation with a DSL or Cable connection. For a T1 or Dedicated connection, a minimum of 60kb per workstation is required.

Recommended Screen Resolution

The recommended screen resolution is 1024 × 768.

Supported Browser

Harris CareTracker supports only Internet Explorer 9, 10, or 11 for desktop devices. Safari for iPad may also be used. Mozilla Firefox and Google Chrome are not yet supported.

Chapter 1

Introduction to the Paperless Medical Office

Key Terms

abstract
Certification
   Commission for
   Health Information
   Technology (CCHIT®)
classification systems
clearinghouse
clinical templates
clinical vocabularies
Computer Physician
   Order Entry (CPOE)
covered entity
Current Procedural
   Terminology (CPT®)
designated record sets
   (DRS)
electronic health record
   (EHR)
electronic medical
   record (EMR)
electronic protected
   health information
   (ePHI)
EncoderPro®
Health Insurance
   Portability and
   Accountability Act
   (HIPAA)
Health Level 7 (HL7)
hybrid conversion
International
   Classification of
   Diseases (ICD)

Logical Observation
   Identifiers Names
   and Codes (LOINC®)
meaningful use
minimum necessary
modifiers
National Drug Code
   (NDC)
nomenclature
notice of privacy
   practices (NPP)
order set
protected health
   information (PHI)
providers
scope of practice
scrub
sequelae
sustainability
Systemized
   Nomenclature
   of Medicine,
   Clinical Terms
   (SNOMED-CT®)
total conversion
treatment, payment,
   and operations (TPO)
Unified Medical
   Language System®
   (UMLS®)
workflow

Learning Objectives

1. Discuss paper records vs. paperless records and the process of converting paper health records to electronic health records (EHRs).

2. Review the CEHRS™ competency and exam outline—administrative and practice management components.

3. Demonstrate knowledge of administrative workflows in Harris CareTracker.

4. Discuss practice management, front office, billing, and administrative functions.

5. Define classification systems.

6. Demonstrate understanding of coding systems such as the International Classification of Diseases (ICD), Current Procedural Terminology (CPT®), and Healthcare Common Procedural Coding System (HCPCS).

7. Illustrate what occurs in an electronic health network.

8. Demonstrate understanding of clinical workflows in Harris CareTracker.

9. List common acronyms and terminology associated with EHRs.

10. Review the CEHRS™ competency and exam outline—clinical components.

Certification Connection

1. Discuss the use of electronic medical records (EMRs) and the effects and implications of federal regulation to the health care industry.
2. Utilize EMR and practice management (PM) systems.
3. Manage data and document accurately in the patient record using the electronic health record (EHR).
4. Manage patient flow (e.g., front office, back office, administrative tasks).
5. Apply electronic technology to maintain effective communication.
6. Communicate in language the patient can understand; articulate the distinction regarding managed care and insurance plans; demonstrate effective and courteous telephone techniques.
7. Identify the impact of the Health Insurance Portability and Accountability Act (HIPAA) for the medical assistant.
8. Adhere to federal, state, and local laws relating to exchange of information and describe elements of meaningful use and reports generated.
9. Access, edit, and store patient information in the EHR database.
10. Perform routine practice management and clinical EHR tasks within a health care environment according to appropriate protocols.
11. Demonstrate ability to use and maintain office hardware and software; keep an inventory of assets.
12. Define clinical vocabularies in a health information management system.
13. Enter live data into an EHR and assist clinicians with charting.
14. Describe how to use and find the most current ICD, CPT®, and HCPCS codes in an EMR.
15. Locate and monitor information in a patient chart for completeness and accuracy; organize patients' health information into a reliable system that promotes accuracy; audit charting to ensure compliance of policies and regulations pertaining to coding, consent forms, release of information (ROI), signature on file, and more.
16. Purge, archive, and secure electronic charts; create an action plan for data recovery in case of downtime or a catastrophic event.
17. Examine the link between accurate charting and the reimbursement received by clinicians.
18. Demonstrate professional standards of care while performing your duties; maintain compliance with confidentiality of protected health information (PHI) and the HIPAA Privacy Rule according to appropriate protocols.

Adapted from national standards of the National Healthcareer Association (NHA), Commission on Accreditation and Allied Health Education Program (CAAHEP), and Accrediting Bureau of Health Education Schools (ABHES)

INTRODUCTION

Welcome to Harris CareTracker PM and EMR, a fully integrated CCHIT® and ONC-ATCB–certified complete practice management (PM) and Electronic Health Record (EHR). You often hear the terms *EMR* and *EHR* used interchangeably, but there is a distinction between the two. **Electronic medical records (EMRs)** are patient records in a digital format. **Electronic health records (EHRs)** refer to the interoperability of electronic medical records, or the ability to share medical records with other health care facilities.

Founded in 2004, the **Certification Commission for Health Information Technology (CCHIT®)** is an independent, not-for-profit group that certifies EHR and networks for health information exchange (HIE) in the United States. Authorized by the Office of the National Coordinator, ONC-Authorized Testing and Certification Bodies (ONC-ATCBs) test and certify that certain types of EHR technology are compliant with the standards, implementation specifications, and certification criteria adopted by the Department of Health and Human Services (HHS). Harris CareTracker PM and EMR is CCHIT® and ONC-ATCB® certified (Figure 1-1), meaning that, among other things, it supports meaningful use, which is discussed later in the chapter.

Harris CareTracker PM is a powerful web-based application that gives medical practices new levels of efficiency, integration, and accountability. Harris CareTracker PM features a sophisticated infrastructure within a simple user experience that:

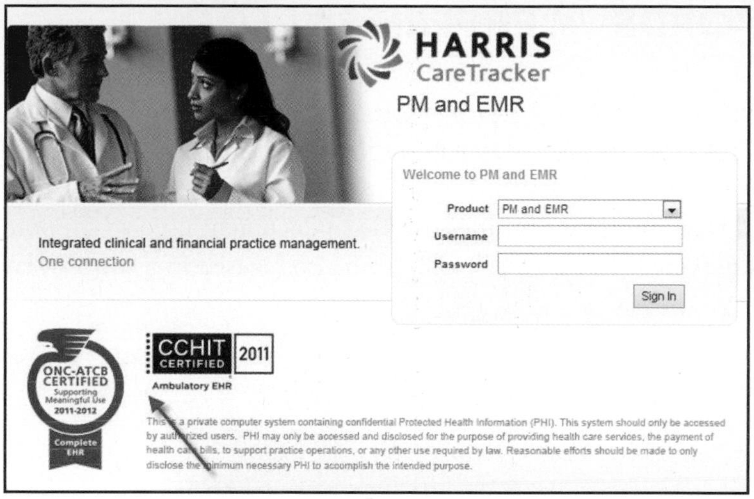

Figure 1-1   Harris CareTracker is CCHIT and ONC-ATCNB Certified.

- Automates patient scheduling and registration
- Verifies eligibility at every step
- Scrubs outgoing claims prior to submission (to **scrub** a claim means
  to verify its technical and coding accuracy before it is filed by identifying potential problems that
  will cause claim rejection or reduction in payment. The claim scrubber provides a comprehensive
  set of coding and technical edits.)
- Maximizes "pay at first pass"
- Returns to payers daily to check claim status
- Monitors contracts for underpayment
- Routes issues to billing staff and managers
- Ensures accountability at all levels

Harris CareTracker EMR is a web-based application that is fully integrated with all the operational functions of a medical practice. Harris CareTracker EMR gives providers a new way to manage tasks, streamline their workflow, and improve the quality of patient care. With Harris CareTracker EMR you can:

- Capture patient visits electronically using *Quick Text*, dictation, and structured templates
- Manage and document patient communications quickly and efficiently
- Generate and process prescription refills
- Complete office workflow tasks with detail or summarize patient information that includes medications, allergies, and more
- Attach patient documents, images, X-rays, or other files in electronic format
- Evaluate patient information using graphs and flow sheets
- Manage medication and allergy interactions
- Generate patient education information

This chapter introduces you to concepts and terminology relating to health information technology (HIT), medical practice workflows, coding systems, and rules implemented by the HHS and the Centers for Medicare and Medicaid Services (CMS). As with all aspects of medical care, the field of EHRs is constantly evolving and improving. As such, medical practices find it desirable to hire employees who are proficient using EHRs, and those who pass the Certified Electronic Health Record Specialist Exam (CEHRS™) will have official certification of their skill and knowledge set.

PAPER RECORDS vs. PAPERLESS RECORDS

Learning Objective 1: Discuss paper records vs. paperless records and the process of converting paper health records to electronic health records (EHRs).

The medical record is an important business and legal document used to support treatment decisions and to document services provided. The medical record can also be used in a court of law.

LEGAL SP●TLIGHT

The release of records requires a written authorization from the patient or a subpoena. Always follow office policy regarding the release of **protected health information (PHI)**. PHI is all individually identifiable health information held or maintained by a **covered entity** or its business associates acting for the covered entity that is transmitted or maintained in any form or medium. Covered entities can include health plans, health care clearinghouses, and health care providers. A **clearinghouse** is any company that processes health information and executes electronic transactions.

Important factors enter into the decision for a medical practice to convert from paper records to electronic records. Primary considerations are improved accuracy and outcomes and coordination of patient care. In addition, the federal government has implemented regulations concerning the adoption and use of EHRs that provide the medical profession financial incentives for using an EHR and penalties if it does not.

Sustainability

There has been a broad consensus among professionals in the medical field and the federal government that changes and developments in technology would better meet the needs of doctors and patients than traditional patient charts. Rising health care costs and persistent errors in patient documentation have led many to advocate for the use of EHRs as an opportunity to improve upon the patient's coordination of care.

EMRs contribute to greater **sustainability** (the responsible use of resources) and coordination of patient care and also cut down on the use of printed resources. Most practices will find the process of electronic charting vs. paper charting to be time-neutral; however, safety, quality, stewardship of resources, and efficiency will be improved.

Sustainability

Consider this . . . Is there a greener way of doing things?
Throughout the text you will be completing Activities in Harris CareTracker PM and EMR. When you are instructed to "Print" the completed activity and place it in your assignment folder, consider saving the page to an electronic file on a thumb drive if this format is preapproved by your instructor.

Government Health Initiatives

Government laws and initiatives outline the roles and responsibilities of the medical assistant. The practice of medicine is governed by the Medical Practice Act and the Board of Medical Examiners. These boards have ruled that physicians are accountable for the actions of medical assistants in their employ. Medical assistants, regardless of their amount of education, training, and experience, must act within their **scope of practice** and within certain laws and limitations. Laws and scope of practice vary from state to state, and it is the responsibility of medical assistants to research the specific requirements and restrictions that apply within their state because there is no single definition of a medical assistant and his or her scope of practice.

LEGAL SP⬤TLIGHT

All medical assistants must work under the direction of a physician or licensed health care professional. The employer is ultimately responsible and accountable for the actions of the medical assistant. A medical assistant is not allowed to independently assess or triage patients, make medical evaluations, independently refill prescriptions, or give out drug samples without the approval of the physician.

Critical Thinking

As a medical assistant at Napa Valley Family Health Associates (NVFHA), log on to the Medical Board of California website and pick a FAQ topic: http://www.mbc.ca.gov/allied/medical_assistants_questions.html. Write a one-page analysis on the subject explaining how you would apply the information learned to your position as a medical assistant. Present the paper to your instructor for class discussion.

There are a number of government initiatives that affect health care professionals and it is important to understand what these laws mean to you as a medical assistant.

HIPAA.   The **Health Insurance Portability and Accountability Act (HIPAA)** law was passed in 1996, providing new directives for protecting patient information and providing security measures as well as specific requirements for electronically transmitting patient data. HIPAA privacy rules apply to all PHI regardless of the method in which the information is acquired, stored, or distributed. Covered entities are required to protect and guard against the misuse of individually identifiable health information. The amount of PHI used or disclosed should be the minimum necessary to do the job.

Title I of HIPAA was intended to protect health insurance coverage for workers and their families when they change or lose their jobs. Title II of HIPAA requires the HHS to establish national standards for electronic health care transactions and national identifiers for providers, health plans, and employers. It also addresses the security and privacy of health data.

LEGAL SP⬤TLIGHT

HIPAA's minimum necessary rule:

- Must provide only PHI in the minimum necessary amount to accomplish the purpose for which use or disclosure is sought
- Does not apply when patients provide a valid, signed authorization for release of PHI
- De-identified information: PHI with all HIPAA identifiers removed

Incentives for EHR Implementation.   In his 2004 State of the Union address, President Bush noted: "By computerizing health records, we can avoid dangerous medical mistakes, reduce costs, and improve care" and set a 10-year goal for all Americans to be using EHRs. Many applauded this statement, recognizing that EHRs represent an enormous opportunity to improve patient care and health system operations. However, efforts to develop the EHR represent a long journey from early visions to today's reality. The EHR is not a simple computer application; rather, it represents a carefully constructed set of systems that are highly integrated and require a significant investment of time, money, process change, and human factor reengineering.

The economic stimulus package of 2009 (the American Recovery and Reinvestment Act) dedicated $19 billion to the cause of accelerating the adoption of progressive health information technologies such as EHRs. Payment incentive funds are distributed in the form of incentives under Medicare and Medicaid. Medicare incentives are provided to physicians in ambulatory medical facilities that use EHRs. The total amount of Medicare incentive is $44,000 per physician, paid out over a period of five years, and paid directly to the health care professional or employer. Incentive bonus payments are also paid to physicians demonstrating they are meaningful users of a certified EHR system.

Medicaid eligible physicians will receive cash incentives of up to $63,750 for purchasing and using qualified EHRs. Under the Medicaid program, $21,250 is offered to every physician to assist in the procurement and implementation of a qualified EHR system. The deadline for purchasing the EHR system is 2016 to be eligible for these incentives. After the adoption of an EHR system, the Medicaid incentive program further provides $8,500 to every physician for persisting with a meaningful use of the EHR configuration.

Meaningful Use.   **Meaningful use** is the set of standards defined by CMS incentive programs that governs the use of EHRs and allows eligible providers and hospitals to earn incentive payments by meeting specific criteria. For EMR software to be certified, it must meet meaningful use. These standards ensure that providers are using their EMR software to its fullest potential, promoting accuracy, access, patient empowerment, and better coordination of care. Chapter 5 expands on meaningful use and its specific stages.

Affordable Care Act.   The Affordable Care Act (ACA) was passed by Congress and then signed into law by President Obama on March 23, 2010. On June 28, 2012, the Supreme Court rendered a final decision to uphold a key provision of the health care law, citing the authority of Congress to impose a tax. The Internal Revenue Service (IRS) is responsible for the collection and taxation provisions of the ACA that will be implemented over the next several years. Many crucial elements of the ACA law are not finalized as of the writing of this book; however, there are expected to be many new rules and regulations written and challenges to the law as it is implemented.

Converting the Practice

The cost to convert a medical practice from paper records to electronic records can be expensive and time-consuming. Costs include the EHR program (software), the technical components (hardware, e.g., computer, scanner, wireless connectivity, etc.), the time to **abstract** data from the paper charts, and to train and provide support to employees and physicians. To abstract data means to condense a record. In the context of medical records, entering data from the patients' paper chart into an EHR is abstracting. For example, the patient's problem list, current medications, allergies, and personal and family history are entered into the electronic chart as a baseline of medical history.

A **total conversion** is when all paper records are converted to electronic records at once. This method can be costly and often would need to be outsourced so as not to interrupt services to patients. Many practices will convert their paper records to electronic in a gradual or incremental process, adding components as the staff becomes familiar with the application. A gradual or incremental conversion tends to lower the initial cash outlay and provides a smooth transition. Some practices will use a combination of paper and electronic data, often referred to as **hybrid conversion**. Regardless of the format used, the provider will need to complete the progress notes.

An analysis of workflow changes and a prearranged schedule can be quite helpful in determining the stages of implementation. For example, once the EHR product has been selected (e.g., Harris CareTracker), the practice will determine a "go-live" date that accounts for acquisition and installation of hardware, training for the staff, and reducing the patient schedule during the initial transition. (Objective 3 more fully addresses workflow in the medical office.)

Critical Thinking

Drawing from your personal experience as a medical assistant and as a patient, describe your present medical office. Has the practice converted from paper to electronic records? If so, when? What advantages/disadvantages have you observed? If not, how would you advocate for the transition? Support your position with facts and personal experience.

INTRODUCTION OF CEHRS™ EXAM OUTLINE

Learning Objective 2: Review the CEHRS™ competency and exam outline—administrative and practice management components.

After witnessing firsthand the poor patient care of his grandmother, entrepreneur Jon S. Brandt founded the National Healthcareer Association (NHA) in 1989, acting on his motivation to create and improve health care training standards, guidelines, and certification for health care professionals. Today NHA provides preparation and certification in 10 allied health professions. NHA certification exams and continuing education resources have helped over 350,000 allied health professionals. Certification can help improve opportunities to secure better jobs, improve pay, and advance your career. Certifications for allied health professions that are available through NHA range from those for people who draw blood, the medical billing specialist, clinical and administrative medical administrative certifications, and the EHR specialist certification (CEHRS™) (Figure 1-2).

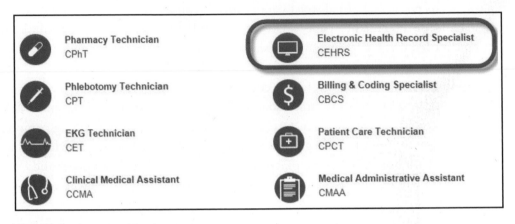

Figure 1-2   NHA Certifications
Source: National Healthcareer Association

The Certified Electronic Health Records Specialist (CEHRS™) is responsible for maintaining the integrity and protecting the privacy and security of patient information. NHA promotes that as a certified EHR specialist, you may perform some or all of the following tasks:

- Audit patient records for compliance with legal and regulatory requirements
- Abstract clinical information for inclusion in reports such as quality improvement studies
- Perform basic coding to submit claims for reimbursement for insurers
- Process Release of Information (ROI) requests for medical records
- Review patient records to ensure they are complete
- Collect patient demographic and insurance information

The CEHRS™ exam consists of 100 scored items and 10 pretest items and is mapped in the CEHRS™ Connection box in each chapter of this textbook. The NHA CEHRS™ Test Plan can be viewed at http://www .nhanow.com/Libraries/pdf/NHA_CEHRS_Test_Plan.sflb.ashx.

To be eligible to sit for the CEHRS™ exam, candidates must be 18 years or older, possess a high school diploma or GED, and have completed a training program or have one year of work experience in the field. Students who are currently enrolled in an allied health program at a school affiliated with NHA can likely take the exam at their school. Study guides are available from ATI Allied Health both in print and online. There is a 30-day waiting period after each failed exam. After three failed attempts, there is a 12-month waiting period before candidates can retest.

CEHRS™ Exam Tip

What are the benefits of NHA certification?

- Many employers prefer and often require employees to obtain certification
- Demonstrates commitment to a chosen profession
- Enables recipients to work anywhere in the country because it is a national certification
- Gives a competitive edge during the job search
- Improves earnings potential, career opportunities, a higher pay scale, job security, and advancement options

The EHR Specialist—Administrative and Practice Management

To promote greater safety, quality, and efficiency in health care delivery, a committee of the Institute of Medicine of the National Academies identified a set of eight core care delivery functions that EHR systems should be capable of performing. The committee's report was sponsored by the U.S. Department of Health and Human Services and is one part of a public and private collaborative effort to advance the adoption of EHR systems. The list of key capabilities will be used by **Health Level 7 (HL7)**, one of the world's leading developers of health care standards for exchanging information between medical applications, to devise a common industry standard for EHR functionality that will guide the efforts of software developers. HL7 is known as a messaging standard used to transfer data between applications. The eight core functions are listed next and described further in Table 1-8:

- Health information and data
- Result management
- Order management
- Decision support
- Electronic communication and connectivity
- Patient support
- Administrative processes and reporting
- Reporting and population health

The certified EHR specialist is expected to know how to input information into an EHR and will commonly find work in physician offices, laboratories, urgent care centers, nursing home facilities, wellness clinics, and hospitals. In addition to traditional occupations, new technology will open many opportunities. The HIT field will provide new, often high-paying, positions such as clinical analyst, health information technician, and records and information coordinator.

A key element of your position as a medical assistant and EHR specialist is to be an active listener and demonstrate respect in your communications, both verbal and nonverbal, with coworkers, patients, providers, and visitors. Always be patient, courteous, and respectful. Refrain from using a negative tone, remark, or expression.

▢ CEHRS™ Exam Tip

The duties of an EHR specialist will vary by practice, size, and specialty of the facility, and range from entry-level positions to more advanced duties including coding, abstracting, HIPAA compliance, or health information management (HIM). A sampling of duties you may perform in the medical practice include:

- Entering Data in the Electronic Chart:
  - Using electronic charts you would enter data, such as demographics, history and extent of disease, diagnostic procedures and treatment into computer.
  - Using the features available in an EHR you would scan, abstract, and organize information and verify the information is complete and accurate.
- Reports and Standards:
  - Using the electronic reports available generate statistical data for analysis and quality improvement measures and assist with special studies and research for public health agencies
  - Compile reports regarding medical care and census data for statistical information on diseases treated, surgery performed, and use of hospital beds for clinical audits; work with National Database Registries as a registrar and contacting discharged patients, their families, and physicians to maintain registry with follow-up information, such as quality of life and length of survival of cancer patients
- Administrative/Regulatory Compliance:
  - Manage data backup and retention of records and maintain a variety of health record indexes, storage, and retrieval systems
  - Coordinate with administrative personnel to review policies and develop new workflows for EHR and organize resources to provide end user training
    - Assist with the daily operations of the front office such as answering the phone; inputting notes into the patient's charts; scheduling appointments, and general reception area duties

For up-to-date information on the CEHRS™ Exam, log on to the NHA website at http://www.nhanow.com/Libraries/pdf/NHA_CEHRS_Test_Plan.sflb.ashx

ADMINISTRATIVE WORKFLOWS IN HARRIS CARETRACKER

Learning Objective 3: Demonstrate knowledge of administrative workflows in Harris CareTracker.

Workflow is defined as how tasks are performed throughout the office (usually in a specific order), for example, the patient is checked in, insurance cards are scanned, and then the patient is taken to the exam room where vital signs are taken/recorded, and so on. Conducting a comprehensive workflow analysis is a critical step in EHR implementation. Workflow analysis allows health care organizations to critically look at how work is currently being done in the practice. In general, workflow analysis should be conducted prior to EHR implementation. This will provide a benchmark of current workflows, which can then be refined during the implementation process. Figure 1-3 is an example of patient flow.

In order to fully document and anticipate workflows, it is helpful to follow a workflow assessment guide and checklist as noted in the appendix. Table 1-1 represents a brief example of front office workflow during a transition from paper to electronic records.

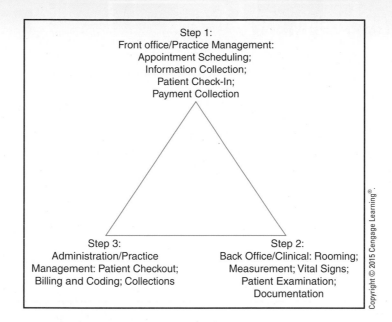

Figure 1-3   Patient Flow

TABLE 1-1	Front Office Workflow	
Workflow	**Actions**	**Paper vs. Electronic Health Record**
Patient registration	How is contact made/information obtained? *Patient calls to establish as patient with practice* *Name/contact information entered* *Registration forms completed by patient*	Phone/in person *Completed registration forms are entered into EHR* *Insurance card is scanned and information populated into insurance demographics fields*
Scheduling	How are appointments made?	How are appointments made?
Pre-visit	Review physician schedule	Review physician schedule
Enter additional front office workflows	Enter additional front office *actions*	Distinguish paper vs. electronic health record *workflows*

Critical Thinking

Review Table 1-1 and the workflow assessment guide and checklist in the appendix and then make additions or corrections to reflect your vision of front office workflow. The first answer has been provided as an example. Expand upon Table 1-1 using the Workflow Assessment Guide and Workflow Assessment Checklist in the appendix.

PRACTICE MANAGEMENT

Learning Objective 4: Discuss practice management, front office, billing, and administrative functions.

Practice management (PM) software runs the business side of health care, from registering a new patient and scheduling patient visits to coding and billing the patient encounter and generating monthly reports. Harris CareTracker PM software can be customized to user preferences. PM software will maximize provider productivity and meets rigorous scheduling demands. Alert messages, a master index, and insurance profiles help reduce error and administrative expenses during registration and charge entry.

Front Office

Front office duties begin with patient demographics (searching for an existing patient, registering a new patient, and editing patient information). Once patient demographics and insurance information are recorded, appointments are scheduled. Much of the patient contact in the front office takes place on the telephone, such as when a patient will call in to the office to make an appointment. Not only must you carefully record the patient's demographics, you must screen the call to determine the most appropriate appointment type and availability. Your knowledge and skills as a medical assistant will be invaluable in determining the urgency of the patient's condition. While operating within your scope of practice, you can take a message for your provider or schedule a routine appointment. If the call is urgent, you must follow office policy and either refer the patient to emergency services or contact the provider for additional instructions.

Accurate documentation in the electronic record is crucial. You must be certain that you are documenting in the correct patient's chart, recording messages for the provider with utmost accuracy, as well as documenting the chief complaint and prescription details. When there is to be a call back to the patient, confirm the telephone number(s) and best time to call. Repeat information you have recorded back to the caller to verify accuracy. Be polite, courteous, and professional at all times.

Your front office duties will also include patient interactions in the office. You will greet the patient upon arrival, accept insurance cards for copying, collect copays, and check the patient in for his or her visit. Each activity or transaction is recorded in Harris CareTracker PM. Once a patient has completed his or her visit, he or she may be asked to schedule a follow-up appointment. Taking instruction from the provider, schedule future appointments and provide any patient education (health information) materials as advised.

The Harris CareTracker PM task sheet (Figure 1-4) provides a quick reference guide to the daily, weekly, and monthly tasks for front office, billing, and administrative duties of the medical assistant.

Billing

Entering a patient's insurance information accurately in the *Insurance* section of the *Demographics* application ensures that insurance companies will pay claims in a timely manner. Accurate and complete information begins with the required fields entered into a patient's demographic screen. Any required information that is missing will prevent a claim from being submitted and/or paid and will affect the revenue cycle of the practice.

Although appointments may be booked for the patient with only the name fields populated, insurance claims cannot be processed until the remainder of the *Demographics* information is complete. If a patient lives

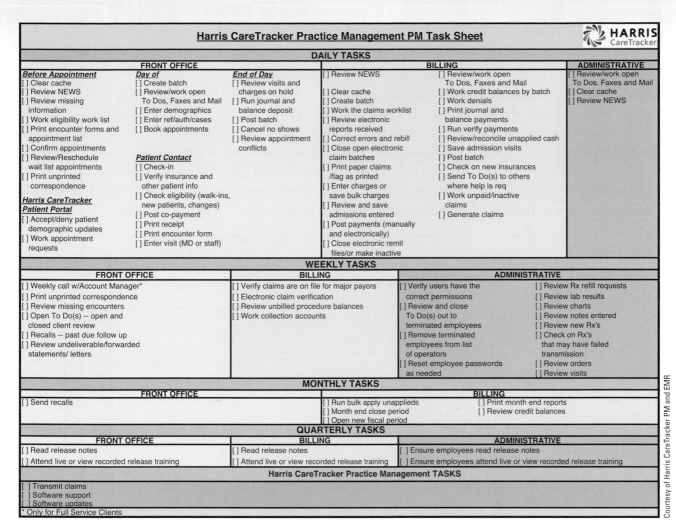

Figure 1-4 Harris CareTracker PM Task Sheet

outside of the United States, his or her address must be entered differently than a patient who lives in the country. Statements will *not* be sent to foreign addresses, but setting up the patient's *Demographics* correctly will prevent the claim from becoming an unbilled claim due to the patient's address. If a patient's gender is not entered, claims for the patient will *not* be electronically transmitted to the insurance company. Any claim lacking a specified gender will become an unbilled claim and will remain as such until an operator specifies a gender and re-bills the claim. The billing functions of Harris CareTracker PM are featured in Chapter 9, describing how to:

- Create a *Batch*
- Manually enter a charge
- Edit an unposted charge
- Generate electronic and paper claims
- Perform activities related to electronic remittance
- Enter and view *Batch* deposits
- Demonstrate understanding and use of the *Claims Manager* feature
- Check status and work *unpaid/inactive claims*
- Generate patient statements

Administrative

The *Administration* module contains the *Administration* application, which is divided into three tabs: *Practice, Clinical,* and *Setup.* Functions of the *Administration/Practice* tab (Figure 1-5) include *Daily Administration, System Administration, Import/Export,* and *Knowledgebase.* These functions contain financial, forms and letters, security logs, messages, and patient security. The *Administration/Clinical* tab (Figure 1-6) includes *Daily Administration, System Administration,* and *Import/Export* functions, which contain forms and letters, security logs, clinical setup, and maintenance. *Administration/Setup* (Figure 1-7) is where you set up PM features. Each tab is organized into sections containing links to other applications in Harris CareTracker PM. Chapter 2 introduces *Administration* features and activities associated with Harris CareTracker.

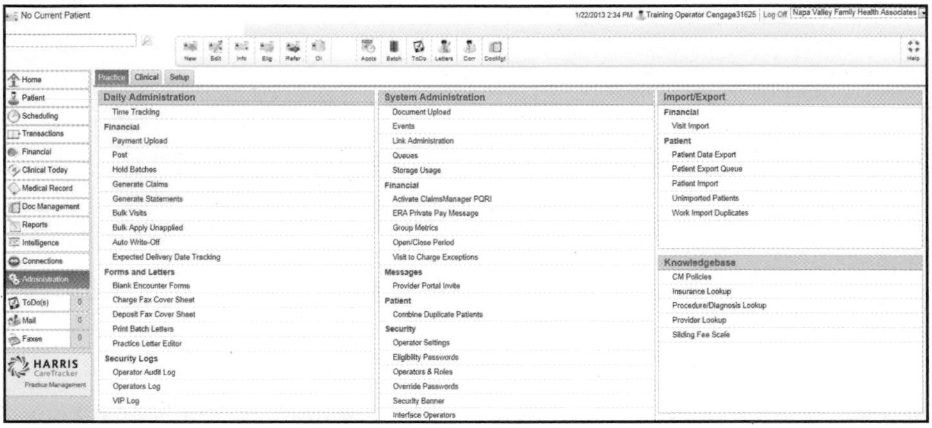

Figure 1-5   Administration/Practice Tab

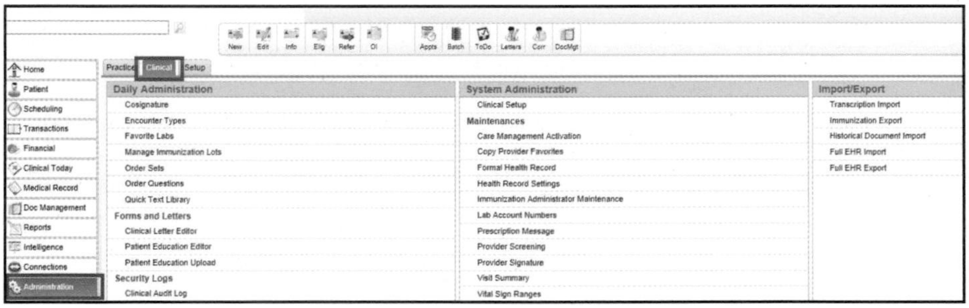

Figure 1-6   Administration/Clinical Tab

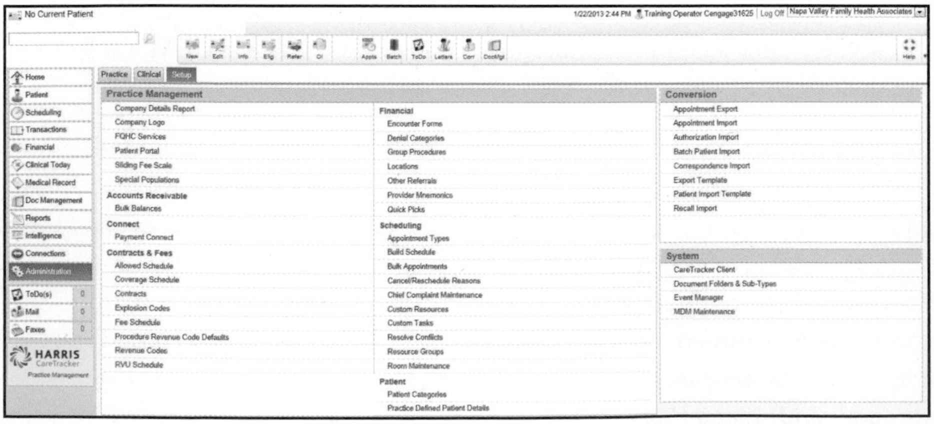

Figure 1-7   Administration/Setup Tab

Every operator must have a user name and a password to log into Harris CareTracker PM and EMR. You are required to change your password every 90 days. Harris CareTracker PM and EMR reminds users seven days before their password expires and gives them the option to change their password at any time after they begin using Harris CareTracker PM and EMR, even prior to the system requirement.

CLASSIFICATION SYSTEMS

Learning Objective 5: Define classification systems.

Classification systems organize related terms into categories for easy retrieval. These classification systems are used for billing and reimbursement, statistical reporting, and administrative functions. There is the expectation with EHRs that the terminology and classification systems work in concert together and support both efficient and effective clinical information and administrative needs for health care organizations. Classifications and terminologies meet diverse user data requirements and are designed for distinctly different purposes. Clinical terminologies are considered the input format, whereas classification systems are the output format.

HIPAA required the HHS to establish national standards, some of which include specific code sets and electronic transactions. The following code set standards were named by HIPAA:

- ICD-9-CM volumes 1 and 2 (diagnosis codes) (Only valid on patient encounters prior to October 1, 2015)
- ICD-9-CM volume 3 (procedure codes) (Only valid on patient encounters prior to October 1, 2015)
- CPT® (outpatient procedure codes)
- HCPCS (items and supplies and non-physician services not covered by CPT®-IV)
- ICD-10-CM/PCS (the new diagnosis coding system developed as a replacement for ICD-9-CM, volumes 1 and 2 [implementated October 1, 2015])
- **NDC (National Drug Code)**—a code that identifies all medications recognized by the Food and Drug Administration (FDA) by vendor (manufacturer), product, and package size.

Examples of output systems would be ICD-9-CM, ICD-10-CM, and ICD-10-PCS. These are typically used for external reporting requirements and are not intended or designed for the primary documentation of clinical care. The input systems, such as SNOMED-CT®, are designed for the primary documentation of clinical care. Together, clinical terminologies and classification systems represent a common medical language that allows data to be shared.

The **Systemized Nomenclature of Medicine, Clinical Terms (SNOMED-CT®)** is the most comprehensive clinical health care terminology in the world, contributing to the advancement of patient care by improving the recording of EHR information, allowing health care facilities to better communicate. **Nomenclature** is a system of terms used in a particular science. SNOMED-CT® is defined as a comprehensive clinical terminology covering diseases, clinical findings, and procedures that allows for a consistent way of indexing, storing, retrieving, and aggregating clinical data across specialties and sites of care. SNOMED-CT® terminology helps structure and computerizes the medical record.

The universal terms and code system for the identification and electronic exchange of laboratory and clinical observations is known as **Logical Observation Identifiers Names and Codes (LOINC®)**. LOINC® enables the exchange and aggregation of electronic health data from many independent systems and includes standardized terms for all kinds of observations and measurements. The **Unified Medical Language System (UMLS®)** is another clinical standard. It is a set of files and software that brings together many health and biomedical vocabularies and standards to enable interoperability between computer systems, that is, a thesaurus database of medical terminology.

CODING SYSTEMS

Learning Objective 6: Demonstrate understanding of coding systems such as the International Classification of Diseases (ICD), Current Procedural Terminology (CPT®), and Healthcare Common Procedural Coding System (HCPCS).

Harris CareTracker features an automatic coding process that checks procedure and diagnosis codes for accuracy. For a provider to receive reimbursement for services, every procedure and diagnosis must be documented in the patient's medical record. Codes are checked for accuracy by a coding specialist. Integrating automated coding with billing facilitates claims processing. Computer-assisted coding in EHRs works a variety of ways, with some systems using keywords or analysis of words, phrases, and sentences. Harris CareTracker features *EncoderPro*®. When all the appropriate CPT® and ICD codes are entered, *EncoderPro*®, Harris CareTracker's partner for online code verification, can be run to verify all the procedures, diagnoses, and modifiers entered for a patient. Clicking on the *EncoderPro.com* button (Figure 1-8) helps to ensure that correct coding information is entered and that claims are processed and paid quickly (Figure 1-9).

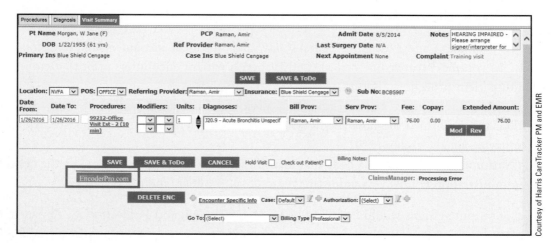

Figure 1-8   EncoderPro Button

Figure 1-9   EncoderPro Defined Code List

International Classification of Diseases (ICD)

Until October 1, 2015, the **International Classification of Diseases** code set of **ICD-9** was the internationally recognizable three- to five-digit code set representing medical conditions or signs and symptoms (standardized categorization of diseases/diagnosis codes) in a health care setting, developed by the World Health Organization (WHO). ICD-9-CM (9th Revision, Clinical Modification) was replaced by the ICD-10 code set on October 1, 2015. Effective January 1, 2012, as a prerequisite for implementing the new ICD-10 codes, health care facilities were required to be ready to submit claims electronically using the X12 Version 5010 and NCPDP Version D.0 standards. CMS later announced that it would not enforce the use of the 5010 transaction standard through June 30, 2012, which made July 1, 2012, the first day enforcement began.

The HIPAA X12 version of 5010 is the new set of standards that regulates the electronic transmission of specific health care transactions including eligibility, claim status, referrals, claims, and remittances. Use of the 5010 version of the X12 standard is required by federal law. All covered entities are required to upgrade to HIPAA 5010 standards. The 5010 standards promise many improvements to Electronic Data Interchange (EDI) transactions including greater clarity in provider loops and National Provider Identifier (NPI) instructions, reduced ambiguity among common data elements, and elimination of unnecessary redundant data elements. HIPAA 5010 also provides for the increase in codes in the new ICD-10 code set. (The ICD-9 code set contained approximately 18,000 total codes, whereas there are over 155,000 ICD-10 codes.)

PM SPOTLIGHT

Characteristics of the ICD-10-CM Coding book format used in the outpatient setting:

- single codebook, with two parts
  - The Index to Diseases and Injuries which is an alphabetic listing of terms and corresponding codes.
  - The two sections of the alphabetic index are the Index to Diseases and Injuries and the Index to External Causes of Injury. A Neoplasm Table and Table of Drugs and Chemicals are also included in the Index.
  - The Tabular List of Diseases and Injuries is an alphanumeric list of codes. The Tabular List is divided into chapters based on body systems (anatomical site) or condition (etiology).

Table 1-2 represents examples of ICD-10-CM codes and descriptions.

TABLE 1-2   ICD-10 Codes Available in the Student Version of Harris CareTracker

Cardiac/Hypertension Codes	Description
I48.91	Unspecified fibrillation
I25.10	Atherosclerotic heart disease of native coronary artery without angina pectoris
I42.8	Other cardiomyopathies

(Continues)

TABLE 1-2   (Continued)

Pediatric Codes	Description
H92.09	Otalgia, unspecified ear
N39.44	Nocturnal Enuresis
R62.51	Failure to thrive (child)
R63.3	Feeding difficulties

Neurology	Description
G56.00	Carpal tunnel syndrome, unspecified upper limb
R42	Dizziness and giddiness
R51	Headache
G43.109	Migraine with aura, not intractable, without status migrainosus

ICD-10, the International Classification of Diseases, 10th Revision, Clinical Modification (ICD-10-CM). The National Center for Health Statistics (NCHS) is the federal agency responsible for the use of the International Classification of Diseases, 10th Revision (ICD-10), in the United States. A clinical modification of the classification has been developed for morbidity purposes: ICD-10-CM. The American Association of Professional Coders (AAPC) is an organization founded in 1988 that provides education and professional certification to physician-based medical coders. Figure 1-10 demonstrates how workflows associated with ICD-10 "will change everything."

ICD-10-CM is the replacement for ICD-9-CM, volumes 1 and 2. On January 16, 2009, the HHS published a final rule adopting ICD-10-CM (and ICD-10-PCS) to replace ICD-9-CM in HIPAA transactions

PM SP⬤TLIGHT

Features of ICD-10-CM are:
- All codes are alphanumeric and all letters are used except "U"
- New diseases and conditions identified with codes
- Injury codes expanded
- Combination codes to identify coexisting diseases added
- Concept of laterality (right and left) added
- Postoperative complications expanded
- Obstetric codes indicate the trimester
- Ambulatory and managed care encounter information added
- Greater specificity in code assignment

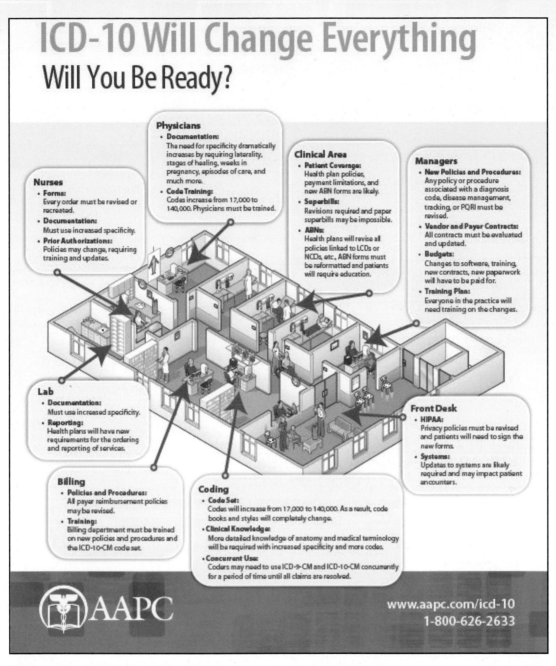

Figure 1-10   ICD-10 Changes Everything
Source: AAPC

with an effective implementation date of October 1, 2013. That date was later changed to October 1, 2015. Prior to October 1, 2015, codes in ICD-10 are not valid for any purpose or use.

Reasons cited for converting from ICD-9-CM to ICD-10-CM is that ICD-9-CM can no longer support many of the HIT and data exchanges targeted in our health care future, including the EHR. ICD-10 is the international classification to the system that contains the most significant changes in the history of ICD. The alphanumeric format provides a better structure than ICD-9. It allows considerable space for future revision without disrupting the numbering system. Experts cite that ICD-10 will provide higher-quality information for measuring health care service, quality, safety, and efficacy.

Developed by the CMS, ICD-10-PCS is intended to replace volume 3 (Procedures) of ICD-9-CM and will be used in the hospital inpatient setting only. Table 1-3 provides a brief comparison between ICD-9 and ICD-10.

TABLE 1-3   Comparison of ICD-9-CM and ICD-10

ICD-9-CM	ICD-10
Title: International Classification of Diseases, 9th Rev., Clinical Modifications	Title: International Statistical Classification of Diseases and Related Health Problems
Contains a chapter titled "Diseases of the Nervous System and Sense Organs"	Divides the chapter into three chapters titled: • "Diseases of the Nervous System" • "Diseases of the Eye and Adnexa" • "Diseases of the Ear and Mastoid Process"
Contains a chapter titled "Mental Disorders"	Renames this chapter "Mental and Behavioral Disorders"
Contains a supplement titled "V Codes"	"V Codes" becomes a chapter rather than a supplement
Contains a supplement titled "E Codes"	"E Codes" becomes a chapter rather than a supplement
Contains numeric codes that require four and five digits	Contains alphanumeric codes that require up to 7 digits and letters
Contains two volumes for diagnosis coding	Contains three volumes for diagnosis coding

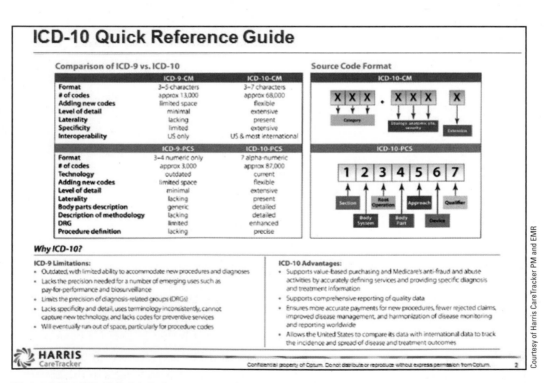

Figure 1-11   ICD-10 Quick Reference Guide/CareTracker Inc.

Figure 1-11 provides a Quick Reference Guide/overview of ICD-10 readiness. Harris CareTracker users are able to select ICD-10 codes from the *Visit* capture, *Diagnosis* tab. (Figure 1-12). If you are completing a Visit (patient encounter) prior to October 1, 2015, you will be able to select the ICD-9 codes

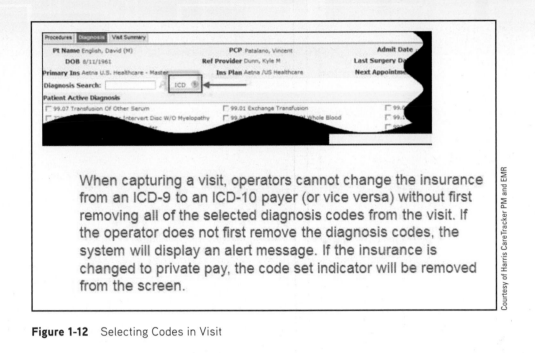

When capturing a visit, operators cannot change the insurance from an ICD-9 to an ICD-10 payer (or vice versa) without first removing all of the selected diagnosis codes from the visit. If the operator does not first remove the diagnosis codes, the system will display an alert message. If the insurance is changed to private pay, the code set indicator will be removed from the screen.

Figure 1-12 Selecting Codes in Visit

- **ICD Mapping Screen**
  - The ICD Mapping screen is accessed by clicking the View Mappings link at the top of the search results. This screen acts as a basic mapping tool, allowing the operator to see which ICD-10 codes map to the current ICD-9 codes and vice versa. Basic mapping is available for:
    - ICD-9-CM Vol. 1 to ICD-10-CM
    - ICD-10-CM to ICD-9-CM Vol. 1
  - The mapping screen contains several columns with information about the relationship between the ICD-9 and ICD-10 codes. The Release notes have a listing of all the mapping descriptions.

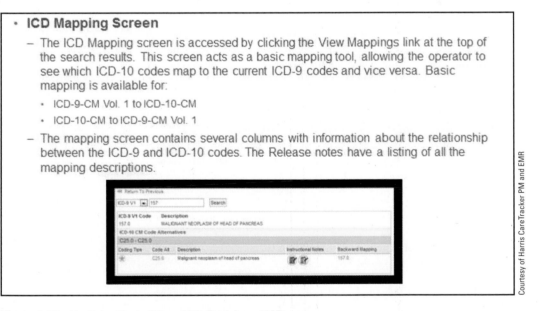

Figure 1-13 Verifying Code 9th or 10th Revision of ICD

based on the date of service. The listing of codes will show in the column whether the selected code is ICD-9 or ICD-10 format (Figure 1-13).

Table 1-4 outlines the types of changes and most of the differences between ICD-10 and ICD-9-CM.

ICD-10 codes consist of up to seven digits, with the seventh digit extension representing the visit encounter or **sequelae** (an aftereffect of disease, condition, or injury; a secondary result) for injuries and external causes. Table 1-5 outlines the features of ICD-9-CM versus ICD-10-CM codes. The change is transformational to the health care industry. As a medical assistant you will be an integral part of the change.

TABLE 1-4 Changes/Differences between ICD-9 and ICD-10

Change	Description
Grouping of codes	Conditions are now grouped in a more logical fashion. This improvement was accomplished by moving conditions from one chapter to another or one section to another. Numerous codes have been added, deleted, combined, or moved.
More complete descriptions	Category titles are usually more complete. The coder does not have to read previous codes to understand the meaning.
Fifth and sixth characters	Fifth and sixth characters are incorporated into the code rather than having common characters listed at the beginning of the chapter, section, or category.
Laterality	Laterality of conditions or injuries are incorporated at the fifth or sixth character.
Increased specificity	Greatly expanded detail on the various conditions are offered.
Use of seventh character	Seven characters will provide additional information.
Combination codes	Numerous codes will group etiology and manifestation.
Terminology used	Many of the titles have been changed to reflect new technology and more recent medical terminology.
Postprocedural conditions	Many codes have been added to describe postoperative postprocedural conditions.
Trimester specificity	Codes in the pregnancy, delivery, and puerperium chapter include those designating the trimester in which the condition occurs.
New codes	Codes for many conditions were not included in ICD-9 and ICD-10 provides for new codes, most notably, codes for blood type and alcohol level.

TABLE 1-5 Features of ICD-9-CM vs. ICD-10-CM Codes

Feature	ICD-9-CM	ICD-10-CM
Number of codes	Roughly 13,000	Approximately 68,000
Code length	Three to five digits	Three to seven characters
Code structure	Three-digit category Fourth and fifth digits for etiology, anatomic site, manifestation	Three-character category Fourth, fifth, sixth characters for etiology, anatomic site, severity Seventh character extension for additional information
First character	Always numeric, except E and V codes	First character is always alphabetic
Subsequent characters	All numeric	Second character is always numeric; all other characters may be alphabetic or numeric

TABLE 1-5 (Continued)		
Feature	**ICD-9-CM**	**ICD-10-CM**
Decimal point	Mandatory after the third character, except E codes where a decimal point is after the fourth character	Mandatory after the third character on all codes
Extensions	None	Some codes use a seventh character as an extension to provide additional information
Placeholders	None	Character "X" is used as a placeholder in certain six- and seven-character codes

Current Procedural Terminology (CPT®)

Current Procedural Terminology (CPT®) is a nationally recognized five-digit numeric coding system maintained by the American Medical Association (AMA) used to represent a service provided by health care providers in an outpatient setting. CPT® is Level I of the Healthcare Common Procedural Coding System (HCPCS). Level I does not include codes needed to separately report medical items or services that are regularly billed by suppliers other than physicians. The CPT® Codebook is divided into sections and code ranges.

SECTION/CODE RANGE of CPT®

- Evaluation and Management   99201-99499
- Anesthesia   00100-01999, 99100-99140
- Surgery   10021-69990
- Radiology   70010-79999
- Pathology and Laboratory   80047-89398
- Medicine   90281-99199, 99500-99607

Table 1-6 represents examples of CPT® codes, fees, and descriptions.

TABLE 1-6 CPT® Codes, Fees, and Descriptions		
Office Visit Established Patients		
99211	$50.00	Office Visit Est - 1 (5 min)
99212	$76.00	Office Visit Est - 2 (10 min)
99213	$112.00	Office Visit Est - 3 (15 min)

(Continues)

TABLE 1-6 (Continued)		
Office Visit Established Patients		
99214	$166.00	Office Visit Est - 4 (25 min)
99215	$245.00	Office Visit Est - 5 (40 min)
Office Procedures		
93000	$46.50	Electrocardiogram (EKG) w/ least 12 Ld W/I&R
G0102	$42.00	Prostate ca screening; dre
94760	$13.00	Noninvasive ear/Pulse Oximetry – single
69210	$135.00	Ear wax removal, impacted cerumen 1/both ears
99173	$15.00	Visual Acuity Screening, Quant, Bilat
J7650	$25.00	Isoetharine HCL, Inhalation, Adm through DME
94620	$25.00	Bronchodilation resp spir; Pre and Post Spir and Oximetry
10061	$337.00	Incision and drainage of Abscess
D7911	$50.00	Complicated sutures up to 5 cm
93225	$50.00	External EKG Recording
V5008	$25.00	Hearing Testing

Source: Current Procedural Terminology © 2012 American Medical Association.

Healthcare Common Procedural Coding System (HCPCS)

In 1983, Medicare developed a new coding system to supplement CPT® Level I, which is currently known as the Healthcare Common Procedural Coding System (HCPCS). HCPCS is divided into two principal subsystems, referred to as Level I and Level II of the HCPCS. Level II of the HCPCS is a standardized coding system that is used primarily to identify products, supplies, and services not included in the CPT®-IV codes (such as ambulance services and durable medical equipment [DME]) as shown in Table 1-7. HCPCS Level II codes are maintained and distributed by the CMS. See Table 1-7 for examples of HCPCS Level II Codes and Descriptions. **Modifiers**, which append the HCPCS codes, are two-digit characters and different from those listed in CPT®. A modifier is a two-character code added to a CPT® or HCPCS code that is used to help in the reimbursement process. For example, a modifier is used to explain that a procedure not normally covered when billed on the same day as another is actually a separate and significant process, or that it is a rural health procedure that gets higher reimbursement. Up to four modifiers can be attached to each CPT® code, although in most cases only one or two are used. Modifiers should be appended to Medicare claims whenever applicable.

TABLE 1-7   HCPCS Level II Codes and Descriptions

Section/Code Range

- Transportation Services Including Ambulance — A0021-A9999
- Enteral and Parenteral — B4034-B9999
- Outpatient PPS — C1300-C9899
- Durable Medical Equipment (DME) — E0100-E8002
- Procedural/Professional Services (Temporary) — G0008-G9147
- Alcohol and Drug Abuse Treatment Services — H0001-H2037
- Drugs Administered Other Than Oral Method — J0120-J9999
- HCPCS Temporary Codes — K0001-K0899
- Orthotic/Prosthetic Procedures — L0112-L9900
- Medical Services — M0064-M0301
- Pathology and Laboratory Services — P2028-P9615
- Q Codes (Temporary) — Q0035-Q9968
- Diagnostic Radiology Services — R0070-R0076
- Temporary National Codes (Non-Medicare) — S0012-S9999
- HCPCS National T Codes (State Medicaid) — T1000-T5999
- Vision Services — V2020-V5364
- Appendix 1 – Table of Drugs
- Appendix 2 – Modifiers
- Appendix 3 – Abbreviations and Acronyms

Section/Code Range

- Appendix 4 – PUB 100 References
- Appendix 5 – New, Changed, Deleted, and Reinstated HCPCS Codes
- Appendix 6 – Place of Service and Type of Service

ELECTRONIC MEDICAL RECORDS

Learning Objective 7: Illustrate what occurs in an electronic health network.

Electronic medical records (EMRs) are patient records in digital format. EMRs can refer to a hospital's electronic patient records, a physician's office electronic patient records, or the EHRs of any other health care establishment. EHR refers to the interoperability of EMRs or the ability to share medical records with other health care entities. Figure 1-14 illustrates what occurs within an electronic health network.

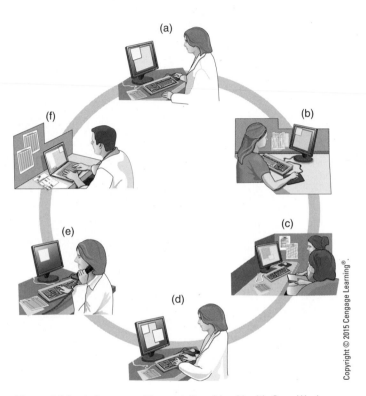

Figure 1-14 A Computer Network Provides Health Care Workers With the Necessary Information With Just a Click of a Button.

- The connection is initiated when the primary care provider (PCP) requests the medical assistant to order diagnostic tests for the patient (a).
- The medical assistant sends electronic orders to the facility where the tests are to be performed (b).
- The testing facility receives the orders, performs the tests, and electronically sends the results back to the PCP (c).
- The PCP reviews the results and officially downloads the results into the patient's medical record (d).
- The patient enters the emergency department with chest pain. The patient alerts the ED physician that he or she just had a physical and diagnostic testing performed at his or her physician's office. A representative from the ED contacts the patient's PCP and requests that all relevant clinical data be sent to the ED physician (e).
- In a matter of minutes, the ED physician has vital information that is needed for determining necessary testing, making a diagnosis, and treating the patient (f).

Core Functions of the EMR/EHR

The electronic record has many features designed to improve patient care and staff efficiency. The type of software that a medical practice selects will depend on many factors including the type of practice, the goals of the practice, the cost of the software, and individual preferences of the clinicians and staff. Following is an overview of the various functions within Harris CareTracker EMR.

- Allows multiple users to access different parts of the chart at the same time
- Creates a chart summary, which identifies key components of the patient's medical history on one screen, including open activities or orders, active problems, active medications, allergy status, immunization status, a listing of the patient's last vital sign measurements, a listing of the patient's progress note history, documents downloaded into the chart, lab results, and correspondence information. This summary can be shared electronically with other providers who see the patient.
- Creates customized progress notes through standardized templates
- Creates customized clinical letters
- Enables the provider and staff members to print, e-mail, or fax progress notes, prescriptions, and other orders directly from the point of care
- Automatically files and displays lab results in a variety of different formats
- Graphs lab values, pediatric growth chart patterns, and vital signs
- Provides electronic tasking features to improve efficiency and communication between staff members
- Provides reporting and benchmarking capabilities that allow users to compare patient outcomes or to track other statistical data
- Interfaces with the practice manager side of Harris CareTracker, making billing more efficient
- Provides full remote access of patient records for those authorized to use them

Through a public and private collaborative effort to advance the adoption of EHR systems, the Institute of Medicine (IOM) and the HHS formed a committee that identified a set of eight core care delivery functions that EHR systems should be capable of performing to promote greater safety, quality, and efficiency in health care delivery. The 2003 report, titled "Key Capabilities of an Electronic Health Record System," enumerated the eight core functions of an EHR system (Table 1-8).

TABLE 1-8 Key Capabilities of an Electronic Health Record System	
Health Information and Data	Designed to have immediate access to essential patient information (e.g., diagnoses, allergies, lab results, and medications). The system holds the information that would be expected in a paper chart—problem lists, medication lists, test results, etc.
Results Management	Has the ability for all health care providers participating in the patient's care to quickly access new and past test results from multiple settings. An EHR enables the importation of lab results, radiology reports, and X-ray images electronically.
Order Management	Contains the ability to enter and store orders in a computer-based system for tests, prescriptions, and other services. Medication order entry and e-prescribing, laboratory, microbiology, pathology, radiology, nursing, and supply orders, as well as ancillary services and consults.

(Continues)

TABLE 1-8 (Continued)	
Clinical Decision Support	Uses technology to improve best clinical practice with reminders, prompts, and computerized decision-support systems to improve compliance, ensure regular screenings and other preventative care practices, identify possible drug interactions, and facilitate diagnoses and treatment. An EHR should warn clinicians about drug–drug and drug–allergy interactions and make available evidence-based guidelines to help providers consider treatment options.
Electronic Communication and Connectivity	Provides access to communications among providers and patients that is efficient, secure, and readily accessible. Providers should be able to efficiently communicate with their staff as well as other care partners (other clinicians, lab, radiology, and pharmacy staff, etc.). EHR systems may also provide options for communicating directly with patients.
Patient Support	Allows patients to access their health records, interactive patient education, and to improve chronic conditions through home-monitoring and self-testing. Patients can access educational materials and enter data themselves through online questionnaires and home-monitoring devices.
Administrative Processes	Improves hospital and clinic efficiency and provides more timely services to patients using computerized administrative tools, such as scheduling systems. The system enhances the overall efficiency of standard practice management functions, aiding with billing and claims management, authorizations, referrals, etc.
Reporting and Population Management	Using electronic data storage with uniform data standards to enable health care organizations to respond quickly to federal, state, and private reporting requirements. An EHR will help organizations adhere to multiple public and private sector reporting requirements at the federal, state, and local levels for patient safety and quality, as well as for public health.

Adapted from the Institute of Medicine.

Advantages of Electronic Medical/Health Records

An EMR system is an electronic platform that facilitates the needs of a medical practice. An advantage of using a fully integrated practice management and EMR such as Harris CareTracker is that it automates the overall workflow to the greatest extent possible to achieve the maximum amount of practice efficiency. Patient care coordination is improved, and there is a demonstrated reduction in errors, which previously resulted from illegible notes or prescriptions. According to information published by the NHA (n.d.), errors in prescribing medicine harm almost one million Americans per year. These errors range from prescribing a drug that interacts with a drug that the patient is already taking to dispensing the wrong medication due to poor handwriting. Although functions vary widely in EHR programs, the ability to e-prescribe is a feature most EHR programs provide. One of the main advantages of e-prescribing is the ability to quickly perform safety checks. EHR programs will send alerts for potential prescription problems.

In 2011, the National Center for Biotechnology Information published an article titled "Benefits and Drawbacks of Electronic Health Record Systems." It was reported that researchers examined the benefits of EHRs by considering clinical, organizational, and societal outcomes. Clinical outcomes include improvements in the quality of care, a reduction in medical errors, and other improvements in patient-level measures that describe the appropriateness of care. Organizational outcomes, on the other hand, have included such items as improvement in financial and operational performance as well as satisfaction among patients and clinicians who use EHRs. Lastly, societal outcomes include being better able to conduct research and achieving improved population health (Menachemi & Collum, 2011).

Duties of an EHR Specialist

The CEHRS™ will perform duties that assist health care facilities and federal government agencies in the proper handling of electronic patient data, including document management, privacy and security, electronic procedures, and compliancy.

According to the U.S. Department of Labor, Bureau of Labor Statistics, medical records and health information technicians (e.g., CEHRS™) organize and manage health information data by ensuring their quality, accuracy, accessibility, and security in both paper and electronic systems by using various classification systems to code and categorize patient information for insurance reimbursement purposes, for databases and registries, and to maintain patients' medical and treatment histories.

CEHRS™ personnel are responsible for documenting patients' health information, including the medical history, symptoms, examination and test results, treatments, and other information about health care provider services. Duties will vary according to the size of the facility in which the specialist works, but typical duties include the following:

- Review patient records for timeliness, completeness, accuracy, and appropriateness of health data
- Organize and maintain data for clinical databases and registries
- Track patient outcomes for quality assessment
- Use classification software to assign clinical codes for reimbursement and data analysis
- Electronically record data for collection, storage, analysis, retrieval, and reporting
- Protect patients' health information for confidentiality, authorized access for treatment, and data security
- Although medical assistants and EHR specialists do not provide direct patient care, they work regularly with physicians and other health care professionals. They meet with these workers to clarify diagnoses or to get additional information to make sure that records are complete and accurate.

With the increasing use of EHRs, job responsibilities of medical records and health information technicians will continue to change and evolve. Specialists will need to be familiar with, or be able to learn, EHR computer software, follow EHR security and privacy practices, and analyze electronic data to improve health care information as more health care providers and hospitals adopt EHR systems. Medical records and health information technicians can specialize in many aspects of health information.

Facilities in Which an EHR Specialist May Work. After achieving the CEHRS™ credential, you can obtain positions in a variety of health care facilities such as a physician office, laboratory, hospital, ambulatory (outpatient) clinic, skilled nursing facility (nursing home), wellness clinic, urgent care center, or various government and private billing agencies. Positions may include file clerk, medical records clerk, document imaging specialist, medical records technician, medical records specialist, or coder.

Most medical records and health information technicians work in hospitals or physician offices. Some work for the government. Table 1-9 lists the industries that employed the most medical records and health information technicians (e.g., CEHRS™) in 2010, as reported by the Department of Labor.

TABLE 1-9 CEHRS™ Employment by Industry	
Hospitals: state, local, and private	39%
Physician Offices	23%
Nursing Care Facilities	7%
Home Health Care Services	3%

Source: U.S. Department of Labor.

Use of EHRs in Ambulatory Care vs. a Hospital. There are distinct differences between the hospital-based EHR and the ambulatory EHR. Dr. Robert Rowley, in his article titled "Ambulatory vs. Hospital EHRs" (2011), identified key elements of each. Ambulatory EHRs address the workflows in the physician's office. These workflows vary (sometimes significantly) from one specialty to another. The Stage 1 criteria for Meaningful Use describe some fundamental elements needed for such systems.

Dr. Rowley describes ambulatory practices as "service nodes" in a larger ecosystem, with much of the work done in concert with other pieces of the delivery system—referring physicians, consultants, pharmacies, outside laboratories, outside X-ray and imaging centers, and so on, focusing on connectivity.

The hospital environment is quite different and tends to be more self-contained as far as the services provided, and the workflows involved are about communication between different hospital departments, generally under the same roof. The EHR in a hospital is extremely important in patient care. The EHR compiles data from multiple clinical systems and provides a single source of information about a particular patient. In addition, the EHR will capture and store information about the patient's care and will assist in managing transactions such as medicine prescribed, tests ordered/test results, and improving the quality of patient care.

Hospital information systems are quite complex. In addition to providing quality care for patients, there are other contributing factors that affect the care the patient receives, such as the financial aspect of a patient's stay, lab tests ordered, pharmacy information, picture archiving, radiology information, and clinical information.

The primary benefits of a hospital EHR are the unlimited access to patients' information, decreased waiting time for medication delivery as well as test results, and increased efficiency and accuracy in overall patient care.

Pitfalls of the Electronic Health Record

EHRs have many benefits as described earlier, but there are also a few pitfalls. In the same article by the National Center for Biotechnology Information (Menachemi & Collum, 2011), it was noted that despite the growing consensus on benefits of EHR functionalities, there are some potential disadvantages associated with this technology. These include financial issues, changes in workflow, temporary loss of productivity associated with EHR adoption, privacy and security concerns, problems that occur when the system goes down, and other unintended consequences.

The financial issues, including adoption and implementation costs, ongoing maintenance costs, loss of revenue associated with temporary loss of productivity, and declines in revenue, present a disincentive for hospitals and physicians to adopt and implement an EHR. These disincentives have been partially offset with the monetary incentives provided by the federal government for providers and health care facilities to adopt EHRs.

Implementation costs for an EHR adoption include purchasing and installing hardware and software, converting paper charts to electronic ones, and training end-users. EHR maintenance can also be costly. Hardware must be replaced and software must be upgraded on a regular basis as technology improves and changes in regulations occur. In addition, ongoing training and support must be available to providers and for the end users of an EHR.

Recently, patients and providers have begun expressing concern over privacy issues related to EHRs and the personal information collected by the federal government. The ACA mandates the IRS as the collection and enforcement arm for the federal government, which troubles many Americans. In addition, as HHS issues more (and new) rules pertaining to the ACA, there is more intrusion into a patient's medical files, and the patient's privacy is being sacrificed. Examples include mental health questions (e.g., "Do you, or have you ever, felt depressed?") and questions regarding relationship status, including number of sexual partners. Data-mining patients' personal health information is made easily accessible through EHRs. Many private citizens and those in the medical field question how these data will be used and by whom.

There are also the unintended consequences from such extensive legislation to overhaul the health care industry. Contrary to the promises that passage of the ACA would lower health care costs and health care insurance costs, insurance premiums have skyrocketed and the law still does not cover most of the approximately 30 million uninsured or underinsured Americans. There is a shift in sentiment with less people favoring the new law as they become familiar with more of the details and regulations involved. During the health care debate of 2009, President Obama promised "First of all, if you've got health insurance, you like your doctors, you like your plan, you can keep your doctor, you can keep your plan" (ABCNews.com, 2009). However, many employers have dropped coverage for employees due to the skyrocketing costs, or in the alternative, find ways to be exempt from the legislation (e.g., reduce hours for employees to less than 30 hours per week). Insurance companies are issuing policy cancellations at an alarming rate, citing ACA mandates in coverage that render existing policies non-compliant. In addition, some providers are retiring or no longer accepting Medicare or Medicaid patients due to the burdensome regulations, reductions in fees paid to them, and restrictions on how providers are able to care for their patients. This is creating a growing shortage of doctors, especially primary care physicians.

Time will tell what the benefits of or the unintended consequences of the ACA will be for the American people and the health care industry.

CLINICAL WORKFLOWS IN HARRIS CARETRACKER

Learning Objective 8: Demonstrate understanding of clinical workflows in Harris CareTracker.

As addressed in the administrative workflow (Learning Objective 3) discussion, it is helpful to follow a workflow assessment guide and checklist. Harris CareTracker *HELP* provides an EHR Task Sheet (Figure 1-15) outlining clinical workflows.

HARRIS CareTracker — **Harris Caretracker EMR Task Sheet**

CLINICAL

Visit	Daily	Weekly and Quarterly
Patient Visit (or Encounter) Activities [ ] Review/Update Patient's Clinical Information [ ] Enter Chief Complaint & Vital Signs [ ] Review/Update History & Immunization Panes [ ] Lab/Imaging Results Committed to Chart & Orders are Linked/Completed [ ] Document Progress Note [ ] Review/Resolve Open Activities [ ] Review/Resolve Pt Care Management Items [ ] Medications (New/Refills) Completed [ ] Lab/Imaging Orders Created [ ] Patient Education, Referrals, Clinical Letters, Recalls, & ToDo's Created [ ] Progress Note Signed [ ] Communication to Referring Provider & Patient as needed (HT&RPP) [ ] Visit Capture Complete [ ] Patient Provided Copy of Chart Summary	*Daily Activities* [ ] Read Harris CareTracker Mail [ ] ToDo(s) Completed(inc.messages from Provider Portal) [ ] Rx Refills Completed Within 48 Hours* [ ] Review/Submit Saved or Failed Rx(s) New & Renewals [ ] Link Lab/Radiology Results to Open Orders [ ] Lab/Radiology Results Committed [ ] Open Encounter [ ] Visits Captured [ ] Progress Notes Signed [ ] Incoming Documents [ ] Scanned or Paper Results Manually Entered [ ] Matched [ ] Signed [ ] Voice Attachments [ ] Untranscribed Notes [ ] Print Scheduled Charts (for next day) [ ] Enter Admissions (if applicable)	*Weekly Activities*** [ ] Print Scheduled Charts (every Friday) [ ] Administrative Review of Quick Tasks (for all providers) [ ] Order Tracking/Run Overdue Orders Report [ ] Repopulate Registries [ ] Read Harris CareTracker News [ ] Clear Your Cache *Quarterly Activities*** [ ] Ensure employees read release notes [ ] Ensure employees attend live or view recorded release training
**Surescript requirement*	**Visit Workflow Responsibilities** / **Which Role?**	***Also see Administrative Tasks related to Clinical Oversight on the PM Task Sheet*

Visit Workflow Responsibilities	Which Role?
Check In	
Take Back	
Vital Signs & Chief Complaint (if done prior to PN)	
Problem List	
Med List	
Allergy	
Update History Pane & Immunizations	
Open Activity/Patient Care Mgmt Review	
Complete Orders/Link/Manual Enter Results	
Progress Note/ Data Entered & Signed	
ePrescriptions/printed scripts	
Clinical Orders (Labs/Referrals/Immunizations)	
Clinical Letters	
Recall Creation or ToDo for Next Appt	
Patient Education Handouts	
Visit Capture	
Check Out Including ToDos	

Courtesy of Harris CareTracker PM and EMR

Figure 1-15 Clinical Workflows — Task Sheet

Critical Thinking

Familiarize yourself with the task sheet of Clinical Workflows (Figure 1-15) and then complete Table 1-10 by identifying the action and describing how the workflow of electronic vs. paper records would differ, and which role would perform visit workflow responsibilities. The first answer has been started for you as an example.

TABLE 1-10 Clinical Workflows and Actions

Workflow	Actions	Paper vs. Electronic Records
Visit	List patient visit (or encounter) activities: *Review/Update Patient's Clinical Information*	Describe how the workflow of electronic vs. paper records would differ: *MA would enter data on a computer into an EMR vs. writing on paper*
Daily Activities	List daily clinical activities	Describe how the workflow of electronic vs. paper records would differ

TABLE 1-10 (Continued)		
Workflow	**Actions**	**Paper vs. Electronic Records**
Weekly Activities	List weekly clinical activities	Describe how the workflow of electronic vs. paper records would differ
Quarterly Activities	List quarterly clinical activities	Describe how the workflow of electronic vs. paper records would differ
Visit Workflow Responsibilities	List visit workflow responsibilities	Which role would perform each of these duties?

COMMON ACRONYMS AND TERMINOLOGY

Learning Objective 9: List common acronyms and terminology associated with EHRs.

Throughout this text and during your career as a medical assistant, you must be familiar with common acronyms and terminology associated with EHRs. In addition to the key terms identified throughout the text, Table 1-11 provides a comprehensive list of acronyms and terminology that are aligned with the CEHRS™ exam. Additional key terms are highlighted in Table 1-11.

TABLE 1-11 Common Acronyms and Terminology Associated with Electronic Health Records	
Terms/Acronyms	**Definitions**
AC (prescription abbreviation)	Take before meals
acute care	Treat patient with urgent problem
ambulatory care	Treatment without admission
clinical standards	Ensure consistency, reliability, safety
clinical templates	Progress notes made within the EHR; allows documentation into EHR; *must be interoperable*
clinical vocabularies	A standardized system of medical terminology; set of common definitions for medical terms
computer based, stand alone	Personal health records that patients can access using a software program that has been downloaded onto a personal patient computer, or by accessing through a secure website
CVX	Vaccine Administered *Immunizations*

(Continues)

TABLE 1-11   (Continued)

Terms/Acronyms	Definitions
designated record sets (DRS)	Any item, collection, or grouping of information that includes PHI and is maintained by a covered entity
DICOM (Digital Imaging and Communication in Medicine)	A standardized system used in the outpatient setting; imaging information to workstations
eMars (electronic medication administration records)	The five rights: right of patient, right of medication, right dose, right time, right route
ePHI (electronic protected health information)	Protected health information that is created, received, maintained, or transmitted in electronic format
general authorization	Required for uses other than TPO
health plan	Insurance plan; provides or pays for medical care
HIT (health information technology)	The use of technology as a resource to manage patient health care information
HS (prescription abbreviation)	Take at bedtime
ICD (International Classification of Disease) • ICD-9 Diagnosis Usage • ICD-9 Procedure Usage	Standards developed by WHO Diagnosis codes used in health care setting Inpatient and outpatient Three to five alphanumeric characters Of the roughly 18,000 ICD-9 total codes, approximately 14,000 codes are associated with diagnosis usage (CM) Inpatient Three to four numeric characters Of the roughly 18,000 ICD-9 total codes, approximately 4,000 codes are associated with procedure usage (PCS)
• ICD-10 Diagnosis Usage	Inpatient and outpatient Three to seven alphanumeric characters Of the approximately 155,000 ICD-10 codes total, there are roughly 68,000 diagnosis codes (CM)
• ICD-10-PCS Procedure Usage	Inpatient Seven alphanumeric characters Approximately 87,000 codes of the total ICD-10 codes are procedure usage (PCS)
IEEE (Institute of Electric and Electronics Engineering)	Device/device connectivity; used to provide communication between medical devices
incremental conversion	Gradual change; smoother; less impact on office; lower cost. Disadvantages: paper still used; not all data available
Internet-based network and interoperable	A networked PHR that allows the transfer of patient information, providers, and health care organizations such as insurance carriers and pharmacies. A networked PHR is continually updated. Potential disadvantage is that networked PHRs do not ensure complete privacy and security

TABLE 1-11 (Continued)	
Terms/Acronyms	**Definitions**
Internet based, tethered	Patients gain access to their PHR through an outside organization (e.g., insurance company or patient's provider). May have limited editing capabilities. Ownership is maintained by the organization that provides access to the patient (user)
Internet based, untethered	Patients granted access to their PHR through a web-based application. After creating a user name and password, patient is able to create and update information as needed
medication reconciliation	Obtain and update list of patients meds
MVX	Manufacturers of Vaccines *Immunizations*
National Health Information Network	Links medical records across the country
NCPDP (National Council for Prescription Drug Program)	Retail pharmacy transactions
NCPDP (National Council for Prescription Drug Program)	Standardized system used to transfer prescription information
NIP	National Immunization Program
Notice of privacy practices (NPP)	Document that describes practices regarding the use and disclosure of protected health information
ONCHIT (Office of the National Coordinator-HIT)	Group that identified standards for electronic exchange
PHR (personal health record)	Patient's life history in electronic format; does not replace legal record; patient owns
PO (prescription abbreviation)	Take by mouth
Providers	People or organizations that furnish, bill, or are paid for health care in the normal course of business
Rights of Individuals	Notice of privacy act given to patient; *right to access and inspect a copy of PHI; request amendment of record; request restrictions on uses and disclosure; file complaint with Office of Civil Rights*
specific authorization	Required for HIV, STD, drug and alcohol abuse
standards	Commonly agreed-upon specification
total conversion	All data converted at once; office still operates; can be outsourced; costly
TPO (treatment, plan, and operations)	Conditions under which PHI can be released without consent of the patient

CEHRS™ CLINICAL COMPONENTS

Learning Objective 10: Review CEHRS™ competency and exam outline—clinical components.

In Objective 1 you were introduced to the CEHRS™ exam outline and components. In addition to the administrative and practice management functions, it is vital to have an understanding of clinical duties and definitions. Table 1-12 provides an explanation of clinical components of the CEHRS™ exam.

TABLE 1-12 Clinical Components of the CEHRS™ Exam	
Allergies	A list of the patient's allergies as well as his or her reactions to each one
Chief Complaint	A verbal account made by the patient describing his or her problems
Diagnosis and Assessment	The physician's conclusion regarding the cause of the patient's problem
Family History	Information regarding the medical problems of the patient's family
HPI (History of Present Illness)	A compilation of information regarding all aspects of the patient's present illness
Medication List	Information regarding the dosage and frequency of the patient's medications
Past Medical History	Information regarding the patient's past medical problems, conditions, or surgeries
Plan and Treatment	The physician's recommended plan of action to cure or manage the patient's condition
Progress Notes	Documentation of the care delivered to a patient along with necessary information regarding diagnosis and treatment
ROS (Review of Systems)	An inventory of body systems in which the patient reports signs or symptoms he or she is currently having or has had in the past
Social History	Information regarding the patient's lifestyle such as smoking and drinking habits, relationship status, and sexual history
Vital Signs	Measurements of the patient's temperature, respirations, pulse, and blood pressure

Computer Physician Order Entry

The EHR improves clinical documentation and orders by use of **Computer Physician Order Entry (CPOE)**. CPOE is an application used by physicians and other health care providers to enter patient care information. EHRs with the CPOE feature also provide support tools that result in improved care and patient outcomes. eMars work with the CPOE system to increase patient safety by electronically tracking medication administration. eMars is Electronic [Customized] Medication Administration Records. The five rights of eMars are:

1. The right patient
2. The right medication
3. The right dose

4. The right time
5. The right route (oral or intravenous)

An **order set** is a grouping of treatment options for a specific diagnosis or condition. Using an order set, rather than individual orders, helps standardize patient care, expedite order entry, and minimize possible delays due to inconsistent or incomplete orders. Order sets are predefined groupings of standard orders for a condition, disease, or procedure. These order sets make it easier to deliver patient care by eliminating errors and providing easy access to clinical content. You must have the appropriate security setting on your user profile to access the *Administration* module in Harris CareTracker to modify order sets.

Medical Terminology

Table 1-11 provides many of the common acronyms and EHR terminology. To further understand health care terminology you must perform word analysis. Words are broken down into word roots, prefixes, suffixes, and combining vowels and forms.

- Word roots, or base words, are the foundation of the health care term.
- A suffix is a word ending.
- A prefix is a word beginning.
- A combining vowel (usually "o") links the root to the suffix or to another root.
- The combining form is word root plus the appropriate combining vowel.

Tip Box

Word analysis example: osteoarthritis (oste/o/arthr/itis)
- oste (bone)
- o (combining vowel)
- arthr (joint)
- itis (inflammation)

Table 1-13 provides examples of some prefixes and their meanings.
Table 1-14 provides examples of some suffixes and their meanings.
Additional suffixes used to describe therapeutic interventions are provided in Table 1-15.
Now that you have learned common prefixes and suffixes, continue with combining forms. Table 1-16 details the framework of combining forms and their meanings.

Positional and Directional Terms.   Familiarize yourself with some common positional and directional terms used in the medical office (Table 1-17).

Action Terms.   Action terms that are helpful to know when working as a medical assistant are referenced and defined in Table 1-18.

TABLE 1-13 Selected Prefixes and Their Meanings

ante-	=	before, in front of
anti-	=	against
brady-	=	slow
dia-	=	through, complete
end, endo-	=	within
epi-	=	above, upon
hyper-	=	excessive, above more than normal
hypo-	=	deficient, below, under less than normal
peri-	=	surrounding, around
pre-	=	before

TABLE 1-14 Selected Suffixes and Their Meanings

-al	=	pertaining to
-algia	=	pain
-dynia	=	pain
-ectomy	=	excision, removal
-emia	=	blood condition
-genic	=	produced by, pertaining to producing
-globin	=	protein
-itis	=	inflammation
-oma	=	tumor, mass, swelling
-osis	=	condition, usually abnormal
-pathy	=	disease condition
-sis	=	state of, condition

TABLE 1-15 Suffixes Used to Describe Therapeutic Interventions

-ectomy	=	excision
-graphy	=	process of recording
-metry	=	process of measurement

TABLE 1-15 (Continued)

-scopy	=	a visual examination
-stomy	=	a new opening
-tomy	=	incision
-tripsy	=	process of crushing

TABLE 1-16 Combining Forms and Their Meanings

arthr/o	=	joint
bi/o	=	life
cardi/o	=	heart
carcin/o	=	cancerous, cancer
cephal/o	=	head
cerebr/o	=	cerebrum (largest part of the brain)
cyt/o	=	cell
dent/l	=	teeth
derm/o	=	skin
electr/o	=	electrical activity
enter/o	=	intestines
fet/o	=	fetus
gastr/o	=	stomach
hepat/o	=	liver
latr/o	=	treatment, physician
leuk/o	=	white
nephr/o	=	kidney
oste/o	=	bone
path/o	=	disease
ren/o	=	kidney
phin/o	=	nose
sarc/o	=	flesh
thromb/o	=	clotting
ur/o	=	urinary tract

TABLE 1-17   Positional and Directional Terms

anterior (ventral)	front surface of the body
deep	away from the surface
distal	far from the point of attachment to the trunk and far from the beginning of a structure
inferior	below another structure
lateral	pertaining to the side
medial	pertaining to the middle or nearer the medial plane of the body
posterior (dorsal)	back side of the body
prone	lying on the belly
proximal	near the point of attachment to the trunk or near the beginning of a structure
superior	above another structure
supine	lying on the back

TABLE 1-18   Action Terms

Action	Description
abduction	movement away from the midline
adduction	movement toward the midline
dorsiflexion	raising the foot, pulling the toes toward the shin
eversion	turning outward
extension	to increase the angle of a joint
flexion	to decrease the angle of a joint
inversion	turning inward
plantar flexion	lowering the foot, pointing the toes away from the shin
pronation	turning the palm or foot downward
protraction	moving a part of the body forward
retraction	moving a part of the body backward
Action	Description
rotation	revolving a bone around its axis
supination	turning the palm or foot upward

Adapted from quizlet.com/2263030/action-terms-flash-cards

Chapter 2
Introduction to Harris CareTracker PM and EMR

Key Terms

accounts receivable
  (A/R)
cache
clearinghouse
event type
fee schedule
Knowledge Base
macros

open order
override
recall
resources
revenue codes
roles
task classes
template

Learning Objectives

1. Log in to Harris CareTracker to begin your training.

2. Use the Help system to become familiar with key features of Harris CareTracker PM and EMR and to access step-by-step instructions on using each aspect of the system to quickly and successfully complete required tasks.

3. Demonstrate knowledge of the Main Menu, Navigation, Home, and Dashboard overview.

4. Discuss Administration features and functions for Practice Management and Electronic Medical Records.

5. Demonstrate understanding and use of the Message Center components.

Certification Connection

1. Perform basic keyboarding skills (e.g., Microsoft Word®, Excel®, etc.).

2. Manage patient flow (e.g., front office, back office, administrative tasks).

3. Access the Internet to obtain patient- and practice-related information and transmit patient data for external use (e.g., insurance, pharmacies, other providers), complying with HIPAA and office protocol regarding security.

4. Operate office machines and devices such as scanners, fax machine, signature pads, and cameras integrated with EHR software.

5. Define clinical vocabularies in a health information management (HIM) system and related patient safety standards regarding abbreviations.

6. Coordinate office workflows regarding patient flow such as scheduling, patient registration and verification, patient referrals, and more.

7. Participate in end-user training of EHR software; provide training to others.

8. Adhere to federal, state, and local laws relating to exchange of information.

9. Identify the impact of HIPAA for the medical assistant and apply security standards related to the confidentiality and release of protected health information (PHI); de-identify PHI.

10. Develop and execute a plan for data recovery in case of downtime or a catastrophic event.

Adapted from national standards of the National Healthcareer Association (NHA), Commission on Accreditation and Allied Health Education Program (CAAHEP), and Accrediting Bureau of Health Education Schools (ABHES)

INTRODUCTION

Welcome to Harris CareTracker PM and EMR, a fully integrated CCHIT® and ONC-ATCB certified complete Practice Management (PM) and Electronic Health Record (EHR). Harris CareTracker Practice Management (PM) is a web-based application that enables physician practices to achieve greater efficiency by streamlining their administrative workflows. Harris CareTracker EMR is a web-based electronic health record application, fully integrated with all the operational functions of the practice.

This chapter introduces the features and function of *Practice Management, Clinical,* and *Billing* activities in a live Electronic Medical Record (EMR) program and the related workflows. You will perform real-world activities, including *Patient Demographics* and *Registration, Appointment Scheduling, EHR Clinical Duties* (patient work-up, completing the visit, and clinical documentation), *Billing,* and *Collections.* Throughout the text there are Applied Learning Case Studies to complete as a "day in the life" of the medical assistant. The text links knowledge and activities to the CEHRS™ credential offered by the National Healthcareer Association (NHA).

Throughout this book you will review the subject matter of the text, follow detailed step-by-step instructions, and refer to associated screenshot(s) to complete activities in your personal Harris CareTracker PM and EMR environment.

Disclaimer

Due to the evolving nature and continuous upgrades of real-world EMRs such as this one, as you log in and work in your student version of Harris CareTracker there may be a slightly different look to your live screen from the screenshots provided in this text.

When prompted, follow the instructions given in the text to complete the activities.

LOG IN TO HARRIS CARETRACKER

Learning Objective 1: Log in to Harris CareTracker to begin your training.

There are system readiness requirements that must be met before logging in to Harris CareTracker. These instructions are found in Activity 2-1. Prior to logging in and working in Harris CareTracker, you must first "clear your cache." The **cache** is a space in your computer's hard drive and random access memory (RAM) where your browser saves copies of recently visited web pages. Following the instructions in Activity 2-1, set your system readiness parameters and clear your cache. The most up-to-date and detailed information on system requirements (including how to clear your cache) can be found in *Help* under the *Contents* tab > *Getting Started > System Requirements & Recommendations.*

Each student will be assigned a user name and password to log in to Harris CareTracker PM and EMR. Your preassigned user name and password can be found on the inside front cover of your book. Your password must be changed the first time you log in to Harris CareTracker PM and EMR. You will also be prompted to change your password every 90 days for security reasons. The password must consist of at least eight characters with one capital and one numeric character.

Before beginning the activities, clear your cache following the instructions in Activity 2-1. If you are using a personal computer (PC), only work in Internet Explorer®. Use Safari® for iPad®. Once the cache has been cleared, you may continue by logging in to your student version of Harris CareTracker (Activity 2-2).

ACTIVITY 2-1: Clear Your Cache

Microsoft Internet Explorer® 11: To clear your cache in Microsoft Internet Explorer® 11:

1. From the Internet Explorer® 11 *Tools* menu, click *Internet Options*. Windows® displays the *Internet Options* dialog box.
2. On the *General* tab, in the *Browsing history* section, click *Delete* (figure 2-1). Windows® displays the *Delete Browsing History* dialog box.

Used with permission of Microsoft.

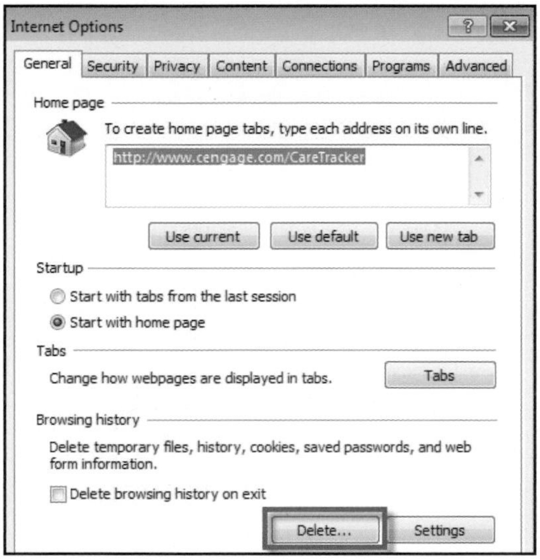

Figure 2-1 IE9 — Delete Browsing History

3. Deselect the *Preserve Favorites website data* checkbox (Figure 2-2).
4. Select the *Temporary Internet Files, Cookies and website data,* and *History* checkboxes.
5. Click *Delete.*
6. Click *OK* when deletion is complete.

Used with permission of Microsoft.

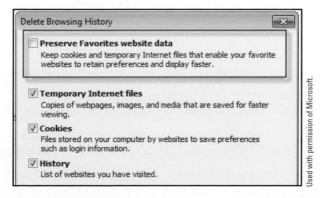

Figure 2-2 Preserve Favorites

Safari® Browser for iPad®: To clear your cache in Safari® for iPad®:

1. Tap *Settings* from your iPad® home screen.

2. Tap *Safari®* from the *Settings* panes on the left. The Safari® Pane displays the *Clear History, Clear Cache*, and *Clear Cookies* at the bottom.

3. Tap *Clear History*.

4. Tap *Clear* in the confirmation window.

5. Repeat steps 3 and 4 to clear your cache and cookies (Figure 2-3).

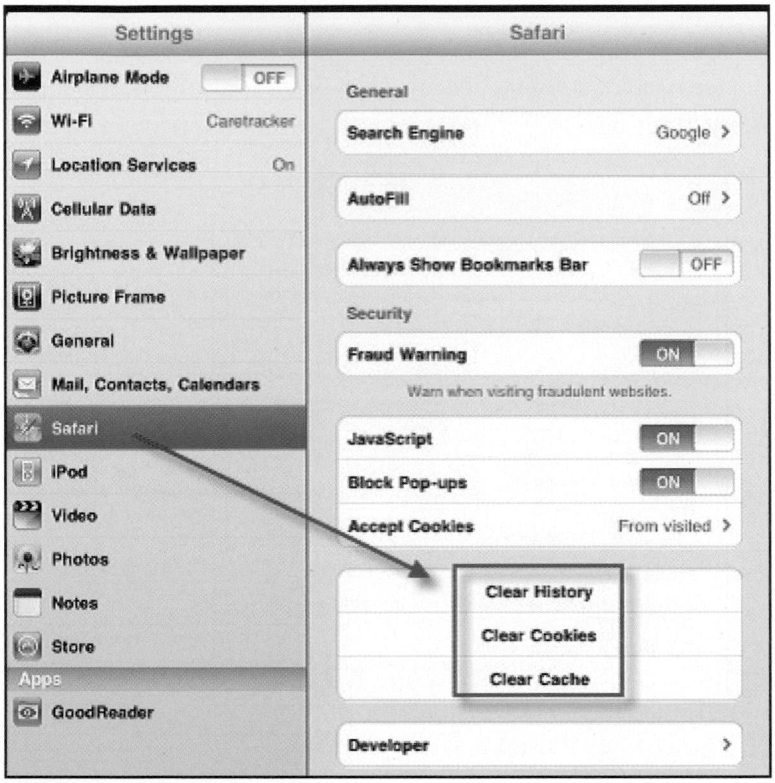

Figure 2-3   Safari Clear Cache

After clearing your cache, begin Activity 2-2 and log in to Harris CareTracker.

ACTIVITY 2-2:   Log in to Harris CareTracker PM and EMR

1. Go to http://www.cengage.com/CareTracker. The product list is set to "Cengage Learning Harris CareTracker Simulation 1.0" by default (Figure 2-4).

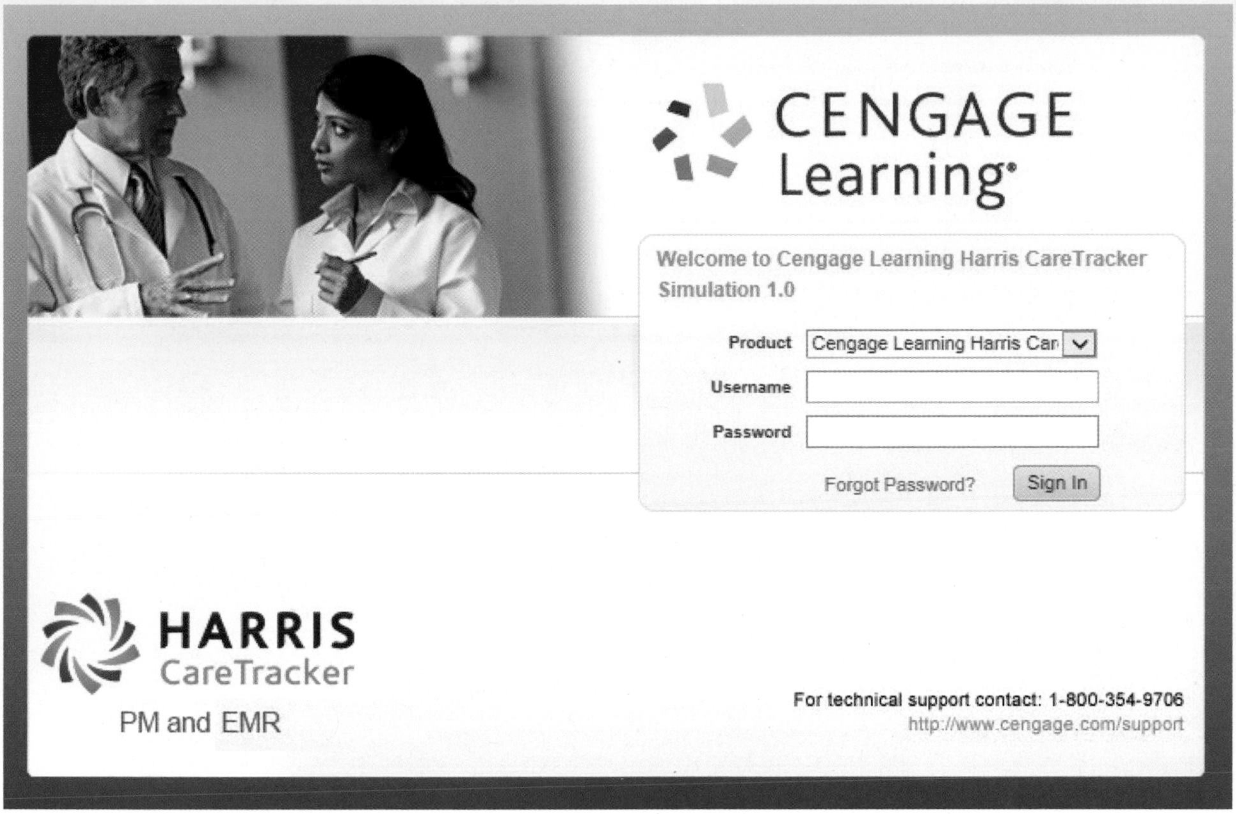

Figure 2-4   Login Screen

2. In the *Username* box, enter the username preassigned to you.

3. In the *Password* box, enter your password. If this is your first time logging in, Harris CareTracker PM and EMR will prompt you to change your temporary password. (**Note:** On subsequent logins, a dialog box called *Operator Encounter Control Batch* will display when you first sign in. Close out of this box by clicking the *Save* button and then clicking the "X" at the top right of the box.)

Tip Box

Both the username and password are case sensitive.
Your new password:

- Must differ from your old password by at least one character
- Must consist of at least eight characters
- Must contain at least one capital letter and one number; for example: Password5
- Must be reentered in the *Verify Password* field

---

4. Click *Save*. A message will display indicating that Harris CareTracker is creating your account and you will receive a notification email when the process is complete. Figure 2-5 is an example of the notification email you will receive. **Note:** You will not be able to log in to Harris CareTracker until you have received the notification email.

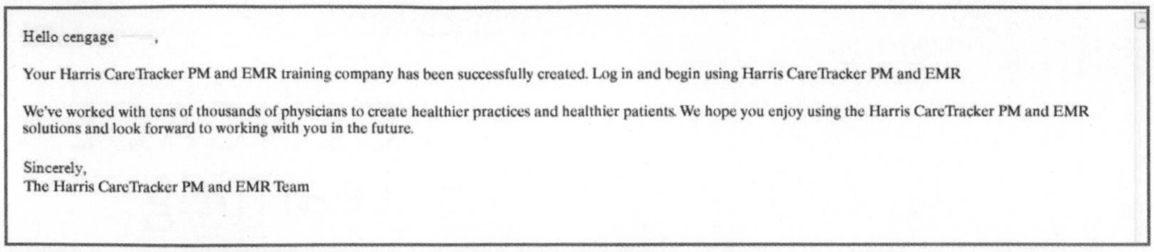

Hello cengage   ,

Your Harris CareTracker PM and EMR training company has been successfully created. Log in and begin using Harris CareTracker PM and EMR

We've worked with tens of thousands of physicians to create healthier practices and healthier patients. We hope you enjoy using the Harris CareTracker PM and EMR solutions and look forward to working with you in the future.

Sincerely,
The Harris CareTracker PM and EMR Team

Figure 2-5   Welcome Login E-mail

Tip Box

To change your password:

- Click the *Administration* module on the left-hand side of the screen and then click *Operator Settings* under the *Security* section (Figure 2-6). Harris CareTracker PM and EMR displays the *Password Maintenance* application.

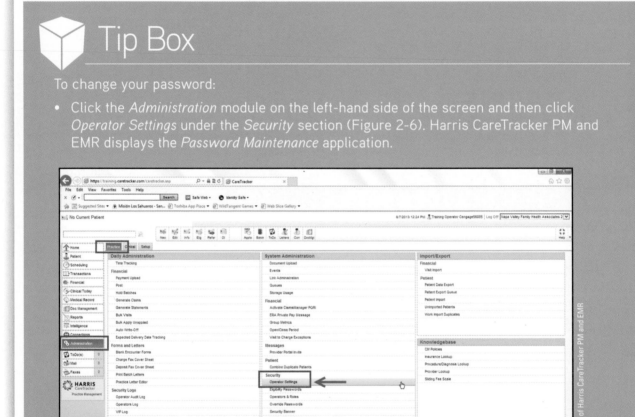

Figure 2-6   Admin-Operator Settings-Security

- Enter your current password in the *Old Password* field (Figure 2-7).

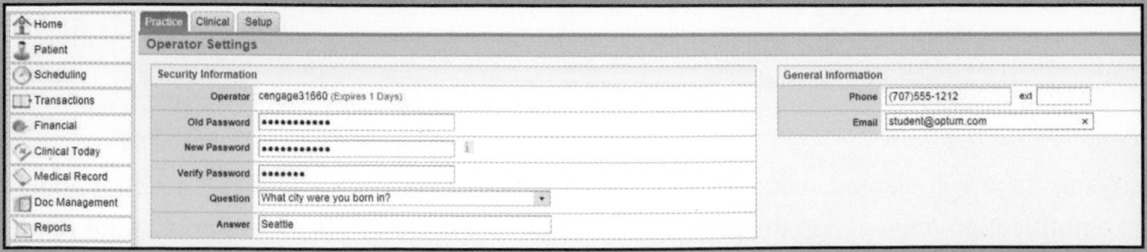

Figure 2-7   Change Password Screen

- Enter your new password in the *New Password* and *Verify Password* fields.
- Select a security question from the *Question* list.
- Type an answer to the security question in the *Answer* field.
- Click *Save*.
- Record your user name and password. You will need this each time you log in to Harris CareTracker. User name _____; Password _____.

HELP SYSTEM

Learning Objective 2: Use the Help *system to become familiar with key features of Harris CareTracker PM and EMR and to access step-by-step instructions on using each aspect of the system to quickly and successfully complete required tasks.*

Harris CareTracker PM and EMR *Online Help* ⊙ integrates product help, recorded training sessions, live webinars, support documentation, and quick reference tools to help you learn about and use Harris CareTracker PM and EMR effectively. The Harris CareTracker PM and EMR *Help* system offers an invaluable one-stop resource for both novice and advanced users. It is designed to familiarize the user with key features of Harris CareTracker PM and EMR, and it provides step-by-step instructions on using each aspect of the system to quickly and successfully complete required tasks.

Harris CareTracker PM and EMR's *Help* system is intended for all staff in the practice with different levels of expertise and job functions. The user can range from front office staff handling appointment scheduling to a physician providing patient care.

Using the Harris CareTracker PM and EMR Help Window

The *Help* system includes left- and right-hand panes (Figure 2-8) and a toolbar (Figure 2-9). Each tool button contains various methods of navigating. The *Help* system is designed to open in the user's default web browser. To become familiar with the *Help* feature, log in to Harris CareTracker, click on *Help* ⊙, and explore the various *Help* topics and materials. This section goes into more detail about the resources available in the *Help* feature.

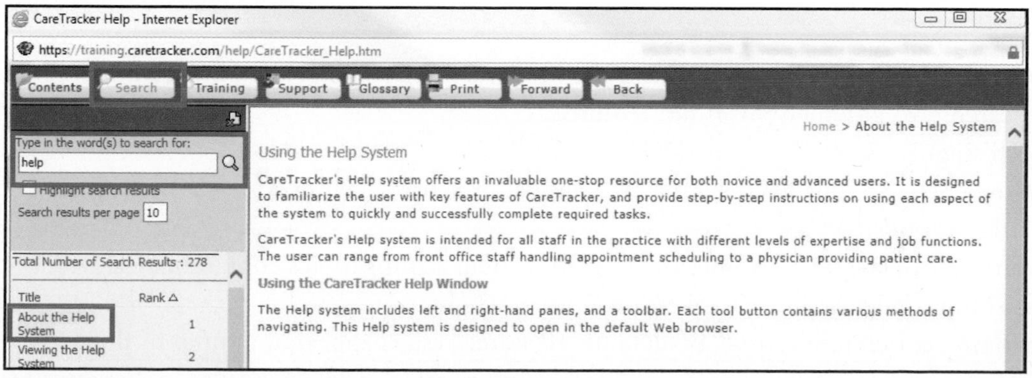

Figure 2-8   Right- and Left-Hand Panes

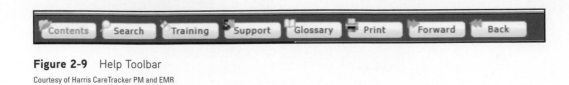

Figure 2-9   Help Toolbar
Courtesy of Harris CareTracker PM and EMR

Figure 2-10 offers a description of conventions used in the *Help* system.

HELP CONVENTIONS	
Convention	**Description**
Text in gray borders	Indicates a note or tip.
Text in red borders	Indicates an important message or warning.
Blue text	Indicates a hyperlink, expanding or pop-up text.
Bold	Denotes the name of a Optum PM & Physician EMR application element, such a module, application or field name.
Italics	Indicates a cross reference or path.

Courtesy of Harris CareTracker PM and EMR

Figure 2-10   Help Conventions

Contents

The *Contents* tab displays the table of contents that includes books and pages in the left-hand pane. Each book or page represents categories of information in the *Help* system. When a closed book 📁 is clicked, it displays sub-books and pages. When an open book 📂 is clicked, it closes. When pages 📄 are clicked, the selected topic displays in the right-hand pane.

Search

The *Search* tab provides a way to explore the content of topics and find matches to user-defined queries. Clicking any topic from the search results list displays the page in the right-hand pane (Figure 2-11). Ways to use the *Search* tab include using a phrase, singular words, a substring, or customizing your search.

- Phrase search—To search for a phrase, the best practice is to enter the phrase in quotation marks in the search box, although this is not required.
- Search singular words—Search using singular instead of plural words to return better results. For example, search for "prescription" instead of "prescriptions."
- Substring search—If you search for "log" the system returns topics containing the words "catalog" and "logarithm." Substring search takes longer than whole-string search.
- Customize search results list—By default, 10 search results appear at a time. In these two outputs, the *Search* pane contains an option for the maximum number of search results to show in a list.

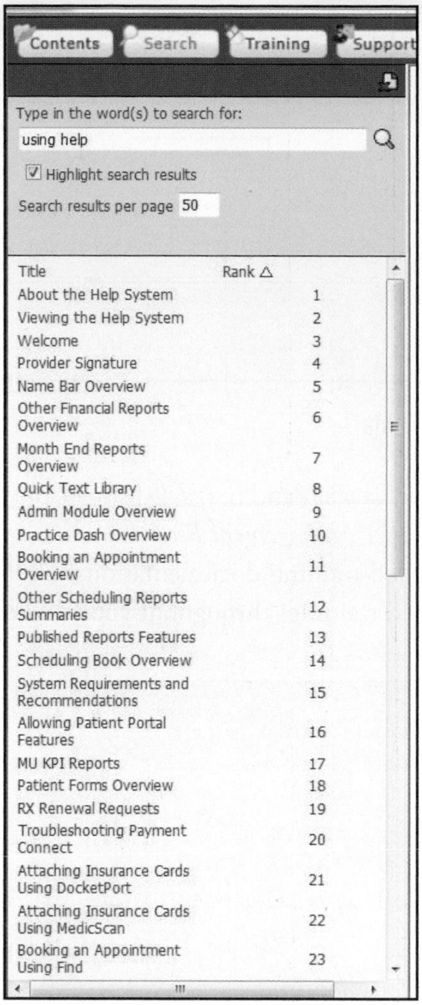

Courtesy of Harris CareTracker PM and EMR

Figure 2-11 Help — Using Search

Training

In addition to the folders in the *Contents* tab, there are also *Live Webinars, Recorded Training,* and *Snipit Training* available in *Help*. *Live Webinars* lists the instructor-led training schedule for the calendar year, registration information, and related webinar material.

Recorded Training. Recorded training sessions are a series of self-paced online trainings that focus on different features in Harris CareTracker PM and EMR. Because these sessions are recorded, you can replay them as often as you need. *Recorded Training* displays a list of recorded web tutorials that give users more information about the features in Harris CareTracker PM and EMR (Figure 2-12). *Recorded Training* provides the flexibility of following each video at your own pace. To become familiar with *Recorded Training* features, click on *Help*, *Training, Recorded Training,* and scroll down through the available topics. You will find the title and description, recorded training, training agenda (in PDF), and training documentation (in PDF).

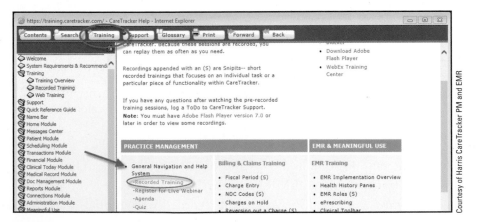

Figure 2-12 Recorded Training

To learn more about Harris CareTracker and the *Help* features provided, click on the *General Navigation and Help System* training under the *Practice Management Recorded Training* header and view the video (Activity 2-3). You may also open the associated training documentation PDF and save it to your computer or print for reference. Refer back to the recorded trainings throughout your studies as needed.

ACTIVITY 2-3: Recorded Training—General Navigation and Help

1. Click on *Help* ⊙.

2. At the top of the screen, click on the *Training* button. (**Note**: The *Training* button is to the left of the *Support* button.)

3. Click on "Learn More" under *Recorded Training*.

4. Scroll down to *Practice Management*.

5. Click on the *General Navigation and Help System* topic (Figure 2-13).

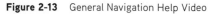

Figure 2-13 General Navigation Help Video

6. Click on the *Recorded Training* link to watch the video.

Print the Recorded Training screen, label it "Activity 2-3," and place it in your assignment folder.

Snipit Training.   A "Snipit" is a short, recorded training that focuses on an individual task or a particular piece of functionality within Harris CareTracker PM and EMR. Snipits are identified with an (S) following the topic header. If you have any questions after watching a Snipit (S) video, you can watch one of the longer recorded training sessions that include the topic. You will view a Snipit (S) in Activity 2-4 by clicking on *Learn More* under *Recorded Training* (Figure 2-14).

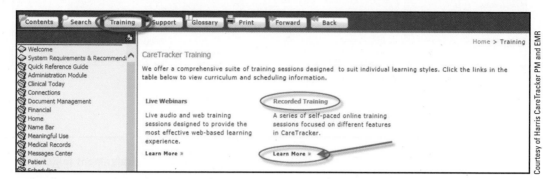

Figure 2-14   Help Snipit Learn More

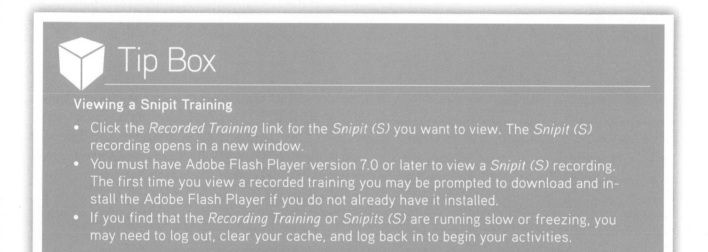

To become familiar with *Snipit (S)* recordings, complete Activity 2-4 to review the *Snipit (S)* on *Fiscal Period*. Refer back to *Snipits (S)* as needed throughout your training for additional reference.

ACTIVITY 2-4:   Snipit (S) Fiscal Period

1. Click on *Help* ⊙.

2. Click on the *Training* button on the toolbar.

3. Click on "Learn More" under *Recorded Training*.

4. Scroll down to the *Practice Management* section. The recorded trainings are grouped by topic area. Any training with an "(S)" at the end of the title is a Snipit training.

5. Click on the *Fiscal Period (S)* topic under "Billing & Claims Training" (Figure 2-15).

Courtesy of Harris CareTracker PM and EMR

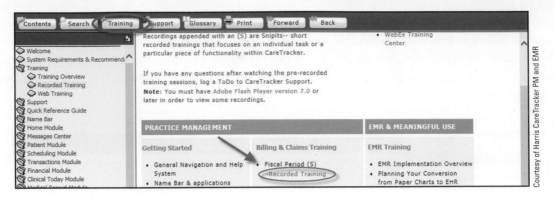

Figure 2-15 Help — Snipit Fiscal Period

6. Click on the *Recorded Training* link to watch the video.

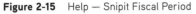

Print the Snipit Fiscal Period screen, label it "Activity 2-4," and place it in your assignment folder.

Support

Support displays a list of innovative and comprehensive resources to assist in performing Harris CareTracker PM and EMR tasks. *Support Knowledge Base* displays a list of documents and articles that include tips and tricks, procedures, trends in the industry, and much more helpful information. The ***Knowledge Base*** is a repository of constantly updated product troubleshooting tips and procedures. The list of support resources available can make all the difference in terms of support, guidance, and inspiration. The support resources are a combination of an online knowledge base and the knowledge and expertise of *CareTracker Customer Service* (Figure 2-16).

Courtesy of Harris CareTracker PM and EMR

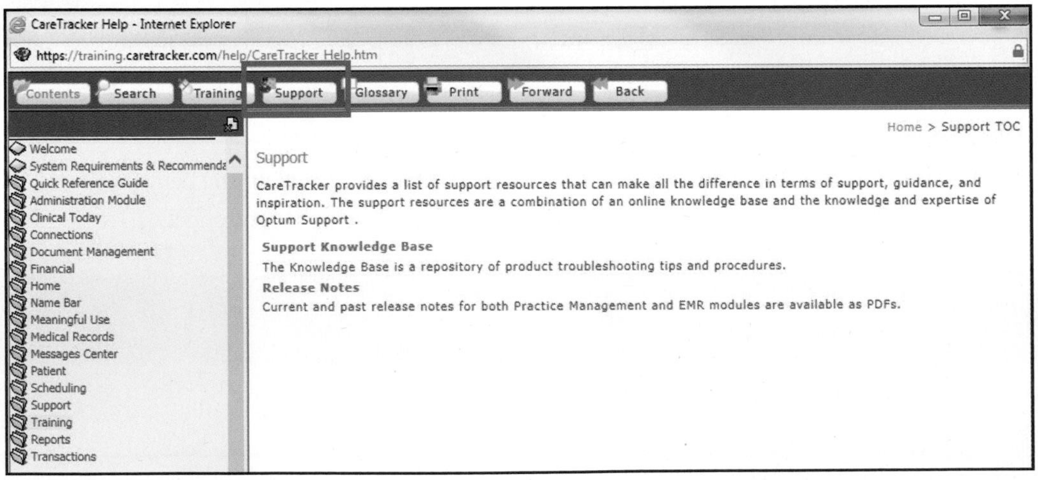

Figure 2-16 Support Tab in Help

PDF Documents can be found online in *Help* on topics for many of the Harris CareTracker applications and modules and are found by clicking on the *Support Knowledge Base* link in the *Support* tab/folder. *PDF Documents* displays a list of available documents in Adobe portable document format (PDF). You have the flexibility and option of viewing, printing, or saving the documents.

Release Notes displays the current and last release notes that include information on new and enhanced features. Current and past release notes for both Practice Management and EMR modules are available as PDFs.

Glossary

The *Glossary* tab displays a *Glossary* in the left-hand pane of the window (Figure 2-17). The *Glossary* is similar to one found in a printed publication and provides a list of words with the associated definition. When a term is selected from the top pane ("Term") of the *Glossary* tab, the corresponding definition displays in the lower pane ("Definition").

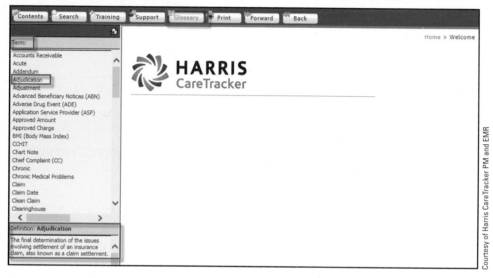

Figure 2-17 Help — Glossary

Print

Print enables printing of the current page that displays in the right-hand pane of the *Help* system (Figure 2-18). An alternate method of printing is to right-click your mouse, then click *Print* on the shortcut menu.

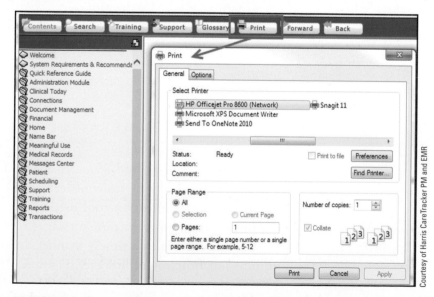

Figure 2-18 Help — Print

Forward and Back

The *Forward* and *Back* tabs guide you through topics based on the history of visited topics. By clicking on the *Forward* or *Back* tabs, your screen will go to the previous topic visited in *Help* (Figure 2-19).

Courtesy of Harris CareTracker PM and EMR

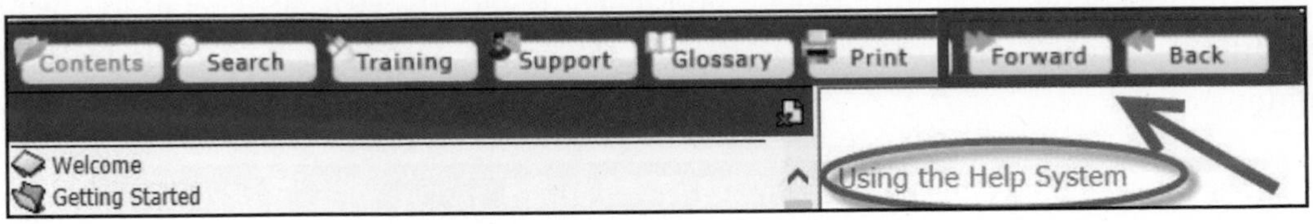

Figure 2-19 Forward and Back Tabs in Help

MAIN MENU AND NAVIGATION

Learning Objective 3: Demonstrate knowledge of the Main Menu, Navigation, Home, and Dashboard overview.

The *Home* module contains the following applications: *Dashboard, Messages,* and *News* (Figure 2-20 and Table 2-1). There are also three tabs: *Practice, Management,* and *Meaningful Use*. Your Harris CareTracker PM and EMR role determines which applications you can access. Your *Home* screen is set to default to the *Home* > *Dashboard* > *Practice* screen.

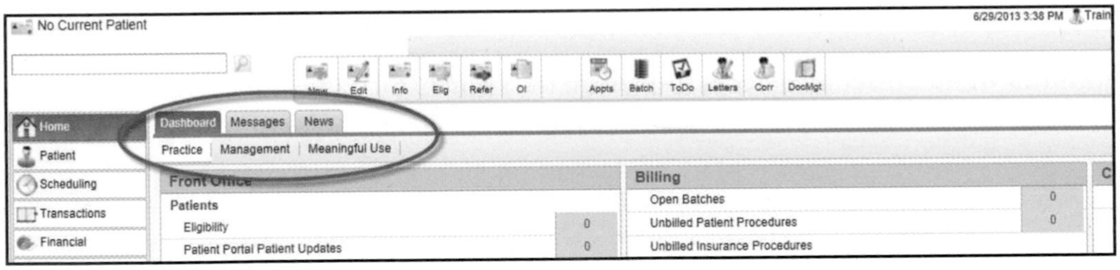

Courtesy of Harris CareTracker PM and EMR

Figure 2-20 Home Application Tabs

Home Overview

The *Home* module contains three applications: *Dashboard, Messages,* and *News*. In Harris CareTracker PM and EMR, the *Dashboard* is where you find your quick links to front office, billing, and clinical functions and features. The *Messages* application is a communication tool used to manage *ToDos*, mail messages, and faxes. The *News* application provides the ability to post messages to patients and employees, ensuring that important information is made available in a timely manner. In your student version of Harris CareTracker, the *News* application is not functional; however, Figure 2-21 represents how *News* would appear in a live practice.

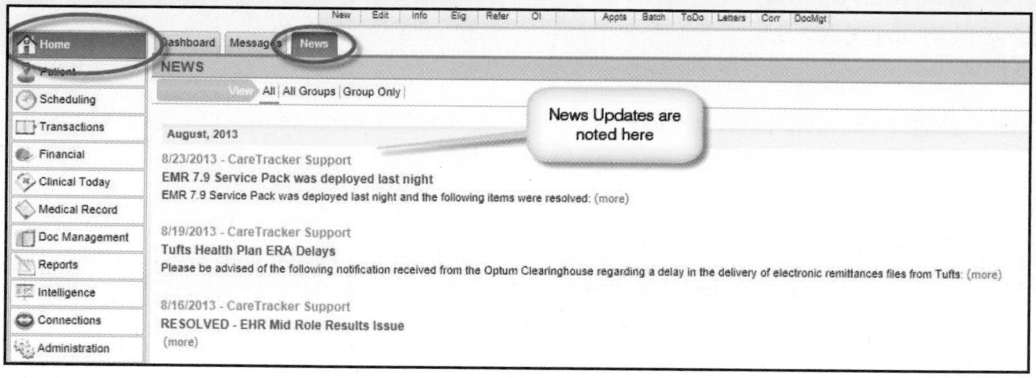

Figure 2-21   News Dashboard

Dashboard Overview

In Harris CareTracker PM and EMR, the *Dashboard* is considered "information central." At a quick glance you can see a summary of what activity has taken place in your practice and you can also see what key indicators need to be addressed, such as inactive claims. The *Dashboard* is divided into three tabs: *Practice, Management,* and *Meaningful Use* (Figure 2-22).

- *Practice.* The *Practice* dashboard includes the practice's front office, billing, and clinical functions.
- *Management.* The *Management* dashboard includes the practice's financial and management functions.
- *Meaningful Use.* The *Meaningful Use* dashboard measures and tracks a provider's progress toward meeting each of the requirements in the Medicaid and Medicare EHR incentive programs.

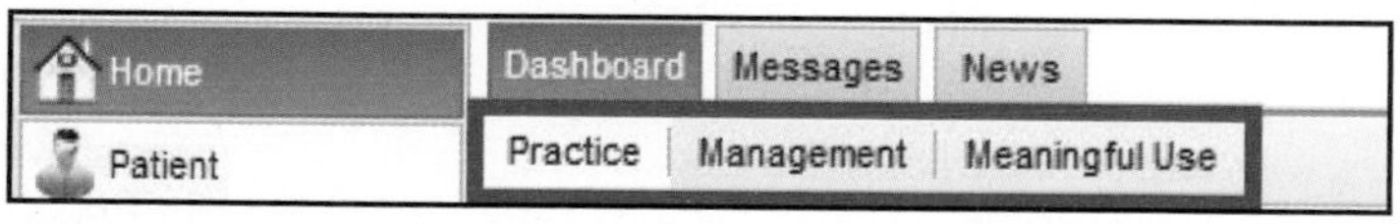

Figure 2-22   Dashboard Tabs
Courtesy of Harris CareTracker PM and EMR

The *Practice* dashboard contains *Front Office, Billing,* and *Clinical* application summaries. Table 2-1 provides a summary of each *Practice* application and description.

The *Management* dashboard contains *Management* application summaries, *Financials* application summaries, and *Staff Measures.* Table 2-2 provides a summary of each *Management* dashboard application and description.

The *Meaningful Use* dashboard is designed to assist providers that are participating in the Medicare and Medicaid EHR Incentive Programs. These programs provide incentive payments to eligible providers that can demonstrate they are using certified EHR technology, such as Harris CareTracker PM and EMR, in ways that can be measured in quality and quantity. Providers must demonstrate meaningful use and then submit report data or self-attest (legally state) to the Centers for Medicare and Medicaid Services (CMS) that they have met the requirements.

TABLE 2-1   Practice Dashboard Application Summaries

FRONT OFFICE APPLICATION SUMMARIES

Application	Description
Show Figures for All Groups	The *Show Figures for All Groups* checkbox is included on both the *Practice* and *Management* dashboards. Select this checkbox to refresh the dashboard and display totals for all of your company's groups.
Links	The *Links* application is included on both the *Practice* and *Management* dashboards. *Links* displays sites that are saved as favorites via the *Link Administration* application in the *Administration* module. This link enables you to quickly access the frequently used sites.
Eligibility	Every evening Harris CareTracker PM and EMR will automatically batch check patient eligibility for the primary insurance saved on each patient's *Demographic* record. This automated eligibility check will be performed for all patients with an appointment scheduled in Harris CareTracker PM and EMR within the next five days. Electronic insurance eligibility checks return a status of *Eligible, Ineligible,* or *Unknown*. The list of *Ineligible* or *Unknown* patients is accessible by clicking on the *Eligibility* link. The application is updated overnight.
Patient Portal Patient Updates	This application allows an operator to approve demographic data changes a patient makes via the *Patient Portal* website.
Missing Patient Information	Any patient with a scheduled appointment whose record is missing or contains inaccurate demographic information essential for billing and submitting insurance claims will be listed in this application. From the *Missing Info* list, you can determine the necessary information to be added to or edited in the patient's record. This application is updated overnight.
New Insurance	Patients who were originally registered in Harris CareTracker PM and EMR without insurance information but have since had insurance information entered onto their account are flagged by this application to ensure that all previously entered charges are billed to the new insurance. The application is updated overnight.
Unprinted Correspondence	By clicking this link you access the *Unprinted Correspondence* application, a queue for form letters generated and saved for patients in Harris CareTracker PM and EMR that need to be printed. These letters can be printed from this application for either all patients or just the patient in context. This application can also be accessed in a window by clicking on the *Corr* button in the *Name Bar*. This application is updated overnight.
Appointments	This link shows the total number of appointments scheduled for the current day for either the entire group or for the specific resource you selected as the resource default when you created your batch. From this screen you can check in patients, take back patients, check out patients, print encounter forms, capture visits, cancel an appointment, view appointment details, and enter copayments. This application is updated in real time.
Wait List	An appointment wait list of patients who would like an appointment with a provider prior to their currently scheduled appointment can be generated by clicking on the *Wait List* link under the *My Lists* section of the *Dashboard*. The *Wait List* link will identify all patients who are currently on the *Wait List* for which an open appointment slot in Harris CareTracker PM and EMR may be available based on a patient's appointment criteria. It will also flag for you the available appointment slot that matches the patient's *Wait List* appointment criteria. The application is updated in real time.
Appointment Conflicts	This link alerts you to any upcoming appointments that are in conflict. From this link you can cancel and reschedule conflicted appointments. This application is updated overnight.

FRONT OFFICE APPLICATION SUMMARIES

Application	Description
Patient Portal Appointment Requests	This link lists all appointment requests submitted by patients via the *Patient Portal* website.
Expired Recurring Appointments	Physical therapy and occupational therapy practices often schedule recurring appointments for their patients. This link identifies patients whose recurring appointments will expire in the near future. Additional authorizations or referrals may be required before future appointments can be scheduled. This application is updated overnight.
Missing Encounters	This link ensures that all appointments scheduled in Harris CareTracker PM and EMR have a visit saved for them and that all visits saved have been turned into charges. From the *Missing Encounters* link, appointments can be canceled, bulk visits can be saved, and bulk charges can be saved. This application is updated overnight.
Admissions	The *Admissions* application is not only a fast and convenient way to keep track of all patients a provider sees during hospital rounds, but will also help boost revenue by ensuring that all your valuable services in a hospital are ultimately billed for. The *Dashboard* represents two values that are refreshed overnight. These values are based on the provider and location selected in the batch. The first value indicates all open admissions. The second value indicates admissions with missing days. It is important to review and work both values daily. This application is updated overnight.
Visits on Hold	The *Visits On Hold* application displays all visits in the "Hold" status. This enables you to work and save the held visits. Held visits do not display in the *Bulk Charges* application and therefore are not billable until the *Claims Manager* screening is passed. This application is updated in real time.
Charges on Hold	The *Charges On Hold* application displays all charges in the "Hold" status, making it easy to work the list to send out the claims. Held charges do not move to *Accounts Receivable* and therefore are not billable to send out as a claim. The held charges are assigned to a *Hold Batch* that is set up when creating a batch for the day. The application is updated in real time.

BILLING APPLICATION SUMMARIES

Open Batches	You must create a batch to enter any financial information into Harris CareTracker PM and EMR (e.g., charges, payments, and adjustments). After running a journal to verify your batch information, click this link to view all open batches and to post your batch into the system. Posting a batch permanently stores all financial transactions linked to it in Harris CareTracker PM and EMR. This application is updated in real time.
Unbilled Patient Procedures and Unbilled Insurance Procedures	*Unbilled Procedures* identifies any procedure that has not been billed. For example, procedures that are paid by Medicare (primary) and then "piggybacked" (crossover claims) to Medex are considered "unbilled procedure balances" (e.g., Medicare paid its portion of the procedure; the remaining balance is transferred to Medex, but the procedure will not be billed because Medicare will notify Medex of its responsibility). This application is updated in real time.
Unapplied Payments	The *Unapplied Payments* link identifies any patient payments entered into Harris CareTracker PM and EMR that have not been applied to a specific date of service. This application is updated in real time.
Electronic Remittances	The total number and sum of remittances received electronically into Harris CareTracker PM displays on the *Dashboard* and a list of the received remittances that need to be posted into the system is accessed by clicking on the *Electronic Remittances* link. They should only be posted after the check is received from the insurance company. This application is updated overnight.

(Continues)

TABLE 2-1 *(Continued)*

BILLING APPLICATION SUMMARIES

Application	Description
Denials	Denials are claims that an insurance company has determined they will not pay due to a specific reason. The number of denials and the total monetary value of the denials for a specific period, batch or group, is identified by the *Denials* link and from this link, denials can be worked accordingly. The application is updated overnight.
Credit Balances	A credit balance is created when either a patient or an insurance company pays more money for a specific procedure for a specific date of service than what was billed. The credit balances that are displayed are for both patients and insurance companies and can be identified for a specific batch, for a specific group, or for all groups. The application is updated in real time.
Verify Payments	*Verify Payments* compares the money an insurance company has paid for a procedure to the allowed amount an insurance company will pay for the same procedure. This feature can only be used for primary payments and is designed to make you aware of instances when you are paid less than the actual allowed amount.
Statements	Harris CareTracker PM and EMR generates and prints patient statements on a weekly basis; however, patients will only receive one statement every 28 days regardless of the number of services they have had. This link identifies the batch of patients who qualify to receive a statement from *ExpressBill* as well as patients who did not receive a statement because of a bad or forwarded address. Once the statements are printed, the status of the batch will be changed to "printed" so they will no longer be identified on the *Dashboard*. This application is updated overnight.
Collections	This link identifies patients eligible to receive different types of collection letters including "Collection Letter 1," "Past Due," "Delinquent," "Final Notice," and "75 Collections." Collection letters are generated from this link as well. Generated collection letters must be printed from the *Print Batch Letters* link under the *Daily Administration* section of the *Administration* module. This application is updated in real time.
Claims Worklist	This link contains all claims identified by Harris CareTracker PM and EMR as those with missing or incorrect information and will not be forwarded to the respective insurance companies until they are corrected accordingly and rebilled, which can be accomplished by clicking on the *Claims Worklist* link. This application is updated overnight.
Open Claims	Open claims are claims that have been submitted to an insurance company but have not been paid yet. An inactive claim would be a claim that not only is unpaid, but has not had any follow-up activity on that claim for the last 30 days. The application is updated overnight.
Unprinted Paper Claim Batches	Harris CareTracker PM and EMR automatically sends all electronic claim batches to the appropriate insurance company or **clearinghouse** and will capture all claims that cannot be transmitted electronically in *Unprinted Paper Claim Batches*. This link identifies the paper claim batches that are ready to be printed. This application is updated overnight. In the medical field, a clearinghouse is a private or public company that provides connectivity and often serves as a "middleman" between physicians and billing entities, payers, and other health care partners (e.g., American Medical Association) for transmission and translation of claims information (primarily electronic) into the specific format required by payers.
Open Electronic Claim Batches	Harris CareTracker PM and EMR sends claims electronically to insurance companies and to clearinghouses. The insurance companies and clearinghouses send an electronic response to Harris CareTracker PM and EMR indicating whether or not they have accepted the claims. All responses must be reviewed and if there are any errors indicated, you must fix and rebill those claims. If the claims have been accepted, the open electronic claim batch may be closed. The application is updated overnight.

BILLING APPLICATION SUMMARIES

Application	Description
Batch Level Rejections	The *Batch Level Rejections* application allows you to view batch level claim rejections received from the Clearinghouse/EDI Services®.

CLINICAL APPLICATION SUMMARIES

Open Encounters	This link identifies patient encounters with missing/unsigned notes and missing/unbilled procedures. *Missing/Unsigned Notes* identifies patients who have an encounter but no encounter note, and *Missing/Unbilled Procedures* identifies patients who have an encounter note but no visit information. **Note:** Operators must have either the "VIP Patient Access" or the "VIP Patient Access Break Glass" override included in their operator profile to access this application for a VIP patient.
Overdue Recalls and Letters	This link identifies patients who have upcoming or overdue recalls. A **recall** is a reminder to the patient to schedule a specific appointment. An overdue recall is a patient who has not yet scheduled a specific appointment and needs to be contacted. From this link, you can generate and print appointment recall letters or labels to send to patients as a reminder that they need to schedule an appointment. This application is updated overnight.
Open Orders	An **open order** is a test that the provider has ordered for a patient, but the practice has not received the results of that test. This link totals all of the open orders for all patients in the group. You can enter and save the test results for all patients by clicking on the *Open Orders* link. *Test Results* for an individual patient can be entered in the *Open Orders* application of the *Clinical* module. The application is updated in real time. **Note:** Operators must have either the "VIP Patient Access" or the "VIP Patient Access Break Glass" override included in their operator profile to access this application for a VIP patient.
Results	Patient lab results transmitted from a laboratory are received into and stored in the *Lab Results* link until the results are reviewed and analyzed by a provider. When a provider has reviewed them, the lab results are saved in the corresponding patient's record. The application is updated in real time. **Note:** Operators must have either the "VIP Patient Access" or the "VIP Patient Access Break Glass" override included in their operator profile to access this application for a VIP patient.
Prescriptions	This link flags all patient prescription refill requests electronically transmitted from pharmacies, and from this link each request should be approved or denied. Approvals and denials of each refill request are in turn transmitted back to the pharmacy. The application is updated in real time. Additionally, this application lists all prescription renewal requests submitted by patients through the *Patient Portal* website. **Note:** Operators must have either the "VIP Patient Access" or the "VIP Patient Access Break Glass" override included in their operator profile to access this application for a VIP patient.
Untranscribed Voice Attachments	This link identifies all audio files, such as dictations, patient interviews, voice mail messages, and more, that require transcription. These audio files are created using the *Attachment* application in the *Medical Record* module. The *Untranscribed Voice Attachment* application supports in-house and third-party transcription by enabling you to directly transcribe through the application or download the file to the computer. The application is updated in real time. **Note:** Operators must have either the "VIP Patient Access" or the "VIP Patient Access Break Glass" override included in their operator profile to access this application for a VIP patient.

TABLE 2-2   Management Dashboard Application Summaries

MANAGEMENT APPLICATION SUMMARIES

Application	Description
Show Figures for All Groups	The *Show Figures for All Groups* checkbox is included on both the *Practice* and *Management* dashboards. Select this checkbox to refresh the dashboard and to display totals for all of your company's groups.
Links	The *Links* application is included on both the *Practice* and *Management* dashboards. *Links* displays sites that are saved as favorites via the *Link Administration* application in the *Administration* module. This link enables you to quickly access the frequently used sites.
Appointments Scheduled	The number that displays here is the total number of appointments scheduled for the month for the entire practice. This is a display-only field. This application is updated overnight.
Accounts Receivable	This link displays the group's total **accounts receivable (A/R)**, which is money that is owed to your group broken out by financial class (e.g., Private Pay, Medicare, Blue Shield, Commercial, etc.), and also by age (e.g., current to 30 days old, 31–60 days old, etc.). You can see the list of patients that comprise a specific financial class A/R by clicking on the *Total* column of the desired financial class. This application is updated overnight.
Visits by Day	Harris CareTracker PM displays the total number of visits that have been entered into the system for the current period. By clicking on this link, you can see a breakdown of the number of visits entered per day for a particular period. This application is updated overnight.
Batch Deposits	The total number of bank deposits made for the current month thus far displays next to this link. By clicking this link, you can view the date and amount of each deposit as well as the source of the money deposited. This application is updated overnight.

FINANCIALS APPLICATION SUMMARIES

Charges	Harris CareTracker PM displays the total amount of charges generated thus far for the entire group and for the current month. Clicking this link will give you charges breakdown by day. This application is updated overnight.
Payments	Harris CareTracker PM displays the total amount of payments received thus far for the entire group and for the current month. Clicking on this link will give a payment breakdown by day. This application is updated overnight.
Adjustments	Harris CareTracker PM displays the total amount of adjustments made thus far for the entire group and for the current month. This link displays adjustments by day. This application is updated overnight.

STAFF MEASURES APPLICATION SUMMARY

User Access Audit	In this link, you can see the total number of operators who worked in Harris CareTracker PM and EMR for a particular date and can drill down to see which operators did what on a specific date. This application is updated overnight.

The *Meaningful Use* dashboard (Figure 2-23) measures and tracks a provider's progress toward meeting each of the requirements in the Medicaid and Medicare EHR Incentive Programs. From the dashboard you can:

- Customize the requirements displayed on the dashboard for each participating provider
- View a status of a provider's progress (percentages are updated nightly) (Figure 2-24)
- Hover over the percentage bar to review the data used to calculate the provider's percentage
- Click the *Menu* icon to download reference documents or run Key Performance Indicator (KPI) reports

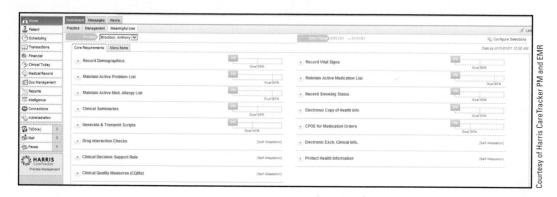

Figure 2-23   Meaningful Use Dashboard

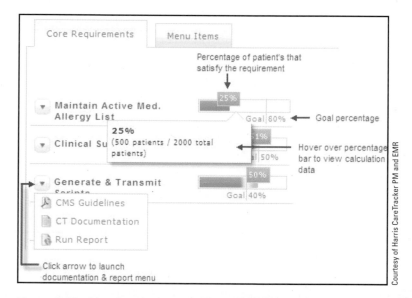

Figure 2-24   Meaningful Use Core Requirements

ADMINISTRATION FEATURES AND FUNCTIONS

Learning Objective 4: Discuss Administration features and functions for Practice Management and Electronic Medical Records.

The *Administration* module contains the *Administration* application, which is divided into three tabs: *Practice, Clinical,* and *Setup*. Each tab is organized into sections containing links to other applications in Harris CareTracker PM.

Practice- Daily Administration

Although there are numerous features in the *Administration* module, we will focus on the applications you will use during the course of your training relative to practice management. In the *Practice* tab, you will find the *Daily Administration, System Administration, Import/Export* (Figure 2-25), and *Knowledgebase* (Figure 2-26) applications. Under each application tab you can perform various functions by clicking on the associated tab. We will explore *Administration > Practice > Daily Administration* features that provide tools for operators to follow that help maintain compliance with HIPAA privacy rules: the *Operator Audit Log, Operator Log,* and *VIP Log*. Figure 2-27 outlines the *Import/Export* tab; however, you will not perform these functions in your student version of Harris CareTracker. The *Knowledgebase* tab (see Figure 2-26) summarizes features that are useful in your daily Practice Management activities.

Operator Audit Log. The *Operator Audit Log* maintains an audit trail of all actions performed in Harris CareTracker PM and EMR by each operator. This log is helpful to monitor each operator's usage. You can customize the log by operator, activity type, and date range. Regardless of the filters you set, the operator log always includes the date, time, operator's log in identification (ID), operator's name, the name of the patient whose record was accessed, the group in which the action was taken, and a comment (the action performed). After you have completed activities in later chapters, you will be asked to generate an *Operator Audit Log* (part of your Applied Learning Case Studies in Chapter 11).

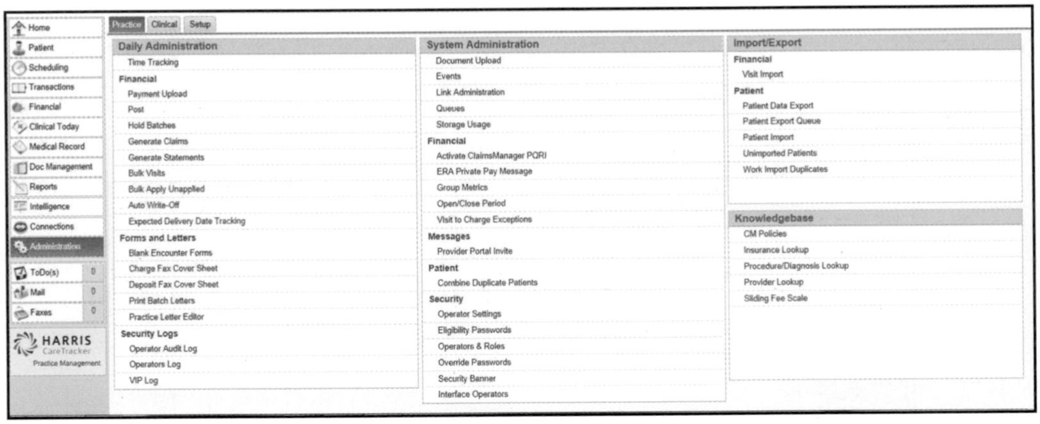

Courtesy of Harris CareTracker PM and EMR

Figure 2-25 Administration Module - Practice Tab

PRACTICE TAB: KNOWLEDGEBASE	
Application	**Description**
CM Policies	The CM Policies application enables you to view and/or search the list of all active, attached policies and/or URLs saved into Optum PM. This will enable the user to click on a mnemonic and view the linked policy if a ClaimsManager edit is triggered during the claim generation process.
Insurance Lookup	A search of all insurance plans compiled in Optum PM's Insurances database can be performed by clicking on this link
Procedure/Diagnosis Lookup	From this link you can search Optum PM's database for a particular procedure or diagnosis code.
Provider Lookup	A search of all providers compiled in Optum PM's Provider database can be performed by clicking on this link.

Courtesy of Harris CareTracker PM and EMR

Figure 2-26 Knowledgebase

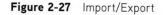

PRACTICE TAB: IMPORT/EXPORT	
Application	**Description**
Visit Import	Through this link you can automatically load visits into Optum PM from a third party system, such as a hospital. Importing visits can either occur as a batch upload (manually) from a file, or can be automatically transmitted from the sending system in either a batch or real time mode.
Patient Data Export	Patient demographics can be exported by clicking on this link. There are numerous filters available with which to limit patient data to export, and data can be exported in HL7 or CSV format.
Patient Export Queue	This queue stores the export data until it is processed in Optum PM.
Patient Import	Through this link you can automatically load patients, either individually or by batch, into Optum PM from a third party system such as a hospital.
Unimported Patients	If your practice utilizes an electronic patient demographic import, you can use the Unimported Patients link under the Patient Setup and Admin section of the Administration Module to update patient records that were not successfully imported for various reasons.
Work Import Duplicates	This application allows you to resolve duplicate patient imports.

Courtesy of Harris CareTracker PM and EMR

Figure 2-27   Import/Export

ACTIVITY 2-5:   Operator Audit Log

1. Click the *Administration* module. The application opens the *Practice* tab.
2. Click the *Operator Audit Log* link under *Security Logs* (Figure 2-28). The application launches the *Operator Audit Log.*

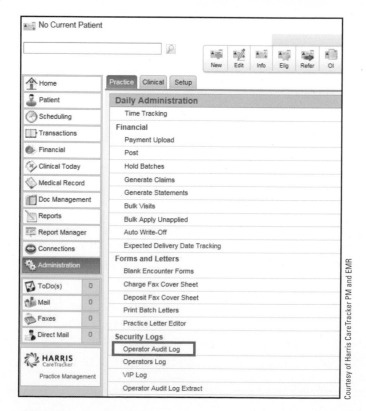

Courtesy of Harris CareTracker PM and EMR

Figure 2-28   Operator Audit Log

3. From the *Operator* list, select the operator for whom you want to generate an audit log (Current Operator). To see a log of all operator activities, you would leave as "-Select-".

4. From the *Type* list, select the type of activity for which you want to view a log. Leave as "-Select-" to view a log of all activities.

5. In the *Date* boxes, enter the dates to include in the audit log. (Leave the dates as they are to run a report for the past seven days.)

6. Click *Show Log*. Harris CareTracker PM displays the log in the bottom half of the screen (Figure 2-29).

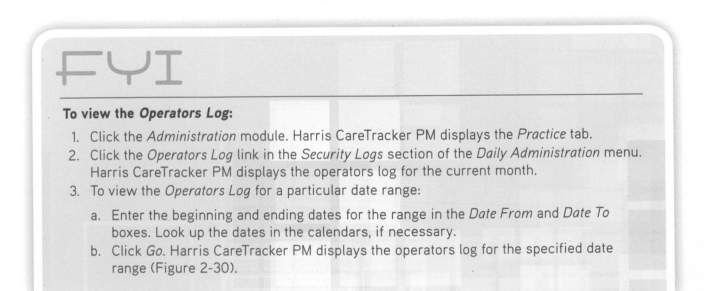

Figure 2-29 Operator Log

To print the log, right-click your mouse on the log and then select Print from the shortcut menu. Label the Operators Audit Log "Activity 2-5" and place it in your assignment folder.

Operators Log. The *Operators Log* tracks the number of operators who log in to Harris CareTracker PM and EMR each day. You can view the log for the current month or for a specific time period.

FYI

To view the *Operators Log*:

1. Click the *Administration* module. Harris CareTracker PM displays the *Practice* tab.

2. Click the *Operators Log* link in the *Security Logs* section of the *Daily Administration* menu. Harris CareTracker PM displays the operators log for the current month.

3. To view the *Operators Log* for a particular date range:

   a. Enter the beginning and ending dates for the range in the *Date From* and *Date To* boxes. Look up the dates in the calendars, if necessary.

   b. Click *Go*. Harris CareTracker PM displays the operators log for the specified date range (Figure 2-30).

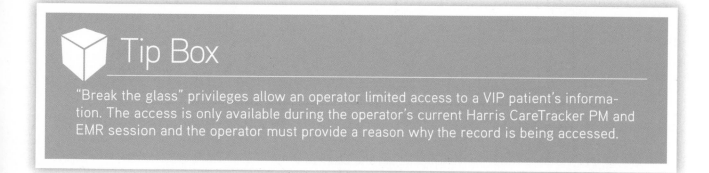

Figure 2-30   Monthly Operators Log

VIP Log. There are many reasons to flag a patient as a VIP. Doing so allows you to restrict operator access to the patient's demographic information. Any operator may flag a high-profile patient as a VIP, but only operators assigned either the "VIP Patient Access" or the "VIP Patient Access Break Glass" override in their profile can access a VIP demographic.

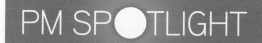

Tip Box

"Break the glass" privileges allow an operator limited access to a VIP patient's information. The access is only available during the operator's current Harris CareTracker PM and EMR session and the operator must provide a reason why the record is being accessed.

Each time an operator accesses a VIP patient demographic, Harris CareTracker PM and EMR creates an entry in the *VIP Patient Log*. The log lists the patient name, the operator who accessed the record, and the date and time the record was accessed. In Chapter 3, Activity 3-5, you will be instructed to register patient(s) and flag them as VIP. You will then view the *VIP Log* using the instructions in the FYI box on page 76.

PM SP●TLIGHT

Important!!

Your operator role must include a *VIP Patient Log* security override to view the *VIP Patient Log*. By default, only the practice administrator ("Fin-Practice Admin" role) is assigned access to view VIP patients and the VIP log. The practice administrator can approve a request for an override.

FYI

Viewing the VIP log

1. Click the *Administration* module. Harris CareTracker PM displays the *Practice* tab.
2. Click the *VIP Log* link under the *Security Logs* section. The application displays the *VIP Patient Log* (Figure 2-31).

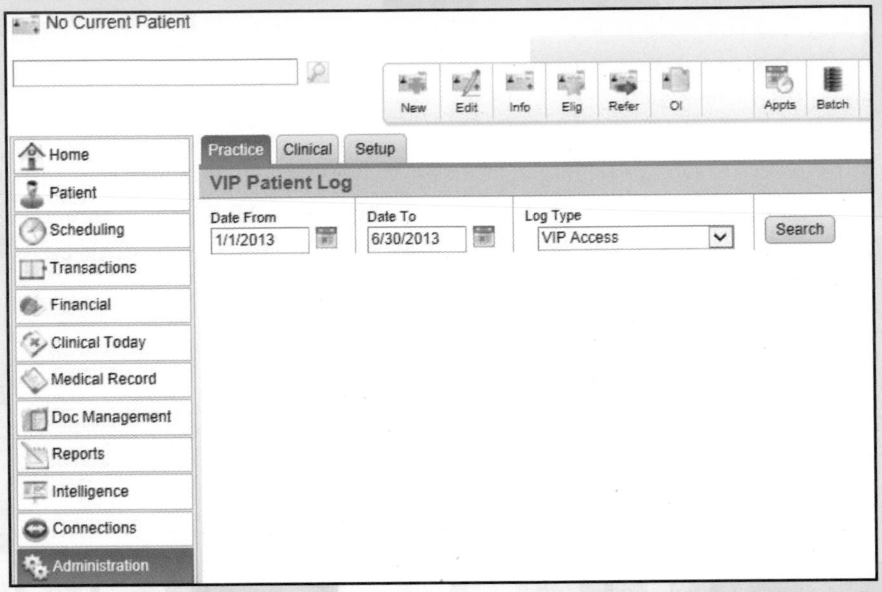

Courtesy of Harris CareTracker PM and EMR

Figure 2-31 VIP Patient Log

3. Select the date range in the *Date From* and *Date To* fields.
4. Select the *Log Type* to view:
   a. VIP Access: displays operators with *VIP Patient Access* override included in their profile.
   b. VIP Break Glass Access: displays the activity of users with the *VIP Break Glass* override included in their profile. (At this point in your text/activities, there will be no activities of users to display. After completing registration and charting on a VIP patient in later chapters, you will be able to generate a log.)
5. Click *Search*. Harris CareTracker PM displays the log (Figure 2-32).

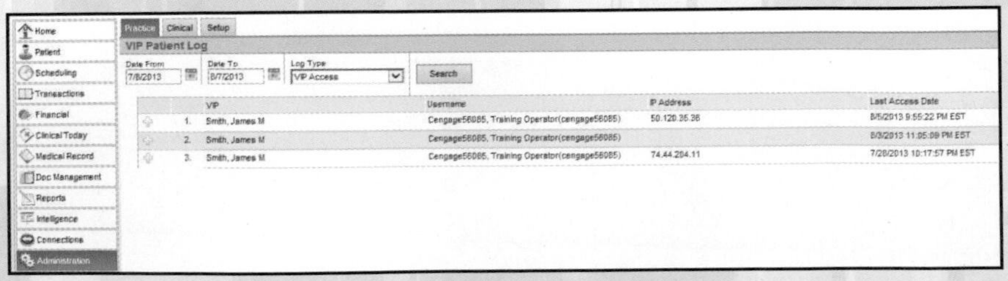

Courtesy of Harris CareTracker PM and EMR

Figure 2-32 VIP Patient Log Created

6. Click the plus sign next to the patient's name to expand the log and view additional details (Figure 2-33).

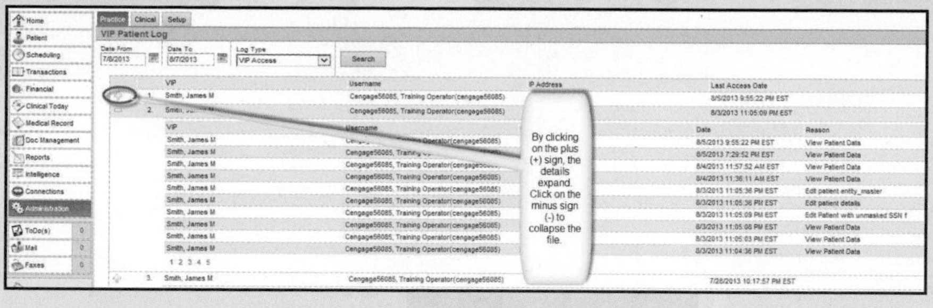

Figure 2-33 VIP Patient Log Expanded

Operator access to both VIP patient demographics and the *VIP Patient Log* is set by the practice administrator in the *Operators & Roles* application in the *Administration* module.

Practice - System Administration

In the *Administration > Practice > System Administration* setting, you will find features including *Financial, Messages* (provider portal), *Patient* (combining duplicate patient accounts), and *Security* sections. Vital *System Administration* functions to be reviewed are the *Open/Close Period, Operator Settings,* and *Operators & Roles.*

Open/Close Period. Working in the correct fiscal period is crucial to the electronic health record. Transactions and entries are permanently linked to a fiscal period and must be accurate. You must define the fiscal periods for your practice before any charges or payments are entered into Harris CareTracker PM and EMR. You can manage the practice's financials by opening and closing each fiscal period. You can post financials to multiple open periods, but you cannot post financials or create a batch for a closed period. The fiscal period and year you are working in displays in all financial transaction applications, such as *Charge, Bulk Charges,* and *Payments on Account.* All reports are linked to the established fiscal periods, not the periods of the calendar year.

Depending on when you begin using this textbook, you may be required to change the fiscal year in addition to opening and closing fiscal periods. Activity 2-6 instructs you how to open a new fiscal year.

ACTIVITY 2-6: Open a New Fiscal Year

1. Click the *Administration* module. Harris CareTracker PM displays the *Practice* tab.
2. Click the *Open/Close Period* link in the *Financial* section (Figure 2-34). Harris CareTracker PM displays all of your fiscal periods for the current fiscal year.

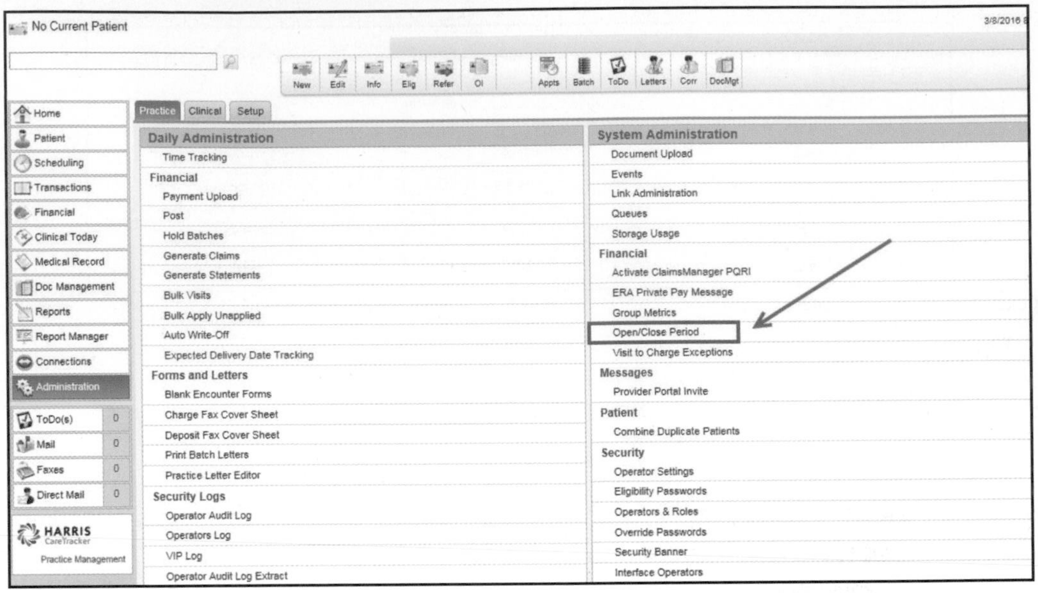

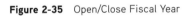

Figure 2-34 Open/Close Period

3. To open a fiscal year for all groups within your company, select *Y* from the *All Groups* list and then click *Go* (Figure 2-35).

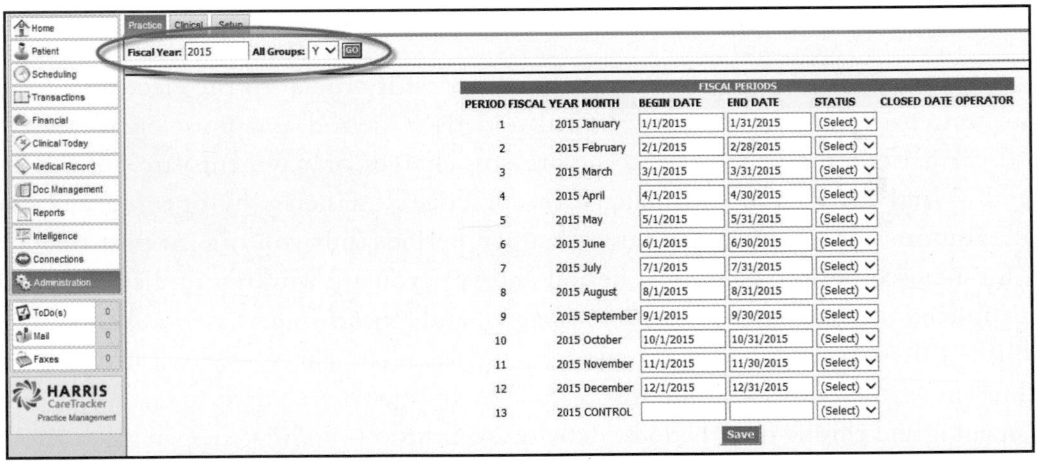

Figure 2-35 Open/Close Fiscal Year

4. By default, the beginning and end date of each period is set to the first and last day of the month. You can change the date range for any month by entering a date in the *Begin Date* and *End Date* boxes for the month.

5. Continue with Activity 2-7 to open a new fiscal period.

Print the Open Fiscal Period screen, label it "Activity 2-6," and place it in your assignment folder.

On the first day of a new period, the practice administrator must change the status of the period to *Open* to begin posting financials to that period. You can also open a period prior to the first day of the period. It is typical for a practice to have multiple periods open.

ACTIVITY 2-7:   Open a Fiscal Period

1. Continue from Activity 2-6. If you had already logged out:

  a. Click the *Administration* module. Harris CareTracker PM displays the *Practice* tab.

  b. Under *System Administration/Financial*, click the *Open/Close Period* link. Harris CareTracker PM displays all of your fiscal periods for the current fiscal year.

  c. For multigroup companies, select *Y* from the *All Groups* list and then click *Go* to open a fiscal period for all groups in the company.

2. From the list in the *Status* column, select "OPEN" for the period you want to open. Select the period (month/year) you are currently working in to open.

Tip Box

You will have to open/close periods while working throughout the text to reflect the current date(s) and activities you are working in.

3. Click *Save*. You can now create batches and post financials for this period (Figure 2-36).

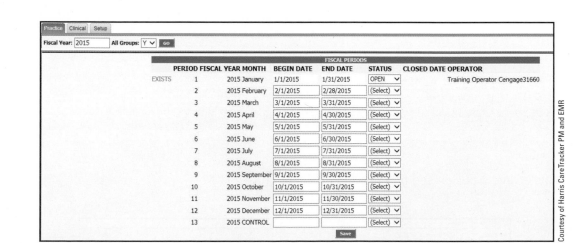

Figure 2-36   Fiscal Period Open

Courtesy of Harris CareTracker PM and EMR

⬤ **Print the Open Fiscal Period screen, label it "Activity 2-7," and place it in your assignment folder.**

When all financials have been posted into a period, your practice administrator will need to change the status of the period to "Closed." Once a period is closed, financials cannot be posted into it.

FYI

Warning!! Do not close a fiscal period until instructed to do so.

To Close a Fiscal Period

1. Click the *Administration* module. Harris CareTracker PM displays the *Practice* tab.
2. Click the *Open/Close Period* link. Harris CareTracker PM displays all of your fiscal periods for the current fiscal year.
3. For multigroup companies, select *Y* from the *All Groups* list and then click *Go* to close a fiscal period for all groups in the company.
4. From the list in the *Status* column, select *Closed* for the period you want to close. You will receive a warning (Figure 2-37) asking, "Are you sure you want to close this period?"

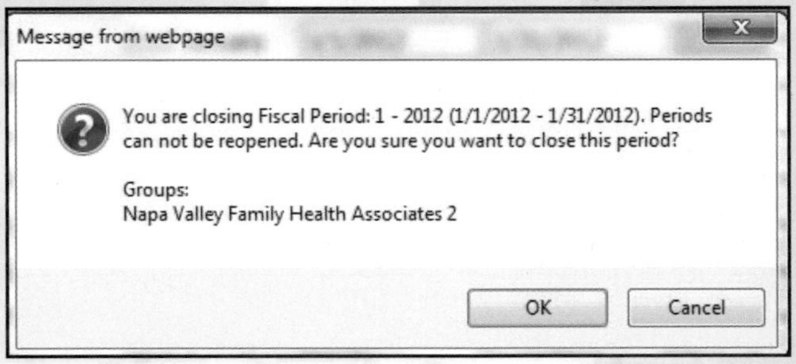

Courtesy of Harris CareTracker PM and EMR

Figure 2-37 Close Period Warning

Tip Box

Do not close a period until all financials for that period have been posted. A closed period cannot be reopened and financials cannot be posted into a closed period.

5. Click *Save*. Your closed period will look like Figure 2-38.

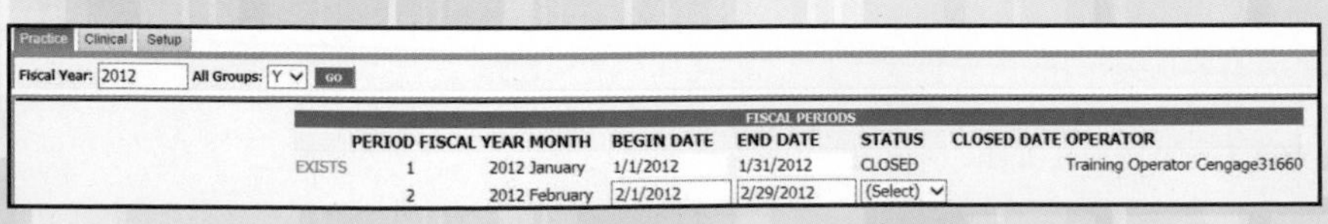

Figure 2-38 Closed Fiscal Period

Courtesy of Harris CareTracker PM and EMR

Operator Settings.   Every operator must have a user name and a password to log into Harris CareTracker PM and EMR. You are required to change your password every 90 days. Harris CareTracker PM and EMR reminds users seven days before their password expires and gives you the option of changing the password at that time. If your password expires, you can reset it without having to log a *ToDo* to *Support*. You can also use *Operator Settings* to change your password at any time after you begin using Harris CareTracker PM and EMR, even prior to being required to by the system.

The *Operator Settings* application is also used to store the operator's contact information. This information is used by *CareTracker Customer Service* to contact operators for support issues or in response to *ToDos*.

Tip Box

It is important to keep the *General Information* section updated with your current phone number and e-mail address.

ACTIVITY 2-8:   Change Your Password

1. Click the *Administration* module. The application displays the *Practice* tab.
2. Click the *Operator Settings* link (Figure 2-39) in the *Security* section. Harris CareTracker PM and EMR launches the *Operator Settings* application.

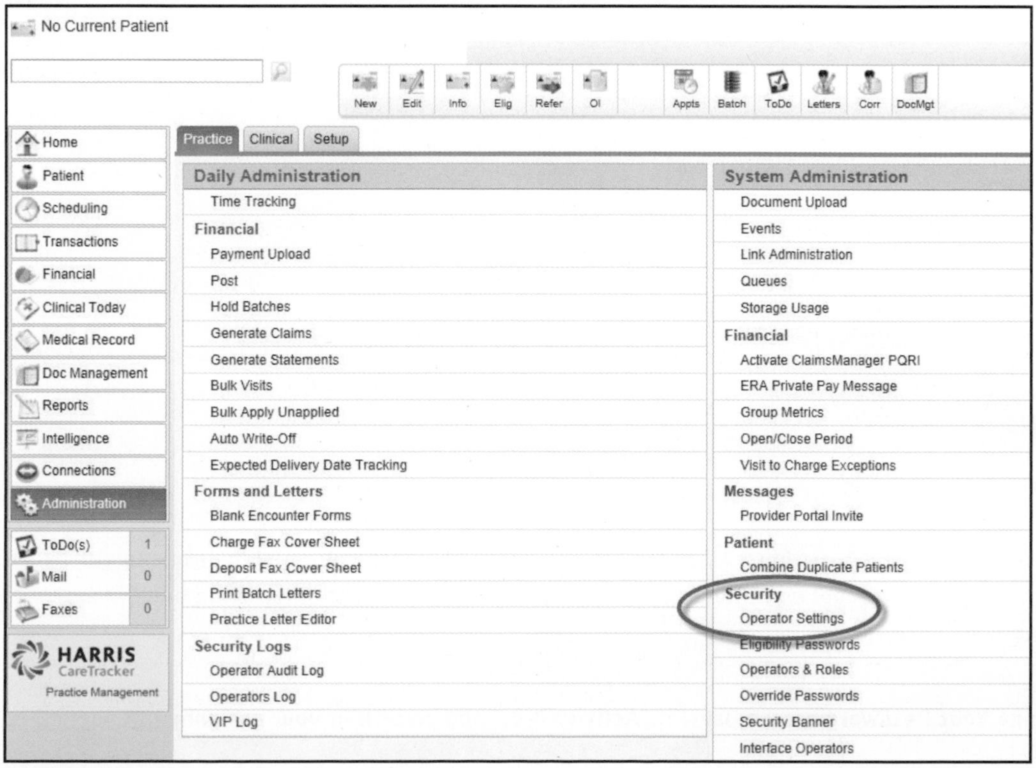

Figure 2-39   Operator Settings

3. In the *Old Password* box, enter your current password (the one you created in Activity 2-1).
4. In the *New Password* field, enter your new password (enter a personal password you will remember). Record your user ID and new password for future reference:
   a. User Name ____________________
   b. New Password: ____________________

The new password must meet the following criteria:

- The new password must differ from your old password by at least one character.
- The new password must consist of at least eight characters.
- At least one of the eight characters must be a capital letter and at least one must be a number. For example: "Password5"

5. In the *Verify Password* box, reenter your new password.
6. From the *Question* list, select a security question.
7. In the *Answer* box, enter the answer to the security question.
8. In the *Phone* and *Email* fields, enter your phone number and e-mail address. It is important to keep this contact information up to date because it is used by *Support* to follow up on support issues or *ToDos*. (See Figure 2-40.)

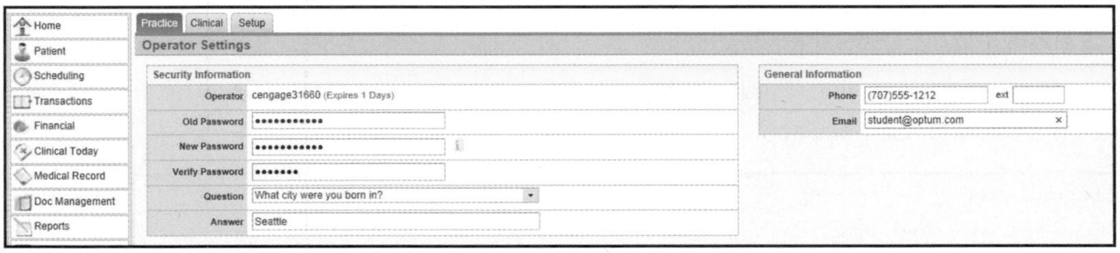

Courtesy of Harris CareTracker PM and EMR

Figure 2-40 Change Password Screen

Tip Box

The application will prompt the operator for an e-mail address if a valid address is not already saved for the operator.

9. Click *Save*. The application redirects you to the login screen where you must log in using your new password. If you do not get an automatic redirect, you may have to log out and log back in again using your new password.

Print the Change Your Password screen, label it "Activity 2-8," and place it in your assignment folder.

Operators and Roles. All Harris CareTracker PM and EMR operators are set up with a user profile based on their responsibilities and duties in a practice. An operator's privileges in Harris CareTracker PM and EMR are determined by the *Role(s)* and *Override(s)* assigned to his or her profile:

- **Roles** determine which Harris CareTracker PM and EMR modules and applications an operator can access.
- **Overrides** are used to either restrict an operator's access to a certain application and functionality, or they can be used to grant an operator additional privileges that may not be included in his or her role. For example, if an operator needs access to only one application within the *Financial* module, you could add an override to the operator's profile to allow him or her to access just a particular financial application.

From the *Operator & Roles* application you can:

- Add an operator
- Edit an existing operator's roles/override
- Remove an operator from your practice
- Monitor operator activities

ACTIVITY 2-9: To Add an Operator

1. Click the *Administration* module. The application displays the *Practice* tab.

2. Click the *Operators & Roles* link in the *Security* section. The application displays the *Group Operators* list.

3. Scroll down to the bottom of the *Operators* list and then click *New*. The application opens the *Add New Operator* form in the lower frame of the screen. (**Note:** Do not click on your operator name. Be sure to click *New* as instructed.)

4. In the *Name* section:

   a. Skip the *Title* box (not used for operators).

   b. In the *First Name* box, enter the operator's first name (enter "Sally").

   c. Skip the *Middle* name box (not used for operators).

   d. In the *Last Name* box, enter the operator's last name (enter "Student").

   e. Skip the *Suffix* box (not used for operators).

   f. In the *Nick Name* box, enter a nickname, if applicable.

   g. In the *Email Address* box, enter the operator's e-mail address. If the operator does not have an e-mail address, he or she should create a free account on any e-mail server, such as Hotmail or Google (enter "student@email.com").

5. In the *User* section:

   a. In the *Login* box, enter the operator's first initial and last name with no space in the middle, followed by the operator number in your username. For example: "sstudent 66694"

   b. In the *Password* box, enter a default password (enter "Password1").

Tip Box

The password must be at least eight characters, containing at least one capital letter and at least one number. For example: "Password1".

---

   c. In the *Verify Password* box, reenter the password.

   d. The *Change Password* checkbox is selected by default to prompt the operator to reset his or her password.

6. In the *Security* section:

   a. In the *Question* and *Answer* boxes, enter a security question and the answer (select "City Born" and enter "Napa").

   b. Skip the *Confirmation Number* box (a confirmation number is not required).

7. In the *Access* section:

   a. The *Active* field is set to *Yes* by default to indicate that the operator is active in the system.

   b. In the *Timeout* box, enter the amount of time (in minutes) that the Harris CareTracker PM system can be idle before the operator is automatically logged out (enter "10").

ADMINISTRATIVE SP⬤TLIGHT

The maximum idle time in Harris CareTracker PM is 180 minutes. For security reasons, it is best practice to keep the idle time short, such as 5–10 minutes.
   The time zone defaults to Eastern Standard Time (EST) if no time zone is set for the operator.

---

   c. From the *Time Zone* list, select the time zone in which the company is located (select "US/Pacific"). The application calculates the check-in, take-back, and check-out time based on the operator's time zone setting. Additionally, the time stamp in the clinical log, progress note, and appointment list are also based on the time zone set for the operator.

   d. (FYI only) The Primary/Secondary IP boxes are used to designate the IP addresses (computers) from which an operator can access Harris CareTracker PM and EMR. Populating these fields means that the operator can only access Harris CareTracker PM and EMR from the designated IP addresses, such as the office or home.

   e. (FYI only) The Single Sign-On feature allows the operator to log on to Harris CareTracker PM and EMR through another system using a single-user ID and password. (This option is only available if single sign-on has been set up for your company.) If the operator will be using single sign-on:

   i. Enter the operator's user ID in the *Single Sign-On* ID box.

   ii. Enter a name for the system the user is logging into in the *Single Sign-On IDP* box. For example: If the operator is accessing Harris CareTracker PM and EMR through the AMA website, then enter "AMA."

Tip Box

If the operator is only allowed to access Harris CareTracker PM and EMR using single sign-on, select *Yes* in the *Single Sign-On Only* field. If the operator is allowed to log on to the application directly, then select *No*.

---

  f. In the *Roles* field, click the [R..] button. The application displays the *Add Operator Role* window. Select the checkbox next to each role you want to assign to the operator (select each role with a check mark).

  g. Then click *Add* (Figure 2-41).

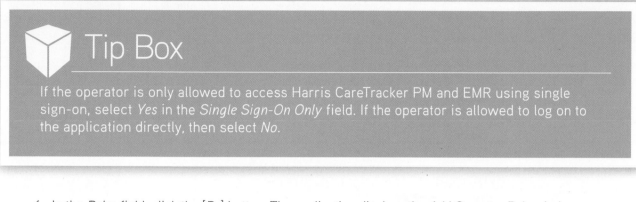

Figure 2-41   Add an Operator

Courtesy of Harris CareTracker PM and EMR

Tip Box

After an operator is added, you can override his or her role to allow access to particular features and applications in Harris CareTracker PM and EMR by accessing *Admin > Practice > Override Passwords*, clicking *Edit*, and updating as needed (Figure 2-42).

(Continues)

(Continued)

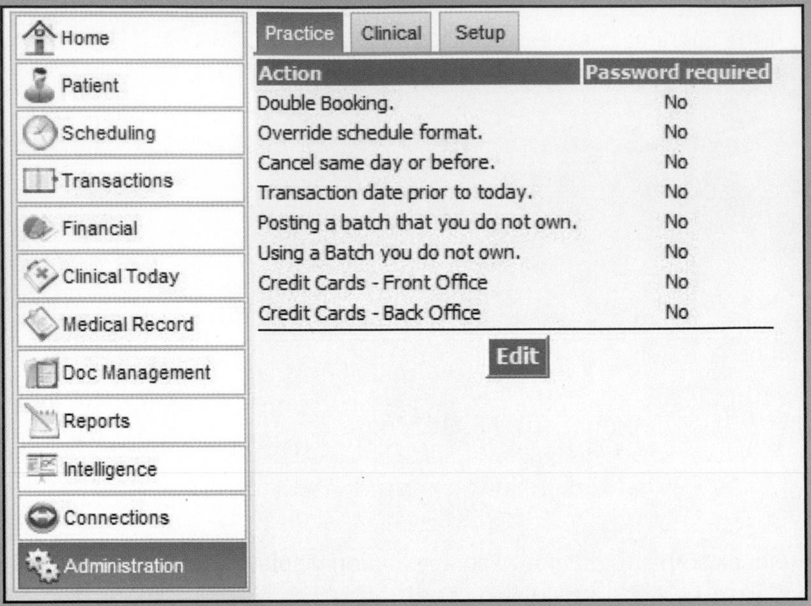
Home
Patient
Scheduling
Transactions
Financial
Clinical Today
Medical Record
Doc Management
Reports
Intelligence
Connections
Administration
Practice
Clinical
Setup
Action
Password required
Double Booking.
No
Override schedule format.
No
Cancel same day or before.
No
Transaction date prior to today.
No
Posting a batch that you do not own.
No
Using a Batch you do not own.
No
Credit Cards - Front Office
No
Credit Cards - Back Office
No
Edit

Figure 2-42 Override Passwords

Courtesy of Harris CareTracker PM and EMR

h. From the *Default Group* list, select a default group for the operator (select "Napa Valley Health Associates 2"). This is the group the operator will enter when logging into Harris CareTracker PM and EMR. From the default group, the operator can access any additional groups to which he or she is assigned.

i. From the *Position* list, select a position for the operator (select "Site Admin").

j. (FYI only) If the operator is a provider, select his or her name from the *Provider* list. This allows the application to identify the operator as a provider in *ToDos*, messaging, etc.

k. (FYI only) In the *Folders* field, click the search [...] button. The application displays the *Operator Folder Access* window. Select the checkbox next to the folder(s) the operator is permitted to access and then click *OK*.

l. (FYI only) In the *ToDo Queues* field, click the search [...] button. Harris CareTracker PM displays the *Operator Queue Access* window. Select the checkbox next to the queue(s) the operator is permitted to access and then click *OK*.

8. Click *Save*. The application adds the operator (Figure 2-43).

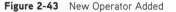

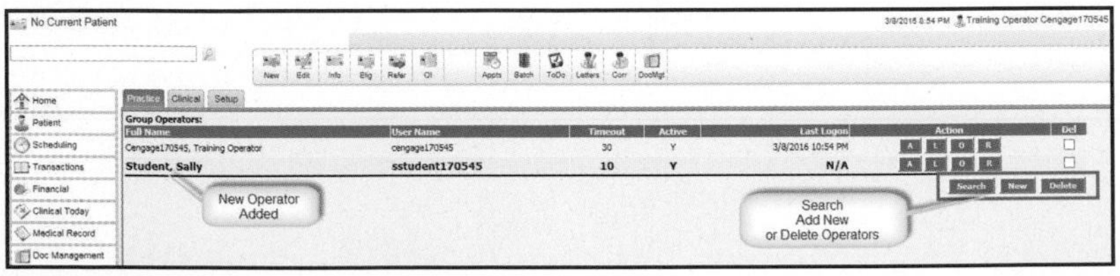
No Current Patient
Student, Sally
sstudent170545
New Operator Added
Search Add New or Delete Operators

Figure 2-43 New Operator Added

Courtesy of Harris CareTracker PM and EMR

Print the New Operator Added screen, label it "Activity 2-9," and place it in your assignment folder.

You can also edit, override, and remove operator settings. Instructions are available in *Help*. In addition to the *Security Logs* link, the *Operator Activity Log* can be accessed from the *Operators & Roles* application, which allows you to monitor each operator's activity. This is an important feature and one more reason never to share your login and password with anyone.

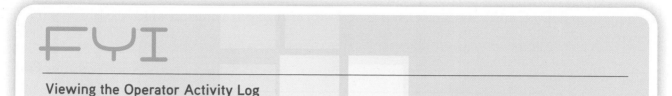

Viewing the Operator Activity Log

Click the *Administration* module. Harris CareTracker PM displays the *Practice* tab.

1. Click the *Operators & Roles* link. Harris CareTracker PM displays the *Group Operators* list.
2. Click the *A, L, O,* or *R* buttons to the right of the operator's name to view the following (Figure 2-44):

- A: generates a list of operator activity for the last seven days
- L: generates a list of operator activity for the last 30 days including the date and time each operator logged in and from what IP address
- O: lists all operator changes
- R: lists each operator's access rights for all Harris CareTracker PM and EMR applications or for all applications of a particular module

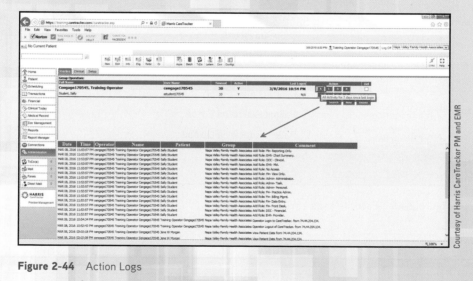

Courtesy of Harris CareTracker PM and EMR

Figure 2-44 Action Logs

Critical Thinking

Identify the buttons in the *Operator Activity Log* and provide a description of their use. In your judgment, rank them in order of importance, explaining your reasons why. Assess the value of the *Operator Activity Log* in maintaining compliance with HIPAA privacy laws. How would you use the *Log* in your duties as a practice manager?

Clinical– Daily Administration

The *Administration > Clinical* module is where you will find EMR features that include *Daily Administration, System Administration,* and *Import/Export.* For example, if you click *Favorite Labs* on the *Administration > Clinical > Daily Administration* column (Figure 2-45), you can view the providers available, the lab name (by using the drop-down feature), add a new lab (Figure 2-46), or change the order in which the labs appear on the screen.

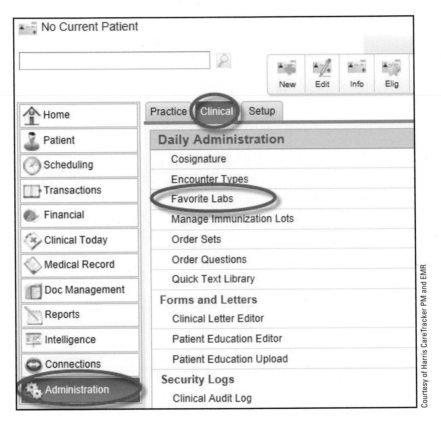

Figure 2-45 Favorite Labs Link

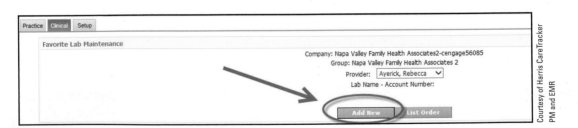

Figure 2-46 Add a New Lab

In the *Favorite Labs* application, you can create a list of commonly used labs. This expedites the ordering process by avoiding the need to go through a long list of facilities supported by Harris CareTracker PM and EMR each time you create an order.

ACTIVITY 2-10:   Add a Favorite Lab

1. Click the *Administration* module and then click the *Clinical* tab.

2. Click the *Favorite Labs* link. The application launches the *Favorite Lab Maintenance* application.

3. Click *Add New*, which will allow you to enter information on a new lab (Figure 2-47).

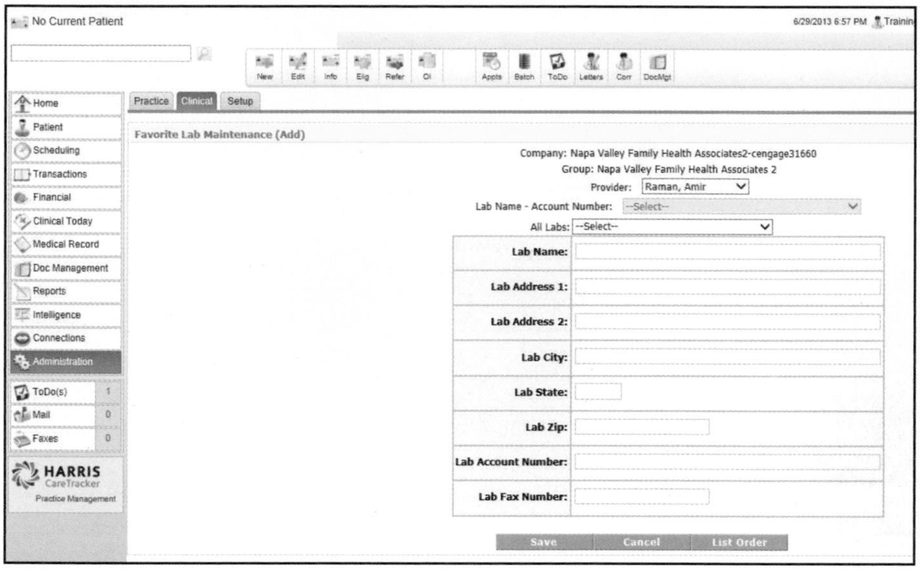

Figure 2-47   Favorite Lab Maintenance

4. Select provider "Ayerick."

5. Select "Test Facility" from the drop-down menu in the *All Labs* list (Figure 2-48). The application automatically populates the lab address fields.

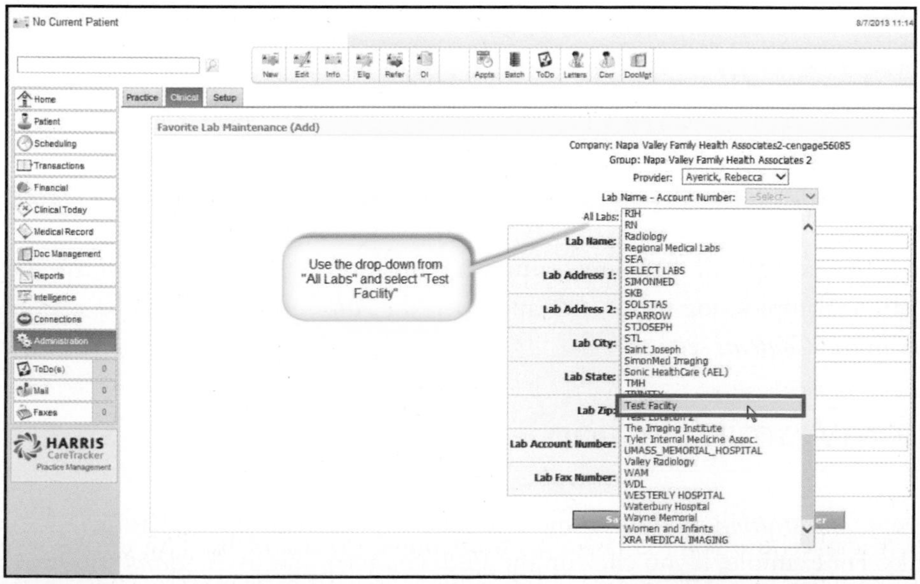

Figure 2-48   Select Test Facility

6. Click *Save*. "Test Facility" has been successfully added to your database (Figure 2-49).
7. Click *Done*.

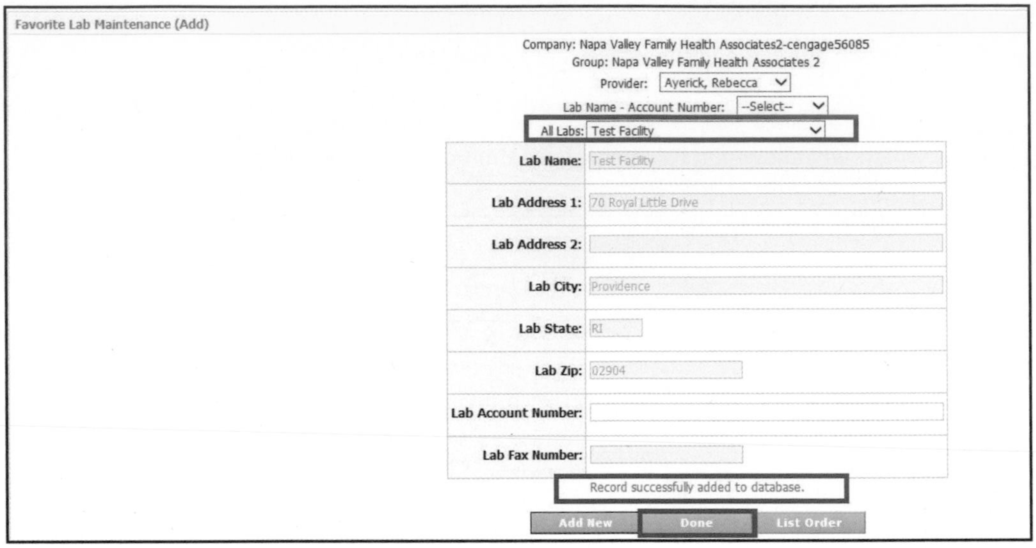

Courtesy of Harris CareTracker PM and EMR

Figure 2-49 New Lab Added - Test Facility

8. Click on the *Lab Name* dropdown menu to see that "Test Facility" has been added to your *Favorite Labs* (Figure 2-50).

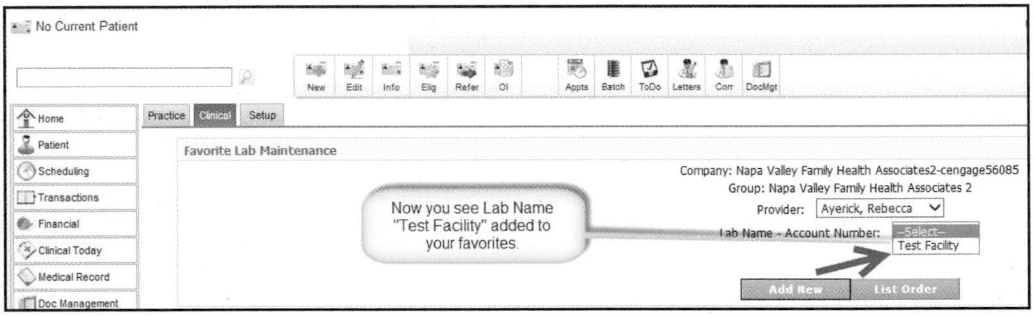

Courtesy of Harris CareTracker PM and EMR

Figure 2-50 New Lab - Test Facility Added

Print the Favorite Labs screen, label it "Activity 2-10," and place it in your assignment folder.

Adding labs is only one example of the many features and functions in the *Daily Administration* > *Clinical* module. To view additional topics, log in to *Help* and open the *Administration Module* > *Clinical* > *Daily Administration* folder in the *Contents* section.

Clinical–System Administration

The *Clinical* > *System Administration* module is where you will find EMR features that include *Clinical Setup* and *Maintenance* links. For example, if you click on the *Visit Summary* link in the *Administration* > *Clinical* > *System Administration* column (Figure 2-51), you can view the checklist for items to include on the *Patient Visit Summary Print Out* (see Figure 2-52). To make changes, you can select *All* or *None*. By selecting *None*, you can choose only the items you want to include on the *Patient Visit Summary Print Out*, or, alternatively, you can deselect items (by clicking on the check mark) to remove them from the list. Complete Activity 2-11 to set up your *Patient Visit Summary* items.

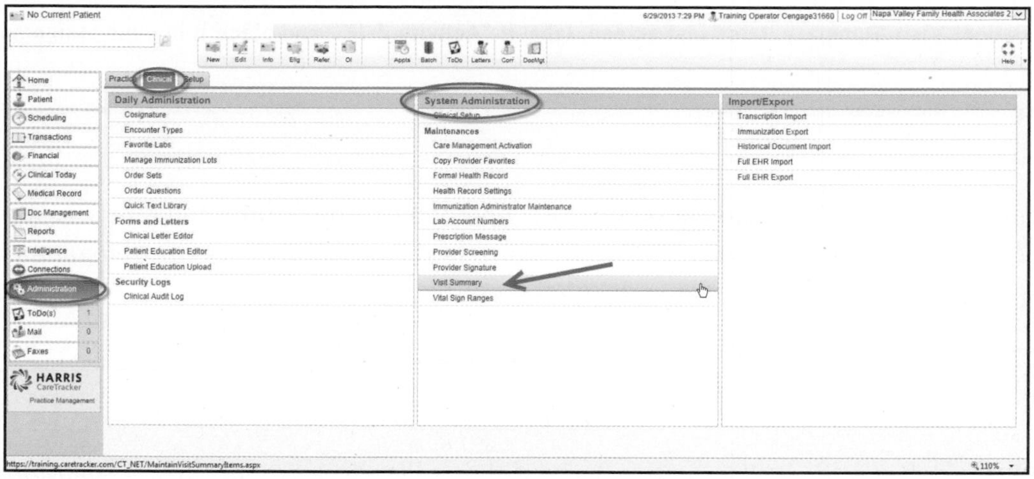

Courtesy of Harris CareTracker PM and EMR

Figure 2-51 Visit Summary Link

ACTIVITY 2-11: Add Patient Visit Summary Items

1. Click the *Administration* module and then click the *Clinical* tab.
2. Click the *Visit Summary* link. The application launches the *Patient Visit Summary* application (Figure 2-52).

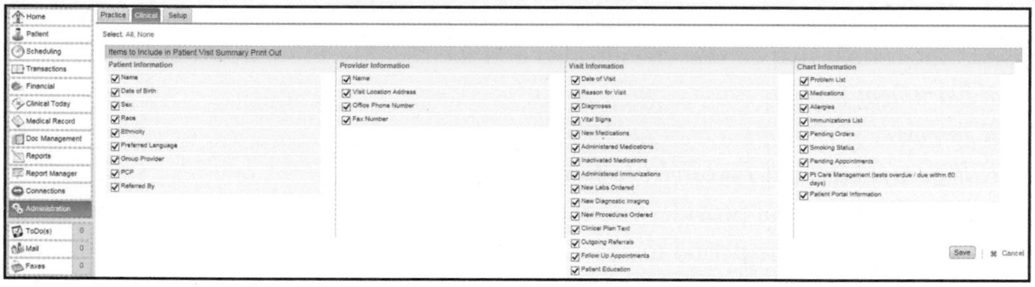

Courtesy of Harris CareTracker PM and EMR

Figure 2-52 Patient Visit Summary

3. Deselect *Inactivated Medications* by clicking on the checkbox (removes the check mark).
4. Deselect *Patient Portal Information* by clicking on the checkbox (removes the check mark) (Figure 2-53).

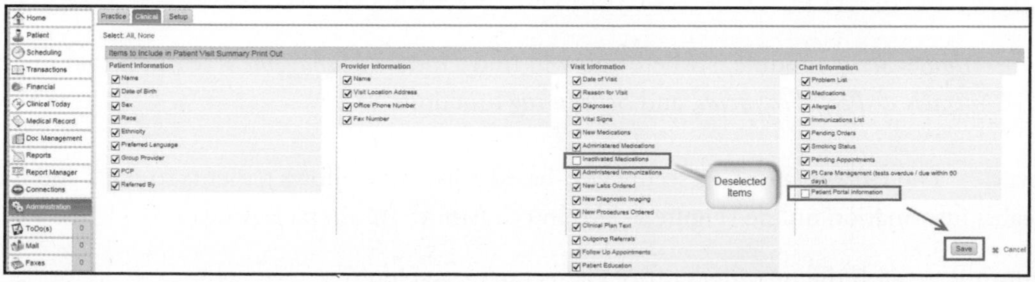

Courtesy of Harris CareTracker PM and EMR

Figure 2-53 Deselect Patient Visit Summary Items

5. Click *Save. Patient Visit Summary Print Out* has been successfully updated.

6. Return to the *Administration > Clinical* tab, click on the *Visit Summary* link, and see that the changes have been saved.

Print the Patient Visit Summary Items List screen, label it "Activity 2-11," and place it in your assignment folder.

Updating patient visit summaries is only one example of the many features and functions in the *Clinical > System Administration* module. To view additional topics, log in to *Help* and open the *Administration Module > Clinical > System Administration* folder in the *Contents* section.

Clinical Import/Export

Although your student version of Harris CareTracker does not allow access to the *Clinical – Import/Export* tabs, in a live environment the following activities would be performed:

- *Transcription Import*
  - In the *Transcription Import* application you can build transcription templates and upload transcription files. Harris CareTracker PM and EMR automatically saves the transcription to the corresponding patient's record. After upload, you can access transcription files in the *Progress Notes* application of the *Medical Records* module.
- *Immunization Export*
  - The *Immunization Export* application allows a practice to generate a record of all vaccinations given during a specified period. The application pulls the Harris CareTracker PM and EMR data into a state-specific format that can be downloaded and then sent to the state's department of health.
- *Historical Document Import*
- *Full EHR Import*
- *Full EHR Export (PDF)* and *Full EHR Export (CDA)*
  - The *Full EHR Export* tool provides you the ability to export a batch of patient clinical data in PDF format. You can select the period to cover and the level of patient information to include.

Log in to *Help* and click on the *Home > Administration Module > Clinical > Import/Export* link to view more information.

Setup

The *Administration > Setup* module is where you will find *Practice Management* features that include the *Patient Portal, Contracts & Fees, Financial,* and *Scheduling* functions.

Patient Portal. The *Patient Portal* is a secure web-based portal that allows patients to track and manage their personal health information online (Figure 2-54). In the *Patient Portal*, patients can:

- Communicate with the provider's office via secure messaging
- Request and confirm appointments

- Update personal information
- View portions of their health record
- Request prescription renewals
- View statements and pay balances
- Download documents and forms

Although this feature is not active in your student version of Harris CareTracker, most medical practices offer a patient portal feature. In the live Harris CareTracker program, you must enable the *Patient Portal* and then configure the site's appearance and features. You can then customize the content, functionality, and colors; upload a logo; and add locations and taglines.

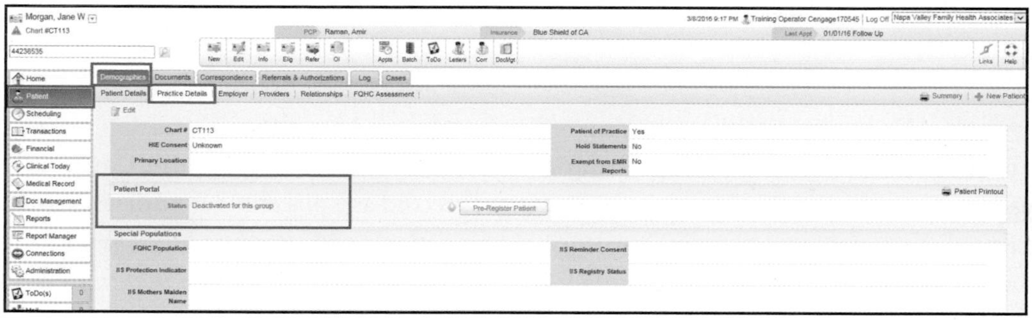

Figure 2-54   Patient Portal feature in Practice Details of Patient Demographics

Critical Thinking

Describe the activities that a patient can perform in the *Patient Portal* feature. Provide an analysis of each of the activities and how might they affect the relationship between patients and providers.

Contracts & Fees.   **Fee schedules** determine the amount charged for each CPT® code entered into Harris CareTracker PM and EMR. Although the fee schedule is initially set up when the practice enrolls with Harris CareTracker PM and EMR, you can edit existing schedules or create new fee schedules for your practice at any time using the *Fee Schedule* application in the *Administration* module.

Revenue Codes.   **Revenue codes** are practice-specific codes that give you an alternative way of reporting financial data in Harris CareTracker PM and EMR. Revenue codes can either be linked to specific CPT® codes on your fee schedule (e.g., "New Patient Office Visits") or be selected during visit or charge entry to represent a specific servicing provider, billing provider, and location combination (e.g., "Evening Clinic").

For reporting purposes, you can group *Month End* reports by revenue codes. When you create a revenue code to use during visit or charge entry, you can link a billing provider, servicing provider, or location you choose to code. However, a revenue code does not have to be linked to a billing provider, servicing provider, or a location.

ADMINISTRATIVE SP◯TLIGHT

If a practice wanted to keep track of its revenue based on groupings of CPT® codes, the following is an example of how a revenue code linked to a specific CPT® code via the fee schedule would be used:

- A revenue code called "New Patient Office Visits" could be created and linked to all new patient office visit CPT® codes (99201–99205).
- Revenue codes are linked to a procedure code via the *Fee Schedule* link under the *Contracts and Fees* section of the *Administration* module. Reports can be generated in Harris CareTracker PM and EMR to include revenue code data.
- When running *Analysis Month End* reports, you can group your report by revenue code.

Pending Insurance.   If a patient's insurance company or plan is not listed in the Harris CareTracker PM and EMR database, you can add *Pending Insurance* to the patient's record as a placeholder until the actual insurance company is created. No statements or claims are generated for patients with *Pending Insurance.* You can identify patients and view charges against *Pending Insurance* in the *Accounts Receivable* and *Financial Class* reports in the *Reports* module.

Financial.   In the *Financial* application of *Setup,* there are commonly used features such as *Encounter Form Maintenance, Locations,* and *Quick Picks,* which will be reviewed later in the textbook.

Encounter Form Maintenance.   The Harris CareTracker PM and EMR Enrollment Department builds encounter forms for clients when they decide to use Harris CareTracker PM and EMR as their practice management system; however, you can use the *Encounter Form Maintenance* application to build a custom encounter form for your practice. You can print the encounter forms based on appointments scheduled in the *Book* application either individually or in a batch.

When a provider uses paper encounter forms to capture CPT® and ICD-10 codes for a patient's visit, you must manually enter the procedure and diagnosis codes into Harris CareTracker PM and EMR via the *Visit* window or the *Charge* application of the *Transactions* module.

Locations.   The *Locations* application allows you to add locations where services are rendered and to search all locations saved in the Harris CareTracker PM and EMR's global database. Global locations are created by Harris CareTracker PM and EMR *Support,* but operators can create new locations specific to their company and group.

ADMINISTRATIVE SP◯TLIGHT

You must have the *Location Maintenance* override included in your operator profile to add and edit locations.

ACTIVITY 2-12: Search for Then Add a New Location

1. Click the *Administration* module and then click the *Setup* tab.

2. Click the *Locations* link (Figure 2-55). Harris CareTracker PM and EMR launches the *Locations* application.

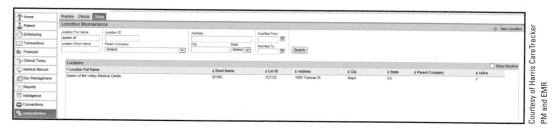

Figure 2-55   Locations Link

3. Enter the search criteria in one or more of the *Name, Modified,* or *Location* fields and then click *Search.* The application displays a list of search results in the bottom half of the screen (enter: "Queen of" in the *Location Full Name* box and "CA" in the *State* box, then click *Search*). The application search will display "Queen of the Valley Medical Center" in Napa, California (Figure 2-56).

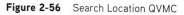

Figure 2-56   Search Location QVMC

Print the Search Location screen, label it "Activity 2-12A," and place it in your assignment folder.

4. Click on the location you want to review (Queen of the Valley Medical Center). The application displays the location details.

You can also add or edit locations from this application. To add a new location:

5. Click on the plus sign next to *New Location* (Figure 2-57).

6. Enter the new location information (Figure 2-57):

   a. Napa State Hospital (NSH), 1234 Grapevine Street, Napa, CA

   b. Click *Save.*

Courtesy of Harris CareTracker PM and EMR

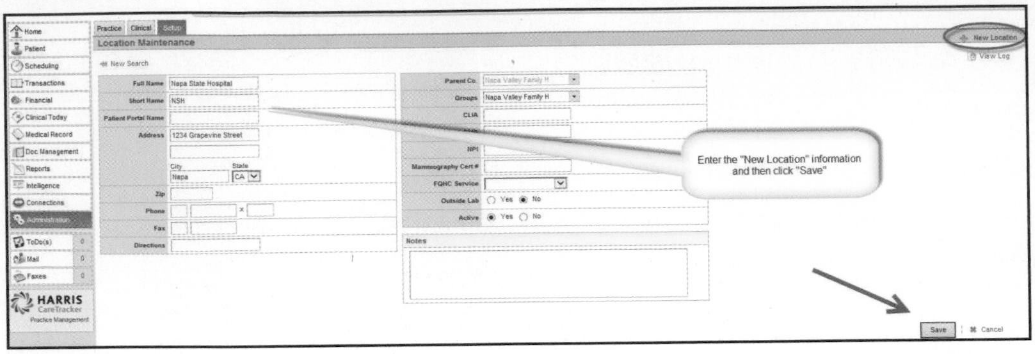

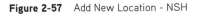

Figure 2-57 Add New Location - NSH

7. Your new location is now saved. Click back on the *Administration* module > *Setup* tab > *Locations* link, enter short name of "NSH", parent company "Napa Valley Family Health Associates 2", and hit *Search.*

8. Your new location is now displayed (Figure 2-58).

Courtesy of Harris CareTracker PM and EMR

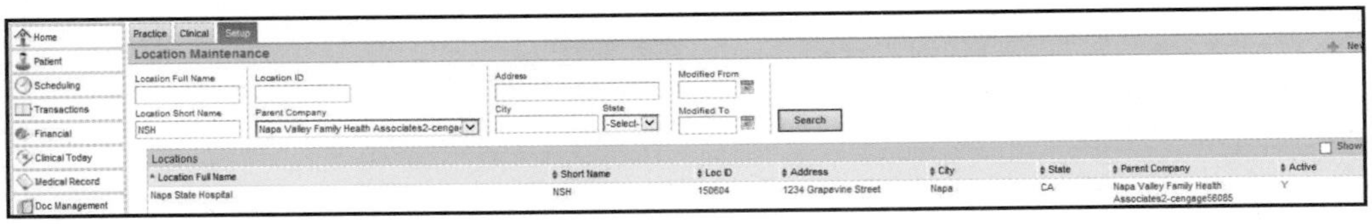

Figure 2-58 New Location Added - NSH

Print the Search Location screen, label it "Activity 2-12B," and place it in your assignment folder.

Quick Picks. Throughout Harris CareTracker PM and EMR, drop-down lists are available from which you can select field-specific data to help create a more efficient work flow, known as *Quick Picks.* Options available in a drop-down list are built for each practice and are group specific. Your practice can build drop-down options for the following data fields:

- Location
- Employers
- Insurance Companies
- Financial Transactions

In order for certain data fields to be available as you work in Harris CareTracker PM and EMR, they need to be added to your "quick picks" list. You can add or remove options from a drop-down list in the *Quick Pick Setup* application.

Tip Box

The *Encounter Procedures* and *Encounter Diagnosis* "quick picks" are only used by clients who have no encounter form set up. These lists populate the diagnoses and procedures in the visit screen when no encounter is linked to the group.

ACTIVITY 2-13:   Add Item(s) to a Quick Pick List

1. Click the *Administration* module and then click the *Setup* tab.
2. Click the *Quick Picks* link (Figure 2-59). Harris CareTracker PM and EMR launches the *Quick Picks* application.

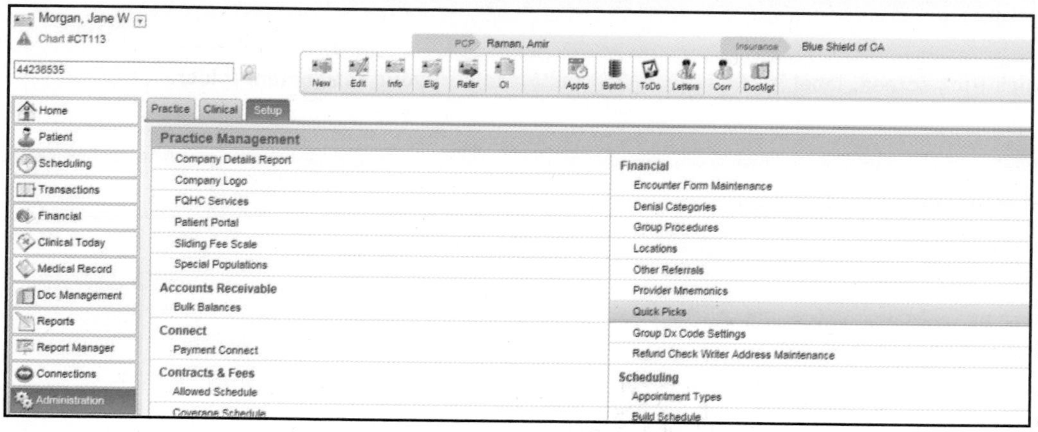

Figure 2-59   Quick Picks link

3. From the *Screen Type* drop-down list, select the quick pick list to which you want to add an item. The application displays the quick pick list (select "Form Letters").
4. Verify that the item you want to add is not already included in the current "quick picks" list.
5. Enter the item you want to add in the *Search* box (enter "No") and then click the *Search* icon. The application displays a search window containing a list of possible matches (Figure 2-60). Click on the desired result to select it (select "No Show fee (pat)"). The application closes the search window and adds the data as an option in the list (Figure 2-61).

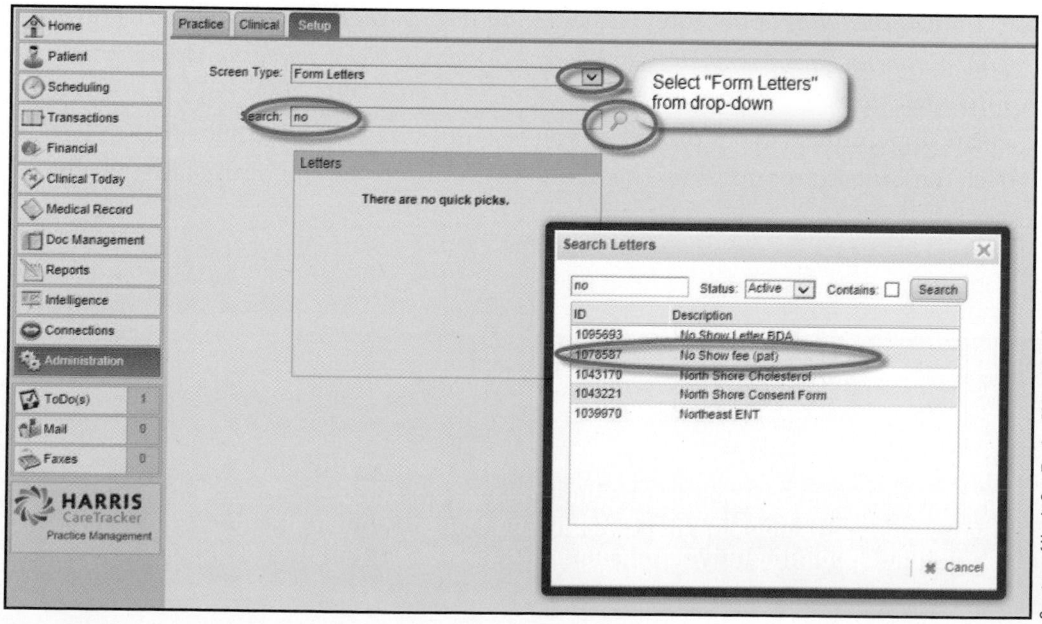

Figure 2-60   No Show Fee Letter

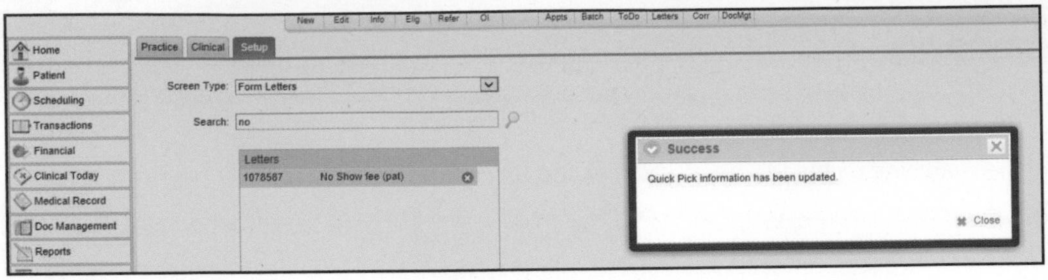

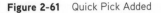

Figure 2-61 Quick Pick Added

Courtesy of Harris CareTracker PM and EMR

Print the Quick Pick screen, label it "Activity 2-13," and place it in your assignment folder.

FYI

To remove item(s) from a *Quick Pick* List:

1. Click the *Administration* module and then click the *Setup* tab.
2. Click the *Quick Picks* link in the *Practice Management* section.
3. From the *Screen Type* list, select the quick pick list from which you want to remove an item. The application displays the quick pick list.
4. Click the *Delete* icon ✖ next to the item you want to remove. The application displays a confirmation dialog box.
5. Click *Yes* to remove the item from the list.

Scheduling. In the *Scheduling* application of the *Administration* module you will use features such as *Building Schedules, Appointment Types, Cancel and Reschedule Reasons, Chief Complaint Maintenance, Room Maintenance,* and *Custom Resources.*

You can create appointment types that allow you to customize your schedule for each resource or group in your practice. You can also set up your schedule so that only certain appointment types can be booked at certain times.

PM SPOTLIGHT

For example, an appointment could be "Established Patient Physical" that has a duration of 30 minutes. This appointment type could then be linked to an "Established Patient" task. Now, when someone is booking an "Established Patient Physical" he or she will only be able to book that appointment type during an "Established Patient" available task time.

After establishing the appointment types, the schedule can be built for each resource. Each day of the week is set up with the appropriate tasks and corresponding availability. Special days, such as holidays, personal days, and vacations, can be set aside with no availability. Also, appointment types can be linked to a specific group or all of the groups in a practice.

You can customize your schedule by color coding appointment types. For example, you can assign a color to help quickly identify new patient visits on the schedule. The color is applied to the border of the appointment in the *Book* application.

Tip Box

The color assigned to an appointment type overrides the default border colors used to identify appointment conflicts (brown/pink) and forced appointments (blue).

The schedule template built in the *Administration* module is the interface used to generate availability for each of the resources in a group. Scheduling is executed at the group level. This means that a parent company, or practice, can have multiple groups with different schedules. A group can customize its own resources, availability, tasks, and appointment types. **Task classes**, which determine what types of appointments can be seen at what times, are the building blocks for a resource's schedule. A day is then built based on the availability of the task classes. Days are built into weeks and then those weeks are used to build the resource's entire schedule.

Cancel/Reschedule Reasons.   The schedule for Napa Valley Family Health Associates has been built into your student version of Harris CareTracker. The practice is responsible for maintaining the schedule template, making changes, and opening future availability, which may be an activity you perform. Refer to *Help* (*Administration Module > Setup > Scheduling*) for steps to make changes in scheduling.

The *Cancel/Reschedule Reasons* application enables you to create company or group-specific cancellation and reschedule reasons. Once a reason is added and made active it is available when cancelling or rescheduling appointments via the *Scheduling* module.

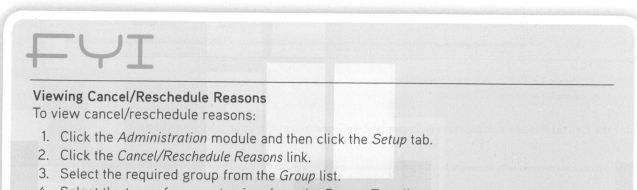

Viewing Cancel/Reschedule Reasons
To view cancel/reschedule reasons:

1. Click the *Administration* module and then click the *Setup* tab.
2. Click the *Cancel/Reschedule Reasons* link.
3. Select the required group from the *Group* list.
4. Select the type of reason to view from the *Reason Type* list.
5. Click *Filter*. Harris CareTracker PM displays a list of reasons. If necessary, you can edit the reason details by clicking the *Edit* button.

ACTIVITY 2-14:   Add a Cancel/Reschedule Reason

1. Click the *Administration* module and then click the *Setup* tab.

2. Click the *Cancel/Reschedule Reasons* link.

3. Select the group to which you want to add the reason from the *Group* list. If a specific group is not selected the reason will be added to all groups in the company (select "Napa Valley Family Health Associates 2").

4. Select the type of reason to add from the *Reason Type* list. There are three options (listed next). For this activity, select "Cancel":

   - (All), which includes both Cancel and Reschedule
   - Cancel: Makes the reason available when cancelling an appointment via the *Scheduling* module
   - Reschedule: Makes the reason available when rescheduling an appointment via the *Scheduling* module.

5. Click *Add Reason*.

6. Enter a description of the reason in the *Reason Name* box (enter "Pt went to emergency room").

7. Enter an abbreviated name for the reason in the *Short Name* box (enter "ER").

8. From the *Active* list, select *Yes* to make the reason available for use (Figure 2-62).

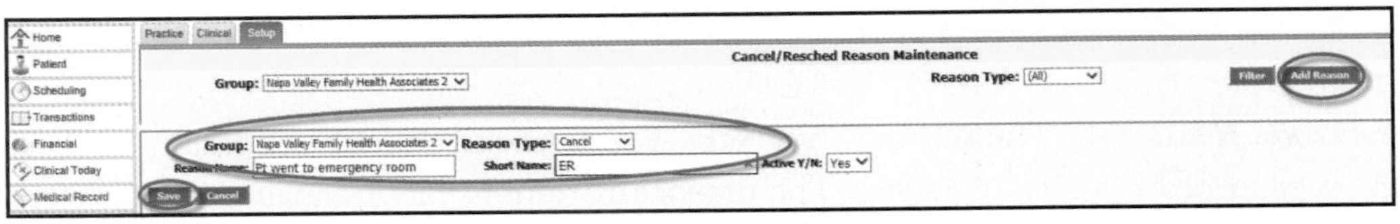

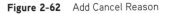

Figure 2-62   Add Cancel Reason

Courtesy of Harris CareTracker PM and EMR

9. Click *Save*.

10. Click on *Filter* and view your cancel reason added (Figure 2-63).

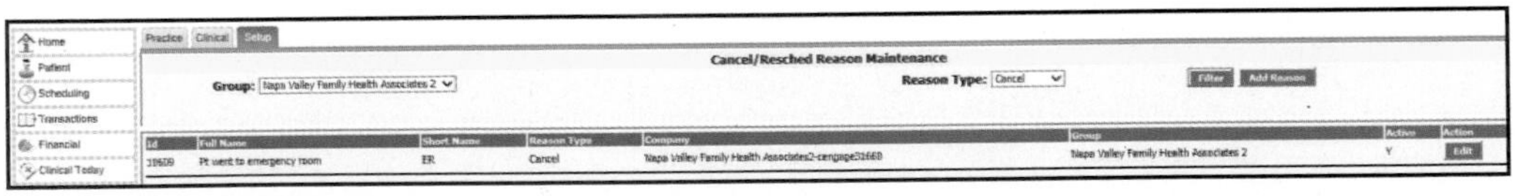

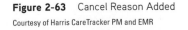

Figure 2-63   Cancel Reason Added

Courtesy of Harris CareTracker PM and EMR

Print the Cancel Reason screen, label it "Activity 2-14," and place it in your assignment folder.

Chief Complaint Maintenance.   The *Chief Complaint Maintenance* application allows you to create a favorite list of Medcin-based chief complaints that are available to select from when booking appointments. You can create a chief complaint that is specific to a group or available to all groups in the company. If the chief complaint is not assigned to a specific group, it is automatically available to all groups in the company.

You can link chief complaints to a progress note template. If the chief complaint is linked to a progress note template, Harris CareTracker PM and EMR will automatically apply the linked template to the *Chief Complaint* section of the progress note for that visit. Harris CareTracker PM and EMR uses the following hierarchy to determine which template is applied to the progress note:

- By default, Harris CareTracker PM and EMR will apply the progress note template linked to the chief complaint selected in the *Book Appointment* window.
- If the chief complaint for the appointment is not linked to a progress note template, then Harris CareTracker PM and EMR will apply the template linked to the appointment type.
- If there is no template linked to either the chief complaint or the appointment type, Harris CareTracker PM and EMR will apply the operator's default template.

ACTIVITY 2-15: Add a Chief Complaint

1. Click the *Administration* module and then click the *Setup* tab.

2. Click the *Chief Complaint Maintenance* link in the *Scheduling* section. The application launches the *Chief Complaint Maintenance* feature.

3. Click the *+ New Complaint* link. The application displays the *Add New Complaint* dialog box.

4. From the *Group* list, select the group for which you want to add a chief complaint (select "Napa Valley Family Health Associates 2").

5. In the *Chief Complaint* field, click the *Search* 🔍 icon. The application displays the *Complaint* search window.

6. Enter the full or partial name of the complaint in the *Search* box, or click on the search 🔍 icon. The application returns the search results.

7. Click on the complaint you want to add (select "New Patient {1000248}", Figure 2-64). The application populates the *Chief Complaint* box with the selected complaint.

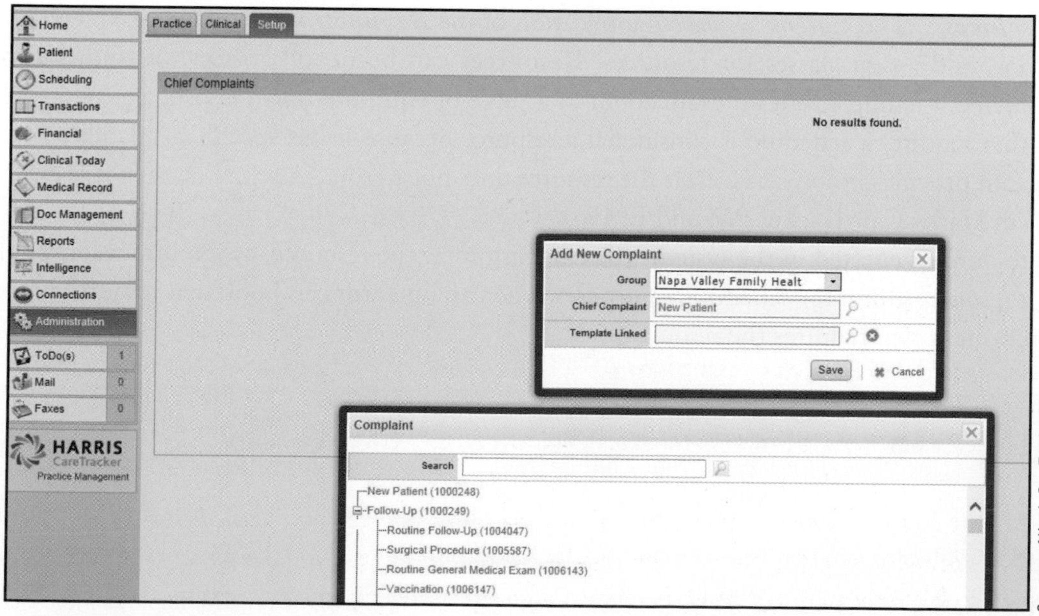

Figure 2-64 Chief Complaint Maintenance

8. (FYI only) In the *Template Linked* field, click the *Search* 🔍 icon. The application displays the *Template* search window.

9. (FYI only) Enter the full or partial name of the progress note template you want to link to the complaint and then click the *Search* button.

10. (FYI only) Click on the template you want to link to the complaint. The application populates the *Template Linked* box with the selected template.

Tip Box

To remove the selected template, click the delete button.

11. Click *Save*. The new complaint is now added to the *Chief Complaint Maintenance* screen (Figure 2-65).

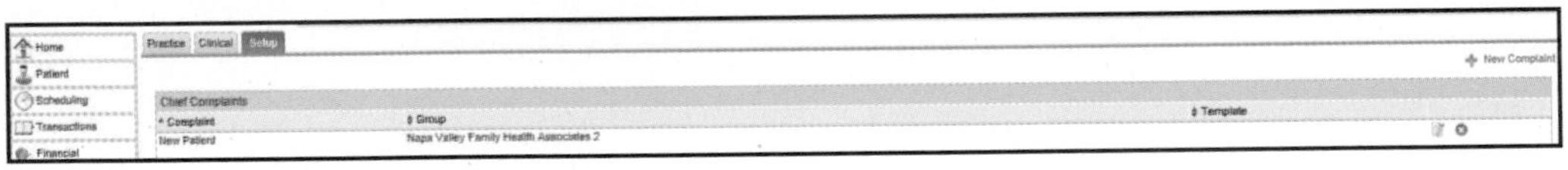

Figure 2-65 New Complaint Saved
Courtesy of Harris CareTracker PM and EMR

Print the New Patient *Chief Complaint* screen, label it "Activity 2-15," and place it in your assignment folder.

You can also edit and delete a *Chief Complaint* in this application. Refer to the instructions in *Help* (*Administration Module > Setup > Scheduling > Chief Complaint Maintenance*).

Custom Resources. The *Custom Resources* application of the *Administration* module is where you can add, define options, and assign classes for resources. **Resources** can be people, places, or things. Providers are always considered a resource, but an exam room or a piece of equipment can also be considered a resource. Something that requires a schedule is considered a resource because it has specific availability with the days and times it can provide certain services. If the resource does not need a set schedule then it is not considered a "resource" in Harris CareTracker PM and EMR.

After a resource is entered in the system, you can customize the resource, assign it to resource classes, and assign it to a resource group for scheduling purposes. Then an operator can book that resource when scheduling an appointment that requires the resource.

ACTIVITY 2-16: Add a Custom Resource

1. Click the *Administration* module and then click the *Setup* tab.

2. Click the *Custom Resources* link in the *Scheduling* section. Harris CareTracker PM displays the *Schedule Resource* page. All providers in the practice are listed as *Available Resources*.

3. (FYI only) If you are adding the custom resource for a particular provider in your group, select the provider from the *Provider* list and then click the left arrow button.
4. Click *New* next to the *Available Resources* list. Harris CareTracker PM displays a dialog box, prompting you to enter a name for the resource.
5. In the dialog box, enter a name for the resource you are creating. Enter "Obstetric 2-D Ultrasound Machine" (Figure 2-66).

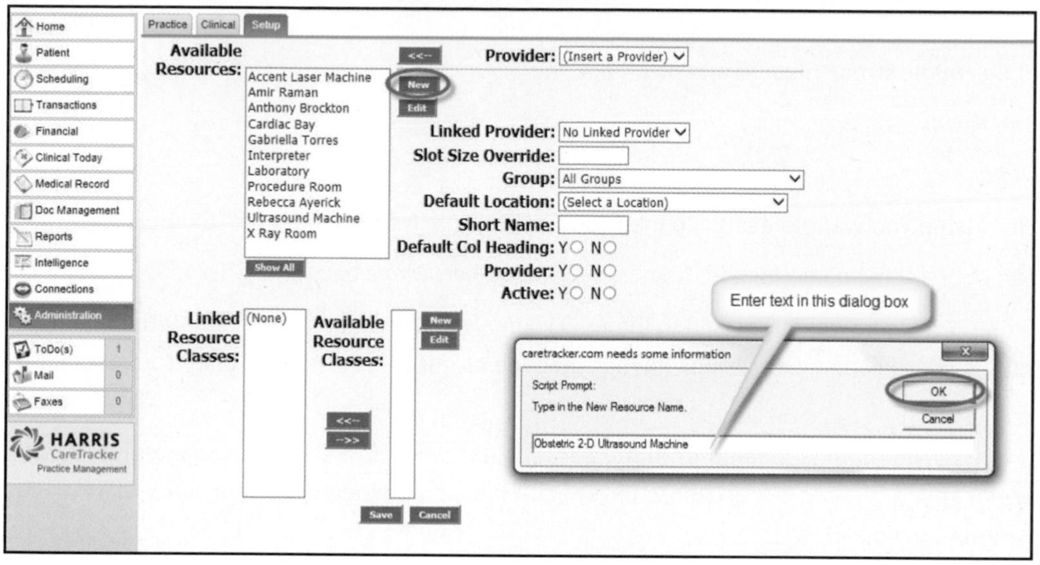

Courtesy of Harris CareTracker PM and EMR

Figure 2-66 Add a Resource

6. Click *OK*. The application adds the resource to the *Available Resources* list (Figure 2-67).

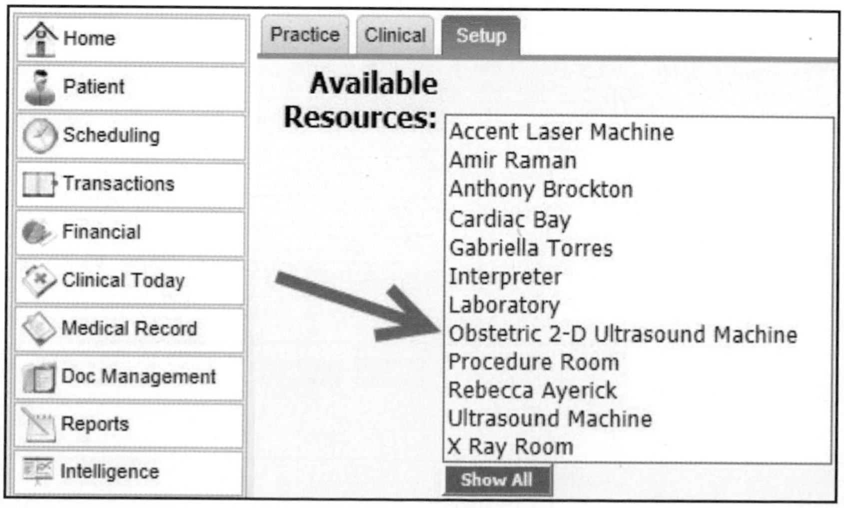

Courtesy of Harris CareTracker PM and EMR

Figure 2-67 Added Resource

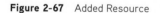

Print the Added Resource screen, label it "Activity 2-16," and place it in your assignment folder.

Room Maintenance. It is important to have an efficient appointment workflow to better serve patients. The *Room Maintenance* feature helps you set up rooms to keep track of where the patients during their visit by updating their location throughout their appointment (e.g., exam room one, nursing station, etc.).

ACTIVITY 2-17: Add a Room

1. Click the *Administration* module and then click the *Setup* tab.

2. Click the *Room Maintenance* link.

3. Click *Add*.

4. Enter the name you want to assign to the room in the *Room Name* box (enter "Exam Room 2").

5. Enter an abbreviated name for the room in the *Room Short Name* box (enter "Ex 2").

6. Select the group you want to assign to the new room from the *Group* list. This determines whether the room is shared among all groups in your practice or if it is only used by one group (select "All Groups").

7. Select where the room is located from the *Location* list. This is useful if you are a multi-location practice or if you want to set up floors for specific hospitals when using the *Admissions* application (select "All Locations").

8. By default, the *Active* field is set to *Y*. This means the room is active (Figure 2-68).

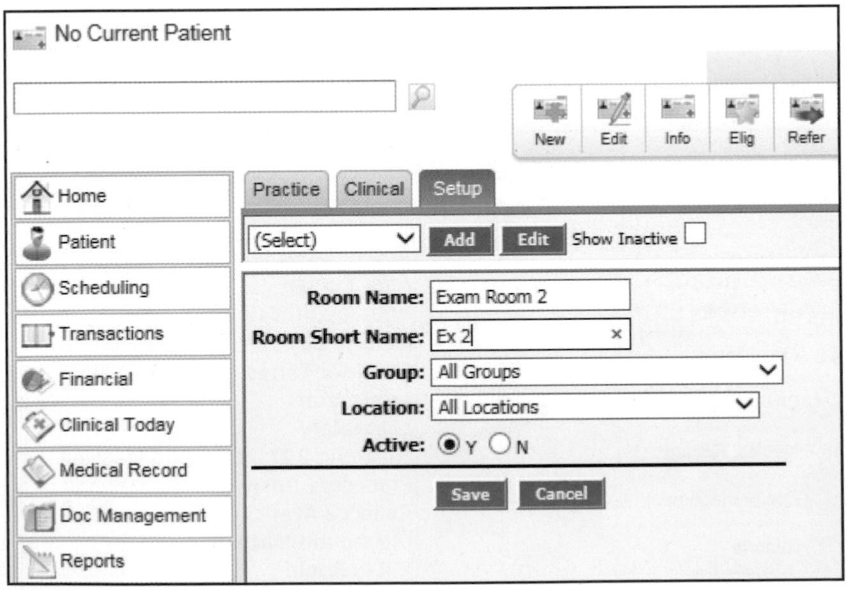

Figure 2-68   Add a Room

9. Click *Save*. The application adds the room.

10. Click back on the *Administration* > *Setup* > *Room Maintenance* link to view the newly added "Exam Room 2" in the drop-down list (Figure 2-69).

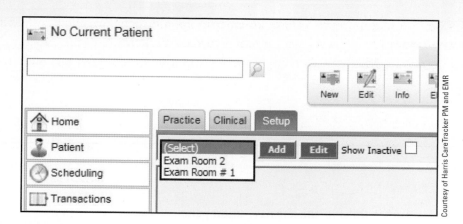

Figure 2-69   Exam Room 3

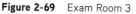 Print the Add a Room screen, label it "Activity 2-17," and place it in your assignment folder.

MESSAGE CENTER

Learning Objective 5: Demonstrate understanding and use of the Message Center components.

The *Message* application is a communication tool that allows you to manage customer, staff, and patient communications. The *Message* application is a combination of the following features:

- *ToDos. ToDos* are Harris CareTracker PM and EMR's internal messaging system that serve two primary functions: assigning a coworker a task and communicating with the Harris CareTracker PM and EMR Support team.
- *Mail.* The *Mail* application is similar to any standard e-mail application and allows you to send, receive, organize, and reply to internal e-mail messages.
- *Queues. Queues* allow you to send *ToDos* to a group of people instead of an individual person.
- *Fax.* The *Fax* feature provides the ability to send and receive electronic faxes through Harris CareTracker PM and EMR.

Accessing the Messages Application

There are several ways to access the *Message Center*:

- Click on the *ToDo* ☑ icon on the name bar.
- Click the *Home* module and then click the *Messages* tab. The *Messages* application displays. By default the application displays all open *ToDos* that pertain to you. You can access and manage other communication methods such as mail, fax, and queues by clicking on the panes on the right-hand side of the window. Each category is further subdivided based on the status. Once you have been entering data in Harris CareTracker, when you click on the *Home-Messages* tab, your messages screen will include information as shown in Figure 2-70 and more.

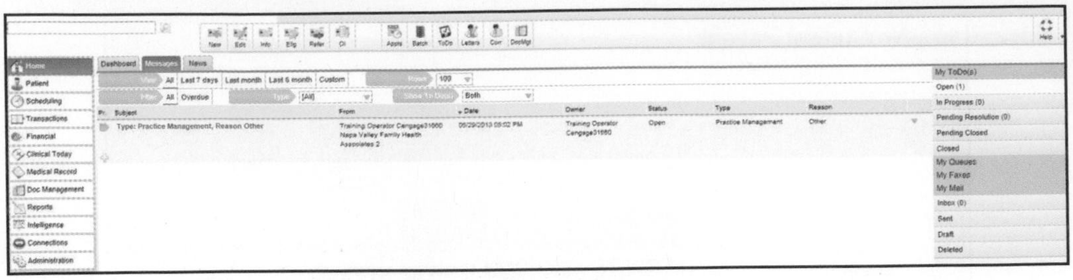

Figure 2-70 Home Messages

- Click the *ToDos* or *Mail* links in the left navigation pane.
- Click the *Clinical Today* module and then click *ToDos* in the *Quick Tasks* menu.

Message Center Templates

You can use templates to create preformatted content for *ToDos*, faxes, and mail messages. For example, you can create a standard mail message used for outgoing referrals. Any time that template is selected the mail message is automatically populated with the text in the **template**.

Templates are created in the *Event Manager* application. The *Event Manager* application is accessed from the *Setup* tab in the *Administration* module. The *Event Manager* application allows operators to create templates and assign them to **macros** that run when certain "events" are triggered throughout Harris CareTracker PM and EMR.

- A *Macro* is a grouping of one or more templates. Macros are assigned to a specific group and *Event Type*.
- A *Template* is a preformatted body of text. Templates are assigned to a specific group and a single macro.
- An **Event Type** is an action that is triggered by a macro such as a *ToDo*, fax, or mail message.

The *Event Manager* application is not available in your student version of Harris CareTracker PM and EMR.

ToDo Application

The *ToDo* application is Harris CareTracker PM and EMR's internal messaging system that allows you to assign administrative and patient-related tasks within your practice as well as communicate with the Harris CareTracker PM and EMR support team. You will know you have an open *ToDo* if a number appears next to the *ToDo* link in the left navigation pane. In the *ToDo* application you can review each *ToDo* that has been sent to you, reply to a *ToDo*, transfer a *ToDo*, take ownership of a *ToDo*, or close a *ToDo*. The application is updated in real time.

ACTIVITY 2-18: Create a ToDo

1. Click the *Home* module and then click the *Messages* tab. The *Messages* application displays all of your open *ToDo*(s).

2. Click on the *ToDo* ✅ icon on the *Name Bar*. The application displays the *New ToDo* window (Figure 2-71).

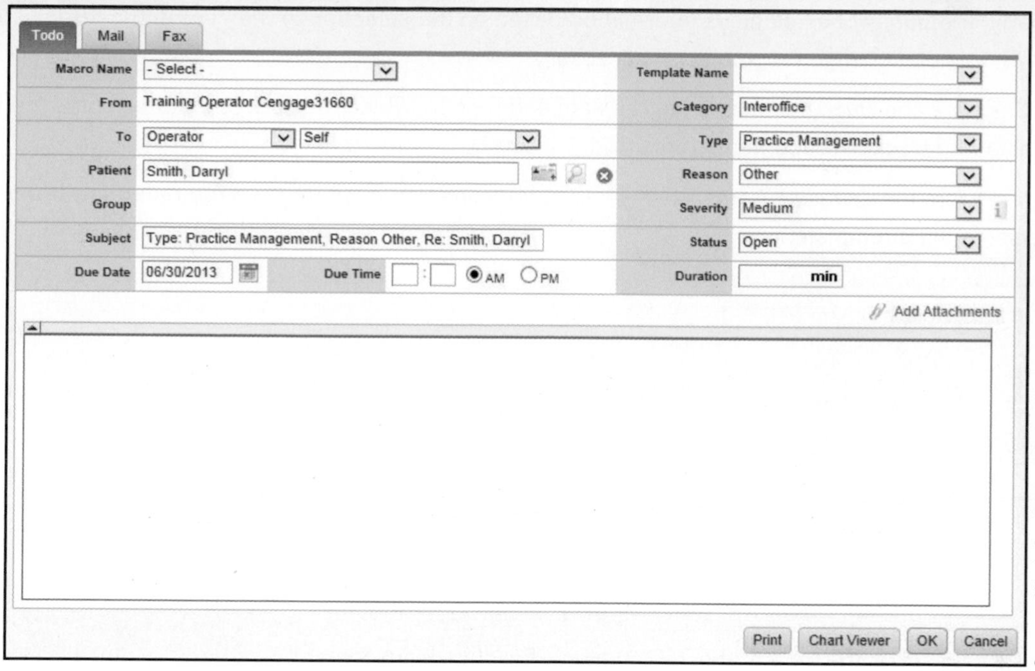

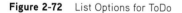

Figure 2-71   ToDo Dialog Box

3. (FYI only) From the *Macro Name* list, you can select the macro you want to use for the *ToDo*.

4. By default, the *From* list displays your name.

5. In the *To* list, click the required options. The *To* list includes the categories described in Figure 2-72. Select "Operator" in the first field and "Self" in the second field.

TO LIST OPTIONS	
Field	**Description**
Operator	Enables you to select a Optum PM and Physician EMR user from your company.
Queue	Enables you to select a work queue set up for the practice. This will redirect the ToDo to the queue. For example, you can send a ToDo to the Support queue and an operator in the queue will respond to the ToDo.
Participant	Enables you to select a participant in the ToDo. This can be a person or a queue that participated in the ToDo.

Figure 2-72   List Options for ToDo

6. If you are sending a *ToDo* to a patient, enter his or her full or partial last name in the *Patient* box and then click the *Search* 🔍 icon. When the search window opens, click on the name of the patient in the search results (search "Smith"; select "Smith, Darryl").

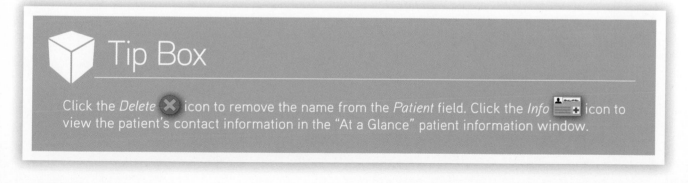

Tip Box

Click the *Delete* ❌ icon to remove the name from the *Patient* field. Click the *Info* 🔳 icon to view the patient's contact information in the "At a Glance" patient information window.

7. By default, the *Subject* box displays information based on the selection in the *Type* and *Reason* lists. However, you can change the subject if necessary.
8. In the *Due Date* and *Due Time* box, enter the date and time by which the *ToDo* should be completed. This is important to track overdue items (enter today's date).
9. (FYI only) From the *Template Name* list, select the template you want to use. (You must select a macro before selecting a template.)

Tip Box

Macros and templates are created in the *Event Manager* application in the *Administration* module.

10. From the *Category* list, select the *ToDo* category (select "Interoffice").
11. In the *Type* list, click the type of the *ToDo* (select "Practice Management").
12. In the *Reason* list, click the reason for the *ToDo* (select "Other").

Tip Box

If the *ToDo* created is for the Harris CareTracker PM and EMR support department, select "Support Center" from the *Category* list. This will automatically populate the *To* field with "Queue" in the first field and "Support Center" in the second field. Use the drop-down menu from the *Type* and *Reason* lists to identify your issue. Free-text a brief message in the body of the *ToDo* (Figure 2-73) and then click *OK*.

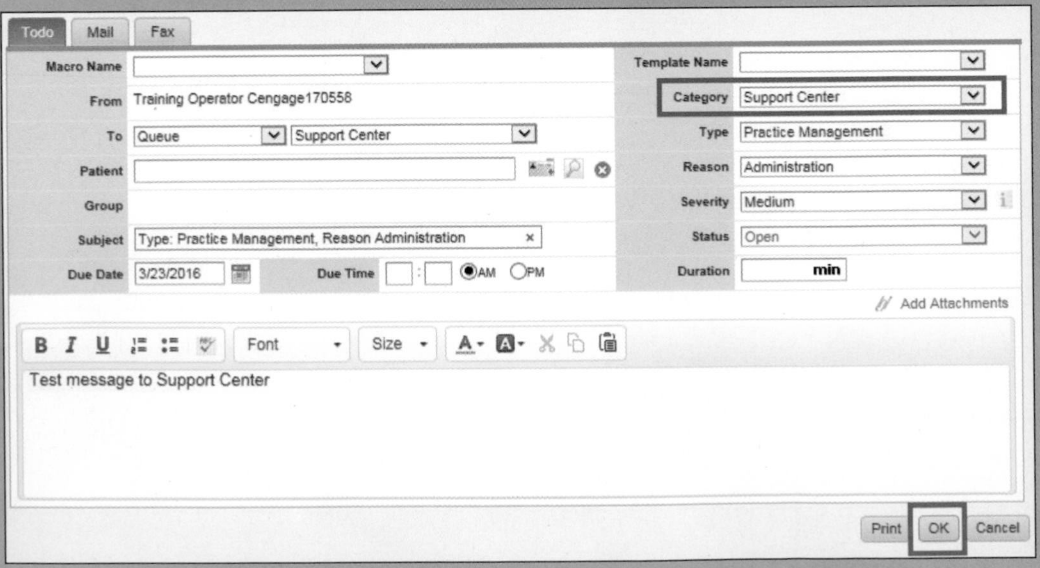

Figure 2-73 Support Center ToDo

Courtesy of Harris CareTracker PM and EMR

13. In the *Severity* list, select the priority level of the *ToDo* (select "Medium").

14. The *Status* list is set to "Open" by default.

15. In the *Duration* box, enter the total time spent working on the *ToDo* (enter "5").

16. (FYI only) The content box is not functional in your student version of Harris CareTracker. However, in the live version you would use it to enter your *ToDo* information. You could format and spell check the note if needed. If you selected a template, this field would be automatically populated with the content in the template. (**Note:** Although this field is not active in your student version of Harris CareTracker, by following the prior steps in this activity you will have created a *ToDo* that will appear in your *ToDo* queue).

17. (Optional) Follow instructions in *Help* to attach documents to a *ToDo*.

18. Click *OK*. The *ToDo* will disappear and show in your *Messages Dashboard* (Figure 2-74).

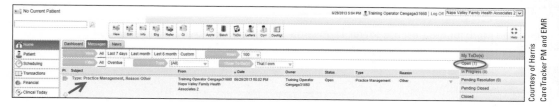

Figure 2-74   Student-Created ToDo

Print the *Messages* dashboard with the completed *ToDo*, label it "Activity 2-18," and place it in your assignment folder.

To view additional information regarding the *ToDo* features of Harris CareTracker, use the *Help* system by going to *Messages Center > ToDos* folder (Figure 2-75).

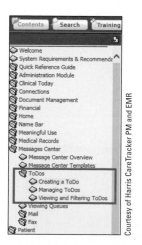

Figure 2-75   Help ToDo Pane

Mail

The *Mail* application allows you to communicate electronically with staff members, providers in your *Provider Portal,* and patients activated in the *Patient Portal.* The mail feature works the same as other e-mail applications, enabling you to open, view, create, send and receive, and delete messages. In addition, you can link attachments such as patient encounter notes, documents, results, referrals and authorization forms, set priorities, and more.

You can use templates to create preformatted content for mail messages. For example, you can create a standard mail message used for outgoing referrals. Any time that template is selected the mail message is automatically populated with the text in the template. Templates are created in the *Event Manager* application in the *Administration* module.

ACTIVITY 2-19: Create a New Mail Message

1. Click the *Home* module and then click the *Messages* tab. The *Messages Center* opens and displays all of your open *ToDos*.
2. Click *Send Mail*, located on the lower right-side *ToDo* pane (Figure 2-76). The application displays the *Message* dialog box.

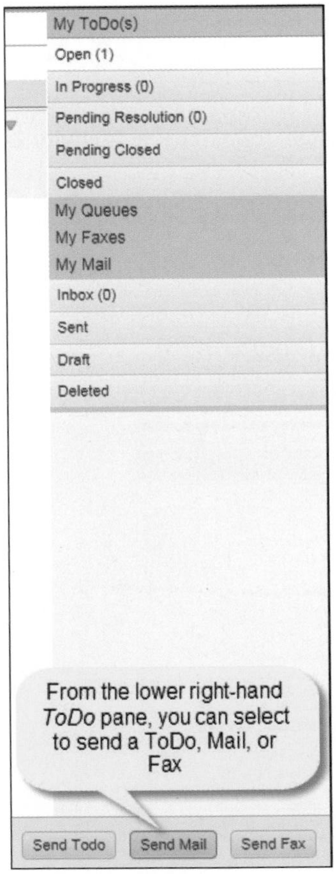

Courtesy of Harris CareTracker PM and EMR

Figure 2-76 Send Mail

3. (FYI only) From the *Macro Name* list, select the macro you want to use.
4. (FYI only) From the *Template* list, select the template you want to use for the mail message. The application populates the *Notes* field with the content from the template. (You must select a *Macro* before selecting a template.)

5. The *From* list defaults to the operator creating the mail message and cannot be edited.

6. In the *To* field, click the *Search* icon. Harris CareTracker PM and EMR opens the *Select Operators* dialog box.

7. Place a check mark in the box by your login name (Figure 2-77).

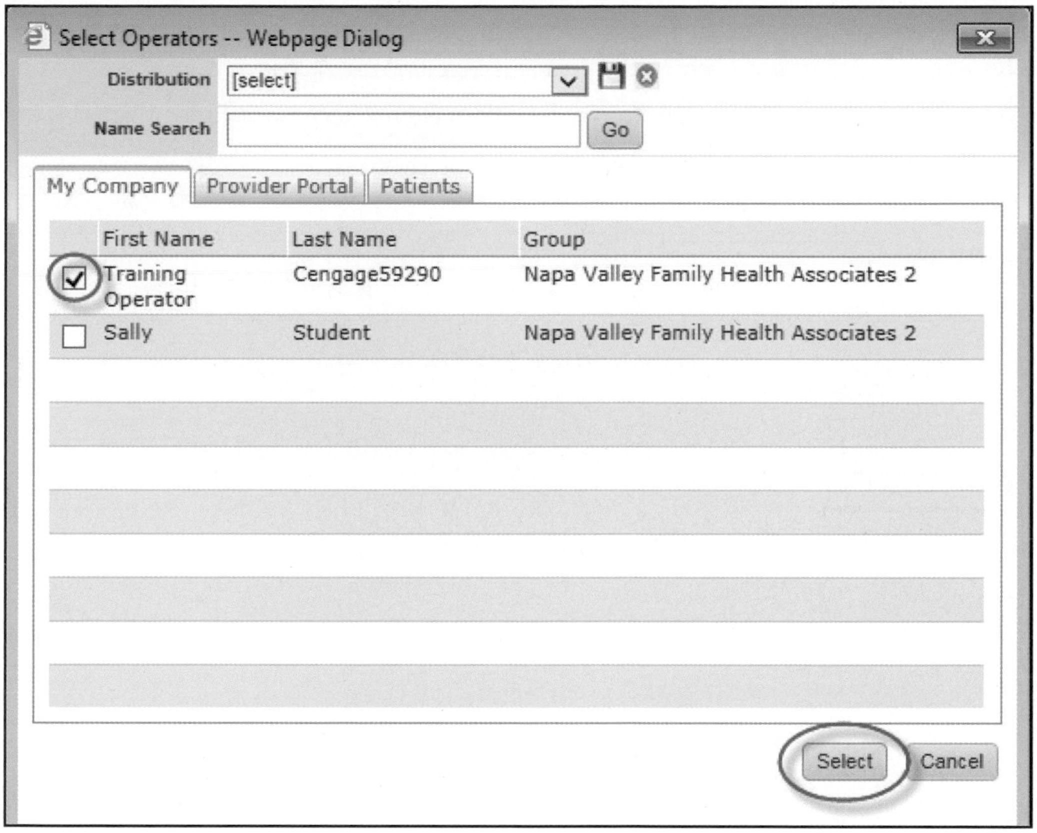

Courtesy of Harris CareTracker PM and EMR

Figure 2-77 Select Operators Dialog Box

FYI

(FYI only) Address the message to one or more recipients using one of the following options:

- To send the message to a group, select the group from the distribution list (if one has been created).
- Select the checkbox next to one or more people on the *My Company* tab.
- To search for an operator, enter the person's name in the *Name Search* box and click *Go*.
- To send a message to a provider in your *Provider Portal*, click the *Provider Portal* tab and select the checkbox next to the provider's name.
- To send a message to a patient registered in the *Patient Portal*, click the *Patients* tab and then select the checkbox next to the patient's name.

8. Click *Select*. The application closes the *Select Operators* dialog box.

9. If a patient is in context, the patient name displays in the *Patient* box. However, you can also send a mail message about a different patient by clicking the *Search* 🔍 icon. For this activity, you will not select a patient.

10. In the *Subject* box, enter the subject of the mail message (enter "Test Mail Message").

11. By default, the *Severity* list displays "Medium". However, you can change the priority of the mail message if necessary. Leave as is.

12. (FYI only) To link a clinical document or chart summary, follow the instructions in *Help*.

13. In the *Notes* box, enter the message and format the information if necessary. Enter "Test Mail Message" (Figure 2-78).

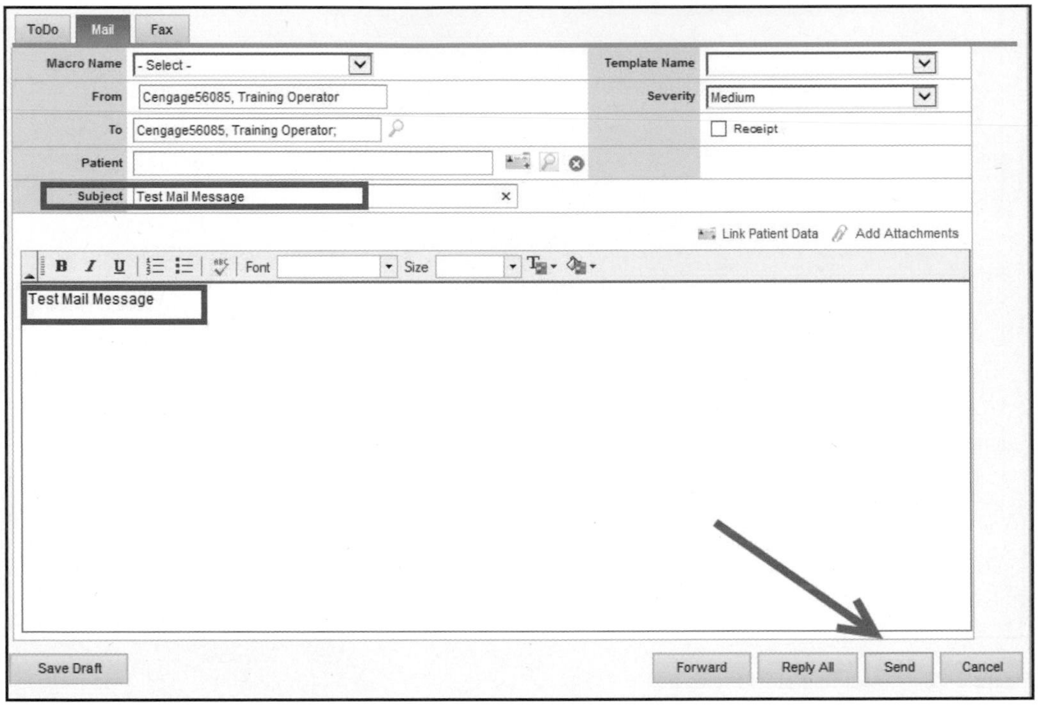

Figure 2-78 Send Test Mail Message

14. Click *Save Draft* to save the message and send later or click *Send* to send the mail message to the selected operators (click *Send*).

15. To view your sent message, click the *Sent* link on the *My ToDo(s)* pane (Figure 2-79).

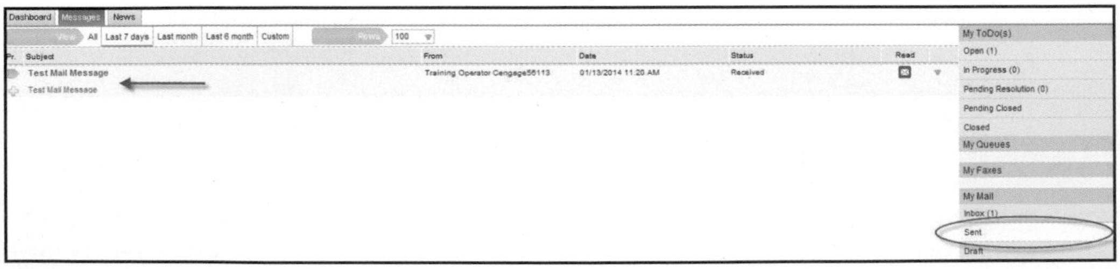

Figure 2-79 Sent Mail Message

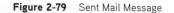

Print the Sent Message screen, label it "Activity 2-19," and place it in your assignment folder.

Queue

Queues are used to organize and group *ToDos*, mail, and faxes in the *Messages Center*. Queues help manage tasks more efficiently by allowing you to route *ToDos* to a group rather than to one individual. At the top of each queue is a set of filters you can use to sort *ToDos*, mail messages, and faxes.

Harris CareTracker PM and EMR provides several global queues, such as the *Support* and *Mail* queues. You can also create custom queues for your company for routing *ToDos* or sending and receiving faxes. Queues are created in the *Queues* application in the *Administration* module.

FYI

View Queues

Once you are working in Harris CareTracker and sending and receiving messages, you will be able to view the activity in *My Queues*. Follow these instructions to view your *My Queues*:

1. Click the *Home* module and then click the *Messages* tab. The *My Queues* section at the right side of the window displays all of your queues. The number next to each queue indicates the number of pending *ToDos* in the queue (Figure 2-80).

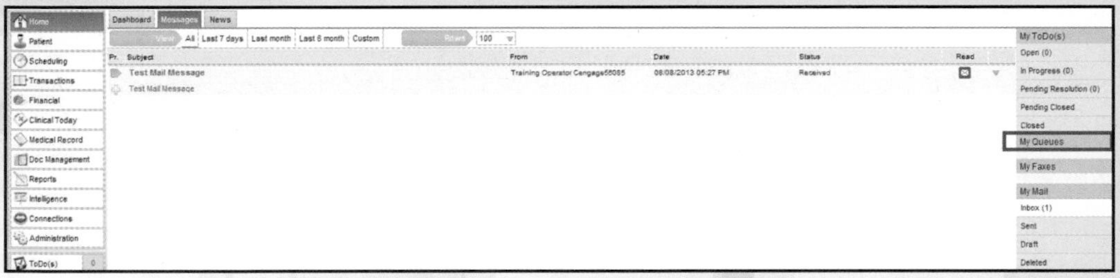

Courtesy of Harris CareTracker PM and EMR

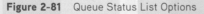

Figure 2-80 My Queues

2. Click the specific queue you want to access. By default, the queue displays all outstanding *ToDos*.
3. By default, the *Type* list displays *All*. Click a different type, such as questionnaires, refill requests, or phone messages.
4. From the *Status* list, click the status of the *ToDo*. All *ToDos* that match the selected type and status will display. The options in the *Status* list are described in Figure 2-81.

QUEUE STATUSES	
Status	**Description**
Open	Indicates the initial state of a ToDo, meaning the ToDo is currently in a queue. It remains open until further correspondence or action is taken.
Closed	Indicates a ToDo that is reviewed and requires no further correspondence or action, meaning completed.
Closed-Client Review	Indicates that the current owner must review the response and change the status to "Closed-Client Review" if satisfied.
In Progress	This status is used to monitor the progress of a ToDo assigned to a queue.

Courtesy of Harris CareTracker PM and EMR

Figure 2-81 Queue Status List Options

(Continues)

5. Figure 2-82 represents how your *My Queues* would look once you have an activity entered and pending.

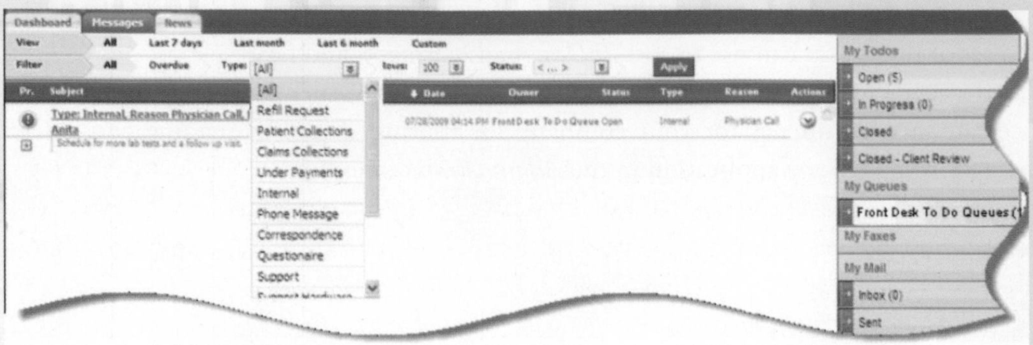

Figure 2-82 Queue Types All

Courtesy of Harris CareTracker PM and EMR

Tip Box

By default, the queue displays all *ToDo*s that are outstanding. To filter *ToDo*s in the queue based on the age, click the *Last 7 days*, *Last month*, *Last 6 month*, or the *Custom* tab. The *Custom* tab enables you to enter a date range to view *ToDo*s for a specified period. In addition, you can also view *ToDo*s that are overdue by clicking *Overdue*. Overdue *ToDo*s are based on the due dates you set for the *ToDo*s to be completed.

Fax Capabilities of Harris CareTracker

In order to utilize the *Fax* feature of Harris CareTracker, you must receive a confirmation e-mail from *Protus* that your *MyFax* number has been linked to your Harris CareTracker PM and EMR account before you can begin faxing. This function is not active in your student version of Harris CareTracker. To check faxing activity, you would log in to your *MyFax* account to view the faxing activity on your account, including the total number of incoming and outgoing faxes.

FYI

To check the faxing activity:
1. Open an Internet browser window and go to http://www.myfax.com.
2. Click *Login* in the upper-right corner of the page. *MyFax* displays the login page.
3. In the *Login ID* box, enter your *MyFax* user ID, fax number, or e-mail address.

4. In the *Password* box, enter your password.
5. Click *Login. MyFax* displays your *MyFaxCentral* account page.
6. *MyFax* displays your fax usage for the month on the right side of the page.

Sending and Viewing Faxes.   Harris CareTracker PM and EMR has integrated *MyFax* technology to enable secure online faxing. Harris CareTracker PM and EMR automatically generates a cover sheet for faxes. The cover sheet displays the name, address, and phone number of the fax sender and recipient, the date, and any text entered in the *Notes* box when the fax was created. You have the option not to include the cover sheet.

FYI

Viewing Faxes

There are multiple ways to view faxes:

- Click the *Faxes* link in the left navigation pane. The number indicates both the new faxes you received and any faxes that failed transmission (Figure 2-83).
- Click the *Home* module and then click the *Messages* tab. Click the *My Faxes* link in the menu on the right side of the page. (You will not be able to click on this link because *MyFax* is not active in your student version of Harris CareTracker.)

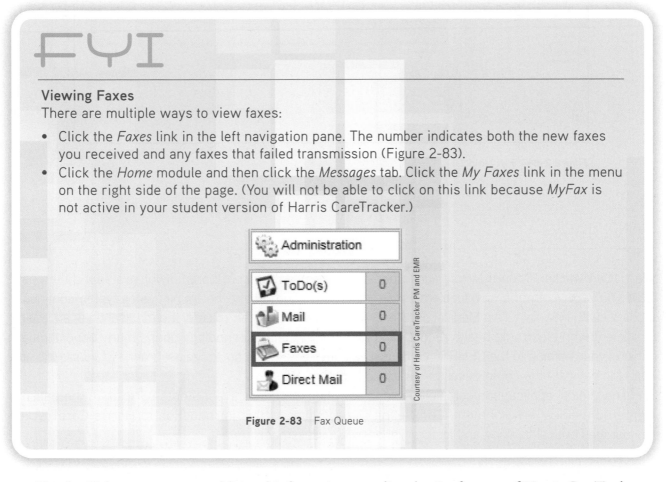

Figure 2-83   Fax Queue

Use the *Help* system to view additional information regarding the *Fax* features of Harris CareTracker at the *Home Module > Messages Center > Fax > Sending and Viewing Faxes* (Figure 2-84).

There you will find instructions on:

- Viewing faxes
- Fax statuses
- Sending a fax
- Resending a fax
- Editing an attachment
- Creating a fax contact list

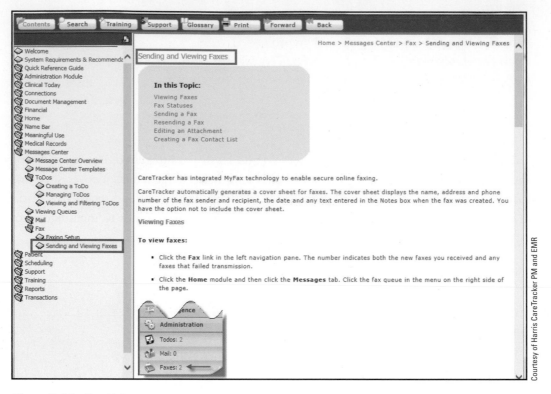

Figure 2-84 Fax Help

SUMMARY

Harris CareTracker PM and EMR provides a robust electronic health record that is fully integrated and interoperable. The *Help* system offers a valuable tool for beginning users and for refresher training as the system continually updates with new features. Medical assistants often advance in their roles in the medical field, and being proficient with electronic health records and health information technology opens many opportunities. Linking your training to the CEHRS™ credential will offer employers an added assurance of your skills and ability to navigate the complexities of electronic health records.

The clinical applications completed mimic activities that medical assistants perform in the patient-centered medical environment. Completing the activities in this introduction to Harris CareTracker encourages critical thinking and fosters higher-level assessment.

Chapter 3
Patient Demographics and Registration

Key Terms

batch
carve-out
context
demographics
edit
eligibility
encryption
explanation of benefits (EOB)
group number
member number
nonparticipating payer

notice of privacy practices (NPP)
Practice Management
primary
protected health information (PHI)
responsible party
secondary
subscriber
subscriber number
tertiary
unknown status
workflow

Learning Objectives

1. Identify components of the Name Bar.
2. Demonstrate knowledge of patient Demographics.
3. Search for a patient within Harris CareTracker PM.
4. Register a new patient in Harris CareTracker.
5. Edit patient information in Harris CareTracker.
6. View and perform Eligibility Checks.

Certification Connection

1. Incorporate electronic technology to prepare patient accounts; retrieve, store, and accurately document information in the patient medical record.

2. Communicate in language the patient can understand; demonstrate effective and courteous telephone techniques; apply electronic technology to maintain effective communication.

3. Search the patient database and retrieve patient accounts.

4. Manage patient flow (e.g., front office, back office, administrative tasks).

5. Manage data and document accurately in the patient record using the EHR.

6. Purge, archive, and secure electronic charts; create an action plan for data recovery in case of downtime or a catastrophic event.

7. Acquire external patient data (labs, radiology reports, patient visit summaries, and more); edit the patient medical record in the EHR within your scope of practice.

8. Perform routine practice management and clinical EHR tasks within a health care environment according to appropriate protocols.

9. Demonstrate time management principles to maintain effective office workflows and patient care follow-up.

10. Adhere to professional standards of care as they pertain to medical records.

11. Identify the impact of HIPAA for the medical assistant; adhere to rules pertaining to the confidentiality and release of PHI.

12. Perform internal audits of medical records, confirming that all signatures have been obtained for consent, release of information (ROI), assignment of benefits, and so on.

Adapted from national standards of the National Healthcareer Association (NHA), Commission on Accreditation and Allied Health Education Program (CAAHEP), and Accrediting Bureau of Health Education Schools (ABHES)

INTRODUCTION

Harris CareTracker **Practice Management** and Physician EMR is a web-based application that enables physician practices to achieve greater efficiency by streamlining their administrative **workflows**. Practice Management (PM) refers to the "front office" of a medical practice: functions that include the patient's financial, **demographic**, and nonmedical information. Workflow refers to how tasks are performed throughout the office (usually in a specific order); for instance, the patient is checked in and his or her insurance cards are scanned, and then taken to the exam room where vital signs are taken/recorded, and so on.

The *Patient* module in Harris CareTracker PM and EMR is where you register patients into the system. The information stored in this module includes the patient's basic and detailed demographics, health insurance information, and referrals and authorizations. *Demographics* comprise the basic patient identifying information, for example, full name, address, phone number, gender, Social Security number, date of birth, and health insurance information; and is defined as relating to the dynamic balance of a population, especially with regard to density and capacity for expansion or decline. Entering accurate patient information is essential because Harris CareTracker PM and EMR pulls the information from the *Patient* module to print insurance claims for billing purposes. The *PM* module makes registration simple and improves service by centralizing billing and demographics details at the first stage of the patient encounter.

PM SPOTLIGHT

Highlights of *Patient Registration* **module:**

- Enter patient demographics
- Enter and record insurance information
- Scan and attach insurance cards and identification cards
- Verify insurance eligibility prior to billing with one click of a button

In this chapter you will learn the role of patient demographics and registration in the paperless medical office. You will complete activities in the PM system such as searching for a patient, registering a new patient, **editing** (modifying the content of the input by inserting, deleting, or moving characters, numbers, or data) patient information, and performing **eligibility** checks (determining whether a person is entitled to receive insurance benefits for health care services). These tasks mimic actual duties you will be performing as a medical assistant. You will learn and discover the many attributes of working in a paperless medical office, along with gaining an understanding of the responsibilities associated with your position.

NAME BAR

Learning Objective 1: Identify components of the Name Bar.

The *Name Bar*, located across the top of the Harris CareTracker window, provides quick access to the most frequently used Harris CareTracker applications (Figure 3-1). A quick reference guide to the various applications launched from the *Name Bar* illustrates each button and a description of the function (Figure 3-2).

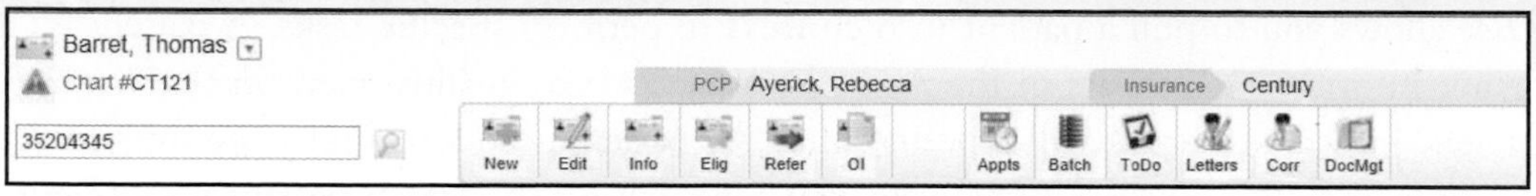

Figure 3-1   Name Bar
Courtesy of Harris CareTracker PM and EMR

NAME BAR	
Button	**Description**
🔍 **Search**	Pulls patients into context by Harris CareTracker PM and EMR ID number, chart number, claim ID or last name. Enter the patient's first name, last name or at least three letters of each name to display the Advanced Search dialog box that enables you to select a patient.
⚠ **Alert**	Displays the Patient Alerts window. The Patient Alerts window notifies the operator when key information is missing from a patient's demographics or if any problems exist with the patient's account.
Edit	Launches the Demographics application in edit mode for the pati ent in context.
New	Launches the Demographics application, enabling you to register a new patient in Harris CareTracker PM and EMR.
Info	Displays a read only summary of the patient's information, including address, contact information, family members, balance information, insurance, etc.
Elig	Displays a history of eligibility checks and enables you to perform an individual electronic eligibility check to ensure that the patient is covered by the insurance company listed as the primary insurance.
Refer	Launches the Referral/Authorization application.
Appts	Displays a list of upcoming patient appointments. In addition, you can view and confirm an appointment, check in/check out a patient, print the encounter form, and perform various other tasks pertaining to the appointment.
OI	Displays information pertaining to dates of service. For example, you can obtain information such as associated procedures, financial transactions and claim activity, and make financial transactions such as payments, adjustments, refunds and more.
Batch	Launches the Batch application, allowing you to create a new batch to enter charges and post payments and adjustments. In addition, you can also set up personal settings when using Harris CareTracker PM and EMR. For example, the main application to launch when logged on to Harris CareTracker PM and EMR.
ToDo	Launches the Harris CareTracker PM and EMR messaging tool, allowing you to communicate with other staff and the Harris CareTracker PM and EMR Support Department.
Letters	Generated and prints letters to send a patient.
Corr	Displays a queue of letters generated and enables you to print the letters to send to patients.

Courtesy of Harris CareTracker PM and EMR

Figure 3-2   Description of Name Bar Applications

The *Name Bar* allows you to pull a patient into **context** to perform specific tasks. A patient is "in context" when his or her information appears in the *Name* list and *ID* box, as illustrated on the *Name Bar* picture. To pull a patient into context you will type in either the patient account number or the first letters of the patient's last name and click *Enter*. Alternatively, you can click on the search patient icon (Figure 3-3) 🔍. When the pop-up screen appears, you will enter the first three letters of the last name and first one to three letters of the first name and click on the *Search* button (see Figure 3-4) to search. Always verify at least two patient identifiers (such as name, date of birth, last four of the Social Security number, etc.) to confirm you have selected the correct patient. Click on the patient, and he or she will be pulled into context. If no patient is found in the search, you will proceed to creating a new account by registering the new patient.

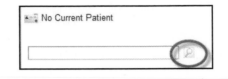

Figure 3-3 Search Patient
Courtesy of Harris CareTracker PM and EMR

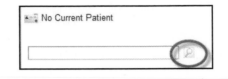

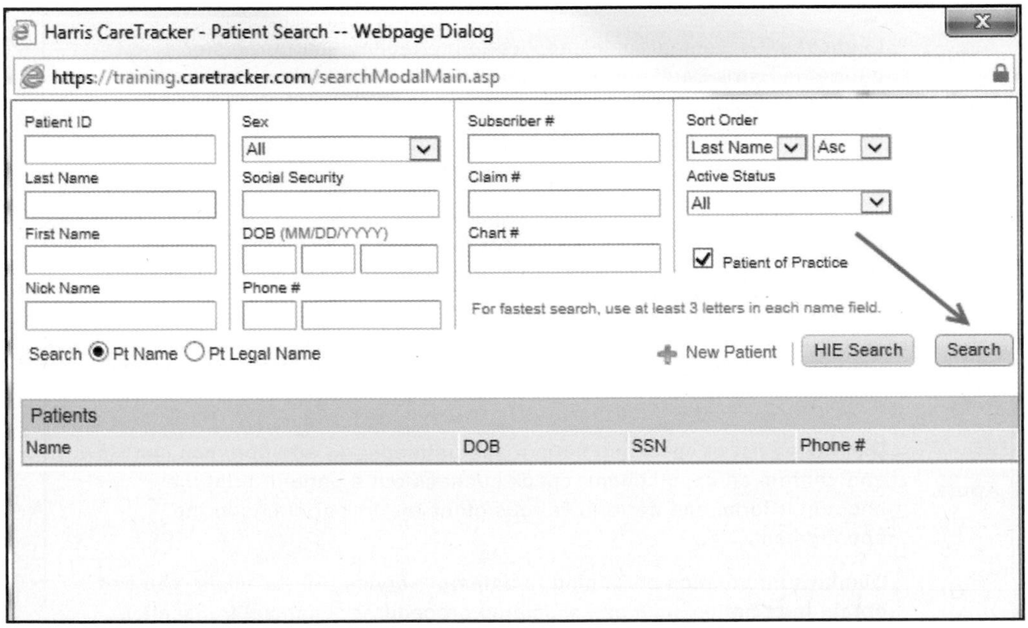

Figure 3-4 Patient Search Window

To access a patient previously in context, click the arrow next to the patient's name (Figure 3-5). To remove the patient from context, select *None*.

Click the *Info* icon next to the patient's name to view patient demographic information, *Patient Portal* status, primary/secondary insurance information, primary/secondary copayment amounts, previous and pending appointment details, and provider information (Figure 3-6). To launch the *Patient Information* window, click the *View Complete Patient Information* link at the bottom.

Your student version of Harris CareTracker will not have access to *Patient Portal* (the Personal Health Record feature of Harris CareTracker). For medical offices that have the fully integrated Harris CareTracker EMR, medical assistants would click the *Patient Portal* tab to launch the *Patient Portal* in the *Patient* module, which allows patients to communicate electronically and securely with their provider. Several types of personal health records (PHRs) are on the market, as described in Table 3-1.

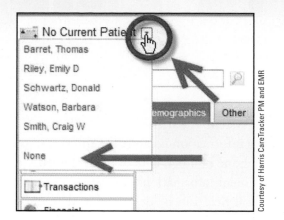

Figure 3-5 Patients Previously in Context

Patient Information		Insurance		
Home Address	998 Corner Rd., Sonoma, CA 95476	Primary Insurance	Proplan Proplan (UNKNOWN)	
Home Phone	(707) 222-5123	Subscriber		
Mobile Phone	NA	Co-Pay	$10.00	
Email	NA	Assignment of Benefits	Yes	
DOB	11/29/1972 (43 yrs)			
Sex	Female	Secondary Insurance	()	
Balance	$0.00	Subscriber		
Patient Portal	Patient not activated	Co-Pay		
Advanced Directive		Assignment of Benefits		
Appointments		**Providers**		
Previous 4	None	PCP		
Pending Appts	None		Ph: Fax:	
Recalls	None			
		Group Provider	Ayerick, Rebecca	
		Referred By	Peretti, Alfred	

View complete Patient Information »

Figure 3-6 Patient Information

TABLE 3-1 Types of Personal Health Records (PHR)

Type of PHR	Description
Stand Alone	Patients access their PHR using a software program that has been downloaded or installed onto their computer. Patients fill in the information from their own records and memories and the data is stored on their computer or on the Internet.
Tethered; Connected	Patients access their PHR through a secure portal of an outside organization (e.g., Harris CareTracker's patient portal *HealthTracker*). Patients can request appointments, prescription renewals, message their provider, and more. May have limited editing capabilities. Ownership is maintained by the organization that provides access to the patient (user).
Internet-based, untethered	Patients access their PHR through a web-based application. After creating a user name and password, a patient is able to create and update information.
Internet-based, networked, and interoperative	An interoperative PHR enables the movement of electronic health information to support patients' health and care needs. A networked PHR is updated continually. Privacy and security of patient information is a challenge.

Source: HealthIT.gov

DEMOGRAPHICS

Learning Objective 2: Demonstrate knowledge of patient demographics.

The *Demographics* application in the *Patient* module is where new patients are registered and added into the Harris CareTracker PM and EMR system. A patient's record will contain basic identifying information and is where pertinent health insurance information is captured. You will record a patient's personal information such as his or her name, address, phone number, date of birth (DOB), Social Security number, marital status, gender, insurance, and employment information necessary to create a patient registration and electronic chart. Demographics in the medical field can be described as defining or descriptive information on the patient (e.g., name, address, phone number[s], gender, insurance information, DOB [age], ethnicity, etc.) (Figure 3-7).

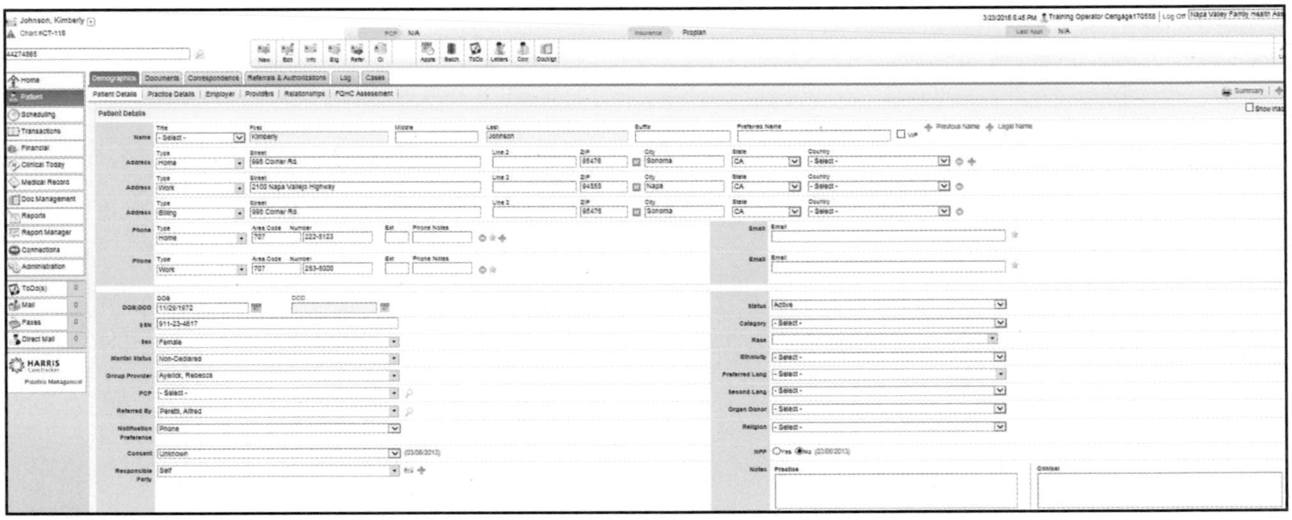

Figure 3-7 Demographics Screen

The minimum required to create a patient record in Harris CareTracker PM and EMR is a patient's first and last names. Harris CareTracker PM and EMR will allow you to save this information and navigate away from the *Demographics* application. However, whenever this patient is pulled into context in the *Name Bar*, an alert will pop up, indicating the patient's record is missing necessary information. Although appointments may be booked for the patient with only the name fields populated, insurance claims cannot be processed until the remainder of the *Demographics* information is complete. In addition, the pop-up alert will notify you if information such as *Primary Language, Race,* and *Ethnicity* are missing when you check the box "Trigger Patient Flash Note" (in the lower right hand corner on the left side of the *Save* button). This information is entered by clicking the *Patient Details* tab, clicking *Edit*, then populating the fields, and then clicking on *Save* (Figure 3-8).

Patient Search

You must take care not to create duplicate patient accounts because it requires significant administrative research and work to confirm patient information and consolidate into one account to maintain chart integrity and patient care coordination. Only use the patient's legal name (e.g., William vs. Bill) and

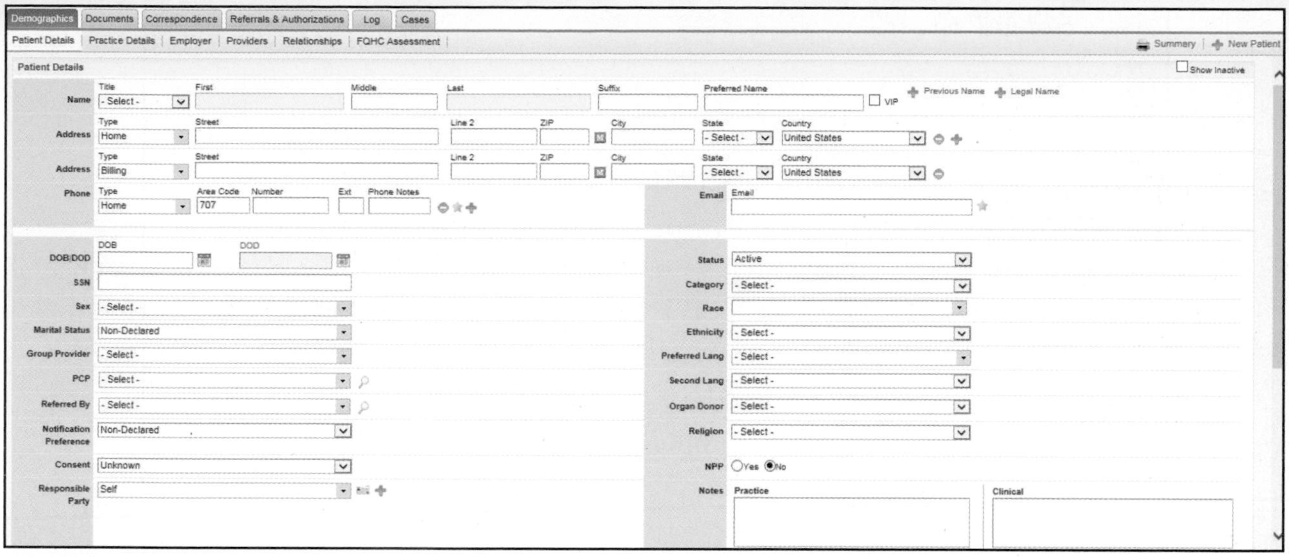

Figure 3-8 Patient Details Window

Courtesy of Harris CareTracker PM and EMR

Critical Thinking

Describe what would happen to the revenue cycle (billing/income to the practice) if a full registration is not completed prior to a patient's visit. Explain how you reached your conclusions.

Tip Box: Navigating

When entering a patient's demographics in the *Demographics* application, the [Tab] key on the keyboard is used to navigate from field to field. When tabbing through the application fields, the field that is active will always be highlighted. When used, the [Tab] key is quick and efficient because the information that is entered is automatically formatted according to the specific field in which the information is being entered. For example, regardless of how a patient's first name or last name is entered, when tabbing out of the name fields, Harris CareTracker PM and EMR will automatically format the name so that the first letter of the name is a capital letter, and the remainder of the letters are lowercase.

verify with the patient's ID and insurance card. Before creating a new patient account, always search for the patient in the database for previous registration by using at least two patient identifiers (e.g., last name [first three letters], first name [first one to three letters], DOB, or Social Security number) (Figure 3-9).

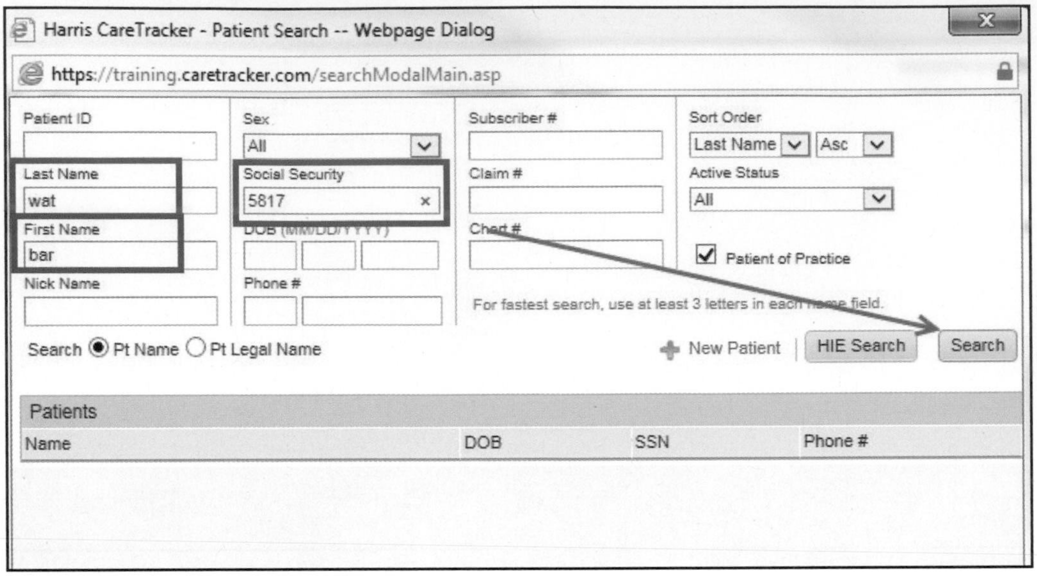

Figure 3-9 Patient Identifiers

Harris CareTracker PM and EMR will alert you if it appears that a duplicate patient record is being created. If duplicate patient records are mistakenly created, those records must be combined into one account using the *Combine Duplicate Patients* application in the *Administration* module.

Patient Alerts

The *Patient Alerts* window notifies the operator when key information is missing from a patient's demographics, or if any problems exist with the patient's account. With a patient in context, you can access *Patient Alerts* by clicking the *Alert* ⚠ icon next to the patient's chart number on the *Name Bar*. Certain conditions trigger Harris CareTracker PM and EMR to display the *Patient Alerts* window. When setting up your **batch** you can set alerts to automatically display. A new batch must be created to enter financial transactions. The *Patient Alerts* window is divided into four sections (Figure 3-10):

1. Patient Demographics
2. Eligibility
3. Other Alerts
4. Notes for this Patient

To launch the application that corresponds to the alert, click the *View* links.

From the *Patient Alert* box, you can edit patient information. It is important to verify accuracy and update information when a patient schedules an appointment or checks in for an appointment. This makes the treatment process faster and avoids unnecessary complications in billing due to outdated information. The pop-up alert will let the operator know what information is missing. In the case of the *View Patient Alerts* example (Figure 3-10), you will see that "Consent" is missing from *Patient Demographics*, and that eligibility is "unknown" from the example provided (Figure 3-11). The *Patient Alert* acts as a form of internal audit of the demographic record. Always confirm in the patient's electronic record that the written registration forms contain the required documentation with a valid signature. These documents include the

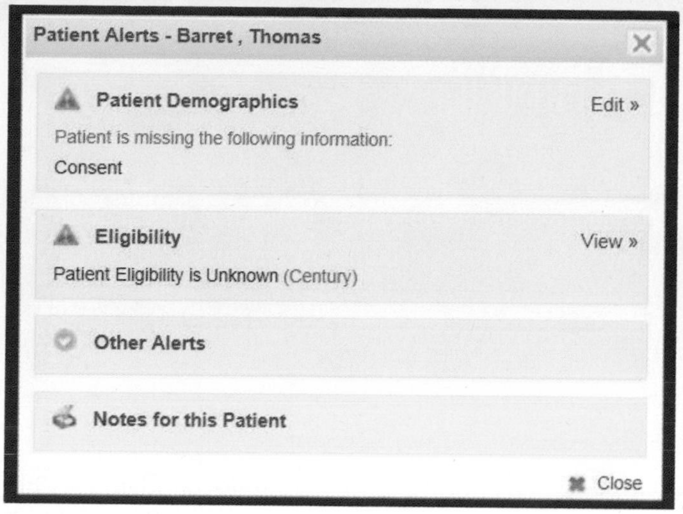

Figure 3-10 View Patient Alerts

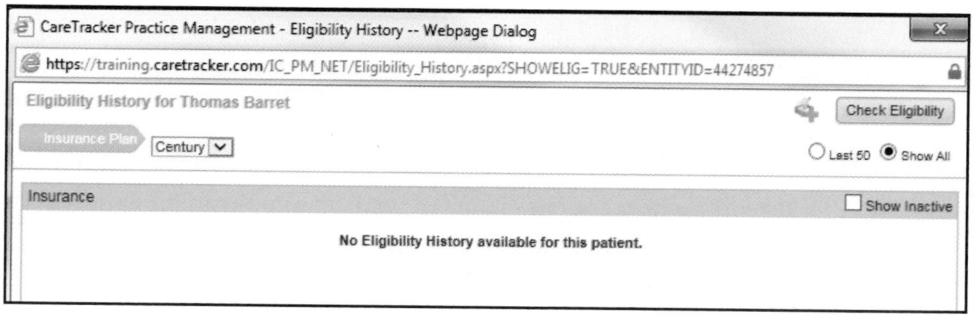

Figure 3-11 View Eligibility

consent form; **notice of privacy practices (NPP)**, a document that describes medical practices policies and procedures regarding the use and disclosure of **protected health information (PHI)**; and a Release of Information (ROI). The Department of Health and Human Services defines PHI as individually identifiable health information, held or maintained by a covered entity or its business associates acting for the covered entity, that is transmitted or maintained in any form or medium (including the individually identifiable health information of non-U.S. citizens). This includes identifiable demographic and other information relating to the past, present, or future; physical or mental health; or condition of an individual; or the provision or payment of health care to an individual that is created or received by a health care provider, health plan, employer, or health care clearinghouse. For purposes of the Privacy Rule, genetic information is considered to be health information (HHS/NIH).

The Rights of Individuals (patients) covered by the NPP regarding the use and disclosure of PHI include the right to:

1. Access and inspect a copy of their PHI
2. Request an amendment of the record
3. Request restrictions on uses and disclosures of PHI, and
4. File a complaint about a violation with the Office of Civil Rights

(*Source:* NHA, Certified Electronic Health Records Specialists)

Critical Thinking

Describe identifiable demographic and other information relating to the past, present, or future; physical or mental health; or condition of an individual that would be considered PHI. How would you assess the information? Provide a comparison of what you would consider PHI and non-PHI.

In addition to documenting patient information, you must de-identify PHI when directed. Methods include **encryption** in the electronic record, shredding paper records, and blacking out information that would identify a patient. Encryption refers to the conversion of letter or numbers to code or symbols so that its contents cannot be viewed or understood.

Name

Registering a new patient begins with entering the patient's name in the *Name* section of the *Demographics* application (Figure 3-12). If you are doing a mini-registration, you can save just the patient's name to create a patient record. Some practices save only a new patient's name to book an appointment and then complete the remainder of the demographic information when the patient comes into the office. Always follow the established office protocol. It is important to review and compare the patient registration form to the demographics as entered into Harris CareTracker to identify any discrepancies.

Patient Name

1. Open an existing patient's demographic record and click **Edit** or click **New** on the **Name Bar** to register a new patient.

2. (Optional) In the **Title** field, select a prefix such as Mr., Mrs., or Dr. It is only necessary to enter a patient's title if the practice would like the title to appear on form letters and statements printed from CareTracker.

3. Enter the patient's name in the **First, Middle** and **Last** name fields. There is no need to capitalize the first letter of the name; tabbing through the fields automatically capitalizes the first letter of each name. A patient can have patient name, a legal name and a previous name. The patient name (entered in the Name fields) is used to submit claims. Operators can search for a patient using either the patient name or legal name.

4. (Optional) In the **Suffix** field, select a suffix such as Jr. or Sr. It is only necessary to enter a suffix if the practice would like it to appear on form letters and statements printed from CareTracker.

5. (Optional) In the **Preferred Name** field you can enter a nickname for the patient. The nickname displays in parentheses next to the patient's proper name whenever it appears in CareTracker. A patient's nickname will not appear on form letters or statements generated in CareTracker.

6. (Optional) Click ✚ **Previous Name** to add the patient's previous name.

7. (Optional) Click ✚ **Legal Name** to add the patient's legal name.

Courtesy of Harris CareTracker PM and EMR

Figure 3-12 Entering a New Patient's Name

Photos

Many practices now require photo identification of their patients to protect against identify theft, ensure the integrity of the patient's chart, and maintain privacy (HIPAA compliance). Harris CareTracker PM provides a means of adding a photo or a copy of a driver's license to the patient's demographic record and is part of the CEHRS™ required knowledge. You will not be able to insert or scan documents in your student version of Harris CareTracker PM, but you will simulate the task as part of Learning Objective 4 (Figure 3-13).

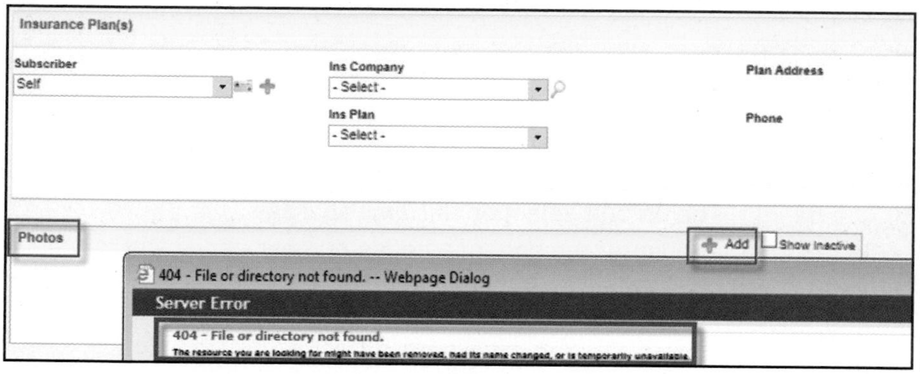

Courtesy of Harris CareTracker PM and EMR

Figure 3-13 Add a Picture in Patient Demographics

Addresses

If the home and the billing addresses are the same, you do not have to enter a billing address. However, if a patient's statements are going to be sent to a different address, add a separate billing address; otherwise the home address becomes the billing address by default. If only a billing address is entered for the patient, the home address defaults to the same address when patient information is saved.

PM SPOTLIGHT

Part of the duties in managing a PM/EHR includes the backup of data, or restoring patient data. Harris CareTracker is a web-based PM and EHR application with automatic system backups, but there are times when it is necessary to deactivate or activate an address, insurance, medication, and so on. To deactivate or activate a patient's address, follow these steps:

- If a patient's address is no longer active, click the *Deactivate* icon at the end of the address line (Figure 3-14). The deactivated address remains in the patient's record but is now grayed out. Additionally, the *Deactivate* icon is changed to *Activate*.
- To reactivate a deactivated address, click the *Activate* icon next to a deactivated address. The address will no longer be grayed out.

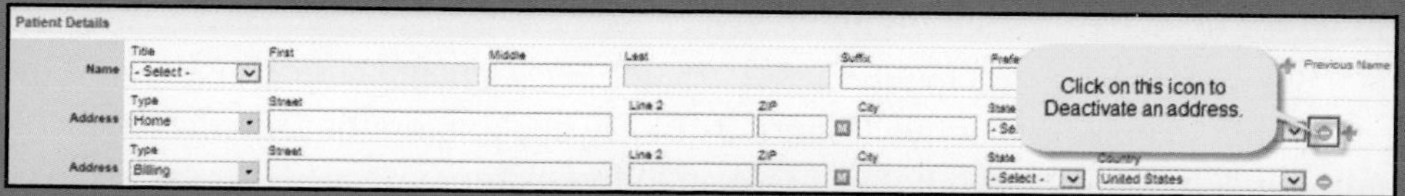

Courtesy of Harris CareTracker PM and EMR

Figure 3-14 Deactivate Patient Address

When a patient lives outside of the United States, his or her address must be entered differently than a patient who lives in the country. Please keep in mind, statements will not be sent to foreign addresses, but setting up the patient's *Demographics* correctly will prevent the claim from being unbilled due to the patient's address.

To enter a foreign address:

- Open an existing patient's demographic record (click *Edit* in the *Name Bar*) or click *New* on the *Name Bar* to register a new patient.
- From the *Type* list in the *Addresses* section, select the type of address you are entering for the patient. The default selection is *Home* address.
- In the Line 1 box enter the patient's house number and street name.
- In the Line 2 box enter the patient's city and state. Depending on the country, this may be a city/town and province.
- In the *City* box, enter the country in which the patient lives.
- From the *Country* list, select the county in which the patient lives. This field does not pull onto the claim and that is why it is necessary to enter the country in the *City* field (Figure 3-15).

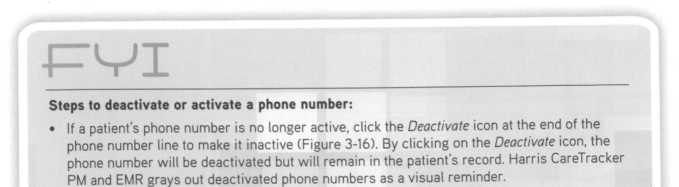

Figure 3-15   Entering a Foreign Address – Foreign

Courtesy of Harris CareTracker PM and EMR

Phones

Entering a patient's phone number into Harris CareTracker PM and EMR is similar to entering a patient's address. A phone number can be deactivated at any time and you can add as many phone numbers as needed. Harris CareTracker PM and EMR prints the patient's *Home* and *Work* phone numbers on the appointment list.

Steps to deactivate or activate a phone number:

- If a patient's phone number is no longer active, click the *Deactivate* icon at the end of the phone number line to make it inactive (Figure 3-16). By clicking on the *Deactivate* icon, the phone number will be deactivated but will remain in the patient's record. Harris CareTracker PM and EMR grays out deactivated phone numbers as a visual reminder.
- Click the *Activate* icon to reactivate a phone number.

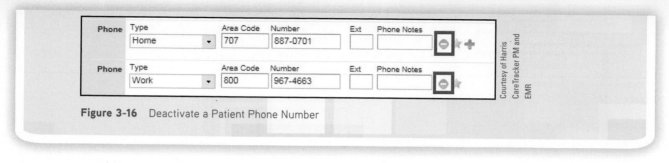

Figure 3-16   Deactivate a Patient Phone Number

Chart Number

When registering a patient, it is not necessary to enter or assign a chart number to the patient in the *Chart Number* field unless the practice prefers that a specific chart number be manually entered for internal purposes. If a practice has converted from another medical management system to Harris CareTracker PM and EMR and chart numbers were previously used, they will cross over and appear in the *Chart Number* field. This makes it possible to search the database for established patients from the previous system (Figure 3-17).

When new patients are registered in Harris CareTracker PM and EMR, the chart number becomes the same as the *ID* number that is automatically assigned by Harris CareTracker PM and EMR.

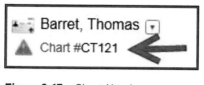

Figure 3-17   Chart Number
Courtesy of Harris CareTracker PM and EMR

Date of Birth

Date of Birth (DOB) displays the patient's date of birth. You can enter the date of birth manually in MM/DD/YYYY format, or click the *Calendar* icon [icon] to select the date. If by error you enter a future date in the *Date of Birth* box, an error message prompts to notify you that a wrong date is entered. To prevent duplicate patient accounts and to speed the patient search option, it is advisable to use the DOB as one of the two patient identifiers. The Date of Death (DOD) field is only enabled when the Status field has been changed to "Deceased."

Social Security Number

The patient's nine-digit Social Security number is entered in the *SSN* field. The application will automatically add the hyphen when you [Tab] to the next field. For security purposes, after saving the patient's demographic, the *SSN* is encrypted and only the last four digits are displayed (Figure 3-18). Encryption is a method of de-identifying PHI.

Gender (Sex)

The *Gender (Sex)* list in the *Demographics* application contains two options: *Male* and *Female*. If a patient's sex is not entered, claims for the patient will not be electronically transmitted to the insurance company. Any claim lacking a specified gender will become an unbilled claim and will remain as such until an operator specifies a sex and re-bills the claim (Figure 3-19).

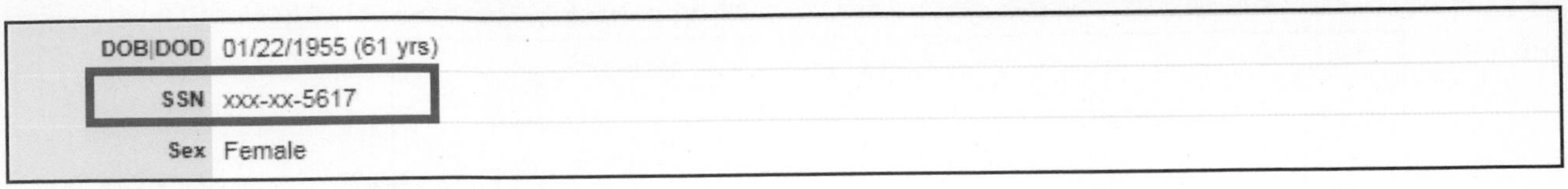

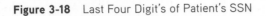

Courtesy of Harris CareTracker PM and EMR

Figure 3-18 Last Four Digit's of Patient's SSN

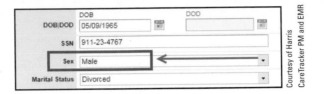

Courtesy of Harris CareTracker PM and EMR

Figure 3-19 Gender (Sex) Field in Demographics Screen

Notes

In the *Notes* field, you can free-type any important patient information to which users may need to be alerted. For example, if a patient is hearing-impaired or does not speak English, you could type that information in the *Notes* field, and the note would be saved in the patient's demographic (Figure 3-20). There is a 249-character limit for the *Notes* field. There are two fields, *Practice* and *Clinical*. Notes entered in the *Clinical Notes* field are displayed in the *Clinical Alert* window when an operator launches a patient's health record.

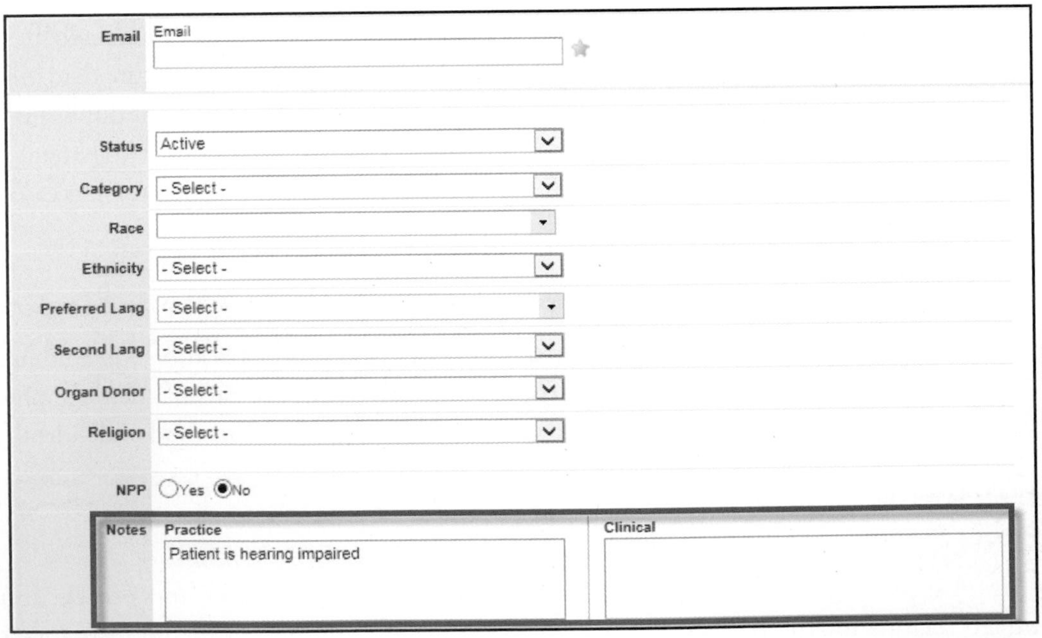

Courtesy of Harris CareTracker PM and EMR

Figure 3-20 Notes Field in Patient Demographics Screen

Tip Box

Flash Note: Select the *Trigger Patient Flash Note* checkbox to create a flash note for the patient. When this checkbox is selected, Harris CareTracker PM and EMR will display the note in an alert each time the patient is pulled into context. The note will also be displayed in the *Notes* field in the *Patient Details* application of the *Patient* module *Demographics* tab.

Critical Thinking

Provide examples of when you would use *Patient Flash Notes*.

Tip Box

Clinical Notes: *Notes* entered in the *Clinical Notes* field are displayed in the *Clinical Alert* window when an operator launches a patient's health record.

VIP Flag

Flagging a patient as a *VIP* allows the practice to restrict operator access to the patient's demographic. Any operator may flag a high-profile patient as a *VIP*, but only operators assigned either the *VIP Patient Access* or the *VIP Patient Access Break Glass* override in their profile can access a *VIP* demographic (Figure 3-21).

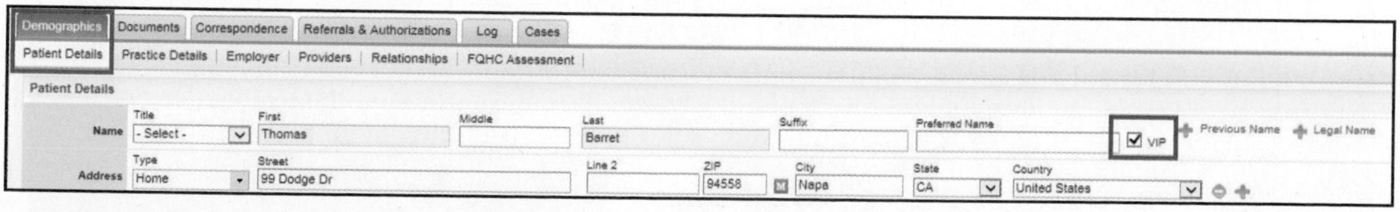

Figure 3-21 VIP Flag

Courtesy of Harris CareTracker PM and EMR

PM SP⬤TLIGHT

Break the glass privileges allow an operator limited access to a *VIP* patient's information. The access is only available during the operator's current Harris CareTracker PM and EMR session, and the operator must provide a reason why the record is being accessed. An operator must have either the *VIP Patient Access* or the *VIP Patient Access Break Glass* override included in his or her operator profile to access a VIP patient. Each time an operator accesses a *VIP* patient demographic, Harris CareTracker PM and EMR creates an entry in the *VIP Patient Log*. The log lists the patient's name, the operator who accessed the record, and the date and time the record was accessed (Figure 3-22).

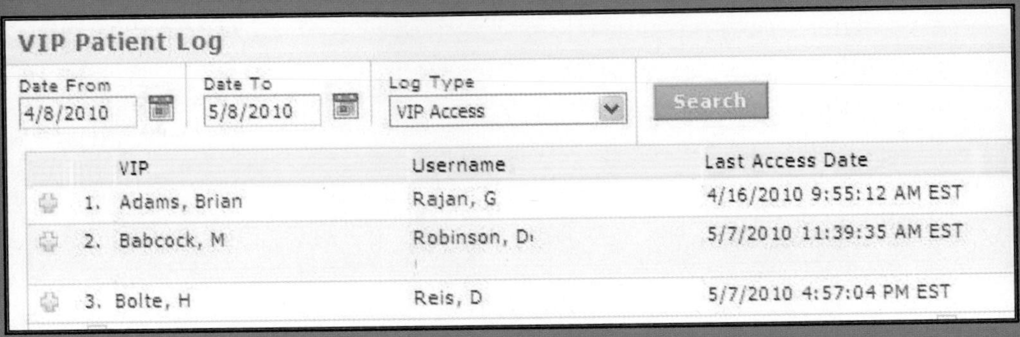

VIP Patient Log

Date From	Date To	Log Type	
4/8/2010	5/8/2010	VIP Access	Search

	VIP	Username	Last Access Date
1.	Adams, Brian	Rajan, G	4/16/2010 9:55:12 AM EST
2.	Babcock, M	Robinson, D	5/7/2010 11:39:35 AM EST
3.	Bolte, H	Reis, D	5/7/2010 4:57:04 PM EST

Courtesy of Harris CareTracker PM and EMR

Figure 3-22   VIP Patient Log

Critical Thinking

Provide examples of when a patient should be flagged as a VIP.

PM SP⬤TLIGHT

Important!!
By default, only the practice administrator ("Fin-Practice Admin" role) is assigned access to the view *VIP* patient demographics and the *VIP Log*. The practice administrator is responsible for assigning access to other operators in the group by adding a security override to their user profile.

Critical Thinking

What law prohibits the unauthorized access of patient charts? What provisions apply? Identify consequences of accessing a patient chart without reason?

Responsible Party

The patient's **responsible party** is the individual who is responsible for any private pay balances; the remaining amount, if any, after insurance has paid its portion. Patient statements are addressed to the person indicated in the *Responsible* field, and *Self* is the default option for the *Responsible* field in the *Demographics* application. Patients over the age of 18 are considered responsible parties. For patients under the age of 18, parents or guardians are usually the responsible parties.

   If the responsible party does not appear in the list, search the database:

1. Click the *Add* icon next to the *Responsible Party* field. The application displays the *Add Responsible Party* window.
2. From the *Type* list, select the type of responsible party.
3. In the *Responsible Party* field, either select the name from the list, or click the *Search* icon to search the database.
4. From the *Relationship* list, select the relationship of the responsible party to the patient. **Note:** This field is only enabled when the responsible party type is "Patient."
5. Click *Save*.
6. Click *Save* on the *Patient Details* tab.

Note: If the responsible party is a patient, but is not found in the search, you can add the patient to the CareTracker database. Click the *Add* icon next to the *Responsible Party* field or the *New Patient* link in the search window and register the responsible party.

Insurance Plan(s)

Entering a patient's insurance information accurately in the *Insurance* section of the *Demographics* application ensures that insurance companies will pay claims in a timely manner. A list of the practice's most frequently accepted insurance companies and plans can be created in the *Quick Picks* application or you can search the Harris CareTracker PM and EMR database (this is not a student task/function). When an insurance company or plan is not listed in Harris CareTracker PM and EMR's database, it can be added using *Pending Insurance* as a placeholder.

Employers

The *Employer* tab of the *Demographics* application is where a practice can track patient employment information. Often, the patient's employment history and insurance history go hand-in-hand. Having a patient's employment information is essential for any work-related injuries covered by workers' compensation, needed to complete paperwork necessary to have the claim paid.

PM SP⬤TLIGHT

A *Deactivate Employer* icon and a *+ New Employer* link are also located in the *Employer(s)* section in addition to the address, phone, and insurance sections. To add an additional employer, click on the *+ New Employer* link and complete the additional employer's information in the same manner in which the information was completed for the initial employer. When a patient is no longer employed by a particular employer, make this inactive by clicking on the *Deactivate Employer* icon located next to the former employer. Employment history usually begins with the patient's current employer(s). To track previous employers, check the "Show Inactive" box. If a previous employer was added, click on the *Deactivate* icon for that employer to save the inactive employer for tracking purposes.

SEARCH FOR A PATIENT

Learning Objective 3: Search for a patient within Harris CareTracker PM.

Now that you have reviewed the patient registration and demographics segment, you will complete activities to demonstrate your knowledge and ability to perform tasks within Harris CareTracker PM. The first activity is to *Search* for a patient (one that is already in the database). Follow the step-by-step instructions to complete the activities for this chapter. Log into Harris CareTracker PM with your user ID and password provided with your materials. Remain logged in as long as you are completing activities.

It is important to have a patient in context for every patient-specific function such as editing demographics, booking an appointment, entering referral/authorization information, and more. The basic methods to pull a patient into context are by the last name, Harris CareTracker PM and EMR ID number, chart number, claim number, and Social Security number. It is recommended that you always use two identifiers to verify that you are viewing the correct chart and do not create a duplicate account.

ACTIVITY 3-1: Searching for a Patient by Name
(currently in the database)

PATIENT: Emily Riley

1. In the *ID* search box on the *Name Bar*, enter the first three letters of the patient's last name ("Ril"), and hit [Enter] (Figure 3-23). The pop-up will list any patient matching your search criteria. Click on patient Emily Riley and the patient will be pulled into context. **Note:** If you receive a pop-up asking if you want to navigate away from this page (Figure 3-24), select "OK" and Harris CareTracker PM will launch the *Patient Demographics* application, displaying the patient's demographics screen.

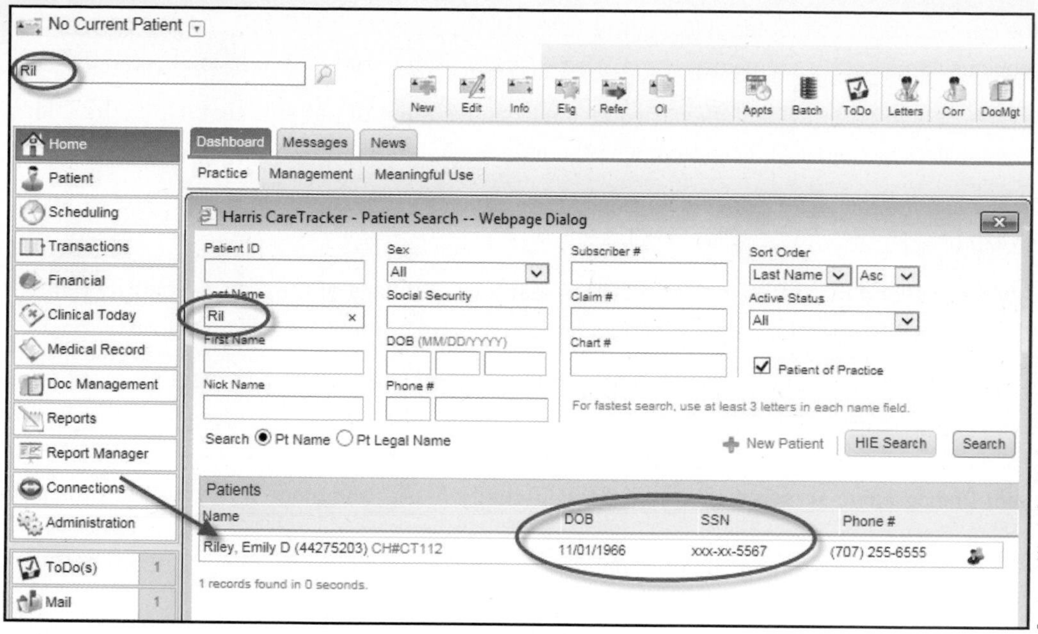

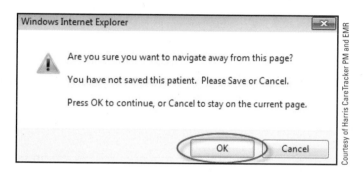

Figure 3-23 Search by First Three Letters of Patient's Last Name

Courtesy of Harris CareTracker PM and EMR

Windows Internet Explorer

⚠ Are you sure you want to navigate away from this page?

You have not saved this patient. Please Save or Cancel.

Press OK to continue, or Cancel to stay on the current page.

[OK]   [Cancel]

Figure 3-24 Leave This Page Pop-up Message

Courtesy of Harris CareTracker PM and EMR

2. An alternate method to search for existing patients is:

a. Remove a patient in context by clicking on the drop-down list at the end of the patient's name (Figure 3-25) and select "None." The name in the patient field will be removed and "No current patient" will display.

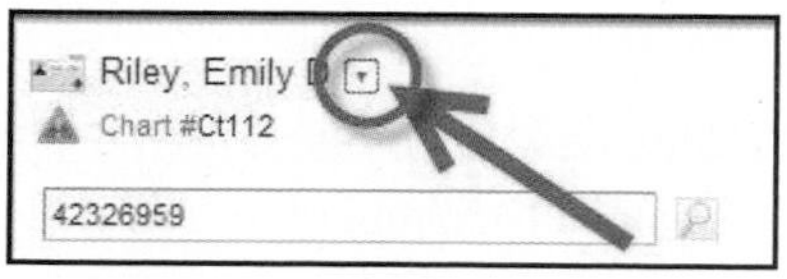

Riley, Emily D ▼
⚠ Chart #Ct112

42326959

Figure 3-25 Remove Patient from Context Drop-Down

Courtesy of Harris CareTracker PM and EMR

b. With "no current patient" in the ID search box, click on the *Search* icon 🔍, which will bring up the *Patient Search* box.

    c. In the *Patient Search* box, enter at least three letters of the patient's last ("Ril") and first name ("Emi"). A previous name such as a maiden name or an alias cannot be used to search for a patient.

    d. Click the *Search* button. The *Patient Search* box displays a list of patients that match the information entered (see Figure 3-23), along with the patient ID and chart number.

    e. Click the *Family* icon 👥 to view the patient's family members registered in Harris CareTracker PM and EMR (if applicable).

    f. Verify the "second identifier" such as DOB or last four numbers of the Social Security number, and then click the specific name to launch the patient into context (see Figure 3-23).

3. Record the patient's ID number, chart number, and Social Security number for additional activities related to searching for a patient.

🖊 **Print the Patient Demographic screen displayed, label it "Activity 3-1A," and place it in your assignment folder.**

4. Repeat Activity 3-1 by searching for four additional established patients by name. Record their ID number and Social Security number for future searches.

    a. Kevin Johnson

    b. Jane Morgan

    c. Kirk Johnson

    d. Abby Zuffante

🖊 **Print the Search Results screen for each patient, label it "Activity 3-1B," and place it in your assignment folder.**

You now have successfully searched for a patient and know the patient's ID number, chart number, Social Security number, and claim number (if applicable) from the record provided. Using that information, practice searching for the same patient using the alternative methods listed next.

ACTIVITY 3-2: Searching for a Patient by ID Number

1. In the *ID* search box (see Figure 3-3), enter patient Emily Riley's ID number (using the ID number obtained from the patient search in Activity 3-1.) **Note:** New ID numbers are assigned to patients for each student version of Harris CareTracker; therefore, patient ID numbers will vary by student.

2. Hit [Enter]. The patient with the corresponding *ID number* launches into context.

3. You can also perform a search by patient ID number by clicking the *Search* icon. In the *Patient Search* box, enter the *Patient ID*, the patient's *Last Name* and *First Name*. Click *Search*. A list of patients that match the information entered will pop up.

🖊 **Print the Search Results screen, label it "Activity 3-2A," and place it in your assignment folder.**

4. Repeat Activity 3-2 by searching for four additional established patients by ID number using the information obtained in your Activity 3-1 search.

   a. Kevin Johnson

   b. Jane Morgan

   c. Kirk Johnson

   d. Abby Zuffante

Print the Search Results screen for each patient, label it "Activity 3-2B," and place it in your assignment folder.

You may also search for a patient by chart number. Typically, the chart number and the Harris CareTracker PM and EMR ID are the same. However, if the practice files paper charts by chart number, Harris CareTracker PM and EMR can assign chart numbers based on your medical record number. In your student version, the chart number and ID number are different for existing patients. New patients will have the same chart number and ID number. (**Note:** If your practice has electronically converted patient demographics to Harris CareTracker PM and EMR from another practice management system, the chart number will be the patient's ID number from your legacy practice management system.)

ACTIVITY 3-3:   Searching for a Patient by Chart Number

1. With no patient in context, click the *Search* 🔍 icon; it will take you to the *Patient Search* pop-up box where you will need to enter the patient's *Chart Number*.

2. Enter the chart number of patient Emily Riley (CT112) and click *Search* (Figure 3-26).

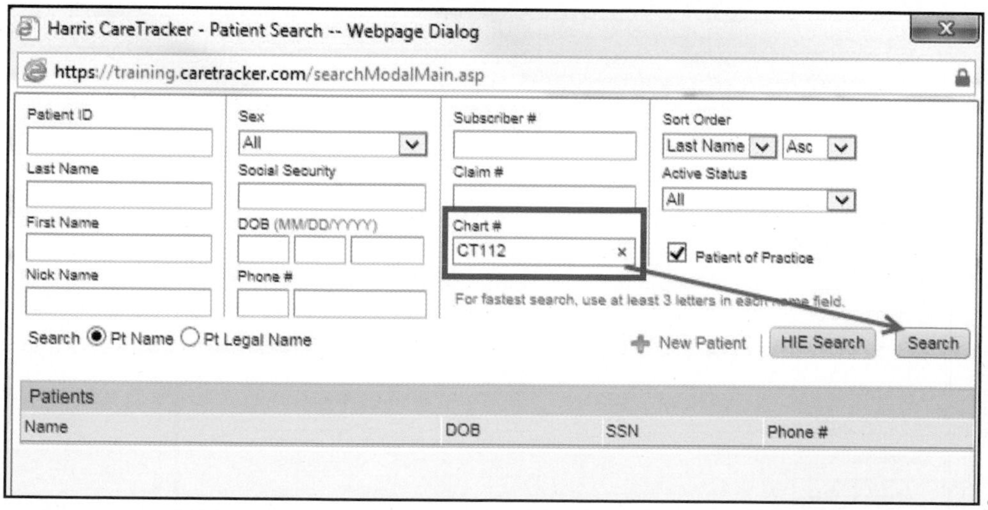

Figure 3-26   Search by Patient Chart Number

Print the Search Results screen, label it "Activity 3-3A," and place it in your assignment folder.

3. Click directly on the patient's name with the corresponding *Chart Number* to launch him or her into context.
   (**Note:** It may take a few moments for Harris CareTracker to "search" and populate the patient demographics.)

4. Repeat Activity 3-3 by searching for four additional established patients using their chart numbers, which were obtained in your Activity 3-1 search.
   a. Kevin Johnson
   b. Jane Morgan
   c. Kirk Johnson
   d. Abby Zuffante

Print the Search Results screen for each patient, label it "Activity 3-3B," and place it in your assignment folder.

Another method of patient search is by *Claim Number*. A claim number is generated when the insurance is billed for the patient encounter and results in an **explanation of benefits (EOB)**. An EOB details the amount of the claim, any discounts for contracted rates, the percentage paid by the insurance, denial reasons (codes), and balance due from the patient. Your student version of Harris CareTracker PM is not able to generate a claim number.

FYI

To simulate this activity/workflow, with no patient in context, click the *Search* icon. In the pop-up screen, enter the claim number and hit *Enter* or *Search*. The steps to search for a patient by *Claim Number* are:

1. With no patient in context, click the *Search* icon.
2. In the *Patient Search* box, enter the claim number. Example: 34052042.
3. Hit [Enter] or *Search*. The application will pull the patient into context (Figure 3-27).

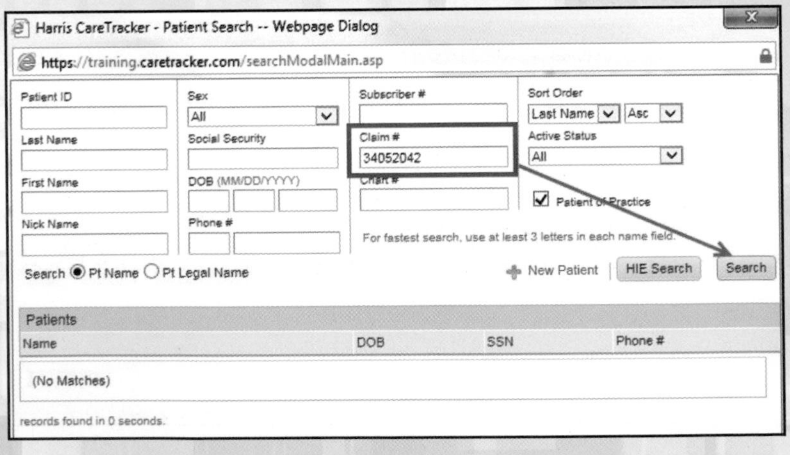

Courtesy of Harris CareTracker PM and EMR

Figure 3-27 Searching by Claim Number

You may also search for a patient by Social Security number using the steps outlined in Activity 3-4.

ACTIVITY 3-4: Searching for a Patient by Social Security Number (SSN)

1. With no patient in context, click the *Search* icon.
2. In the *Patient Search* pop-up, enter the last four digits of patient Emily Riley's Social Security number (5567), obtained in Activity 3-1, and hit [Enter] (or click on the *Search* button).

Print the Patient Search pop-up screen, label it "Activity 3-4A," and place it in your assignment folder.

3. Click on the corresponding patient (Figure 3-28).

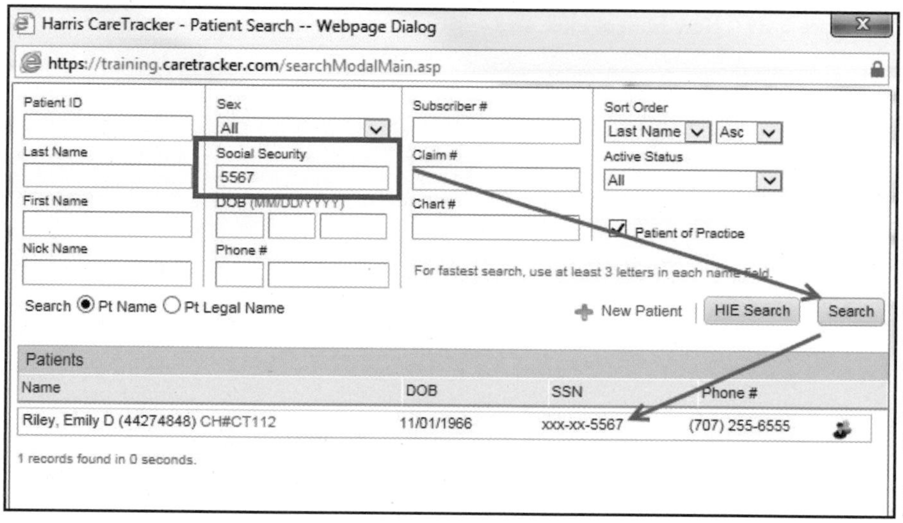

Courtesy of Harris CareTracker PM and EMR

Figure 3-28 Search by Social Security Number

4. The application pulls the patient into context and launches the *Patient Demographics* application.
5. Repeat Activity 3-4 by searching for the four additional established patients using their Social Security numbers obtained in your Activity 3-1 search.
   a. Kevin Johnson
   b. Jane Morgan
   c. Kirk Johnson
   d. Abby Zuffante

Print the Patient Search pop-up screen for each patient, label it "Activity 3-4B," and place it in your assignment folder.

REGISTER NEW PATIENTS

Learning Objective 4: Register a new patient in Harris CareTracker.

Your next activity is to register a new patient, one who is not in the current database (Figures 3-29 and 3-30). It is important to register all patients in the Harris CareTracker PM and EMR system with their demographics information such as name, contact information, date of birth, insurance and employer information, and more. This information is required to ensure proper treatment as well as to facilitate billing. Prior to registering a new patient, always search the database to be certain that the patient has never been registered. Use two patient identifiers when searching to avoid creating a duplicate account.

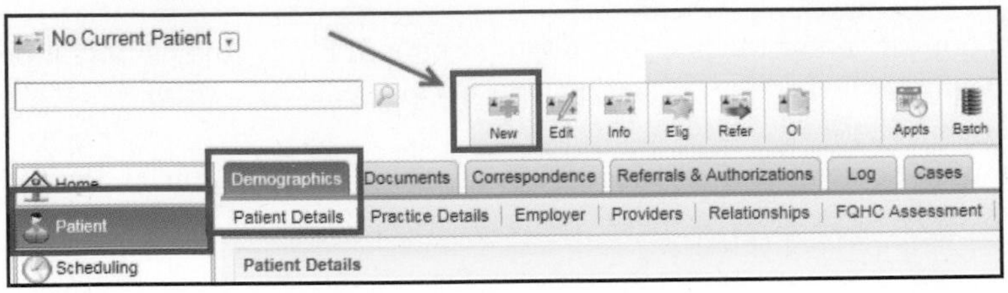

Courtesy of Harris CareTracker PM and EMR

Figure 3-29 New Patient Link

Tip Box

Navigate through each field by pressing the [Tab] key and Harris CareTracker PM and EMR will automatically format the entry, regardless of the way it is entered. For example, by tabbing through the *First Name* and *Last Name* boxes, Harris CareTracker PM and EMR automatically applies title case to the name, meaning the first letter of each name is capitalized. To navigate back to a field, press [SHIFT+TAB].

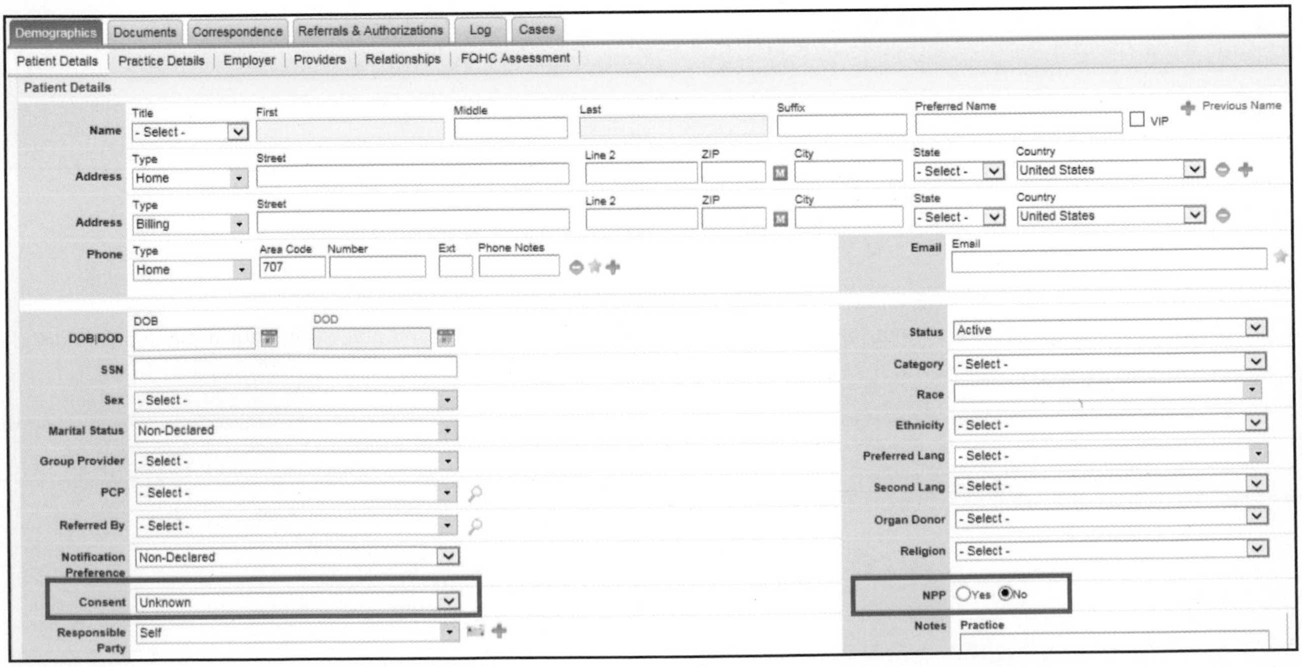

Courtesy of Harris CareTracker PM and EMR

Figure 3-30 New Patient Demographic Screen with Consent Fields Highlighted

ACTIVITY 3-5: Register a New Patient

Search the existing database to confirm the patient (new patient James M. Smith) has never been registered. After confirming he is not in the system, click *New* on the *Name Bar*. Harris CareTracker PM displays the *Patient Details* window. Register "New Patient" James M. Smith's demographic information, responsible party, insurance, and employer information from his patient registration form. When finished, click *Save*. To register new patient James M. Smith, please refer to Source Documents 3-1 (Registration Form) and 3-2 (NPP).

1. *Name:* Enter the patient's name (including nickname if used, for example, Jim for James).
2. *Address:*
   a. In the *Line 1* box, enter the patient's street address (house number + street name).
   b. In the *Line 2* box, enter the patient's apartment or condominium number, if applicable.
   c. In the *Zip* box, enter the patient's zip code (Figure 3-31).

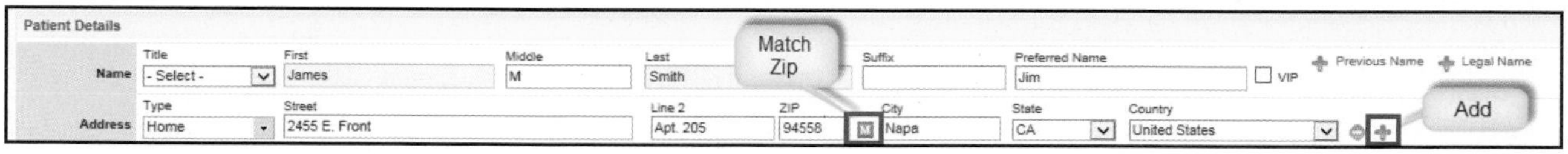

Courtesy of Harris CareTracker PM and EMR

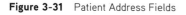

Figure 3-31 Patient Address Fields

   d. Press the [Enter] key. Harris CareTracker PM automatically populates the *City, State,* and *Country* fields based on the zip code. **Note:** Unless a separate billing address is entered, the patient's home address becomes the billing address by default.
   e. If needed, click the + icon to add additional address fields.
3. *Phone:*
   a. The phone number field will default to the patient's home phone number. You can also use the drop-down feature from the *Type* list to select the type of phone number you are entering (Figure 3-32).

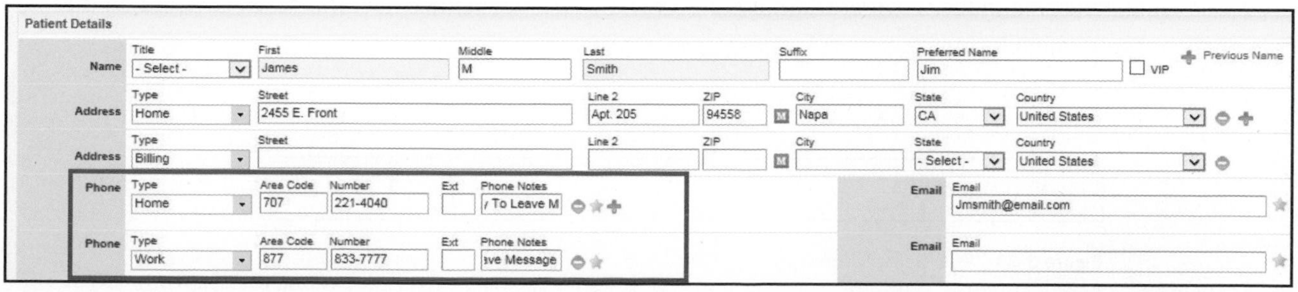

Courtesy of Harris CareTracker PM and EMR

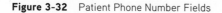

Figure 3-32 Patient Phone Number Fields

b. In the *Area Code* field, enter the area code if not already populated.

c. In the *Number* field, enter the phone number. You do not need to enter a hyphen (it will automatically be added as you enter the phone number).

d. (Optional) If the phone number entered requires an extension, enter the extension in the *Ext* field.

e. In the *Phone Notes* field, enter any notes related to the patient's contact information, for example, "OK to leave message, do not call after 8 P.M." and so on. (Enter whether okay to leave detailed message as noted in Source Document 3-1 here.)

f. Click on the *Set as Preferred Contact* ☆ icon at the end of the line. Click the + icon to add additional phone number lines to the demographic record, as indicated in Source Document 3–1.

g. In the *Email* field, enter the patient's email address on the same line as the patient's home phone number. Enter the email address exactly as you would if you were sending an email. Harris CareTracker PM will validate the email address format when the record is saved.

Tip Box

Although email is listed as an optional field, most practices require the collection of the patient's email address to establish online, secure communications, and appointment reminders.

4. *Date of Birth* (DOB) (Age): Enter the date of birth in MM/DD/YYYY (or mm/dd/yy—six-digit) format, or click on the *Calendar* icon ▦ to select a DOB.

5. *SSN* (Social Security Number): Enter the patient's Social Security number. Do not include dashes. This field must contain the nine digits or be left blank. Once you save your edits, the first five digits will be encrypted and only the last four digits display.

6. *Sex:* Enter the patient's sex. If no sex is entered, a claim cannot be sent.

7. *Marital Status:* Enter the patient's marital status, if known or declared. Choose the status from the drop-down list.

8. *Group Provider:* Select from the drop-down list the provider listed on the patient registration form.

9. *PCP* (Primary Care Provider): Select the PCP for the patient noted on the registration form from the drop-down list. (**Note:** If you were searching for a provider who is not on the list, you would click the Search icon 🔍 to the right of the field, type in as much information as you have [minimally last name and state], and search for providers) (Figure 3-33). You would normally select the provider listed on the patient registration form.

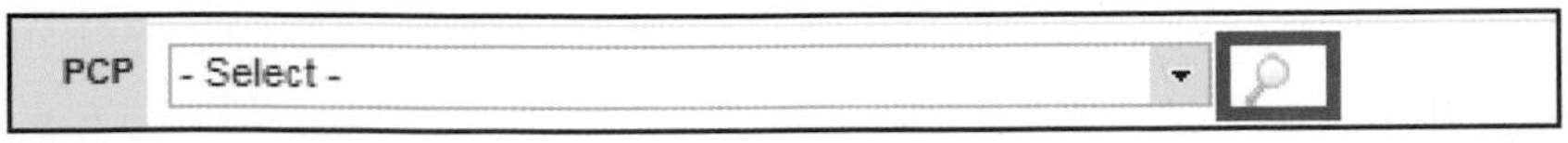

Courtesy of Harris CareTracker PM and EMR

Figure 3-33 PCP Search Icon

10. *Referred By:* From the drop-down list, select the most appropriate. If you do not find the referring physician in the drop-down list, you can search the National Provider Identifier (NPI) database. For this activity, the referring providers are in your quick-pick drop-down list.

11. *Notification Preference:* From the drop-down list, select the preferred method of communication noted in Source Document 3-1.

12. *Consent:* From the drop-down box, select from the options: Unknown, Yes, No, or Revoked. Review Source 3-1 and 3-2 in Appendix A and determine if Consent and NPP have been given. Enter the appropriate response in each field (see Figure 3-30).

13. *Responsible Party:* Enter the responsible party information from the patient registration form and insurance card. The only option available from the drop-down list is "Self." If you click on the + icon to the right of the field, the *Add Responsible Party* dialog box will pop up, and you can add a responsible party if it is other than "Self." Using the *Search* icon 🔍 in the *Add Responsible Party* box allows you to search the practice's database. There is also a *Relationship* field, and from the *Relationship* list you can select the patient whose demographic information is being completed. When a relationship is selected, the patient's name is displayed in the *Responsible Party* field.

FYI

Add New: To enter a responsible party who is not a patient of the practice, click the + icon to the right of the *Responsible Party* drop-down list. Once the + icon is selected, the *Add Responsible Party* dialog box will open in which you can add the information for the responsible party (Figure 3-34).

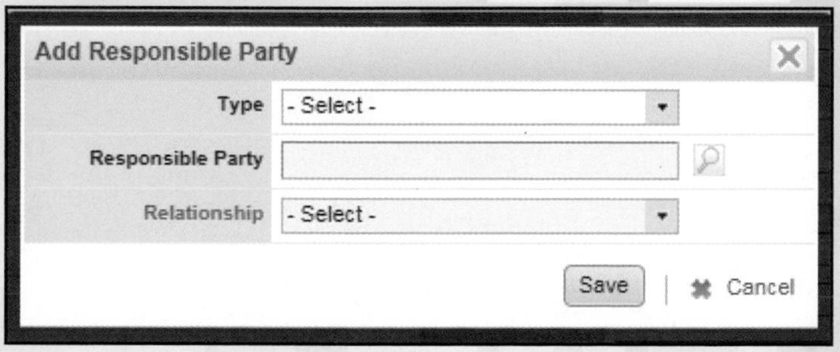

Add Responsible Party	
Type	- Select - ▾
Responsible Party	🔍
Relationship	- Select - ▾
	Save	✖ Cancel

Courtesy of Harris CareTracker PM and EMR

Figure 3-34   Add New Responsible Party

14. *Status:* This field is used to note the patient's status. Choose "Active" for new patients. (Other choices from the drop-down list would be used as appropriate, for example, Deceased, Discharged, Followed by Another M.D., Inactive, Moved Out of Area, or Not a Patient of Practice.)

15. *Category:* From the drop-down list, select the most appropriate category (if any). Categories available are Bad address, Collections, and High deductible. Leave Category as "-Select-" when registering a new patient. (**Note:** Additional categories can be added through the *Administration* module if the practice chooses to do so.)

16. *Race:* In the drop-down menu, select from the following options: American Indian or Alaskan Native, Asian, Black or African American, Native Hawaiian or other Pacific Islander, Patient Refusal, or White.

17. *Ethnicity:* In the drop-down menu, select from the following options: Hispanic or Latino, Not Hispanic or Latino, or Patient Refusal.

18. *Preferred Lang:* Select the preferred language of the patient from the drop-down menu.

19. *Second Lang:* Select the patient's second language from the drop-down menu, if applicable.

20. *Organ Donor:* Identify whether the patient is an organ donor (if noted on the patient registration form).

21. *Religion:* Select the patient's religion from the drop-down menu (if noted on the patient registration form).

22. *NPP* (Notice of Privacy Practices): Select the radio dial button. Referring to the Patient Registration packet, select the radio dial button "Yes" or "No" indicating whether the NPP has been signed/recorded.

Tip Box

Always confirm if the *Consent* and *NPP* were signed by the patient, and check "Yes" on the demographics screen. Harris CareTracker will automatically "date stamp" when the *NPP* and *Consent* information were entered.

23. *Notes* (*Practice* or *Clinical*): Enter any notes that you want to include for this patient. In the lower right-hand corner of the demographics screen, check the box *Trigger Patient Flash Note* which will activate the notes to flash when you pull the patient into context. For example, "requires interpreter," etc.

24. *Insurance Plan(s):* Click on the + Insurance link on the right side of the screen and complete the fields with information from the patient registration form (Source Document 3-1).

    a. The *Subscriber* field defaults to "Self." Leave this selection if the patient is the **subscriber**. (James Smith is the subscriber, so leave as "Self.") If an individual other than the patient or the responsible party is the subscriber, click on the + icon at the end of the *Subscriber* field.

Tip Box

A subscriber is an individual who is a member of a benefits plan. For example, in the case of family coverage, one adult is ordinarily the subscriber. A spouse and children would ordinarily be dependents.

FYI

To add a new *Subscriber*

1. Click the + icon next to the *Subscriber* field (Figure 3-35). Harris CareTracker PM displays the *Add Subscriber* window.
2. In the *Add Subscriber* dialog box, you will select the appropriate *Type, Subscriber,* and *Relationship*. (In your end-of-chapter Case Study 3-1, you will use patient Justin Riley [Emily Riley is his mother] for this activity.)
3. To search for the *Subscriber*, click on the *Search* icon. (**Note:** Only search the database if the subscriber was ever a patient of the practice.) If the subscriber is not found in the database, close the *Search Patients* window and click the + icon in the *Add Subscriber* window. Harris CareTracker PM displays demographic fields for the new subscriber information.
4. Complete the demographic information for the subscriber in the fields provided. You must enter the subscriber's *SSN, DOB, Sex,* and *Insurance* information.

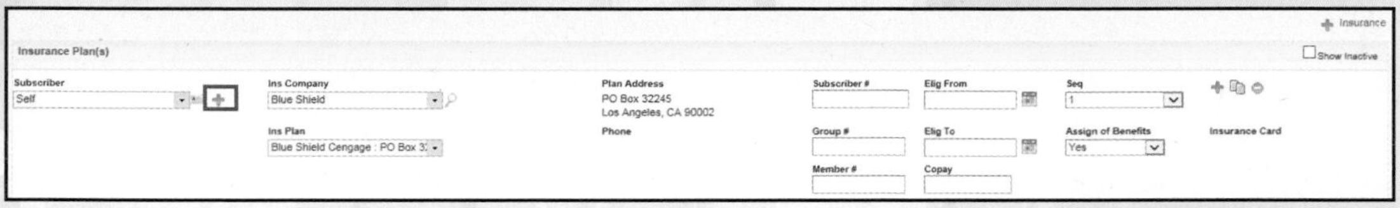

Courtesy of Harris CareTracker PM and EMR

Figure 3-35 Search Icon in the Subscriber Field

b. In the *Ins Company* field, select the subscriber's insurance company from the drop-down list (Figure 3-36). Verify that you have the correct insurance plan by double-checking the address displayed next to the insurance plan name. The insurance plan will populate with the name and address if you select a plan from the drop-down list. If the plan name is not in the list, search the Harris CareTracker PM database.

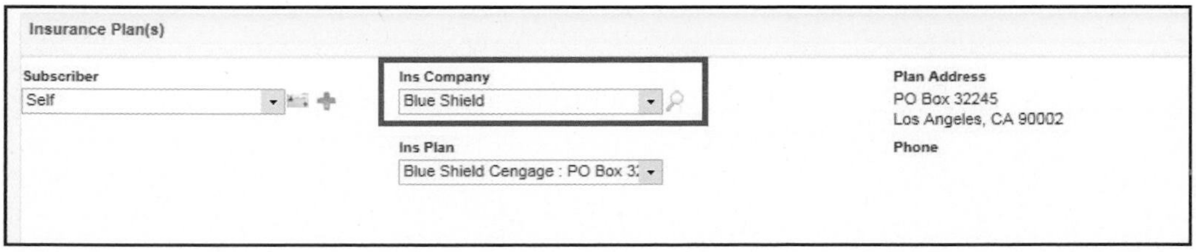

Courtesy of Harris CareTracker PM and EMR

Figure 3-36 Select Subscriber's Insurance Plan

FYI

To Search for an Insurance Plan

1. Click on the *Search* 🔍 icon next to the *Ins Company* field. Harris CareTracker PM displays the *Insurance Plan Search* window.
2. You can search by *Plan* name, *Keyword, Address, Company,* and *State*. However, the easiest search is by PO Box. Enter the plan's PO Box number (including the words "PO Box") in the *Address* box and then click the *Search* button.
3. Click the plan you want to select in the search results. Harris CareTracker PM pulls the plan information into the demographic record.

Tip Box

If the subscriber's insurance plan is not listed in the Harris CareTracker PM database, the medical practice will send a *ToDo* to *Support* requesting that the new plan be added to the database and include the insurance company name, complete address, and telephone number. (This is not a student task/function.) Adding *Pending Insurance* to the patient's record will serve as a temporary placeholder until the actual insurance plan is added to the database.

c. In the *Subscriber #* field, enter the subscriber number listed. The **subscriber number** refers to the insurance policy number.

d. (If applicable) Enter the group number in the *Group #* field. The **group number** typically identifies the employer.

Tip Box

The use of group numbers varies among insurance carriers, so be sure to enter the numbers in accordance with each carrier's numbering policy.

e. (If applicable) Enter the member number in the *Member #* field. (There is no member number for this patient.) The **member number** is typically assigned to individual family members on the policy.

f. In the *Elig From* and *Elig To* fields, enter the subscriber's effective dates of coverage with a particular insurance carrier. Often the date entered in the *Elig From* field will match the patient's employment start date if the patient is covered through that employer. The *Elig To* field remains blank until the patient changes insurance plans. To complete the eligibility fields, you can either enter the dates manually in MM/DD/YYYY format, or you can click the *Calendar* ⊞ icon and select a date.

g. If the subscriber is required to pay a copayment, enter the copayment amount in the *Copay* field. Do not use dollar signs. When charges are entered for the patient, Harris CareTracker PM will automatically calculate and **carve-out** the co-payment amount for private pay (the amount for which the patient is responsible).

Tip Box

The carve-out occurs only if the copay amount is entered in the *Copay* field.

h. The *Sequence* field indicates whether the insurance plan entered for the patient is the **primary** (first in order), **secondary** (second in order), or **tertiary** (third in order) insurance. The number of insurance plans entered on a patient's demographic determines the numbers that display on the *Sequence* list. Select "1" for the primary insurance, select "2" for the secondary insurance, and so on. For example, if the secondary insurance plan saved on a patient's demographic becomes the primary insurance, you would then change the plan's sequence to "1" instead of "2". (Select "1".)

i. Confirm that the patient has signed the Assignment of Benefits/Financial Agreement, and select "Yes" from the *Assignment of Benefits* drop-down menu (other options from the drop-down list are "No" or "Patient Refused"). It is imperative that patients sign the Assignment of Benefits authorization so the practice may bill the insurance company for reimbursement.

PM SPOTLIGHT

Adding Multiple Insurances

- To add additional insurance plans, click the + *Insurance* link in the *Insurance Plan(s)* section of the *Demographic* record. Harris CareTracker PM displays additional insurance fields. Complete the insurance fields and then click *Save*.

Activating and Deactivating Insurances

- If an insurance plan is no longer active, click the *Deactivate* icon next to the plan you want to deactivate. Clicking the *Deactivate* icon will deactivate the insurance plan and highlight it in orange to indicate that the plan has been deactivated. It is important to keep track of deactivated insurance plans because the information can be useful in resolving unbilled or denied claims.

- To reactivate a deactivated insurance plan, click the *Activate* icon next to the insurance plan you want to activate.

Copying an Insurance

- To add a new insurance by copying an existing insurance, click the *Copy Insurance* icon next to the insurance you want to copy (Figure 3-37).

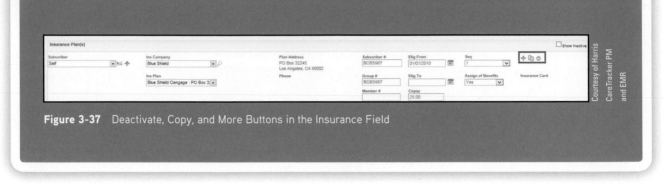

Figure 3-37 Deactivate, Copy, and More Buttons in the Insurance Field

25. The last field in the *Patient Details* tab is where photos are added. This feature is not active in your student environment.

26. Prior to navigating to another tab or application, be sure to scroll down and click *Save* to save your entries.

27. At the top of the *Demographics* screen, click on the *Employer* tab, to the right of the *Patient Details* tab.

28. Click on the *+ New Employer* link on the left side of the screen and complete the fields with information from the patient registration form (Source Document 3-1).

   a. A list of the practice's most common patient employers is available from the *Employer* field drop-down list. Select the appropriate employer choice from the drop-down list. When an employer is selected from the list, the employer's work address information will be populated in the *Address* fields.

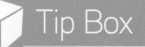

Tip Box

In the *Administration* module, the employer can also be added to your quick pick list if necessary by going to the *Administration* module > *Setup* tab > *Financial* header > *Quick Picks* link (this is not a student task/function).

FYI

To Search for an Employer

1. If the patient's employer is not an option in the *Employer* drop-down list, search Harris CareTracker PM's employer database. This can be done by clicking the *Search* 🔍 icon next to the *Employer* field (Figure 3-38). This will open the *Search Employers* window. If the employer is not listed, you can click the + *New Employer* link and add the employer information.

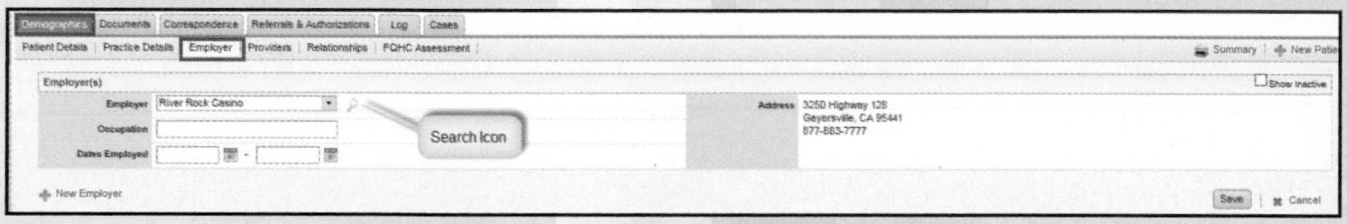

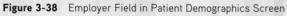

Figure 3-38   Employer Field in Patient Demographics Screen

Courtesy of Harris CareTracker PM and EMR

2. Enter the name of the employer in the *Employer Name* field. In addition, you can narrow the search by entering the employer's city and state. Click on the *Search* button to display a list of the employers that match the information entered.
3. By clicking on the appropriate selection, the employer's name, address, phone number, and fax number are entered into the respective fields.

b. The patient's occupation should be entered in the *Occupation* field, for example, "IT Support."

a. Enter the start and end dates in the *Dates Employed* fields. If the patient is presently an employee, no ending date is entered. A date can be entered into either of the fields manually in MM/DD/YYYY format, or by clicking on the *Calendar* 📅 icon and selecting the appropriate date.

d. Click *Save*.

Tip Box

Harris CareTracker PM and EMR saves the patient and assigns a unique identification number. The newly registered patient is also pulled into context. After completing the new patient registration activity, you may receive a pop-up alert advising you of missing information (Figure 3-39).

(Continues)

(Continued)

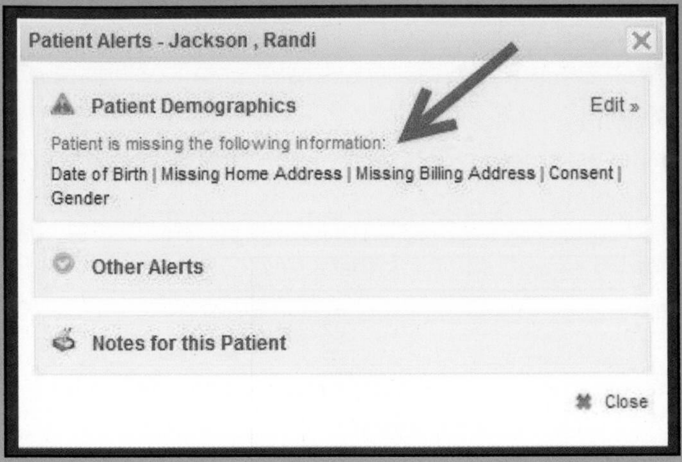

Courtesy of Harris CareTracker PM and EMR

Figure 3-39 Patient Alerts Pop-up Box

29. Click *Edit* and continue the full registration process for any missing information. It is important to know that all fields should be completed, although they are not required. The pop-up will also alert you to missing information such as primary location (should be "Napa Valley Family Associates [NVFA]"), primary language, secondary language, ethnicity, race, organ donor status, and religion. Click *Save* to save any changes.

30. (FYI) There are additional tabs in the *Demographics* application which may or may not be used by the practice.

Print the completed *Patient Details* and *Employer* screens, label them "Activity 3-5," and place them in your assignment folder.

As part of your end-of-chapter Case Studies, you will repeat Activity 3-5 (Register a New Patient) for an additional four new patients.

After a patient's demographic information has been saved, you can click *Edit*, and review the link to scan/attach insurance cards.

Scan/Attach Insurance Card(s)

In the Harris CareTracker PM and EMR *Demographics* application, you can scan and attach a copy of the patient's insurance card to the patient's medical record. Your student version of Harris CareTracker PM does not have scanning capabilities; however, it is important that you understand the workflow and reasoning for scanning/attaching insurance cards. After a scanned insurance card is saved in Harris CareTracker PM and EMR, you can view the image whenever the patient is pulled into context. This is helpful when questions arise regarding the patient's insurance information and eliminates the need to photocopy the insurance card.

Even though a patient's insurance card is scanned and saved in Harris CareTracker PM and EMR, the insurance information must be entered into the insurance fields. A scanner must be attached to your computer to scan documents and images into Harris CareTracker PM and EMR.

FYI

Attach an Insurance Card Scan

1. Pull into context the patient for whom you want to attach a scanned insurance card image. Patient: Emily Riley
2. Click the *Patient* module and then click the *Demographics/Patient Details* tab. Harris CareTracker PM displays the patient's demographic record.
3. Click *Edit*. Harris CareTracker PM displays the page in edit mode.
4. In the *Insurance Plan(s)* section, click the *Add Insurance Card icon* (Figure 3-40). **Note:** You will not be able to scan insurance attachments in your student version of Harris CareTracker.

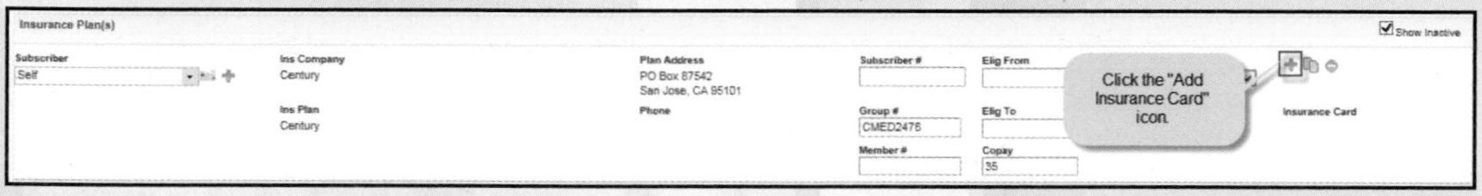

Figure 3-40   Add Insurance Attachment

There are additional features in Harris CareTracker for uploading documents. Although there is no *Document Management* feature in your student version of Harris CareTracker PM, it is best to have an understanding of the functions. Additional information and references to *Document Management* can be found in *Help*. You would access *Documentation Management* under *Doc Management Module > Uploading Documents*.

The steps to attach a photo are similar to attaching documents or insurance cards, but there are slight deviations. Figure 3-41 shows where you would attach a photo in the *Patient Details* tab of the *Demographics* application. This feature is not functional in your student version of Harris CareTracker and you will receive an error message when attempted.

Figure 3-41   Add Picture Link in Patient Details Screen

Print Patient Demographics Report

Medical practices may find it useful to print a patient's demographic report for a variety of reasons. Some practices will give a copy of the printed report to a patient at check-in to verify information and to make any necessary corrections/updates. Following this workflow will help identify inconsistencies between the patient information and information stored in your practice management software.

However, for practices that are trying to stay "paperless," you could use the *At-a-Glance* button for quick verification of demographics, balance due, appointments, and so on. To access *At-a-Glance*, click the *Info* ![icon] icon next to the patient's name to view the patient's demographic information, *Patient Portal* status, primary/secondary insurance information, primary/secondary copayment amounts, previous and pending appointment details, and provider information.

You can generate (print) a *Patient Demographics* report for the patient in context, which includes:

- Some of the detailed demographic information entered in the *Patient Details* tab of the *Patient* module
- The patient's previous four and pending appointments and recalls
- Primary and secondary insurance information
- Provider information

ACTIVITY 3-6: Print the Patient Demographics Summary

1. Pull a patient into context (New Patient #1 – James Smith).

2. Click the *Patient* module. Harris CareTracker PM and EMR displays the *Demographics* tab.

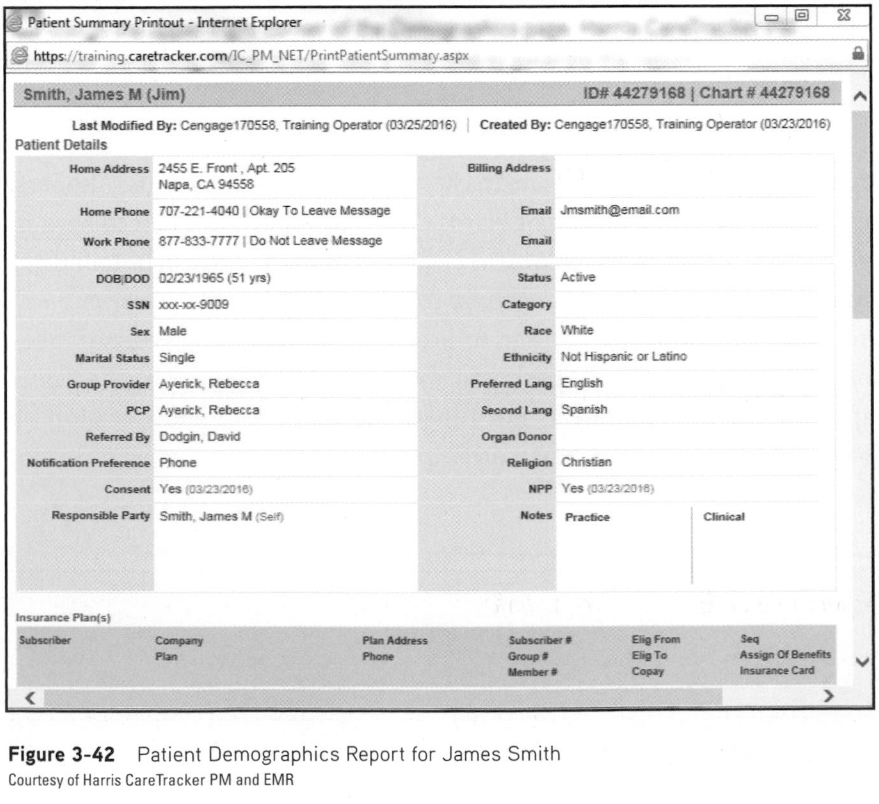

Figure 3-42 Patient Demographics Report for James Smith
Courtesy of Harris CareTracker PM and EMR

3. Click the *Print* icon to the left of the *Summary* link in the upper-right corner of the *Demographics* application. Harris CareTracker PM displays your printing options, along with a *Patient Summary Printout* screen (Figure 3-42). (**Note:** It may take a little time to generate the report.)
4. Choose a printer listed in the *Print* dialog box to print the patient demographics summary (Figure 3-43). (Alternatively you can close the print prompt box and take a screenshot of the report, or right click on the report and select *Print*.)

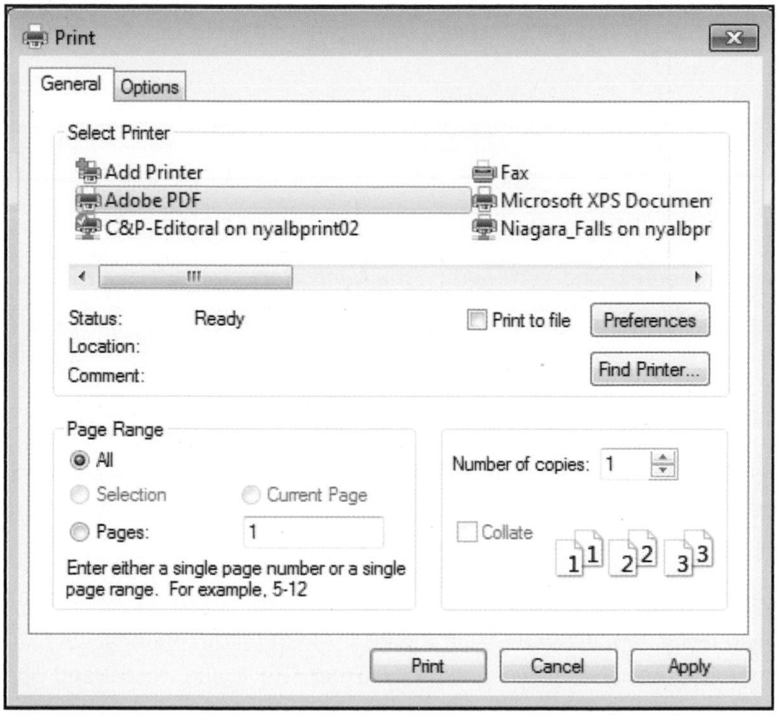

Courtesy of Harris CareTracker PM and EMR

Figure 3-43 Print Prompt Screen

Print the *Patient Demographics* report, label it "Activity 3-6" and place it in your assignment folder.

As part of your end-of-chapter Case Studies, you will print the demographics *Summary* (using the instructions in Activity 3-6) for each new patient you register.

EDIT PATIENT INFORMATION

Learning Objective 5: Edit patient information in Harris CareTracker.

It is important to verify accuracy and update information when a patient schedules an appointment or checks in for an appointment. This makes the treatment process faster and avoids unnecessary complications in billing due to outdated information (Figure 3-44).

Courtesy of Harris CareTracker PM and EMR

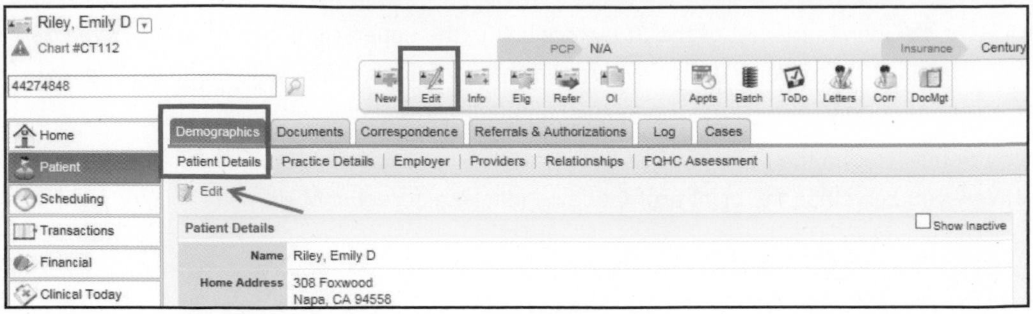

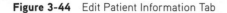

Figure 3-44 Edit Patient Information Tab

ACTIVITY 3-7: Editing Patient Information

1. Pull patient Emily Riley into context and click *Edit* on the *Name Bar*.
2. Harris CareTracker PM displays the *Patient Details* window. Click on the *Employer* tab at the top of the screen.
3. Click the *Edit* link at the top left of the screen.
4. Deactivate Ms. Riley's current employer (Napa State Hospital) by clicking on the *Deactivate Employer* icon. Then, click on the + *New Employer* link at the bottom left of the screen. (**Note:** You may receive a pop-up window asking if you want to leave the page. Click on "Leave this page.")
5. You can select a new employer from the *Employer* drop-down menu. Ms. Riley's current employer, Silverado Resort and Spa in Napa, CA, is not listed in the drop-down menu. Instead, click on the *Search* icon, which will open the *Search Employers* window. Enter "Silverado Resort and Spa" in the *Employer Name* field and click *Search*. Click on the appropriate result. The new employer information, including address, will populate in the *Employer* window.
6. Update the *Employer* window with *Occupation* ("Massage Therapist") and *Dates Employed* (use today's date as the start date, and leave the ending date blank) (see Figure 3-45). (**Note:** If applicable, the work telephone number would be added in the *Patient Details* tab.)
7. Click *Save*.

Print the updated *Demographics/Employer* screen, label it "Activity 3-7," and place it in your assignment folder.

Courtesy of Harris CareTracker PM and EMR

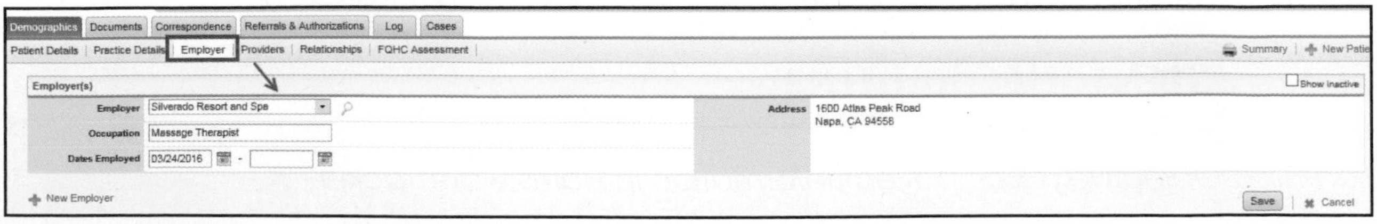

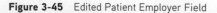

Figure 3-45 Edited Patient Employer Field

ELIGIBILITY CHECKS

Learning Objective 6: View and perform eligibility checks.

The *Eligibility* application enables you to view a history of eligibility checks. It also enables you to electronically check eligibility with the primary insurance as well as the secondary insurance saved in *Patient Demographics*. Harris CareTracker PM and EMR automatically performs eligibility checks every evening for all patients scheduled for appointments for the next five days. Automated batch eligibility checks are performed for a patient once every 30 days regardless of the number of appointments scheduled for the patient during that month. However, it is sometimes necessary to perform individual eligibility checks periodically throughout the treatment and payment cycle or for any walk-in patients. The eligibility check helps to identify potential payer sources, reducing the number of denied claims or bad debt write-offs, and decrease staff hours required for performing manual eligibility checks.

Your student version of Harris CareTracker PM does not have the electronic eligibility feature. To perform the simulated workflow of an eligibility check, you would click the *Elig* button on the dashboard, and then access payer website or call the insurance company to verify eligibility when electronic access is not available (Figure 3-46).

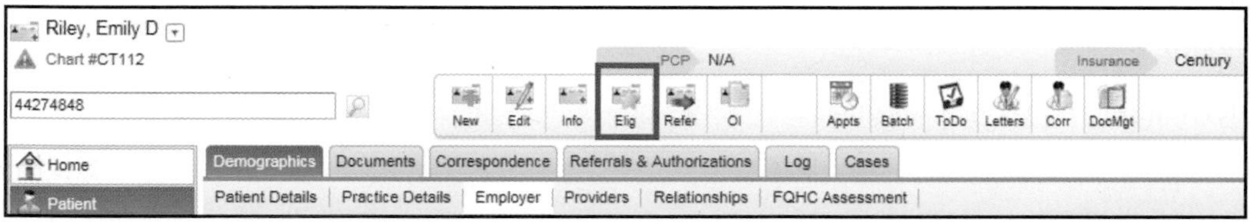

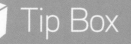

Figure 3-46 Patient Eligibility Icon

PM SP🔵TLIGHT

If a patient's primary insurance is a non-participating payer and your practice has not signed up to check eligibility for the payers, the *Elig* button is disabled, preventing you from performing electronic checks. This feature is not available on your student version of Harris CareTracker PM.

Tip Box

For up-to-date information on participating and non-participating payer information, refer to the Harris CareTracker PM and EMR Eligibility Payer List in the *DOC* link. (This feature is not enabled in your student version of Harris CareTracker PM.)

An eligibility check can result in one of three statuses that include *Eligible, Ineligible,* or *Unknown.* An **unknown status** results when the patient's primary insurance is a **non-participating** (non-par) payer. A non-participating payer is a payer who chooses not to enter into a participating agreement to provide electronic eligibility checks for free. A service fee applies to eligibility checks with non-participating payers.

ACTIVITY 3-8: View and Perform Eligibility Check—Electronic Eligibility Checks

1. Pull patient Emily Riley into context and then click *Elig* on the *Name Bar*. Harris CareTracker PM displays the *Eligibility History* dialog box. In the professional version of Harris CareTracker, this box would contain a list of eligibility checks performed for the patient and additional details about the most recent eligibility check. In your student version of Harris CareTracker, you will receive a message stating "No Eligibility History available for this patient."

2. In a live environment, you would click the *Check Eligibility* button in the top right corner to check eligibility. For this activity, you will have to manually simulate checking for patient eligibility. To do this, click the *+ Add Notes* icon to the left of the *Check Eligibility* button. This will open the *Manual Eligibility* box.

3. Enter information into the *Manual Eligibility* box as shown in Figure 3-47A.

   a. *Status:* Select "Eligible."

   b. *Verification:* Enter today's date.

   c. *Mark Reviewed:* Select "No."

   d. *Note:* Enter "Patient is eligible."

   e. Click *Save.*

4. The manual eligibility check will now show in the *Eligibility History* window (Figure 3-47B).

Courtesy of Harris CareTracker PM and EMR

Chapter 4
Appointment Scheduling

Key Terms

batch
chief complaint (CC)
copayment
history of present
  illness (HPI)
multi-resource
  appointment

nonverbal
  communication
recall
receipt
resource
TeleVox®
verbal communication

Learning Objectives

1. Book, reschedule, and cancel appointments.
2. Schedule non-patient appointments.
3. Add a patient to the Wait List.
4. Perform activities managing the daily schedule.
5. Check in patients.
6. Create a batch, accept payments, print patient receipts, run a journal, and post the batch.

Certification Connection

1. Utilize EMR and practice management (PM) systems.
2. Describe scheduling guidelines; recognize office policies and protocols for scheduling appointments; manage appointment schedules using established priorities.
3. Schedule patient appointments; collect updated patient information to record in the EHR.
4. Post payments and copayments to patient accounts at the time of visit; generate a receipt.
5. Operate office machines and devices such as scanners, fax machine, signature pads, and cameras integrated with EHR software.
6. Acquire external patient data (labs, radiology reports, patient visit summaries, and more); edit the patient medical record in the EHR within your scope of practice.
7. Communicate in language the patient can understand; demonstrate effective and courteous telephone techniques; apply electronic technology to maintain effective communication.
8. Coordinate office workflows regarding patient flow such as scheduling, patient registration and verification, patient referrals, and more.
9. Access, edit, and store patient information in the EHR database.
10. Identify the impact of HIPAA for the medical assistant; adhere to rules pertaining to the confidentiality and release of PHI.

Adapted from national standards of the National Healthcareer Association (NHA), Commission on Accreditation and Allied Health Education Program (CAAHEP), and Accrediting Bureau of Health Education Schools (ABHES)

INTRODUCTION

All appointment information is entered and saved in the *Scheduling* module. The *Book* application is where you schedule, reschedule, and cancel both patient and non-patient appointments (e.g., meetings). To find future appointment availability, you can set specific appointment search criteria, for example, provider, location, and day of the week. Conveniently, the *Book* application is set up so that through a patient's scheduled appointment, you can access several other applications and functions in Harris CareTracker PM and EMR. This makes it possible to edit patient demographics, print encounter forms, save visits, and enter patient **copayments** without having to navigate away from the *Book* application.

Appointment history is tracked in Harris CareTracker PM and EMR. Any time an appointment is rescheduled or canceled, the information is saved in the *Scheduling* module. A reason for rescheduling or canceling the appointment must be entered and will always be linked to the appointment. All previous, rescheduled, and canceled appointments can be accessed in the *History* application. In addition, scheduled, rescheduled, and canceled appointments can also be linked to **recalls**. Recalls are reminders to patients that an appointment needs to be booked.

There are a few different ways to view appointments in the *Scheduling* module besides the *Book* application. The *Month* and *Calendar* applications allow you to view all patient scheduled appointments in a calendar, bar chart, or date book format. When a patient is in context, all upcoming appointments for any family member linked to that patient can be viewed in the *Family* application. The list includes the patient's upcoming appointments as well.

Within the *Scheduling* module there are eight applications: *Book*, *Month*, *Calendar*, *Family*, *Advanced*, *Recalls*, *History*, and **TeleVox®**, outlined in Table 4-1. *TeleVox®* is an optional application of an automated appointment reminder and confirmation system that can be used to notify patients of upcoming appointments.

TABLE 4-1 Application Summaries

	Description
Book	In this application you will schedule, reschedule, and cancel patient appointments. You can access several other applications and functions within Harris CareTracker PM and EMR through the mini-menu that displays when you click on a patient's appointment.
Month	At a glance, this application displays the number of appointments scheduled for each day of a particular month. You can choose the month, the resource, and the location for which to view a month calendar. In this application you can also view a month's appointments in bar chart format instead of a calendar view. **Resources** can be people, places, or things. Providers are always considered a resource, but an exam room or a piece of equipment can also be considered a resource. Something that requires a schedule is considered a resource because it has specific availability with days and times it can provide certain services. If the resource does not need a set schedule, then it is not considered a "resource" in Harris CareTracker PM and EMR.
Calendar	This application allows you to view appointments in a small date book calendar.
Family	You can view all upcoming appointments for any family members linked to the patient in context and the patient's upcoming appointments are listed in this application as well.
Recalls	An appointment recall for the patient in context is entered in this application and any pending recalls for the patient are listed in this application as well.

TABLE 4-1	(Continued)
History	This application shows all pending, previous, canceled, and rescheduled appointments for the patient in context. Canceling a patient's upcoming appointments should be completed from this application as well.
Advanced	This application enables you to book and reschedule appointments in accordance with predetermined parameters and criteria established by your practice. The *Advanced* method of booking appointments prevents overbooking and scheduling conflicts and also maintains consistency in terms of the days and times that different services and procedures are provided. The patient's existing appointments, pending recalls, and referrals are listed in this application as well.
TeleVox®	This is an automated appointment reminder and confirmation system that can be used to notify patients of upcoming appointments. Two major steps are involved in the *TeleVox®* interface: sending an electronic appointment list and viewing the results of the automated calls made by *TeleVox®*. This is an optional feature of Harris CareTracker PM and EMR.

Courtesy of Harris CareTracker PM and EMR

BOOK APPOINTMENTS

Learning Objective 1: Book, reschedule, and cancel appointments.

Building upon activities in Chapter 3, you will now learn how to book (schedule) appointments. The most common method of initiating an appointment booking is when the patient calls on the phone. At times you will also book appointments while the patient is in the office (commonly when booking a follow-up appointment). You must demonstrate excellent communication skills, both verbal and nonverbal. **Verbal communication** is the use of language or actual words spoken. **Nonverbal communication** consists of body language, gestures, eye contact, and expressions to communicate a message. Because most patient appointments are made over the phone, it is important that medical assistants develop positive telecommunication skills. The patient's impression of the practice will be strongly influenced by the medical assistant's phone etiquette.

PM SP⬤TLIGHT

Examples of proper phone etiquette:

- Answer promptly (within three rings when possible).
- Speak clearly into the phone (and do not forget to smile).
- Identify the medical practice and yourself.
- If you must place a caller on hold, ask permission first, and thank the caller.
- If the wait time is going to be long, it is often better to ask the patient if you can return the call rather than keep the patient on hold. Do not forget to return calls as you promised. Always get the best number (and an alternate) and the best time to call, especially if a manager or another team member must return the call.
- Never interrupt the patient while he/she is talking to you.
- Never engage in an argument with a caller or allow an angry or aggressive caller to upset you. Remain calm and composed, and ask for your supervisor's assistance if necessary.

(Continues)

(Continued)

- Maintain privacy. Do not handle an unhappy caller's concern openly at the check-in/check-out desk.
- Be patient, and do not give the impression that you are rushed or unconcerned. Learn how to handle several callers simultaneously with ease and grace.
- Always make collection calls in private and away from the patient flow or public areas.
- Make sure that the caller, or the person called, hangs up first.

Booking appointments in Harris CareTracker PM and EMR takes place in the *Book* application of the *Scheduling* module. Both patient and non-patient appointments (e.g., meetings) are booked in this application. You must have a patient in context in the *Name Bar* to book a patient appointment. Three methods are used to book appointments (Figure 4-1):

1. Schedule directly in *Book*: This allows you to book patient and non-patient appointments by manually moving the schedule to a specific day and clicking on a specific time. You can use the *Book* filters to view the schedule for a specific time, day, location, and provider. Scheduling appointments directly from *Book* gives you the advantage of seeing appointment times that can be double-booked.
2. Using *Find*: This allows you to search for the next available appointment time based on specific appointment criteria you set. When searching appointment availability, you can filter your search by provider, location, appointment type, date, day, and time.
3. Using *Force*: This allows you to double-book appointments and to book an appointment during a different appointment-type time slot. Forced appointments appear outlined in blue on the schedule.

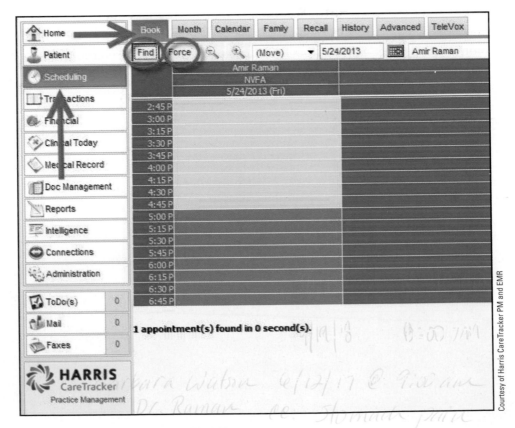

Figure 4-1   Screenshot of Book, Find, Force

Harris CareTracker offers the versatility of customizing appointment types. In your student version, the physician and practice schedules have been built in Harris CareTracker PM and EMR so that only certain appointment types can be scheduled during certain times, at certain locations, or for certain providers. Further customization of *Appointment Types* for your practice is done in the *Setup* tab of the *Administration* module. The schedule can also be customized by color coding appointment types. For example, you can assign a color to help quickly identify new patient visits on the schedule. The color is applied to the border of the appointment in the *Book* application. The color assigned to an appointment type overrides the default border colors used to identify appointment conflicts (brown/pink) and forced appointments (blue).

When booking an appointment there is an option to either select a **chief complaint (CC)** from a list of favorites or manually enter a complaint in a free text field. A chief complaint is the patient's reasons for being seen for the visit in the patient's own words. You can only use one of the fields to enter a chief complaint. The chief complaint is displayed on the schedule and carried over to the progress note for the visit associated with the appointment in certain templates.

If the chief complaint is linked to a progress note template, Harris CareTracker PM and EMR will automatically apply the associated progress note template and select the chief complaint that is linked to the appointment. If the complaint is entered manually this text will appear on the schedule in brackets [[ ]] and for a limited amount of templates, the text can be pulled into the CC/HPI (Chief Complaint/**History of Present Illness**) text box (Figure 4-2).

You can create a list of favorite complaints for your group in the *Chief Complaint Maintenance* application in the *Administration* module. HPI is the patient's account of related symptoms for today's visit. The HPI is generated with the use of problem-focused templates, voice dictation, or handwriting and voice recognition (Figure 4-2).

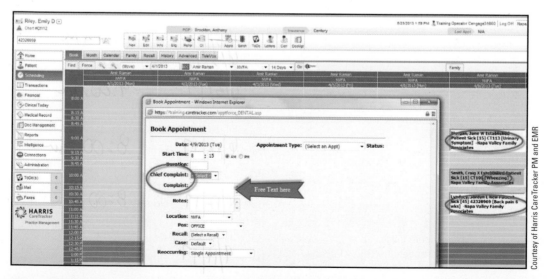

Figure 4-2   Chief Complaint

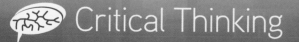

Critical Thinking

Identify when and why documenting a chief complaint would be critical in your role as a medical assistant and the importance of accuracy.

Using established patients in your database as well as building upon your previously registered new patients (from Chapter 3), schedule an appointment for each of the patients in Table 4-2 using *Book*.

> ⚠️ **Alert**
>
> You will need to schedule appointments for Activities 4-1 through 4-8 approximately one week in the future because certain features will not work on "past dates"; that is, you cannot reschedule an appointment on a day that has already passed. Scheduling patient appointments approximately one to two weeks in the future should give you enough time to complete all of the activities in this chapter. Avoid booking too far in advance because that would affect future patient visit and billing activities. For example, if today's date is May 15, it would be best to book your appointments sometime between May 22 and May 29.
>
> **Note:** In order to make ICD-10 diagnosis code selections in later activities, all patient appointments must be scheduled for after January 1, 2016.

TABLE 4-2 Patient Appointments to Be Scheduled

Patient Name / Provider	Complaint	Type of Appointment: Record Date/Time Selected
Jane Morgan / Dr. Raman	Urinary symptoms	1st available next week/Est. Pt. Sick Date: ~~5/1~~ 6/5/17 Time: 9:30 AM
Ellen Ristino / Dr. Brockton	Sore throat and nasal congestion	1st available next week/Est. Pt. Sick Date: 6/5/17 Time: 9:00 AM
Craig X. Smith / Dr. Raman	Wheezing	1st available next week/Est. Pt. Sick Date: 6/12/17 Time: 8:00 am
Adam Thompson / Dr. Brockton	Productive cough	1st available next week/Est. Pt. Sick Date: 6/12/17 Time: 8:00 am
James Smith / Dr. Ayerick	Three-month follow-up exam/consultation; review lab and EKG	Book three months from today/Follow-up Date: 9/11/17 Time: 9 am
Sonia Ramirez / Dr. Ayerick	Annual comprehensive physical exam (CPE)	Book out one year, plus one day/Est. Pt. CPE Date: 9/12/18 Time: 8:45 am
Jordyn Lyndsey / Dr. Raman	Back pain, six weeks, discuss possible MRI and referral to orthopedist	1st available next week/New Pt. Sick Date: 9/19/18 Time: 8:00 am

Barbara Watson 6/12/17 @ 9:00 am
Dr. Raman   cc: Stomach pain

ACTIVITY 4-1:   Book an Appointment

1. Using patient data in Table 4-2, schedule an appointment for each patient.

2. Pull the patient for whom you are booking an appointment into context on the *Name Bar*.

3. Click the *Scheduling* module. Harris CareTracker PM and EMR opens the *Book* application by default.

4. Display the desired date using one of the following options:

   a. Select an option from the *Move* list to display the schedule for specific time increments such as Next Day, Next Week, 2 Months, and so on.

   b. Manually enter a date in MM/DD/YYYY format or click the *Calendar* ⊞ icon to display the schedule for a specific date.

5. Select the provider, location, and the number of days to display, and then click *Go* (Figure 4-3).

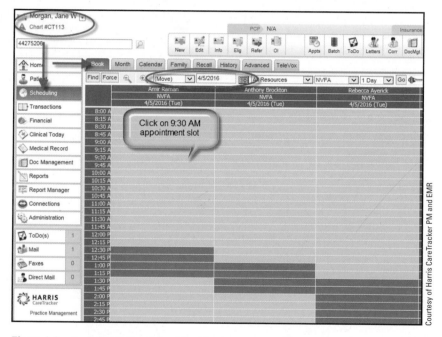

Figure 4-3   Book Appointment for Jane Morgan

6. Click on the *time slot* for which you are booking the appointment. (If the schedule is displayed for multiple providers and locations, be sure to click the *time slot* in the appropriate column.) The application displays the *Book Appointment* window.

▢ Tip Box

If the patient has existing appointments scheduled, the application displays the *Existing Appointments* window. Click *Book Appointment* at the bottom of the window to book a new appointment.

7. From the *Appointment Type* list, select the appointment type. When you select an appointment type, Harris CareTracker PM and EMR automatically populates the *Task* and *Duration* fields (Figure 4-4).

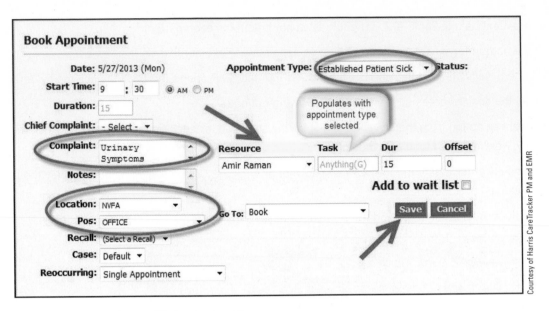

Figure 4-4   Book Appointment Window for Jane Morgan

8. From the *Resource* list, select the resource (i.e., provider) needed for the appointment.

9. There are two options for entering a *Chief Complaint* (you can only use one):

a. From the *Chief Complaint* list, select a chief complaint from the drop-down list. This list is populated with the favorite complaints selected in the *Chief Complaint Maintenance* application in the *Administration* module. (This is not available in your student version. You will use the "free text" option.)

b. Free text the chief complaint (as noted in Table 4-2) in the *Complaint* box (see Figure 4-2). (The application will display the complaint in brackets [[ ]] next to the patient's name on the schedule.)

PM SP⬤TLIGHT

If *Chief Complaints* have not been set up for your groups, this list is disabled. If the chief complaint is linked to a progress note template, Harris CareTracker PM and EMR will automatically apply the associated progress note template and select the chief complaint that is linked to the appointment. If the complaint is entered manually, this text will be pulled into the CC/HPI text box in certain templates.

10. In the *Notes* box, enter any notes about the appointment (there are no notes associated with the patients in Table 4-2). (Notes appear in parentheses next to the patient's name on the schedule and also appear when you move your mouse over the appointment on the schedule.)

Tip Box

Do not use any symbols when entering appointment notes or patient complaints. Using symbols will cause an error when you try to print encounter forms.

11. From the *Location* list, select "NVFA".

12. From the *Pos* (Place of Service) list, select "OFFICE".

13. (Optional): To link the appointment to an open recall for the patient, select the recall from the *Recall* list. (Do not link an appointment in this activity.)

FYI

If you want to link the patient's appointment to a specific case, you would select the case from the *Case* list. This feature is not available in your student version.

14. Click *Save*. The application schedules the appointment (Figure 4-5).

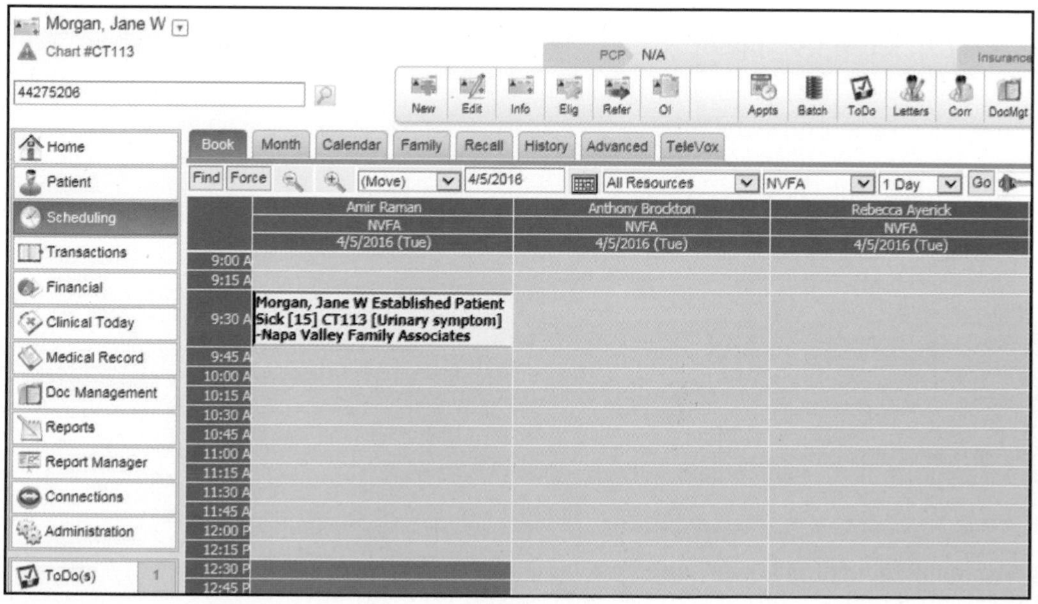

Figure 4-5   Scheduled Appointment for Jane Morgan

Courtesy of Harris CareTracker PM and EMR

Print the Schedule/Booking screen for each patient scheduled (from Table 4-2), label them "Activity 4-1," and place them in your assignment folder.

Booking an Appointment Using Find

Often when scheduling an appointment, you will need to find the next available open time slot for that particular encounter (e.g., CPE, same day/urgent, procedure, follow-up). The *Find* feature allows you to search for the next available appointment time based on specific appointment criteria you set. When searching appointment availability, you can filter your search by provider, location, appointment type, date, day, and time.

Tip Box

When using *Find*, Harris CareTracker PM and EMR will search for appointments from the current day forward.

Building upon your previous scheduling practice (see Activity 4-1), schedule an appointment on the most appropriate date for the following patient using the *Find* button (Table 4-3). Record the date and time of the appointment scheduled for future reference.

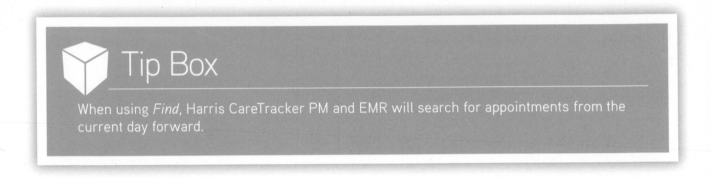

TABLE 4-3 Patient Appointment to Be Scheduled Using *Find*		
Patient Name *Provider*	**Chief Complaint**	**Type of Appointment: Record Date/Time Selected**
Barbara Watson *Dr. Raman*	Fever – 103F	Find 1st available/Est. Pt. Sick Date/Time: _____

Copyright © 2015 Cengage Learning®.

ACTIVITY 4-2: Book an Appointment Using the Find Button

1. Pull patient Barbara Watson into context.

2. Click the *Scheduling* module. Harris CareTracker PM displays the *Book* application.

3. Click the *Find* button in the top left corner of the *Book* application. Harris CareTracker PM displays the *Appointment Criteria* window (Figure 4-6).

4. Select the parameters of the appointment, including *Provider* (Raman), *Location* (NVFA), *Appointment* type (Established Patient Sick), date, day, and time (any 15-minute appointment the next day).

Tip Box

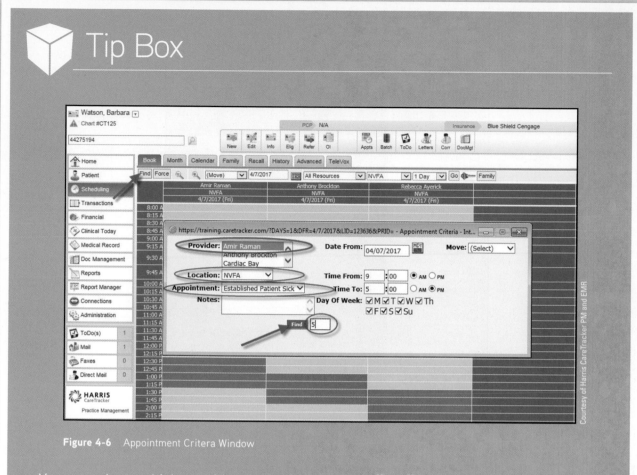

Figure 4-6   Appointment Critera Window

You can select multiple providers by holding down the [[Ctrl]] key on your keyboard while clicking on each provider name.

5. *Find* will default to display the first 20 appointments that match the search criteria. Change the number to "5" and click *Find* (Figure 4-6).

6. To select an available appointment, click in the *Appointment/Task Class* column or anywhere on the row that corresponds to the desired date and time for that particular appointment. Harris CareTracker PM re-displays the *Book* application for the selected appointment date, highlighting the selected time in red (Figure 4-7).

7. Click the selected time slot. The application displays the *Book Appointment* window.

8. Select the *Appointment Type* (Established Patient Sick). When you select an *Appointment Type*, the application automatically populates the *Resource, Task,* and *Duration* fields.

9. Enter the *Complaint* by entering the free text description (Fever 103F).

10. From the *Location* list, select the location "NVFA".

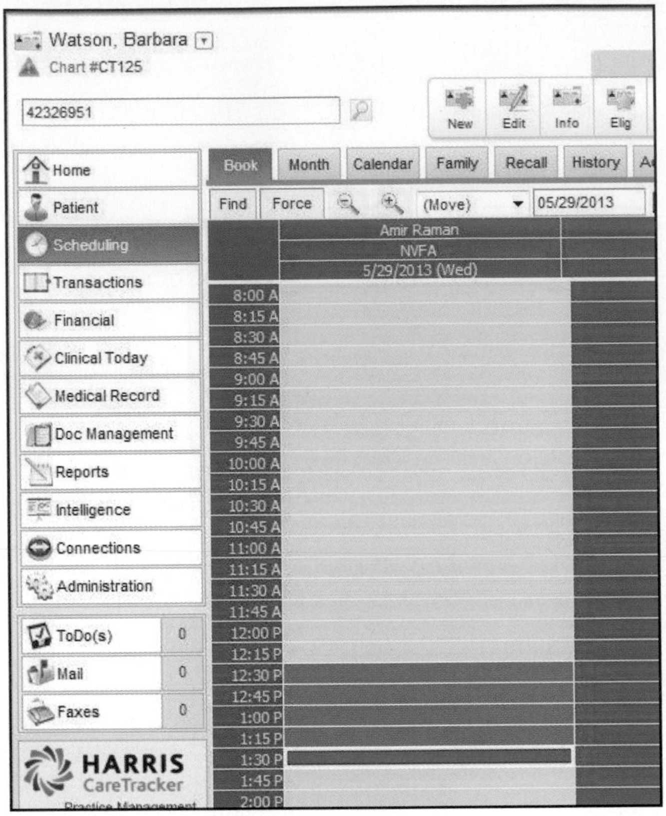

Courtesy of Harris CareTracker PM and EMR

Figure 4-7 Find Appointment-Red Highlight

11. From the *Pos* list, select the place of service (OFFICE).

12. Click *Save*. The application schedules the appointment (Figure 4-8).

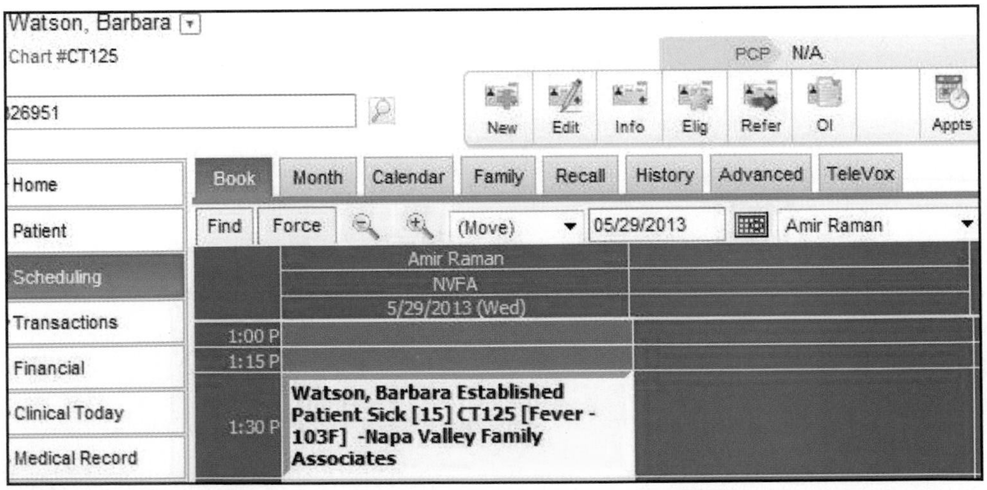

Courtesy of Harris CareTracker PM and EMR

Figure 4-8 Scheduled Appointment for Barbara Watson

Print the Booked Appointment screen, label it " Activity 4-2," and place it in your assignment folder.

Forcing an Appointment

Using *Force* allows you to double-book appointments and to book an appointment during a different appointment-type time slot. You can also double-book appointments by left-clicking on the appointment time slot from the drop-down mini-menu. *Forced* appointments appear outlined in blue on the schedule. Using the patient in Table 4-4, force an appointment at the same time slot as the previous patient in Activity 4-2, Barbara Watson.

TABLE 4-4 Patient Appointment to Be Scheduled Using *Force*		
Patient Name *Provider*	**Chief Complaint**	**Type of Appointment: Record Date/Time Selected**
Thomas Barret *Dr. Raman*	Fell – swollen wrist	Find 1st available/Est. Pt. Sick Date/Time: _____

ACTIVITY 4-3:   Book an Appointment Using the Force Button

1. Pull patient Thomas Barret into context.

2. Click the *Scheduling* module. Harris CareTracker PM displays the *Book* application.

3. Click the *Force* button in the top left corner of the *Book* application. Harris CareTracker PM displays the *Book Appointment* window.

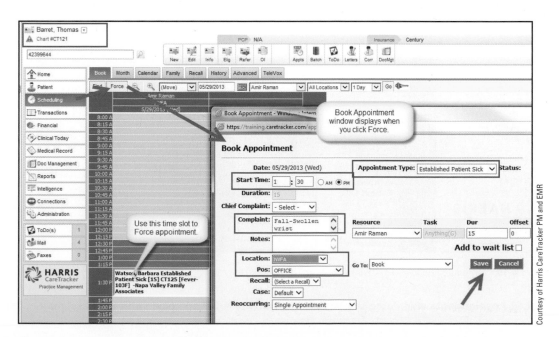

Figure 4-9   Force Appointment for Thomas Barret

4. From the *Appointment Type* list, select the appointment type "Established Patient Sick". When you select an appointment type, Harris CareTracker PM automatically populates the *Task* and *Duration* fields (Figure 4-9).

5. From the *Resource* list, select the resource needed for the appointment (Dr. Raman).

6. In the *Start Time* field, enter the start time for the appointment. (Use the same date and time as for the patient booked in Activity 4-2, Barbara Watson.)

7. Enter *Complaint* by entering free text (Fall – swollen wrist).

8. From the *Location* list, select "NVFA".

9. From the *Pos* list, select "OFFICE".

10. Do not link the appointment to an open recall for the patient.

11. Do not link the patient's appointment to a specific case.

12. Do not select reocurring appointment.

13. Click *Save*. The application schedules the appointment (Figure 4-10).

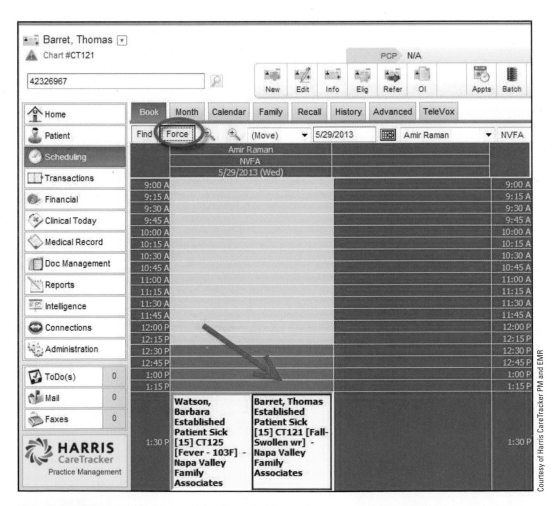

Figure 4-10 Scheduled Appointment Using Force for Thomas Barret

Print the Booked Appointment using Force screen, label it "Activity 4-3," and place it in your assignment folder.

Reschedule Appointments

There are two ways to reschedule patient appointments in the *Book* application: either directly from the schedule or by using the *Find* button. In either instance, the patient needs to be in context so the existing appointments will display. Harris CareTracker PM and EMR saves the rescheduled appointment in the *History* application in the *Scheduling* module.

ACTIVITY 4-4: Reschedule Appointments

Reschedule an appointment to the following day:

1. Pull into context the patient for whom you are rescheduling an appointment. (Use Jane Morgan from Activity 4-1.)
2. Click the *Scheduling* module. The application displays the *Book* application by default.
3. *Move* the schedule to display the date, provider, and location for the new appointment (Figure 4-11). (From the date of Jane's current appointment, *Move* to "Next Day", same provider, same location.)

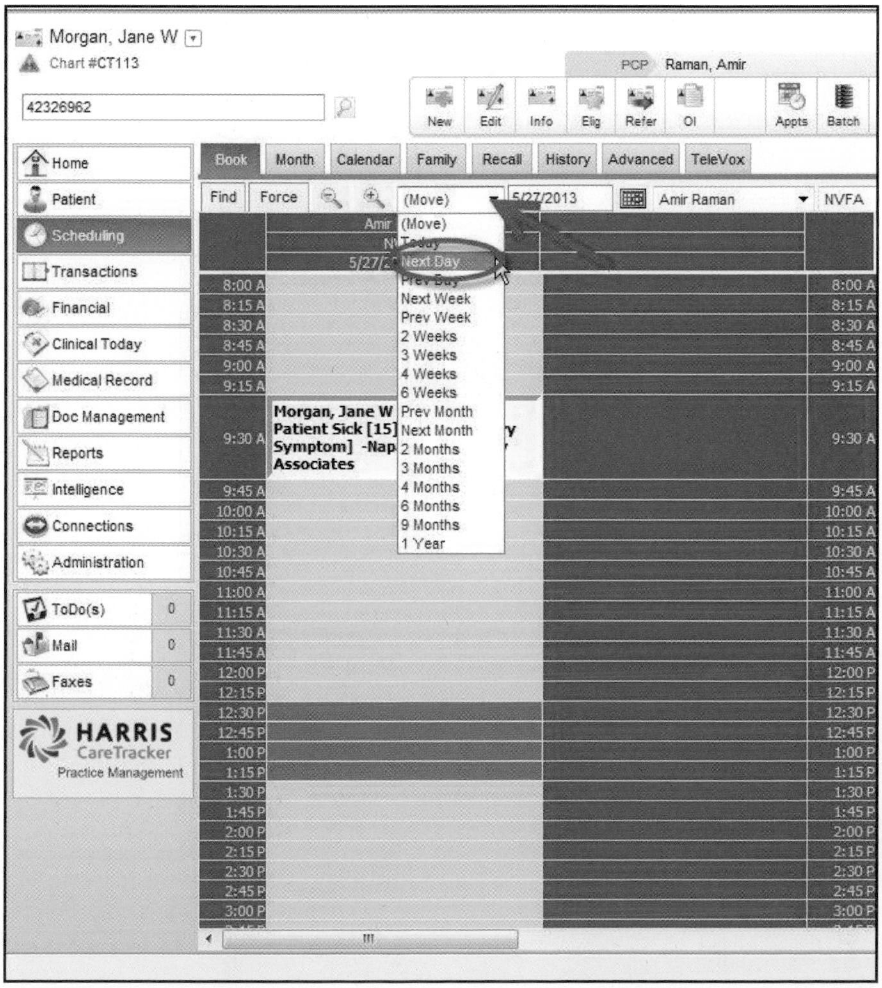

Courtesy of Harris CareTracker PM and EMR

Figure 4-11 Reschedule Appointment for Jane Morgan

4. Click on the time slot in which you want to reschedule the appointment (same time slot as previous appointment). The application displays the patient's existing appointment(s) (Figure 4-12). (**Note:** You cannot reschedule an appointment that has an encounter created or that has already passed.)

5. From the *Action* list, select "Reschedule" and then click *Go*. The application displays the *Reschedule Appointment* window.

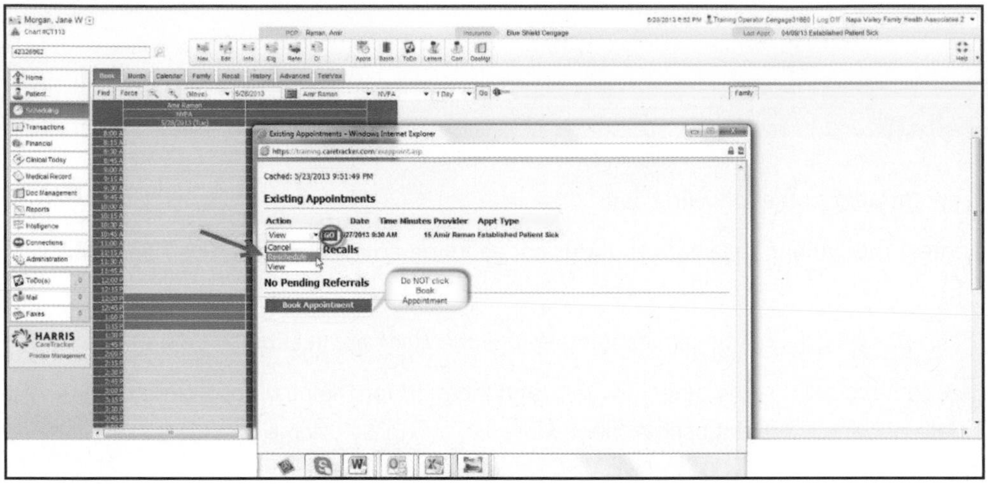

Courtesy of Harris CareTracker PM and EMR

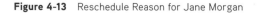

Figure 4-12 Existing Appointments Window

Tip Box

Do not click the *Book Appointment* button. If you do, you will book an additional appointment instead of rescheduling the existing appointment.

6. From the *Reschedule* list, select a reason for rescheduling the appointment (Figure 4-13). (Select "Entry Error.")

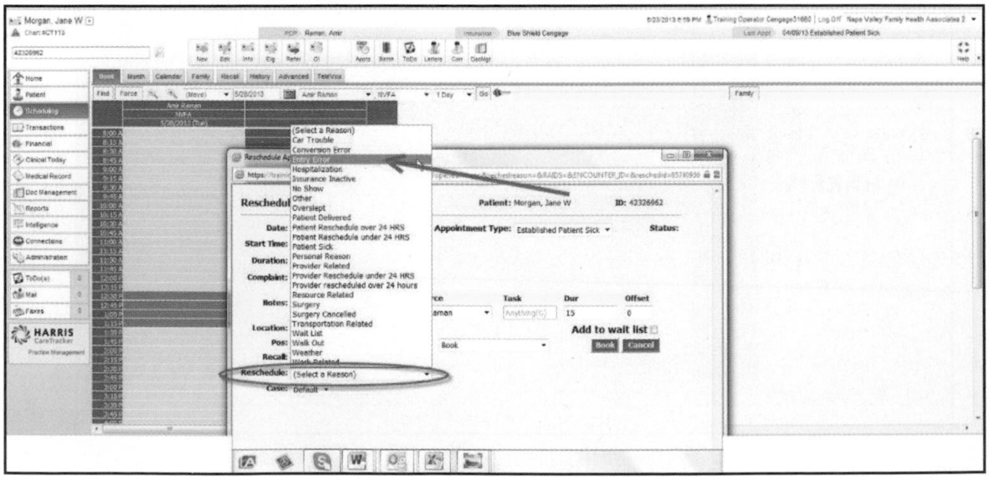

Courtesy of Harris CareTracker PM and EMR

Figure 4-13 Reschedule Reason for Jane Morgan

Print the Rescheduled Appointment screen, label it "Activity 4-4," and place it in your assignment folder.

7. Click *Book*. The application cancels the original appointment and adds the rescheduled appointment to the calendar. Record the rescheduled appointment date/time in Table 4-2.

As mentioned, the *Find* button can also be used to reschedule an appointment.

ACTIVITY 4-5: Reschedule Appointments Using the Find Button

Using the same patient you rescheduled in Activity 4-4 (Jane Morgan), reschedule the appointment to the next available day using the *Find* button.

1. Pull patient Jane Morgan into context.

2. Click the *Scheduling* module. Harris CareTracker PM displays the *Book* application by default.

3. Click *Find* in the top left corner of the *Book* application. Harris CareTracker PM displays the *Appointment Criteria* window. Select the search parameters for the appointment you want to find. Select the same provider, location, date, time, and appointment type as the patient's original appointment (from Activity 4-1).

4. Click *Find* (Figure 4-14). Harris CareTracker PM displays the *Search Results* window containing the first 20 appointments that match the search criteria.

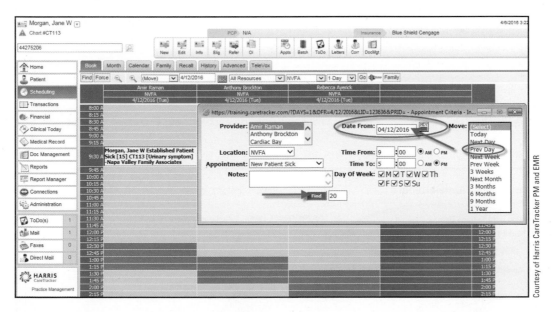

Figure 4-14   Reschedule Appointment for Jane Morgan Using Find

5. Click on an appointment in the *Appointment/Task Class* column to select it. (Select the same time slot as previous appointment.) The application displays the selected appointment in the *Book* application.

6. A red bar on the schedule marks the available appointment time you selected from the *Search Results* list. Click on the red bar in the selected time slot. Harris CareTracker PM displays the patient's existing appointment(s) (Figure 4-15).

7. From the *Action list* select "Reschedule" and then click *Go*. The application displays the *Reschedule Appointment* window.

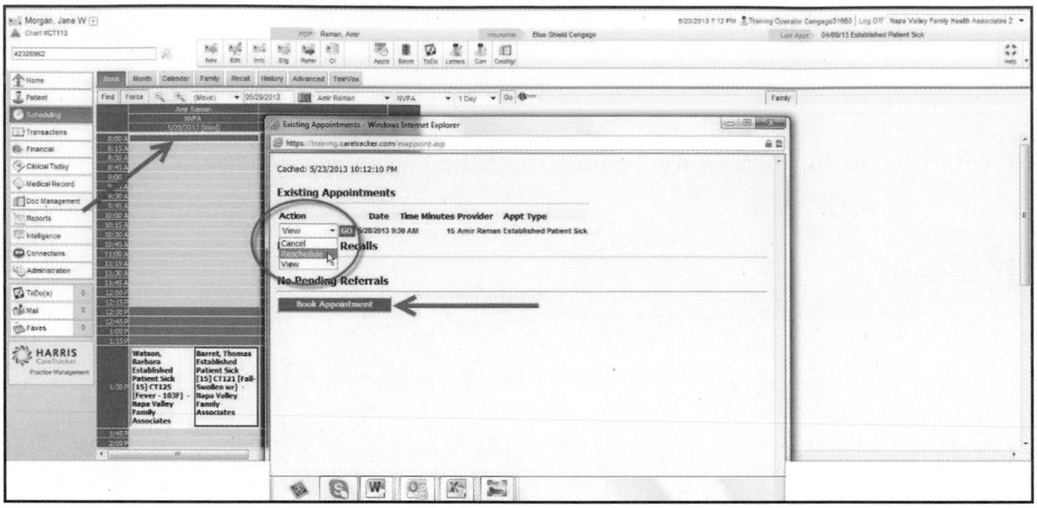

Courtesy of Harris CareTracker PM and EMR

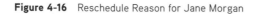

Figure 4-15 Existing Appointments Window for Jane Morgan

Tip Box

Do not click the *Book Appointment* button. If you do, you will book an additional appointment instead of rescheduling the existing appointment.

8. From the *Reschedule* list, select a reason for rescheduling the appointment (Figure 4-16). (Select "Entry Error.")

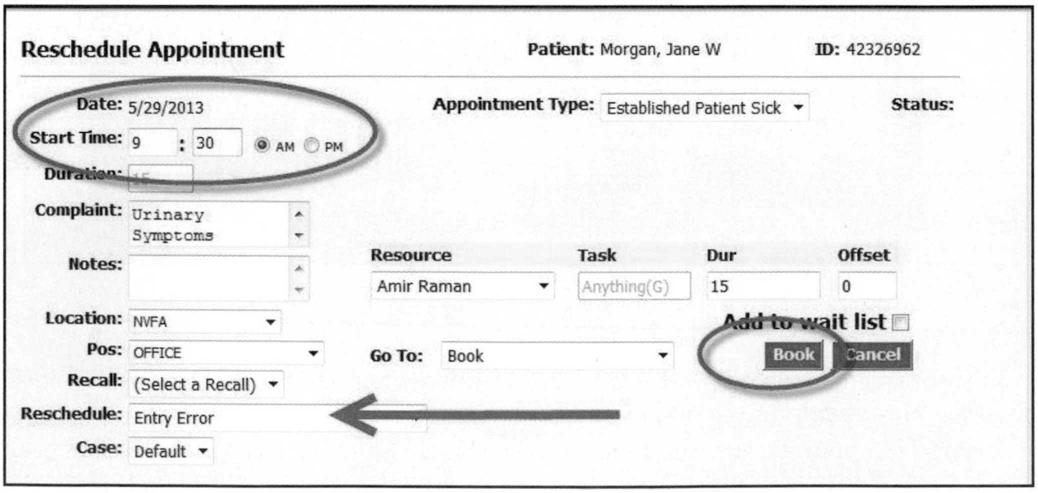

Courtesy of Harris CareTracker PM and EMR

Figure 4-16 Reschedule Reason for Jane Morgan

Print the Rescheduled Appointment screen, label it "Activity 4-5," and place it in your assignment folder.

9. Click *Book*. Harris CareTracker PM cancels the original appointment and adds the rescheduled appointment to the calendar (Figure 4-17). Record the rescheduled date/time in Table 4-3.

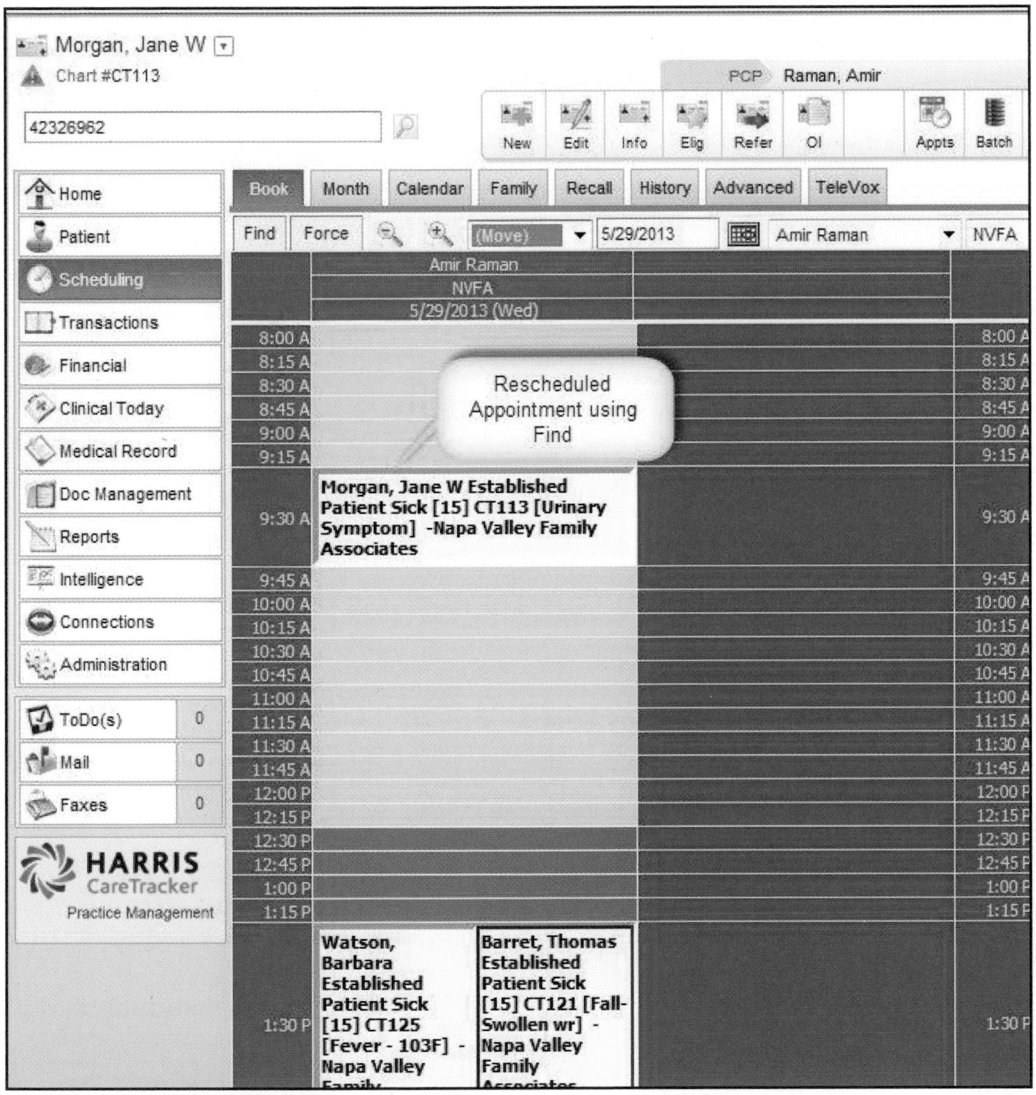

Figure 4-17 Rescheduled Appointment for Jane Morgan Using Find

Cancel Appointments

Upcoming appointments are canceled in the *History* application. You can click on the appointment you wish to cancel and select *View Appointment*, and then cancel it from the *Appointment Detail* window that appears. If the patient's canceled appointment was attached to a recall, the recall will become active again once the appointment is canceled. You can also click on the appointment you wish to cancel and select *View Appointment*, and then cancel it from the *Appointment Detail Window* that appears.

ACTIVITY 4-6: Cancel Appointments

Using the appointment you scheduled for Thomas Barret in Activity 4-3, cancel the appointment in the *History* application.

1. Pull the patient for whom you are canceling an appointment into context (Thomas Barret).
2. Click the *Scheduling* module and then click the *History* tab (Figure 4-18).

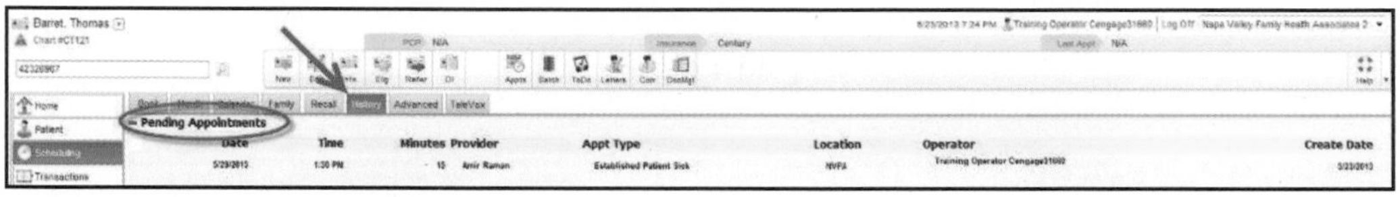

Figure 4-18 History Tab in Scheduling Module
Courtesy of Harris CareTracker PM and EMR

3. Under the *Pending Appointments* heading, click on the appointment you want to cancel (the appointment scheduled in Activity 4-3). Harris CareTracker PM displays the *Appointment Detail* window (Figure 4-19).
4. (Optional) Enter a note regarding the canceled appointment in the *Notes* box. (Free text note: "Patient went to Urgent Care.")
5. Click the *Cancel Appointment* button.

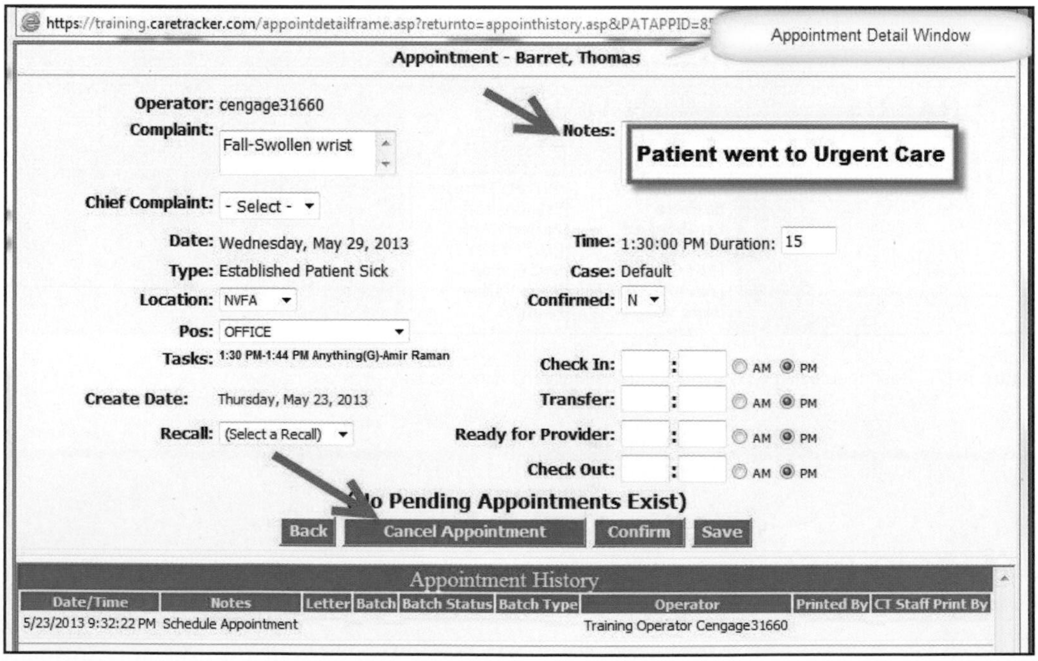

Figure 4-19 Appointment Detail Window

Courtesy of Harris CareTracker PM and EMR

6. From the *Cancel Reason* list, select the reason for canceling the appointment (Figure 4-20). (Select "Hospitalization.")

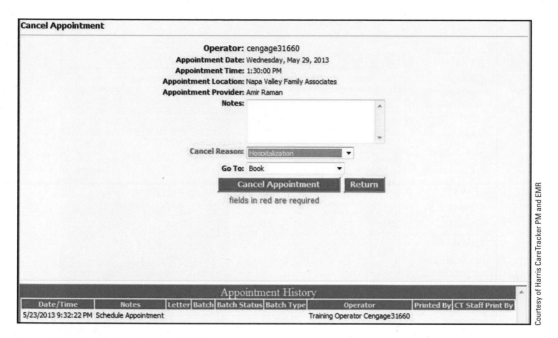

Figure 4-20   Cancel Appointment Window

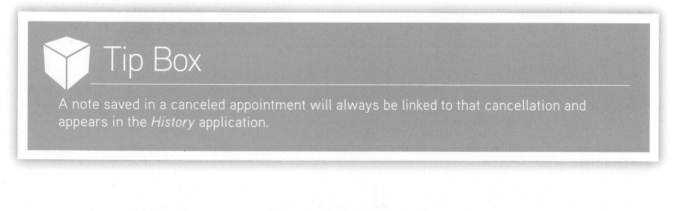

Tip Box

A note saved in a canceled appointment will always be linked to that cancellation and appears in the *History* application.

7. (For recurring appointments only) In the *Cancel Remaining Visits* field:

   a. Select *No* (default) to cancel one appointment in the series.

   b. Select *Yes* to cancel all of the recurring appointments in the series.

8. The *Go To* field defaults to "(Select)." From the drop-down menu you can select an application so that when the appointment is canceled, Harris CareTracker PM opens that application. (Select "Book.")

Print the Canceled Appointment screen, label it "Activity 4-6," and place it in your assignment folder.

9. Click *Cancel Appointment.* Harris CareTracker PM cancels the appointment and removes it from the schedule (Figure 4-21).

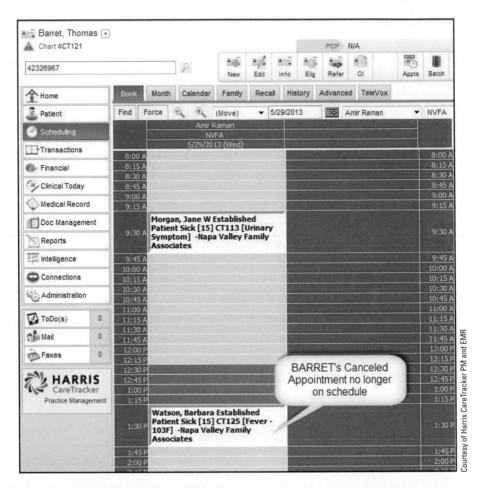

Figure 4-21 Canceled Appointment for Thomas Barret

PM SP⬤TLIGHT

A password may be required to cancel same-day appointments or appointments prior to the current day. The password is not a widely used feature; you will not create a password in your student version of Harris CareTracker.

Appointment Conflicts

Other reasons to cancel or reschedule an appointment occur when there is an appointment conflict. Appointment conflicts occur if an appointment is forced or booked into an unavailable time slot, booked at a location where the provider is not scheduled, or if the provider changes his or her schedule. Appointments remain in conflict until they are canceled or rescheduled. The steps to cancel an appointment due to conflict are slightly different than a cancellation by a patient.

FYI

1. Click the *Home* module and then click the *Dashboard* tab. Harris CareTracker PM displays the *Practice* dashboard tab by default.
2. Click *Appointment Conflicts* in the *Front Office* section of the *Dashboard*, under the *Appointments* header (Figure 4-22). Harris CareTracker PM displays the *Appointments List*.

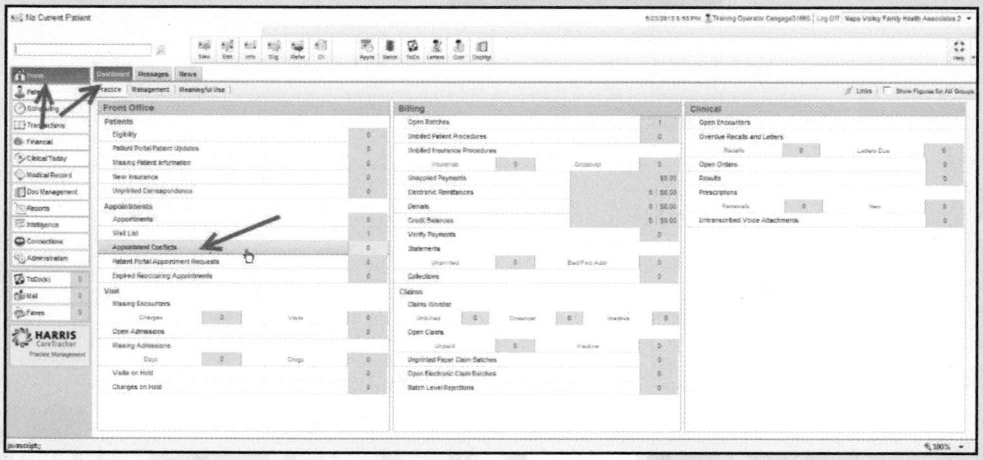

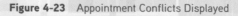

Figure 4-22 Appointment Conflicts Link

Courtesy of Harris CareTracker PM and EMR

3. By default, Harris CareTracker PM displays any appointment availability conflicts for all providers at every location with scheduled appointments for the next 30 days. If needed, you can use the filters to select a specific conflict type, time period, provider, or location, and then click *Go*. Harris CareTracker PM displays a list of conflicted appointments (Figure 4-23). (**Note:** You may have to scroll down the page to view conflicts because they may appear on the lower portion of the screen.)

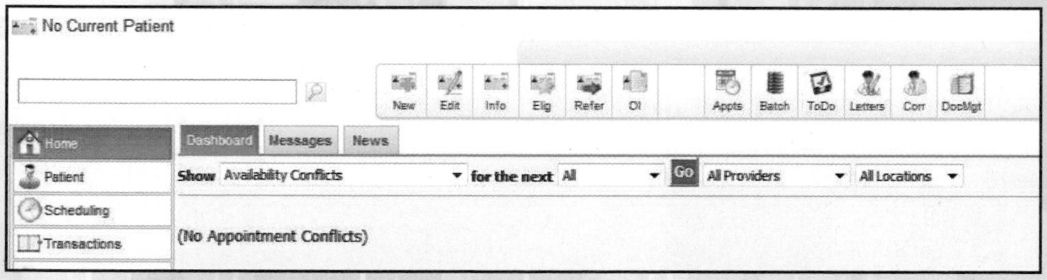

Figure 4-23 Appointment Conflicts Displayed

Courtesy of Harris CareTracker PM and EMR

4. Click the *Cancel* link in the *Action* column for the appointment you want to cancel. Harris CareTracker PM displays the *Cancel Appointment* screen.
5. (Optional) Enter a note regarding the canceled appointment in the *Notes* box. A note saved in a canceled appointment will always be linked to that cancellation and appears in the *History* application.
6. From the *Cancel Reason* list, select the reason for canceling the appointment.

(Continues)

(Continued)

7. (For recurring appointments only) In the *Cancel Remaining Visits* field:
   a. Select *No* (default) to cancel one appointment in the series.
   b. Select *Yes* to cancel all of the recurring appointments in the series.
8. The *Go To* field defaults to *Book*, which means that when the appointment is canceled, Harris CareTracker PM and EMR opens the *Book* application. You can select a different application if desired.
9. Click *Cancel Appointment*. Harris CareTracker PM and EMR cancels the appointment and removes it from the schedule.

NON-PATIENT APPOINTMENTS

Learning Objective 2: Schedule non-patient appointments.

Non-patient appointments, such as meetings or out-of-office times (i.e., provider vacation or training), are scheduled in the *Book* application of the *Scheduling* module. You can book a non-patient appointment with or without a patient in context on the *Name Bar*. A non-patient appointment can be scheduled for multiple providers at one time. However, you cannot search non-patient appointment availability using the *Find* button or the *Advanced* application.

ACTIVITY 4-7:   Booking a Non-Patient Appointment with No Patient in Context

1. Select "None" from the *Name* list on the *Name Bar* so that there is no patient in context (Figure 4-24).

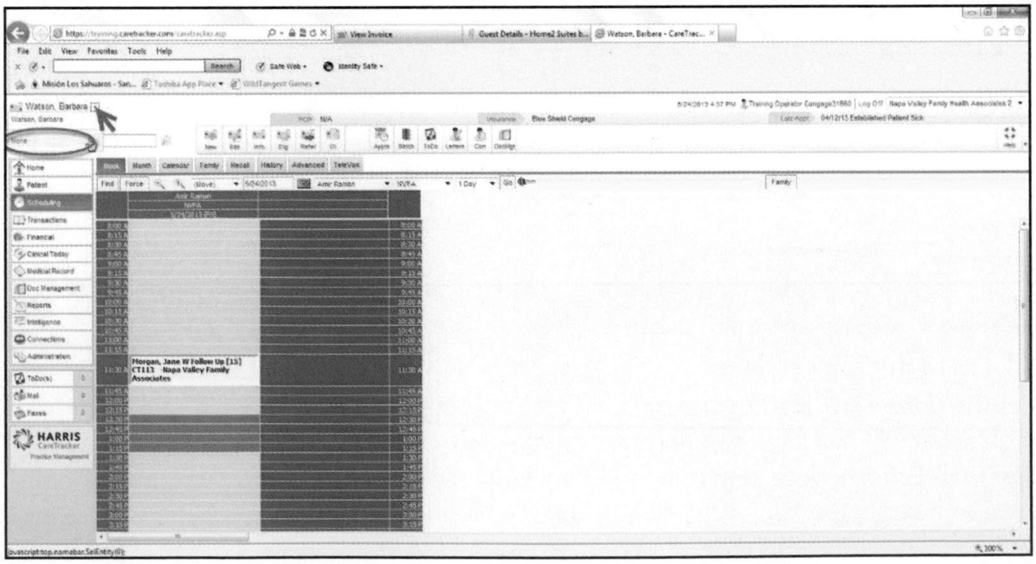

Courtesy of Harris CareTracker PM and EMR

Figure 4-24   No Patient in Context

2. Click the *Scheduling* module. Harris CareTracker PM opens the *Book* application by default.

3. Display the desired date using one of the following options:

   a. Select an option from the *Move* list to display the schedule for specific time increments such as Next Day, Next Week, 2 Months, and so on. (Select "Next Month" [Figure 4-25])

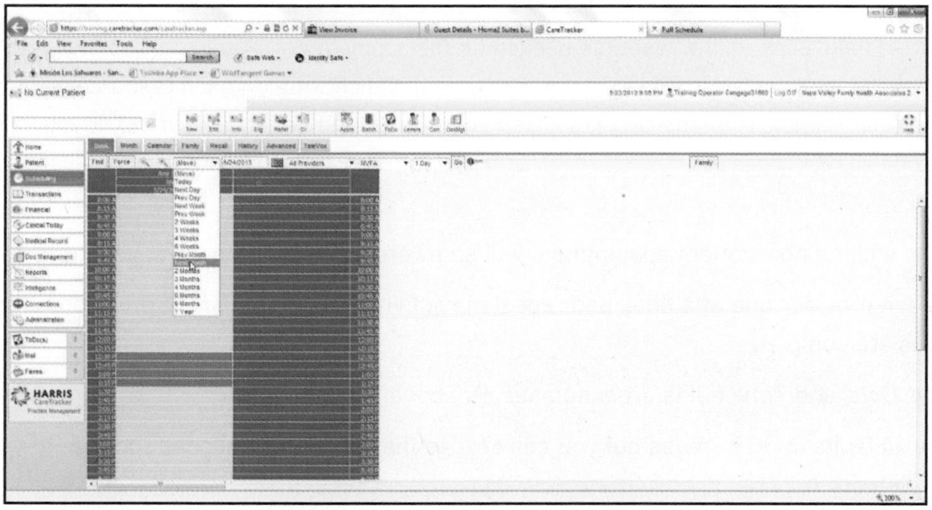

Figure 4-25   Move Schedule to Next Month

   b. Manually enter a date in MM/DD/YYYY format or click the *Calendar* icon to display the schedule for a specific date.

4. Select the resources (All Resources), location (All Locations), and the number of days (1 Day) to display and then click *Go* (Figure 4-26).

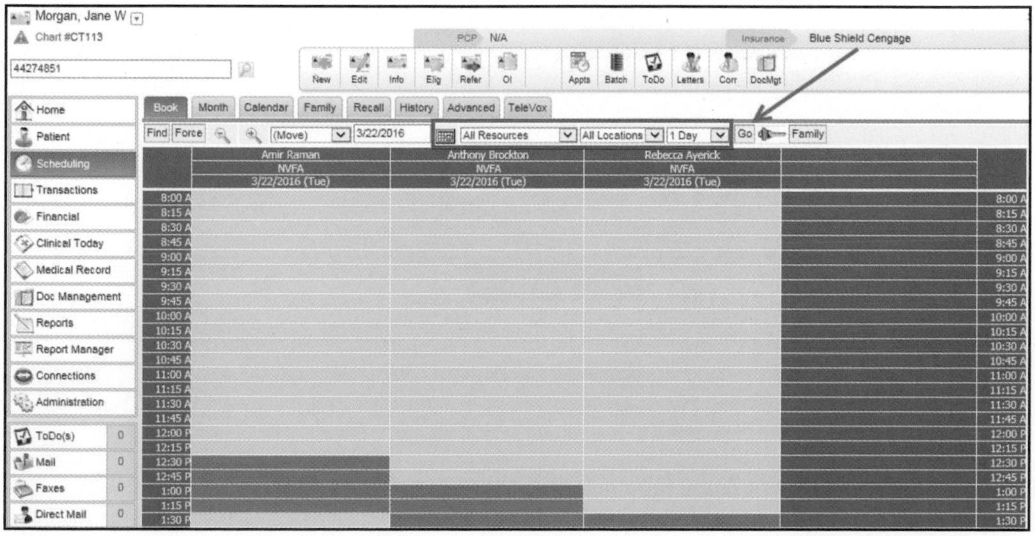

Figure 4-26   Set Schedule for Non-Patient Appointment

5. Click on the time slot in any provider's schedule for which you are booking the appointment (1:00 PM). Harris CareTracker PM displays the *Non-Patient Appointment* window (Figure 4-27).
6. In the *Description* field, enter a brief description of the appointment. (Monthly Providers Meeting)
7. In the *Notes* field, enter any additional information about the appointment. (Guest Speaker, Cardiology Group)
8. In the *Resources* field, click on the resource needed for the appointment. You can select multiple resources by holding down the [Ctrl] key on your keyboard and clicking on each resource (select all providers: Amir Raman, Anthony Brockton, Gabriella Torres, and Rebecca Ayerick). If you select *All* you will include all resources such as lab, cardiac bay, and so on. If you cannot select only the providers, you can:
   a. Select *All* and the non-patient appointment will show on each schedule, or
   b. Select each provider one at a time, and repeat the activity for the remaining providers until all schedules are complete.
9. The *Location, Date,* and *Time* fields are automatically populated.
10. The *Duration* defaults to 30 minutes but you can change the duration as needed (change to 60 minutes) (Figure 4-27).

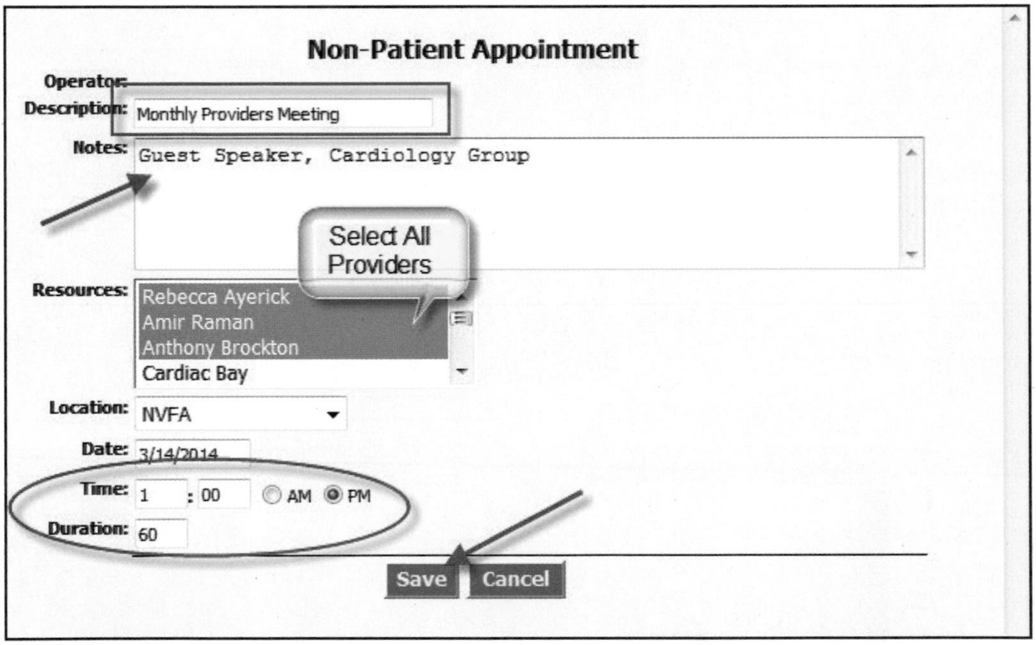

Courtesy of Harris CareTracker PM and EMR

Figure 4-27 Non-Patient Appointment Window

11. Click *Save*. The application schedules the appointment for all of the selected resources.

Print the Book screen with the Non-Patient appointment scheduled, label it "Activity 4-7," and place it in your assignment folder.

ADD PATIENT TO THE WAIT LIST

Learning Objective 3: Add a patient to the Wait List.

Patients who would like an appointment with a provider sooner than their currently scheduled appointment can be added to the *Wait List* in Harris CareTracker PM and EMR. A patient must have a currently scheduled appointment in Harris CareTracker PM and EMR to be added to the *Wait List*.

When adding a patient to the *Wait List*, you must provide information about the appointment the patient needs, such as the appointment type, provider, and location. Harris CareTracker PM and EMR will only flag available appointments that match the appointment criteria selected for the patient.

There are several places you can add a patient to the *Wait List* in Harris CareTracker PM and EMR:

- From the scheduling mini-menu in the *Book* application (see Figure 4-32 and Activity 4-8)
- From the *Book Appointment* window in the *Book* application (Figure 4-28)
- From the *Actions* menu in the *Appointment List* (Figure 4-29)
- From the *Appointments* tab in *Clinical Today* (Figure 4-30)

The *Wait List* is managed in the *Wait List* application accessed from the *Wait List* link under the *Appointment* section of the *Dashboard* (Figure 4-31). The *Wait List* identifies any patient on the *Wait List* and any available appointments that match the appointment criteria. From the *Wait List*, you can reschedule a patient's appointment or remove the patient from the *Wait List* after his or her scheduled appointment date has passed.

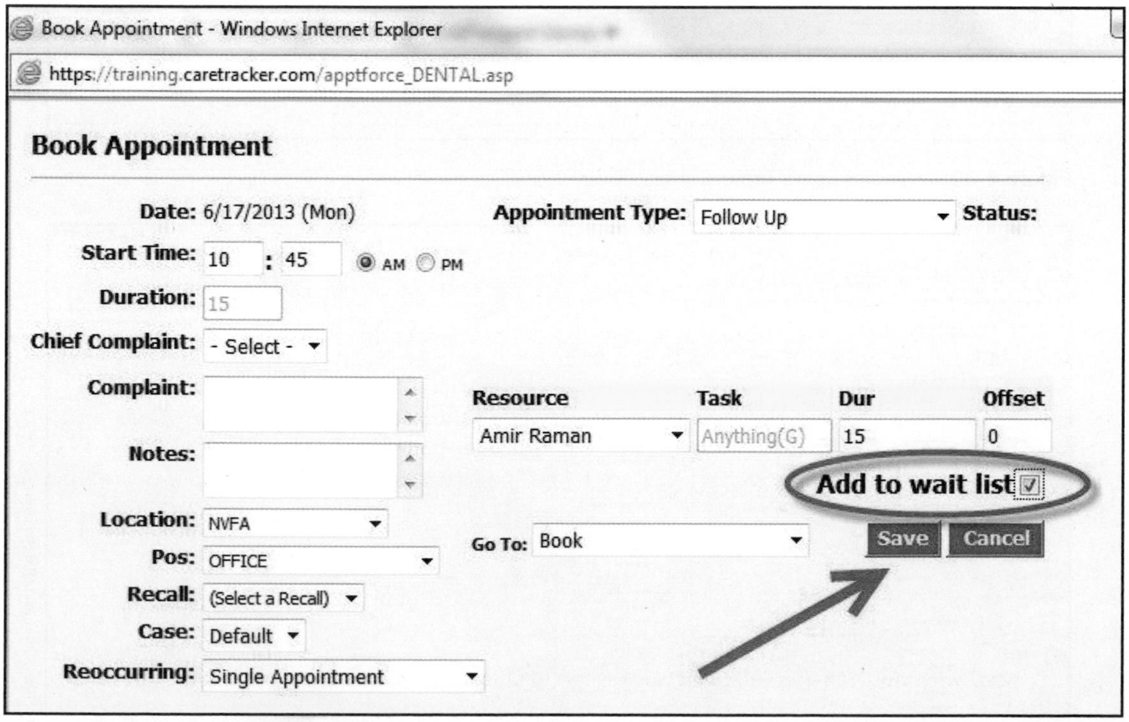

Courtesy of Harris CareTracker PM and EMR

Figure 4-28 Book Appointment Window - Add to Wait List

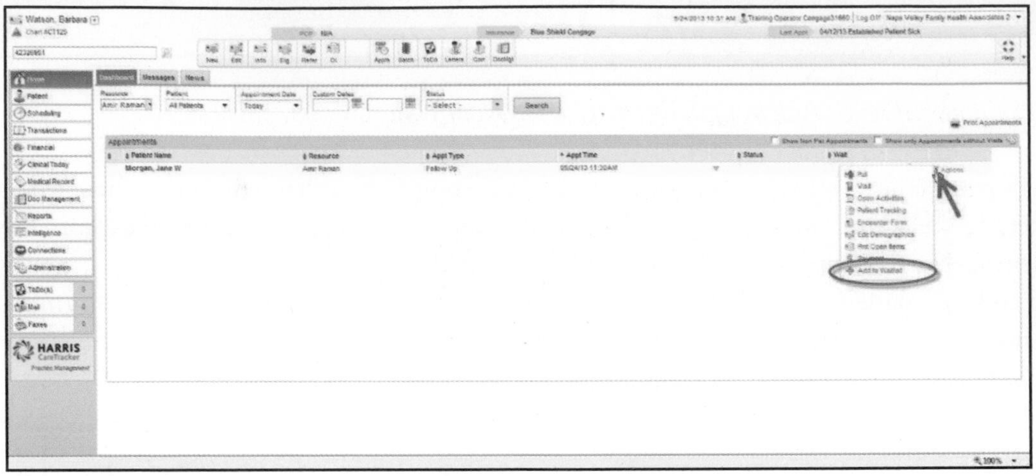

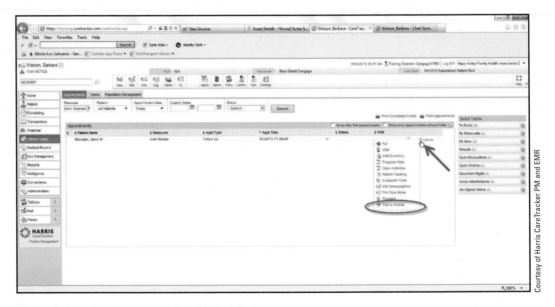

Figure 4-29 Appointments Actions Drop-Down

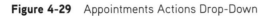

Figure 4-30 Appointments Tab in Clinical Today

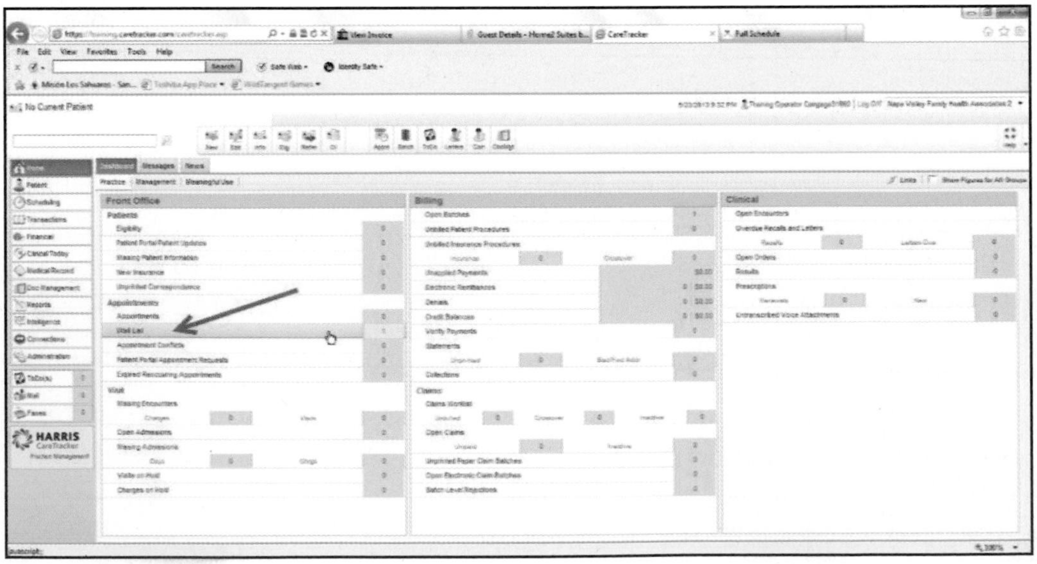

Figure 4-31 Wait List Link

Mini-Menu

When you left-click on a patient's name in the schedule, Harris CareTracker PM displays a convenient mini-menu (Figure 4-32) that contains a list of shortcuts. From this menu you can access several applications in Harris CareTracker PM and EMR that help create a more efficient workflow.

After you left-click on a patient's name, the mini-menu displays on the screen for only 8 seconds. If the mini-menu disappears before you make your selection, left-click on the patient's name again.

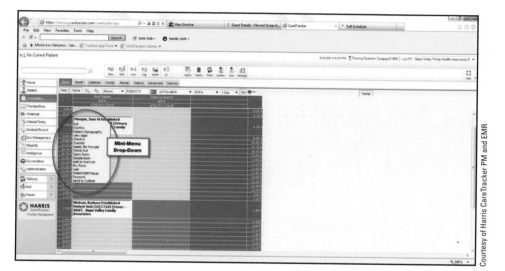

Figure 4-32 Scheduling Mini-Menu

Courtesy of Harris CareTracker PM and EMR

Tip Box

In the *Scheduling* module, *VIP* patient appointments are visible to all operators, but an operator cannot use the scheduling mini-menu for a *VIP* patient unless the operator's profile contains either the "VIP Patient Access" or the "VIP Patient Access Break Glass" override.

ACTIVITY 4-8: Add Patient to the Wait List from the Mini-Menu

1. Click the *Scheduling* module. Harris CareTracker PM displays the *Book* application by default.

2. *Move* the schedule to display the appointment for the patient you want to add to the wait list (select the appointment you created for Adam Thompson in Activity 4-1). This can be done by manually entering the date in the *Date* box by clicking the *Calendar* ▦ icon, or by selecting a time period from the *Move* list. (**Note:** If the appointment scheduled has already passed, you will need to first enter a new appointment for the patient scheduled out one week from today.)

3. Left-click on the appointment and select *Add to Wait List* from the mini-menu. The application displays the *Appointment Wait List* window (Figure 4-33).

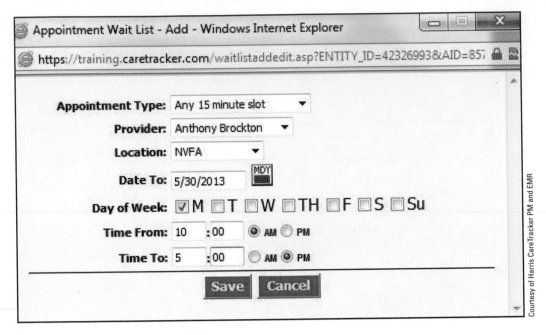

Figure 4-33   Appointment Wait List Window

4. From the *Appointment Type* list, select the type of appointment the patient needs or select "Any 15 minute slot" to book the first available appointment type. (Select "Any 15 minute slot.")

5. From the *Provider* list, select the provider the patient wants to see (Anthony Brockton). You would select "Any Provider" to book the first available provider.

6. From the *Location* list, select the location where the patient wants to be seen. (Select "NVFA.")

7. In the *Date To* field, click the *Calendar* icon and select the last date before which the appointment must fall (select the day the original appointment was scheduled for patient Adam Thompson in Activity 4-1, or the day of the rescheduled appointment if the original appointment has passed).

8. In the *Day of Week* field, select the checkbox next to each day the patient is available for an appointment (select "Monday" only, unchecking the other days).

9. In the *Time From* and *Time To* fields, select the desired time for the appointment. (Select "10:00 AM" through "5:00 PM.")

10. Click *Save*. The application adds the patient to the *Wait List*. (The *Wait List* is managed from the *Wait List* link in the *Front Office* section of the *Dashboard*, under *Appointments*.)

11. Return to the *Dashboard* and click on the *Wait List* link (see Figure 4-31).

12. Select *Resource* (Anthony Brockton).

13. Review the *Date From* and *Date To* displayed. If they are within the range you wish to wait list the appointment, click *Go*.

14. The wait-listed appointment will appear with a *Possible Match* (Figure 4-34).

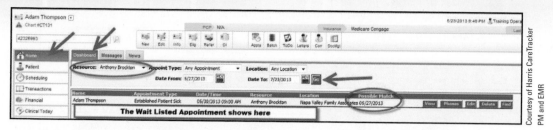

Figure 4-34   Wait List Dashboard Display

Print the Patient Wait List screen, label it "Activity 4-8," and place it in your assignment folder.

DAILY SCHEDULE

Learning Objective 4: Perform activities managing the daily schedule.

Now that you have completed the *Book* activities, you can further manage the daily schedule using the other seven applications in the *Scheduling* module: *Month, Calendar, Family, Recall, History, Advanced,* and *TeleVox®.*

Month Application

The *Month* application displays at a glance the number of appointments scheduled for each day of a particular month and for a particular resource. This is a useful application for quickly viewing the number of scheduled appointments. You can choose the month, resource, and location for which to view the *Month* calendar, or you can choose to view the month's scheduled appointments as a bar chart.

ACTIVITY 4-9:   View Appointment Totals for a Month

1. Click the *Scheduling* module. Harris CareTracker PM opens the *Book* application by default. This can be done with or without a patient in context.

2. Click the *Month* tab. Harris CareTracker PM displays the *Month* application.

3. Select the month. (Choose the month you have entered appointments for in this chapter.)

4. Select a *Resource* for which to view appointments. (Select "Amir Raman.")

5. The *Location* field defaults to "(Locations)", which displays appointment totals for all the resource locations. You can also select a specific location. (Select "NVFA.")

6. (Display Options): The default display is *Calendar* format. (You also have the option of selecting *Bar Chart*.)

   a. Click *Go.*

   b. Repeat the activity for both *Calendar* (Figure 4-35) and *Bar Chart* (Figure 4-36).

   c. Harris CareTracker PM displays the appointment totals for each day of the month.

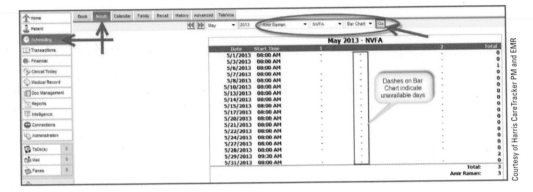

Figure 4-35   Appointment Totals for Month – Calendar View

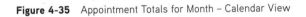

Figure 4-36   Appointment Totals for Month – Bar Chart View

Print both the Calendar and Bar Chart screens, label them "Activity 4-9," and place them in your assignment folder.

Calendar Display

On the *Calendar* screen (in the *Month* tab), gray days represent days on which the provider has no availability at the location selected (see Figure 4-35). In the *Calendar* format, you can drill down into any day of the month by clicking on the *Date Link* for that day.

The *Calendar* application allows you to view appointments in the format of a small date book calendar. The *Date Book* is more concise than the schedule in the *Book* application but contains fewer appointment details. For each scheduled appointment, the *Calendar* shows the appointment time, the patient's name, his or her Harris CareTracker PM and EMR ID number, the appointment type, duration, and any saved patient complaint. *Calendars* can be generated for multiple providers for either one day or one week.

ACTIVITY 4-10:   Generate a Calendar

1. Click the *Scheduling* module. Harris CareTracker PM opens the *Book* application by default.

2. Click the *Calendar* tab. Harris CareTracker PM displays the *Calendar* application.

3. In the *Date* field, enter the date in MM/DD/YYYY format for which you want to generate a calendar (select the date for the appointments you scheduled in Activity 4-1) or click the *Calendar* MDY icon and select the date.
4. From the *Display* list, select either a one day or one week calendar. (Select "1 week.")
5. In the *Provider* field, select the provider(s) for which you want to generate a calendar. (Select "All.")
6. By default, the appointment information will display in multiple lines. Select the *1 Line* checkbox to display the appointment information in a single line.
7. From the *Location* list, select the location for which you want to generate a calendar. (Select "All.")

Courtesy of Harris CareTracker PM and EMR

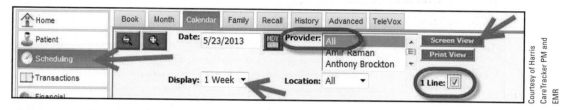

Figure 4-37 Generate Calendar – Screen View

8. To view the calendar on the screen, click *Screen View* (Figure 4-37). Harris CareTracker PM displays the calendar (Figure 4-38).

Courtesy of Harris CareTracker PM and EMR

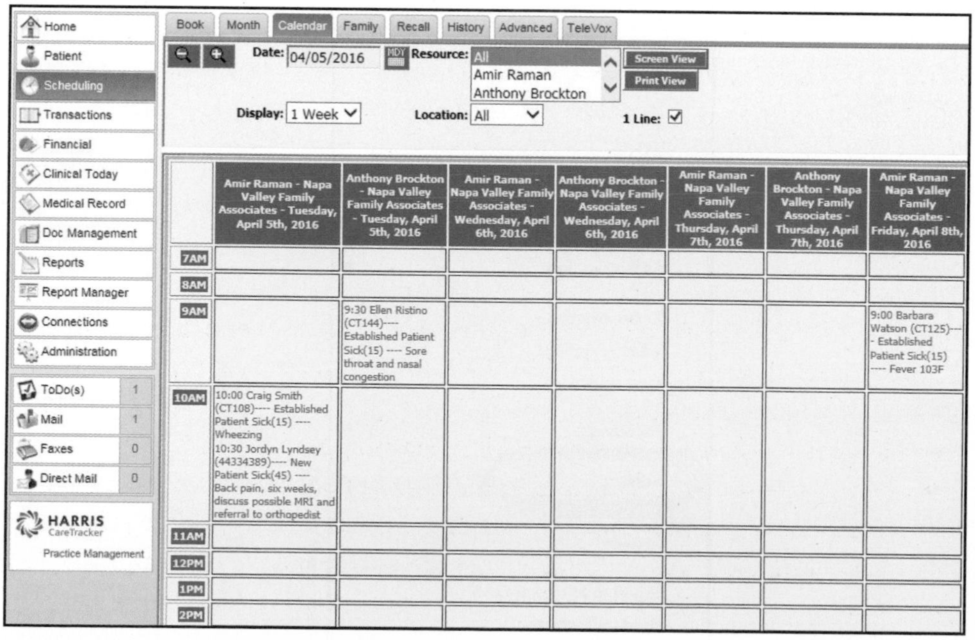

Figure 4-38 Generated Calendar for All Providers

9. To *Print* the calendar:
   a. Click *Print View*. Harris CareTracker PM displays the calendar (Figure 4-39).
   b. Right-click on the calendar and select *Print* from the shortcut menu (Figure 4-40).

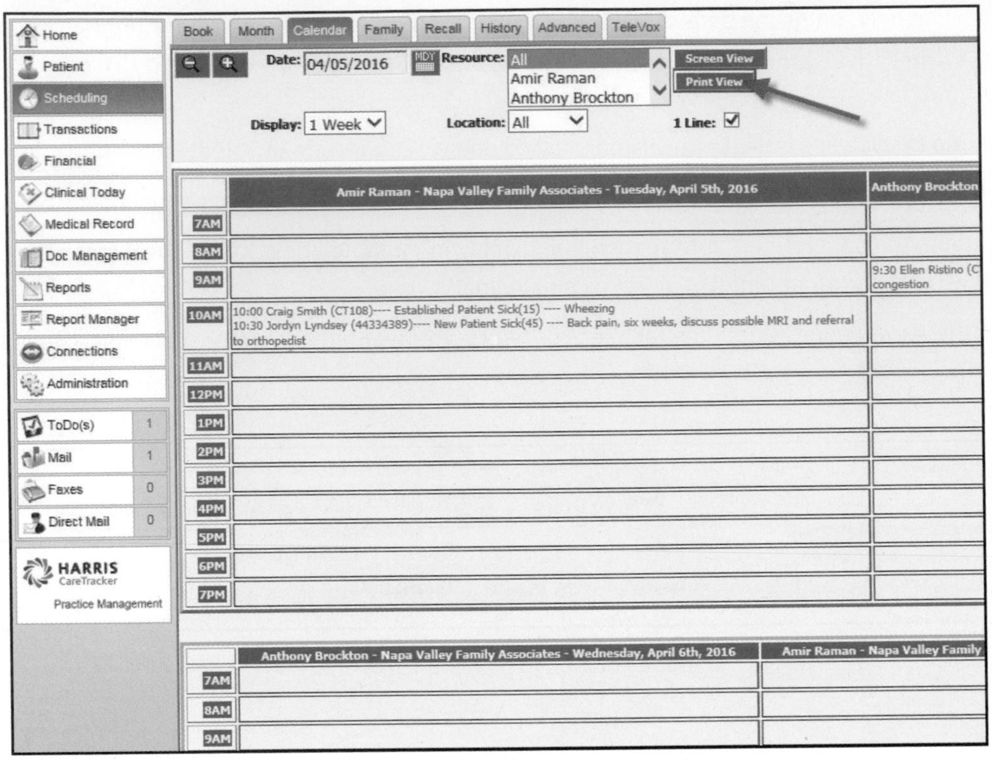

Courtesy of Harris CareTracker PM and EMR

Figure 4-39 Generate Calendar – Print View

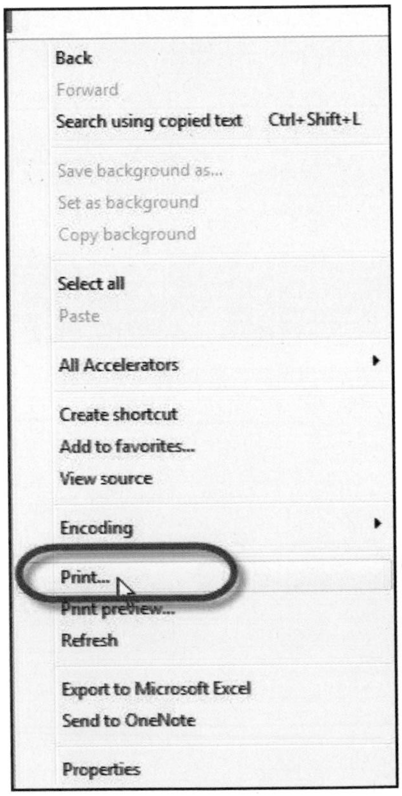

Used with permission of Microsoft®

Figure 4-40 Right-Click to Print

Print the Calendar screen, label it "Activity 4-10," and place it in your assignment folder.

Bar Chart Display. Unavailable days on the *Bar Chart* (in the *Month* application) are indicated with dashes rather than the name of the resource. You cannot access the schedule from the *Bar Chart* format (see Figure 4-36).

> ## Tip Box
>
> In the *Calendar* format, you can drill down into any day of the month by clicking on the date link for that day. Harris CareTracker PM displays the schedule for the selected resource in the *Book* application.

Family

When multiple family members see the same provider, it is common for them to request appointments on the same day. The *Family* tab in the *Scheduling* module lists all upcoming appointments for family members as well as for the patient in context. With a patient in context you can access the *Book* application from the *Family* tab by clicking on the appointment line.

The *Family* application is used to store the patient's family information and emergency contacts and link the patient's family members. This is especially useful in family billing situations, such as a pediatric practice, because multiple patients can be linked to one responsible party. When a common responsible party is indicated, Harris CareTracker PM and EMR generates one statement for all the patients linked to the responsible party. In addition, when in the *Scheduling* module, you can view upcoming appointments for all family members that are linked together.

ACTIVITY 4-11: Linking Existing Patients as Family Members

1. Pull into context the patient (Justin Riley) for whom you want to add a family member. (Justin was added as a new patient in Case Study 3-1).

2. Click the *Patient* module and then click the *Relationships* tab under the *Demographics* tab.

3. In the *Add Relationship* drop-down menu at the top right of the screen, select "Family Member." The *Add Patient Relationship* dialog box will display.

4. In the *Add Patient Relationship* dialog box, click on the *Search* 🔍 icon next to the *Patient* field.

5. In the *Search Patients* window, enter "Riley" in the *Last Name* field and "Emily" in the *First Name* field. Click *Search*.

6. Click on the radio button next to Emily Riley's name. In the drop-down menu that appears to the right of the *SSN* field, select "Mother." Click the *Select* button at the bottom of the screen.

7. In the *Add Patient Relationship* dialog box, Emily Riley's name will now appear, along with her relationship to the patient. Click *Save*.

8. Emily Riley is now listed as Justin Riley's mother on the *Relationships* screen (Figure 4-41).

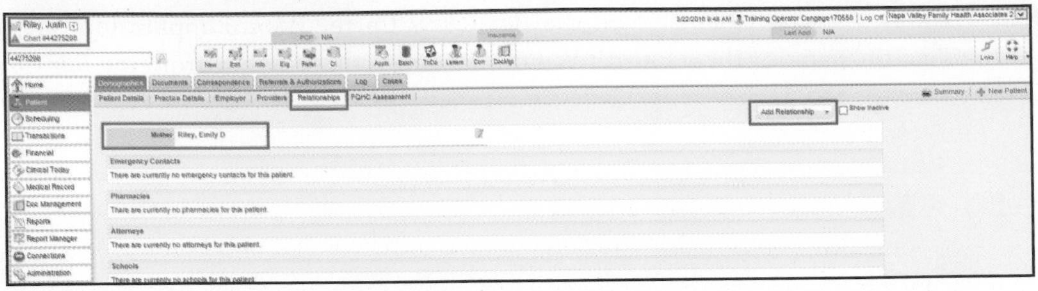

Courtesy of Harris CareTracker PM and EMR

Figure 4-41 Link Existing Patients as Family Members

Print the linked Patient/Family Member screen, label it "Activity 4-11," and place it in your assignment folder.

Deleting and Editing Family Members. At times it may be necessary to delete or edit a family member from a patient's record. To delete a family member, you would select the checkbox in the *Delete* column next to the family member you want to remove and then click *Update*. To edit a family member, click the *Edit* button next to the family member you want to edit.

> **Critical Thinking**
>
> List times when it may be necessary to delete or edit a family member from a patient's record and why. Explain what the consequences might be for not deleting or editing the record and how you reached your conclusion.

Advanced

The *Advanced* application in the *Scheduling* module (Figure 4-42) enables you to book appointments in accordance with predetermined parameters established by the practice. The *Advanced* method of booking appointments prevents overbooking and scheduling conflicts and helps to maintain consistency in terms of

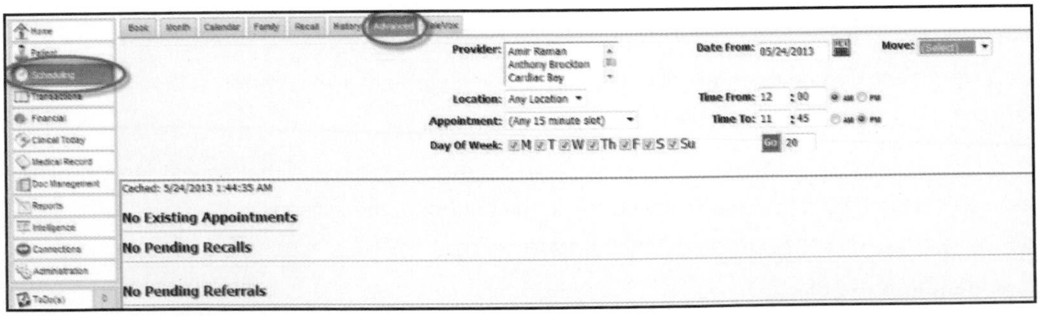

Courtesy of Harris CareTracker PM and EMR

Figure 4-42 Advanced Application in the Scheduling Module the days and times when services and procedures are provided. In addition, the existing appointments, pending recalls, and active referrals for the patient in context appear in the *Advanced* screen.

The use of the *Advanced* application is recommended if your practice books **multi-resource appointments**. A multi-resource appointment is an appointment that requires two or more resources. For example, if a patient is to be seen by a provider but also needs an ultrasound at the same visit, the *Advanced* application allows you to book one appointment for both resources.

You can also reschedule and cancel existing patient appointments in the *Advanced* application. When you reschedule an appointment in the *Advanced* application, you can search future appointment availability and be assured that you are rescheduling the appointment with the same criteria as the original appointment. If necessary, additional appointment search parameters can be added or removed from the *Advanced* fields. Canceling an appointment from the *Advanced* application functions the same way as when canceling an appointment from *Book*. Before you are allowed to cancel an existing appointment, you are required to select a reason for the cancellation. Any scheduled, rescheduled, or canceled appointment made in the *Advanced* application is saved in the patient's record and can be viewed in the *History* application of the *Scheduling* module.

Recalls

Recalls are reminders to patients that an appointment needs to be booked. Rather than scheduling a future appointment, a recall (reminder) date is set for the appointment. You can generate patient recall letters for any recall tracked in Harris CareTracker PM and EMR.

You can manually link an appointment to recalls when booking the appointment. In the case where a recall already exists, and a patient schedules an appointment for the same type as the existing recall, this recall will also be linked to the appointment. After a recall is linked to an appointment, it becomes inactive rather than open, but should the patient cancel the appointment, the recall becomes open again.

Tip Box

You can access the *Recalls* application from one of the following locations:

1. *Scheduling* module > *Recall* tab
2. *Medical Record* module > *Recall* link on the *Clinical Toolbar* (Figure 4-43)

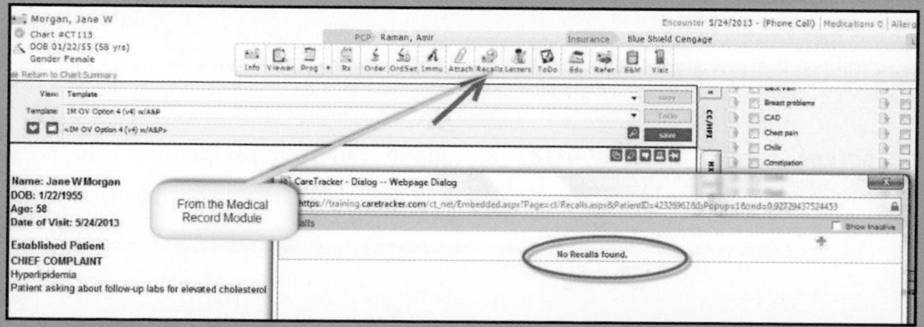

Figure 4-43   Patient Recalls in the Visit Window via Recalls Link

ACTIVITY 4-12: Entering an Appointment Recall

1. Pull patient James Smith into context.
2. Click the *Scheduling* module and then click the *Recall* tab.
3. Click *+ New Recall.* Harris CareTracker PM displays the *Add Patient Recall* box (Figure 44-4).
4. Select the time frame for the recall from the *Time Frame* list (select "1 Year"). When Days, Weeks, Months, or Years is selected, you must also enter a numeric value to correspond to the selected time unit.
5. Select the type of appointment from the *Appointment Type* list. (Select "Lab.")
6. Select the provider from the *Resource* list. (Select "Amir Raman")
7. Select the location from the *Location* list. (Select "Napa Valley Family Associates")
8. If the recall appointment needs to be linked to a case, select the appropriate case from the *Case* list (not applicable here).
9. (Optional) Select an alert type from the *EMR Alert Status* list. (Select "Soft Alert.")
10. (Optional) Enter a note about the recall in the *Recall Notes* field. (Free text note: "Annual CPE Labs")

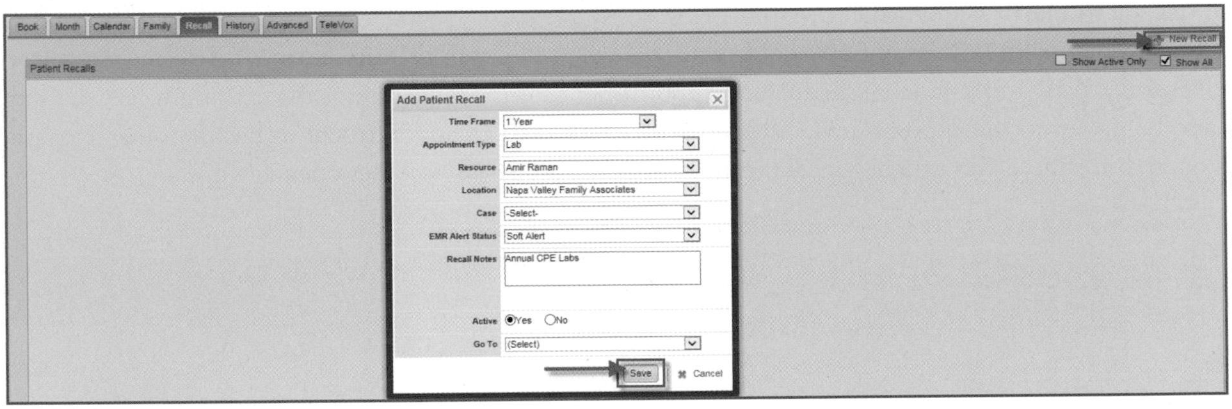

Courtesy of Harris CareTracker PM and EMR

Figure 4-44 Entering an Appointment Recall

11. Click *Save* (Figure 4-44).

Print the Patient Recalls screen, label it "Activity 4-12," and place it in your assignment folder.

FYI

When you need to inactivate an appointment recall:

1. Pull a patient into context.
2. Open the *Scheduling* module and click the *Recall* tab.
3. Click the *Edit* icon next to the appointment recall you want to inactivate (Figure 4-45). In the *Edit Patient Recall* box, change the *Active* status to "No" and click *Save*. Harris CareTracker PM changes the recall status from Active to Inactive.

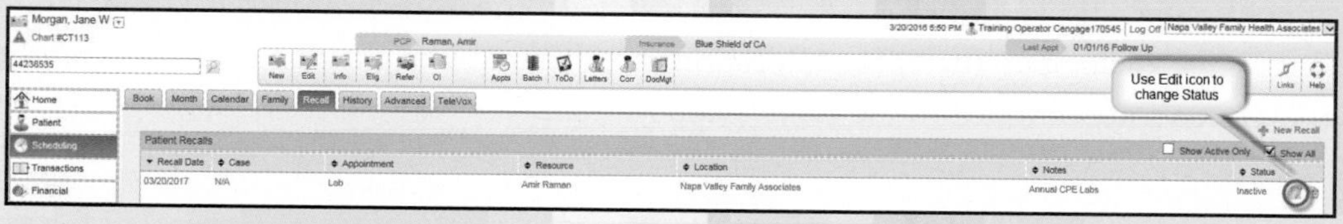

Courtesy of Harris CareTracker PM and EMR

Figure 4-45 Pending Recall

To activate an appointment recall previously inactivated:

1. Pull a patient into context.
2. Open the *Scheduling* module and click the *Recall* tab.
3. Click *Show All*. Harris CareTracker PM displays all active and inactive appointment recalls.
4. Click the *Edit* icon in the *Status* column to open the *Edit Patient Recall* box (Figure 4-46). Change the *Active* status to "Yes" and click *Save*.

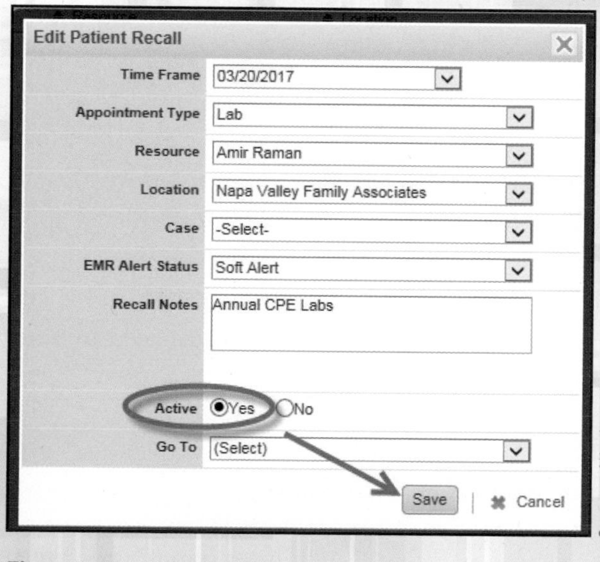

Courtesy of Harris CareTracker PM and EMR

Figure 4-46 Activate Recall

History

Harris CareTracker PM and EMR maintains a detailed history of all appointments, including those that are canceled or rescheduled, in the *History* tab of the *Scheduling* module. The *History* tab has four different sections: *Pending Appointments, Previous Appointments, Cancelled Appointments,* and *Rescheduled Appointments* (Figure 4-47).

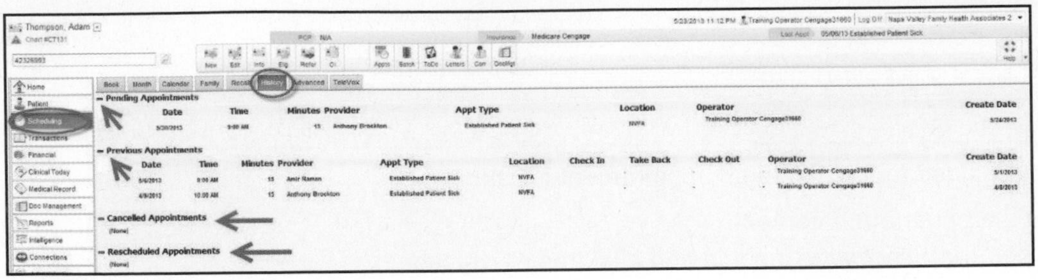

Figure 4-47 Appointment History

Pending appointments display from oldest to newest to keep them in chronological order. You can view the *Appointment Details* dialog box (date, time, location provider, etc.) by clicking on the *Appointment Line*. Upcoming appointments are canceled in the *History* application.

Tip Box

If the patient's canceled appointment was attached to a recall, the recall will become active again once the appointment is canceled.

TeleVox®

Missed appointments are a significant concern for medical practices. Not only is revenue lost for the missed appointment, but continuity of care may be compromised. In addition, missed appointments do not afford the opportunity for another patient to be seen in that time slot. Therefore, most practices have initiated some form of appointment reminder system. In Harris CareTracker, *TeleVox®* is an optional application of automated appointment reminder and confirmation system that can be used to notify patients of upcoming appointments. There are two main steps involved in using *TeleVox®*:

- Sending an electronic appointment list to *TeleVox®*
- Viewing the results of the automated calls made by *TeleVox®*

When the appointment list is received at *TeleVox®*, reminder phone calls are transmitted during calling hours that are chosen by your practice. If the reminder call does not go through to a patient, answering machine, or voice mail, *TeleVox®* continues to try and reach the patient.

You can review the *TeleVox®* results the day after the appointment list was sent. From the results list you can either confirm or cancel patient appointments, depending on the result of the call. There are nine *TeleVox®* call results. The practice is only charged for calls that go through (any status except Called-No Answer and Invalid Phone Number). The practice will be charged a standard rate per successful call as stated in the contract (Table 4-5).

TABLE 4-5 *TeleVox*® Call Results	
Answered—Yes	Person answered the phone and pressed the touch tone key to indicate "Yes" as the response.
Answered—No	Person answered the phone and pressed the touch tone key to indicate "No" as the response.
Answered—No Response	A person answered the phone and listened to the entire message but did not use the touch tone keys to indicate a response.
Answered—Left Message	A person answered the phone and pressed the "touch tone key" to leave a message.
Answered—Repeated Message	A person answered the phone and pressed the "touch tone key" to have the automated message repeated.
Answering Machine	A message was delivered on an answering machine.
Called—No Answer	Last calling attempt had no answer.
Invalid Phone Number	The number dialed did not pass the Metro Tables, meaning the call was not completed.
Out of Order	A special information tone was received, meaning a call was attempted but it was not a person or a machine that received the message.

Courtesy of Harris CareTracker PM and EMR

Tip Box

Multiple calls are restricted when using *TeleVox*®. This means that *TeleVox*® cannot call two people who have the same phone number and have an appointment on the same date of service (such as siblings).

Critical Thinking

Identify issues that a missed patient appointment causes for a medical practice. What steps can and should be taken to avoid missed appointments?

Activate Appointment Reminder System. To activate the appointment reminder system, you need to submit an appointment list to *TeleVox*® 2 to 3 days prior to the service date you are confirming. Your student version of Harris CareTracker is not enrolled in *TeleVox*® (Figure 4-48).

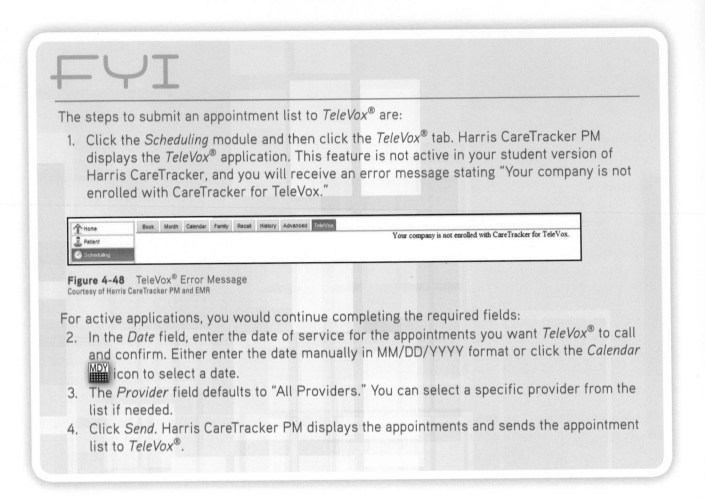

ⵎⵎⵉ

The steps to submit an appointment list to *TeleVox*® are:

1. Click the *Scheduling* module and then click the *TeleVox*® tab. Harris CareTracker PM displays the *TeleVox*® application. This feature is not active in your student version of Harris CareTracker, and you will receive an error message stating "Your company is not enrolled with CareTracker for TeleVox."

Figure 4-48 TeleVox® Error Message
Courtesy of Harris CareTracker PM and EMR

For active applications, you would continue completing the required fields:

2. In the *Date* field, enter the date of service for the appointments you want *TeleVox*® to call and confirm. Either enter the date manually in MM/DD/YYYY format or click the *Calendar* icon to select a date.
3. The *Provider* field defaults to "All Providers." You can select a specific provider from the list if needed.
4. Click *Send*. Harris CareTracker PM displays the appointments and sends the appointment list to *TeleVox*®.

If a patient does not want to get a confirmation call from *TeleVox*®, you must update his or her demographic information on the *Patient Details* tab in the *Patient* module/*Demographics* tab by updating the patient's *Notification Preference* field to "Patient Refusal."

ACTIVITY 4-13: Remove a Patient from the Call List

1. Pull patient James Smith into context.
2. Click the *Patient* module, which will default to the *Demographics/Patient Details* tab.
3. Click *Edit*.
4. Scroll down to the *Notification Preference* field. Click on the drop-down menu and select "Patient Portal" (Figure 4-49).
5. Scroll down and click *Save*. The patient's notification preference is now listed as "Patient Portal" (Figure 4-50).

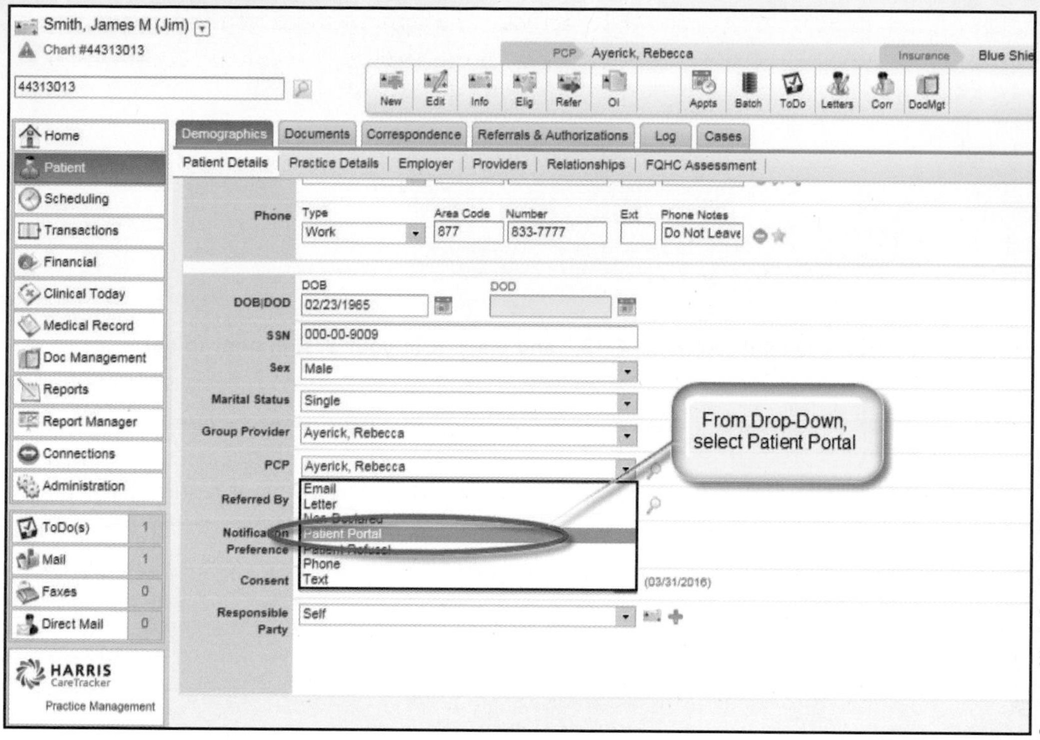

Figure 4-49 Remove Patient from Call List

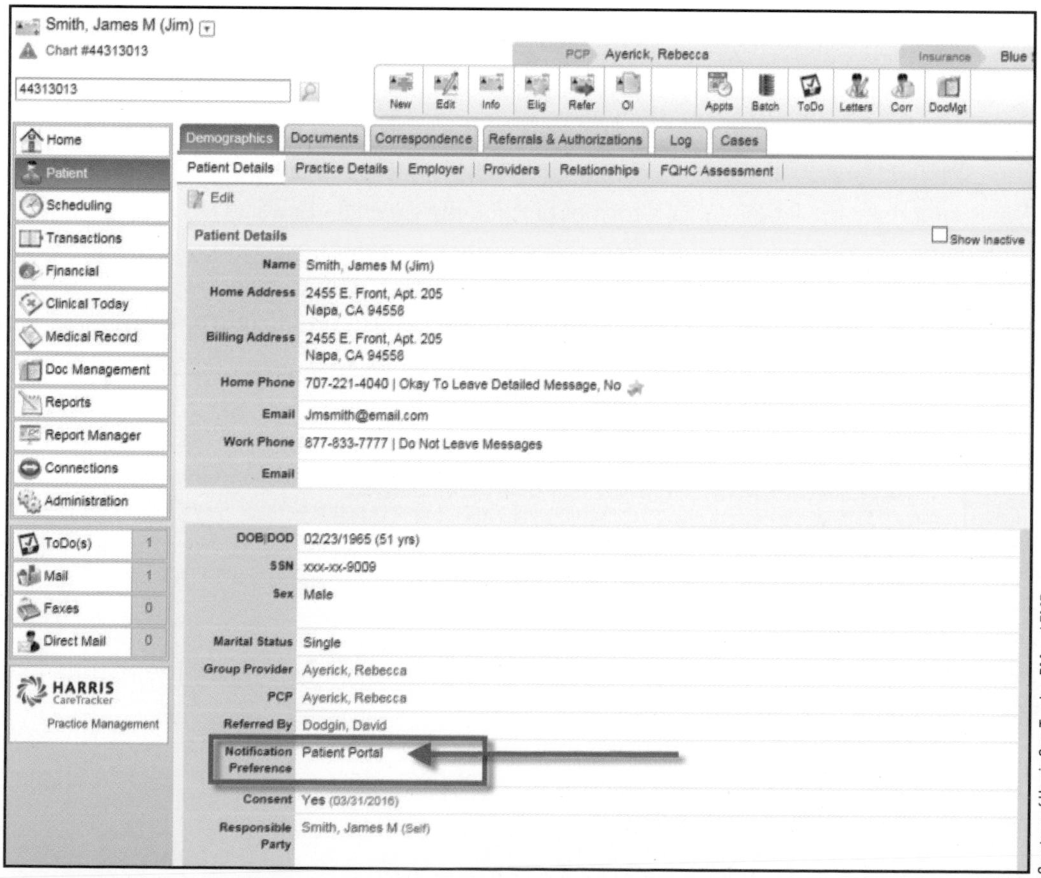

Figure 4-50 Patient's Notification Preference

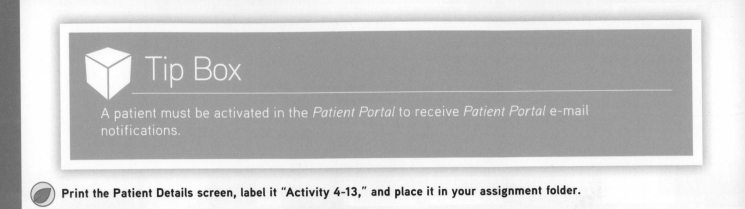

Tip Box

A patient must be activated in the *Patient Portal* to receive *Patient Portal* e-mail notifications.

Print the Patient Details screen, label it "Activity 4-13," and place it in your assignment folder.

Viewing *TeleVox®* **Call Results.**   As a best practice, you should review the call results list the day after you sent the appointment list to *TeleVox®*; however, your student version of Harris CareTracker is not enrolled in the *TeleVox®* feature so you will be unable to use this function.

FYI

Steps to view and work *TeleVox®* call results (in a live environment):

1. Click the *Scheduling* module and then click the *TeleVox®* tab. Harris CareTracker PM displays the *TeleVox®* application. If you attempt this activity in your student environment, you will receive a message stating:

    "Your company is not enrolled with CareTracker for TeleVox."

2. In the *Date* field, enter the date of service for which you want to view call results. Either enter the date manually in MM/DD/YYYY format or click the *Calendar* 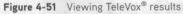 icon to select a date.

3. The *Provider* field defaults to "All Providers." You can select a specific provider from the list if needed.

4. Click *Look Up*. Harris CareTracker PM displays the call results (Figure 4-51).

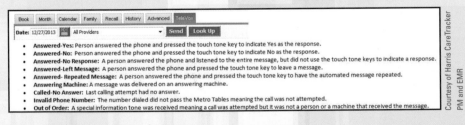

Figure 4-51 Viewing TeleVox® results

5. Review the call results list. To confirm or cancel an appointment from the results list, click on the patient's name.
    a. To confirm an appointment:
        i. Click on the appointment you want to confirm. Harris CareTracker PM displays the *View Appointment* window.
        ii. From the *Confirm* list, select "Y."
        iii. Click *Save*. Harris CareTracker PM confirms the patient's appointment.

b. To cancel an appointment:
   i. Click on the appointment you want to cancel. Harris CareTracker PM displays the *View Appointment* window.
   ii. Click *Cancel Appointment*. Harris CareTracker PM and EMR displays the *Cancel Appointment* window.
   iii. From the *Cancel Reason* list, select the reason for canceling the appointment.
   iv. Click *Cancel Appointment*. Harris CareTracker PM cancels the patient's appointment.

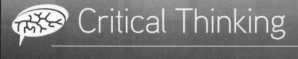

Critical Thinking

What do you think is the reasoning behind the instruction to submit an appointment list to *TeleVox*® 2 to 3 days prior to the service date you are confirming? What should you do with the results of the *TeleVox*® report?

CHECK IN PATIENTS

Learning Objective 5: Check in patients.

For a patient encounter to be generated in the electronic medical record (EMR), the patient must be checked in when he or she arrives for an appointment. Checking in a patient changes his or her Harris CareTracker PM and EMR status to "Checked in," and Harris CareTracker PM and EMR verifies that the patient's billing and demographic information is complete. Harris CareTracker PM and EMR will display the *Patient Alert* dialog box if the patient is missing important billing or demographic data.

Tip Box

Patient Alerts will only display if the *Show Alerts* feature is activated in your batch.

You can check in a patient in Harris CareTracker PM and EMR in the following places:

- In the *Book* application of the *Scheduling* module, using the mini-menu drop-down feature (see Figure 4-53)
- From the *Appts* button in the *Name Bar*
- From the *Appointment List* on the *Dashboard*
- From the *Appointment* tab in *Clinical Today*

ACTIVITY 4-14: Check in Patient from the Mini-Menu

1. Click the *Scheduling* module. Harris CareTracker PM opens the *Book* application by default.

2. With or without the patient in context, move the schedule to display the appointment for the patient you want to check in (check in patient Craig X. Smith for his appointment scheduled in Activity 4-1). This can be done by manually entering in the date in the *Date* box, by clicking the *Calendar* 🔲 icon, or by selecting a time period from the *Move* list.

3. Left-click the name of the patient you want to check in and select *Check In* from the mini-menu (see Figure 4-53). Harris CareTracker PM and EMR changes the patient's status to "Checked In" and highlights the patient's appointment in green in both the *Book* application and the *Appointments* link in the *Front Office* section of the *Dashboard*. Additionally, Harris CareTracker PM and EMR records the check-in time and displays the patient's wait time in the *Appointments* link (Figure 4-52). Checking in a patient from the mini-menu will pull the patient into context.

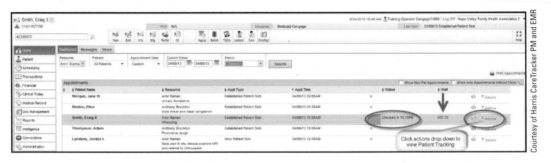

Courtesy of Harris CareTracker PM and EMR

Figure 4-52 Check-in Wait Time

Tip Box

Harris CareTracker PM and EMR allows you to view the patient tracking log that tracks the progress of the patient's appointment. You can track the progress by logging an entry each time the patient's status changes and each time a patient is moved to a different location. The log displays a time stamp next to each activity and calculates the total time of the visit, beginning at check-in and ending at check-out. To view the patient tracking log, access the *Appointments* application from one of the following locations:

- The *Appts* button 📅 on the *Name Bar*
- The *Appointments* link on the *Practice* tab of the *Dashboard*
- The *Appointments* tab in the *Clinical Today* module

In the *Appointments* list, locate the appointment for which you want to view the *Patient Tracking* log. Click the *Arrow* ▼ icon next to the *Actions* ▼ Actions menu along the appointment row, and click *Patient Tracking*. Harris CareTracker PM and EMR displays the *Patient Tracking* log.

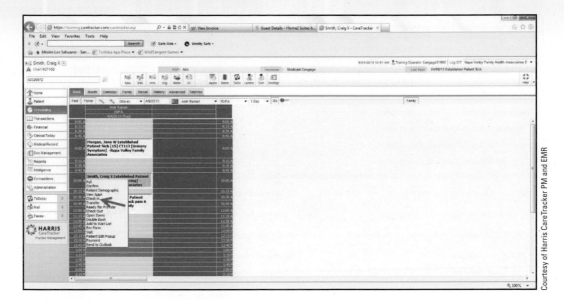

Figure 4-53   Mini-Menu Check-In

Print the Schedule screen with the patient checked in, label it "Activity 4-14," and place it in your assignment folder.

CREATE A BATCH

Learning Objective 6: Create a batch, accept payments, print patient receipts, run a journal, and post the batch.

The *Batch* application is used for setting defaults for both "Financial" and "Clinical" components. The "Financial" portion of the **batch** establishes defaults and assigns a name to a batch (group) of financial transactions you will be entering into Harris CareTracker PM and EMR. A new financial batch is created daily to enter financial transactions into Harris CareTracker PM and EMR, for example, charges, payments, and adjustments. This helps identify transactions linked to the batch, the date of each transaction, and the operator who entered it into the system. Setting up the financial batch helps identify a group of charges or payments and helps run reports to balance against the actual charges or payments entered.

The "Clinical" batch settings are typically set up only once and are used to set preferences and prepopulate fields common to your workflow (Figure 4-54). The "Clinical" batch settings are in the middle and lower sections of the *Operator Encounter Batch Control* dialog box. Setting the defaults here can speed up scheduling by having default *resource* and *location* defined.

For this learning objective, you will create a batch, accept copays, and print a **receipt**. Once you have created your batch, you will run a journal to verify your batch information, click the link to view all open batches, and then post your batch (later activity) into the system. Posting a batch permanently stores all financial transactions linked to it in Harris CareTracker PM and EMR. The application is updated in real time. Receipts in Harris CareTracker PM can identify a patient's previous balance, the activity of charges and payments for that date of service, and the new patient balance.

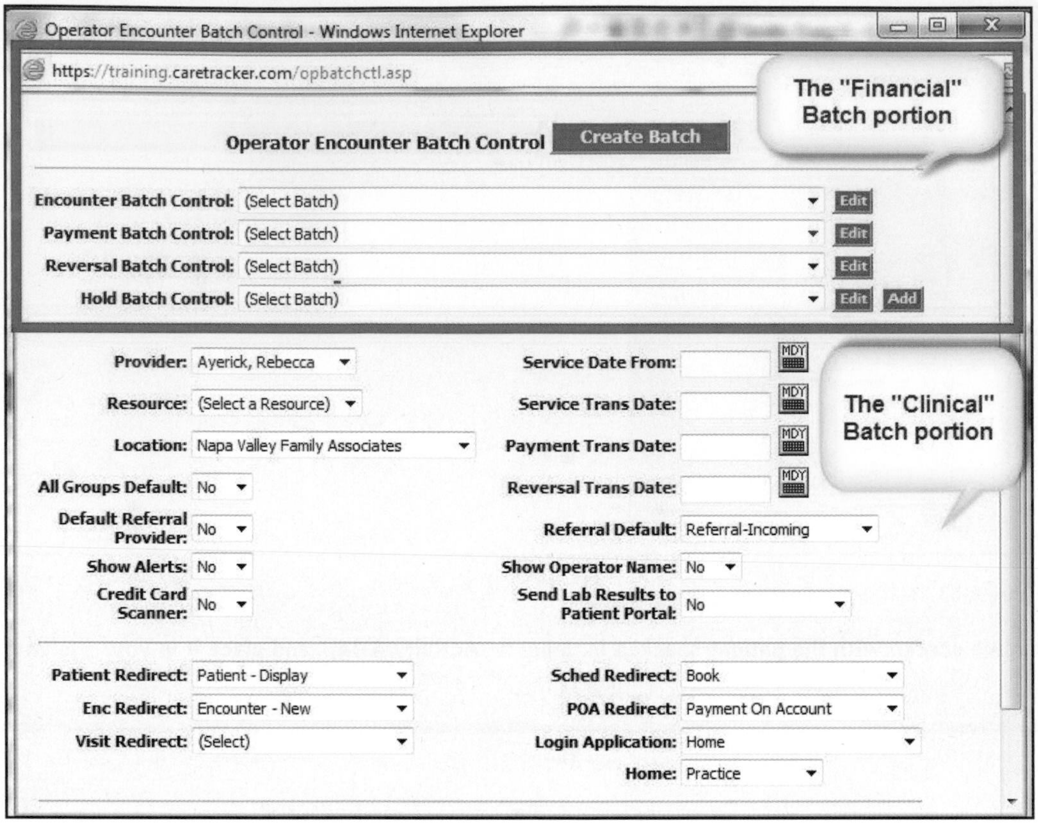

Figure 4-54   Financial and Clinical Components of a Batch

Tip Box

A real-world best practice is to close out batches at the end of each day; however, for student activities do not close out until instructed to do so. If you have already closed your batch, when you log in again, hit *Save* in the *Batch* pop-up.

Setting Operator Preferences

The *Batch* application enables you to set up operator preferences based on the workflow for your role. This reduces the number of clicks required to get from one application to the other, making navigation through Harris CareTracker PM and EMR easy. Set your operator preferences in Activity 4-15.

The first time you log in to Harris CareTracker you will be prompted to create a batch. Activities related to searching for a patient or scheduling a patient do not require that a batch be created. For the activities related to financial and clinical workflows, you will need to have a batch open. You begin by setting your operator preferences (Activity 4-15).

ACTIVITY 4-15: Setting Operator Preferences

1. With no patient in context, click *Batch* on the *Name Bar*. Harris CareTracker PM and EMR displays the *Operator Encounter Batch Control* dialog box.

2. By default, Harris CareTracker PM and EMR assigns redirects, making it easy to navigate from different applications within Harris CareTracker PM and EMR. The default redirects are based on the most commonly used workflow.

3. Click *Edit* if the fields are grayed out. Otherwise, enter (or confirm if already populated) the information, following the instructions for the available redirects described in Table 4-6. These are located in the lower section of *the Operator Encounter Batch Control* dialog box (Figure 4-55).

TABLE 4-6 Batch Redirects

Redirects

Field	**Description**
Patient Redirect	Launches the selected application after editing a *Demographic* record in the *Patient* module. You can also change this setting in the *Demographic* application if necessary. (Select "Patient – Display")
Enc Redirect	Launches the selected application after saving a *Charge* in the *Transactions* module. (Select "Encounter – New")
Visit Redirect	Launches the selected application after a visit is saved in the *Visit* application. (Select "Select")
Sched Redirect	Launches the selected application after an appointment is booked via the *Book* application of the *Scheduling* module. (Select "Book")
POA (Payment on Account) Redirect	Launches the selected application after a payment is entered via the *Payment on Account* application of the *Transaction* module. (Select "Payment on Account")
Login Application	Launches the selected application when you log in to Harris CareTracker PM and EMR. (Select "Home")
Home	If the *Log in Application* is set to "Home," you can select which *Home* module application to display by default. For example, the Management, Meaningful Use, Messages or News applications. (Select "Practice")
Click *Save*	Screen will be saved with selections made

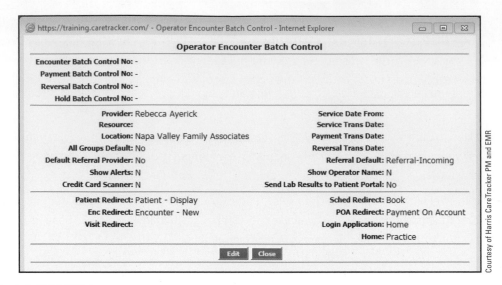

Figure 4-55 Operator Encounter Batch Control

Print the Operator Encounter Batch Control screen, label it "Activity 4-15," and place it in your assignment folder.

A provider's paperless desk is incorporated in the *Clinical Today* module. Therefore, selecting the *Clinical* module from the *Login Application* list takes you directly to the *Clinical Today* module each time you log in to Harris CareTracker PM and EMR, streamlining workflow (Figure 4-56).

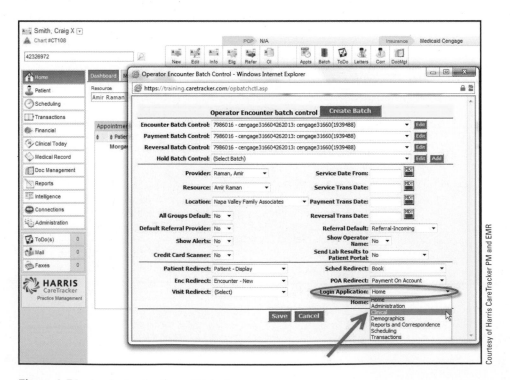

Figure 4-56 Login Application - Clinical

Table 4-7 outlines the fields and related instructions to complete your batch details. You will finish creating a batch in Activity 4-16, referencing instructions in Table 4-7. After entering the copayments as assigned in Activity 4-17, you will print a receipt (see Activity 4-18), run a journal (see Activity 4-19), and post your batch (see Activity 4-20). Posting a batch permanently stores all financial transactions linked to it in Harris CareTracker PM and EMR. The application is updated in real time.

TABLE 4-7	Batch Details Field and Instructions
Batch Details Field	**Instructions**
Provider	From the *Provider* list, select the name of the billing provider associated with the batch. **Note:** The *Admissions* application accessed via the *Dashboard* and the *Charges* application in the *Transaction* module display the billing provider set up in the batch.
Resource	From the *Resource* list, select the servicing provider. In most instances, the billing provider and the resource are the same. **Note:** The *Book* application in the *Scheduling* module and the *Appointment* application in the *Clinical Today* module display the resource set up in the batch.
Location	From the *Location* list, select the location associated with the batch. **Note:** The *Admissions* application accessed via the *Dashboard* and the *Book* application in the *Scheduling* module display the location set up in the batch.
All Groups Default	By default, the *All Groups Default* list is set to "No." Change the list to "Yes" if necessary. This displays patient financial information for the current group or all groups in the practice based on the setting selected. If *Yes* is selected, you can only see the financial transactions for the groups that you have access to as an operator. This setting mostly benefits multi-group practices and also determines the default value in the *Open Items* application of the *Financial* module and *Edit* application of the *Transactions* module.
Default Referral Provider	By default, the *Default Referral Provider* list is set to "No." Change the field to "Yes" if there is no referring provider in the patient's demographics or if there is no active referral/authorization for the patient. This sets the billing provider as the referring provider.
Show Alerts	In the *Show Alerts* field, select "Yes" to enable Harris CareTracker PM to display the *Patient Alert* window; otherwise select "No." The *Patient Alerts* window notifies users when key information is missing from a patient's demographics or when there are other issues with a patient's account.
Credit Card Scanner	The *Credit Card Scanner* field is set to "No" by default. Your student version of Harris CareTracker will NOT have this feature. In a real practice setting, select "Yes" if your group uses a credit card scanner to process payments by credit card.
Service Date From	Click the *Calendar* icon and select the start of the service dates included in the batch.
Service Trans Date	Click the *Calendar* icon and select the service transaction date included in the batch.
Payment Trans Date	Click the *Calendar* icon and select the payment transactions date included in the batch.
Reversal Trans Date	Click the *Calendar* icon and select the reversal transactions date included in the batch.

(Continues)

TABLE 4-7 *(Continued)*

Batch Details Field	Instructions
Referral Default	By default, the *Referral Default* list is set to "Referral-Incoming." Select a referral type based on your practice specialty. The selected option will display as the default option when the *Ref/Auth* application is accessed via the *Name Bar* or *Patient* module.
Show Operator Name	Select "Yes" to display the operator's name on the Harris CareTracker PM and EMR interface. Select "No" if you do not want the operator's name displayed.
Click *Save*. The batch information is saved.	
Note: Click *Edit* to make changes if necessary.	
Click *X* on the right-hand corner to close the dialog box.	

Courtesy of Harris CareTracker PM and EMR

Having set up your operator preferences in the *Operator Encounter Batch Control* in Activity 4-15, you will now create a batch. Reference the instructions in Table 4-7 when creating your batch.

ACTIVITY 4-16: Create a Batch

With the *Operator Encounter Batch Control* dialog box in display from Activity 4-15:

1. Click *Edit* and then click *Create Batch*. The *Batch Master* dialog box displays (Figure 4-57).

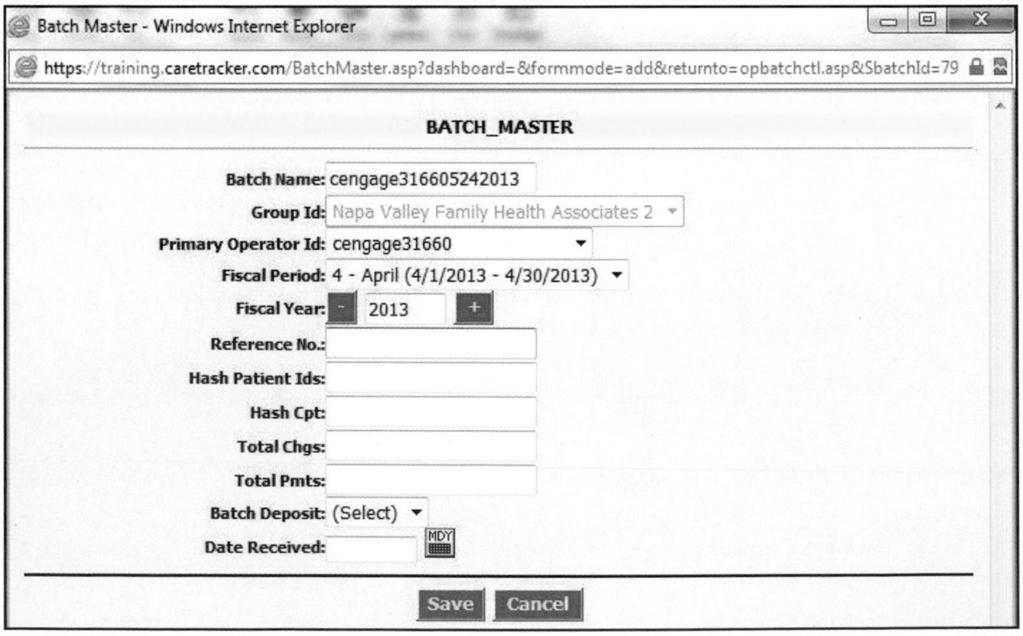

Figure 4-57 Batch Master Dialog Box

Courtesy of Harris CareTracker PM and EMR

2. By default, the *Batch Name* box displays a batch identification name. The name consists of your user name followed by the current date. (**Note:** You can edit the batch name if necessary to identify the types of financial transactions associated with the batch; for example,"copayment5132014.") Do not use symbols when editing the name. Name this Batch "FrontOfficeCopayment" (Figure 4-58).

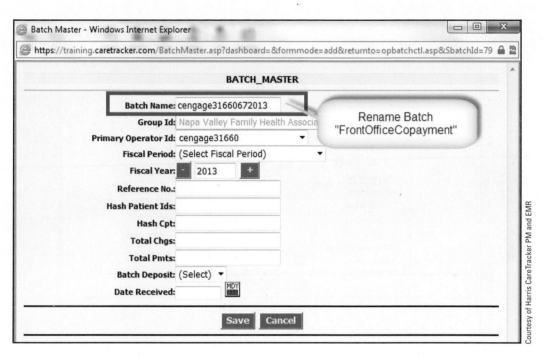

Figure 4-58   Rename Batch FrontOfficeCopayment

3. By default, the *Group Id* displays the name of your group.

4. By default, the *Primary Operator Id* displays your user name.

5. In the *Fiscal Period* list, click the period (period/year/month) in which you scheduled patients in Activity 4-1 to post related financial transactions. The list will only display fiscal periods that are currently open. If the desired *Fiscal Period* does not display or no *Fiscal Period* displays, you must first open the period to continue creating your batch (refer to Tip Box below).

Tip Box

To open a fiscal period, click the *Administration* module and then click the *Open/Close Period* link in the *Financial* section under *System Administration*. Select the period/year/ month you want to open by selecting "Open" under *Status*, and then click *Save*.

6. By default, the *Fiscal Year* displays the current financial year set up for your company.

Tip Box

Entering information for steps 7 through 12 helps to ensure that you post all payments and/or charges into Harris CareTracker PM and EMR correctly and prevents you from posting a batch until the monies match the data entered (Figure 4-59).

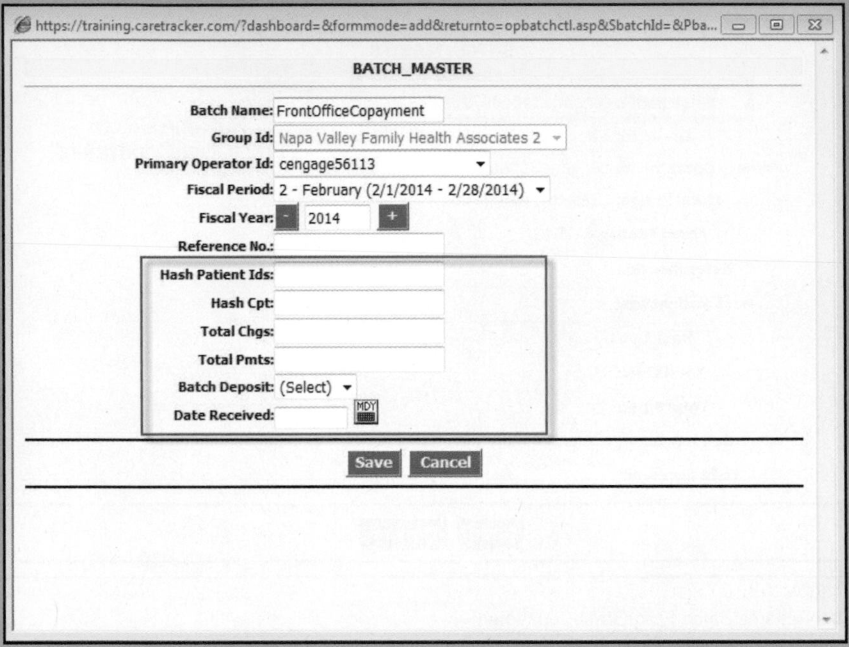

Courtesy of Harris CareTracker PM and EMR

Figure 4-59 Batch Master Selections for FrontOfficeCopayment

7. (Optional – Leave Blank) In the *Hash Patient Ids* box, enter the sum of all patient Harris CareTracker PM and EMR ID numbers pertaining to the charges associated with the batch. This is to ensure that a charge is entered for all patients associated with the batch.
8. (Optional – Leave Blank) In the *Hash Cpt* box, enter the sum of all CPT® codes pertaining to the charges associated with the batch. This is to ensure that a charge is entered for all procedures. Example: If two patients are seen for the day, and the CPT® codes selected on the encounter form for the first patient are 71101 and 99213, and the second patient are 71101 and 99203, calculate the *Hash CPT* by adding 71101 + 99213 + 71101 + 99203 = 340618.
9. (Optional – Leave Blank) In the *Total Chgs* box, enter the sum of all charges that are associated with the batch.
10. (Optional – Leave Blank) In the *Total Pmts* box, enter the sum of check(s) that are associated with the batch.
11. (Optional – Leave Blank) In the *Batch Deposit* list, select the *Deposit ID* to link to a deposit number, if using the *Batch Deposit* application. (This feature is not active in your student version.)
12. In the *Date Received* box, enter the date the encounter was received in MM/DD/YYYY format or click the *Calendar* MDY icon and select the date. (Leave Blank)
13. Click *Save*. Harris CareTracker PM and EMR displays the *Operator Encounter Batch Control* dialog box with the new batch information (Figure 4-60).

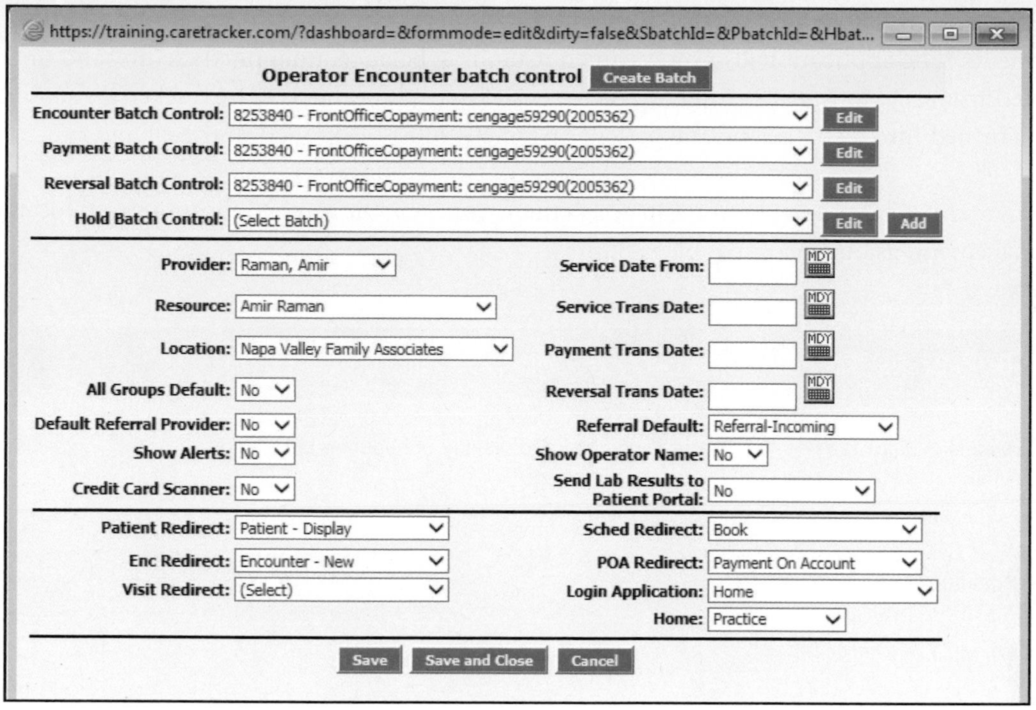

Courtesy of Harris CareTracker PM and EMR

Figure 4-60 Operator Encounter Batch Control Dialog Box

14. Now, further edit your batch by updating the provider, resource, location, and so on (the middle section of the *Operator Encounter Batch Control box*). Select the *Provider* (Amir Raman), *Resource* (Amir Raman), and *Location* (Napa Valley Family Associates).

15. Click *Save*.

16. Write down your "Encounter Batch Control No." for future reference. (Should include "FrontOffice-Copayment") ______________________.

Print the Batch screen, label it "Activity 4-16," and place it in your assignment folder.

17. Click "*X*" in the right-hand corner to close the dialog box.

Accept a Payment

Certification Connection

In Harris CareTracker PM and EMR there are many ways to record both patient and insurance payments. Payments may be processed electronically or manually. All payments entered into Harris CareTracker PM and EMR must be associated with a batch and should be verified using a journal before the batch is released for posting. All payments entered are associated with a billing period for financial reporting purposes.

Entering Payments on Account.   The *Payments On Account (Pmt on Acct)* application is used to record patient payments. The application also shows any outstanding balance, unapplied credits, and unposted payments accrued from previous visits. After a patient's visit is saved in Harris CareTracker PM and EMR, that visit must be turned into a charge and the patient's payment must be applied to the charge.

Accessing Payments on Account.   You can access the *Payments on Account* application from locations within practice management, as outlined in Table 4-8.

TABLE 4-8   Access the Payments on Account Application
Scheduling module > *Book* tab > left-click on *appointment* to display Scheduling Mini-Menu > Select *Payment* link
Name Bar > *Appts* button > *Actions* menu > *Payment* link
Transactions module > *Pmt on Acct* tab
Transactions module > *Charge* tab

Courtesy of Harris CareTracker PM and EMR

ACTIVITY 4-17:   Accept/Enter a Payment

1. Pull patient Jane Morgan into context.

2. In the *Transactions* module, click on the *Pmt on Acct* tab (see Table 4-8).

3. From the drop-down list at the top of the screen, select whether the payment is being made by the *Patient* or *Responsible Party*. (Select "Patient.")

4. If a patient is paying a portion of his or her balance, enter the dollar amount of the payment in the *Amount* box. (Enter "$20.00")

   Note: If the patient is paying his or her entire balance, click *Pay Bal*. Harris CareTracker PM and EMR automatically pulls the patient's balance into the *Amount* box.

5. From the *Payment Type* list, select the payment method. (Select "Payment - Patient Check.")

   Note: If the payment type is credit card, you would select the *Process Credit Card* checkbox.

6. If the payment method is a check, enter the check number in the *Reference #* box. (Enter "5013" as the check number.) The reference number will print on the patient's receipt.

7. From the *Method* list, select how to apply the payment to the patient's account:

   a. If you are collecting a copayment for a patient who does not have an outstanding balance, select "Force Unapplied." Harris CareTracker PM and EMR creates an unapplied balance for the patient that is applied to the patient's private pay balance when their charges are saved. (Select "Force Unapplied" and check the *Copay?* box)

Tip Box

If the patient has an outstanding balance:

- Select *Today's First* to apply the money starting with the most current balance and then back toward the oldest date of service for which the patient has an outstanding balance.
- Select *Oldest to Newest* to apply the money to the oldest date of service for which the patient has an outstanding balance and then forward toward the most current date of service.

8. In the *Trans. Date* box, enter the transaction date to which you want to link the payment. (Select the date of the financial batch you created.) This date will pre-populate if you selected the date in your batch defaults.

PM SPOTLIGHT

Transaction Date Defaults:

- If a transaction date was selected when you created your batch, Harris CareTracker PM and EMR pulls that date into the *Trans. Date* box.
- If a transaction date was not selected, the transaction date defaults to the date in your batch name.
- If there is no date in your batch name, the transaction date defaults to the date the payment is entered in Harris CareTracker PM and EMR.

9. In order to override the copayment amount recorded in the patient's demographic record for a specific appointment:

a. Select the *Copay?* checkbox.

b. In the *Appt* box, select the appointment date to which the copay applies. (**Note:** You cannot link a copay to a future appointment date.)

Tip Box

The *Plan Name* and *Copay Amt* fields display the insurance plan and copay amount saved in the patient's demographics, if applicable. These fields are read-only.

10. The *Go To* field defaults to the redirect option selected in the operator's batch. You can select a different option if needed (Figure 4-61). (Select "Payment on Account.")

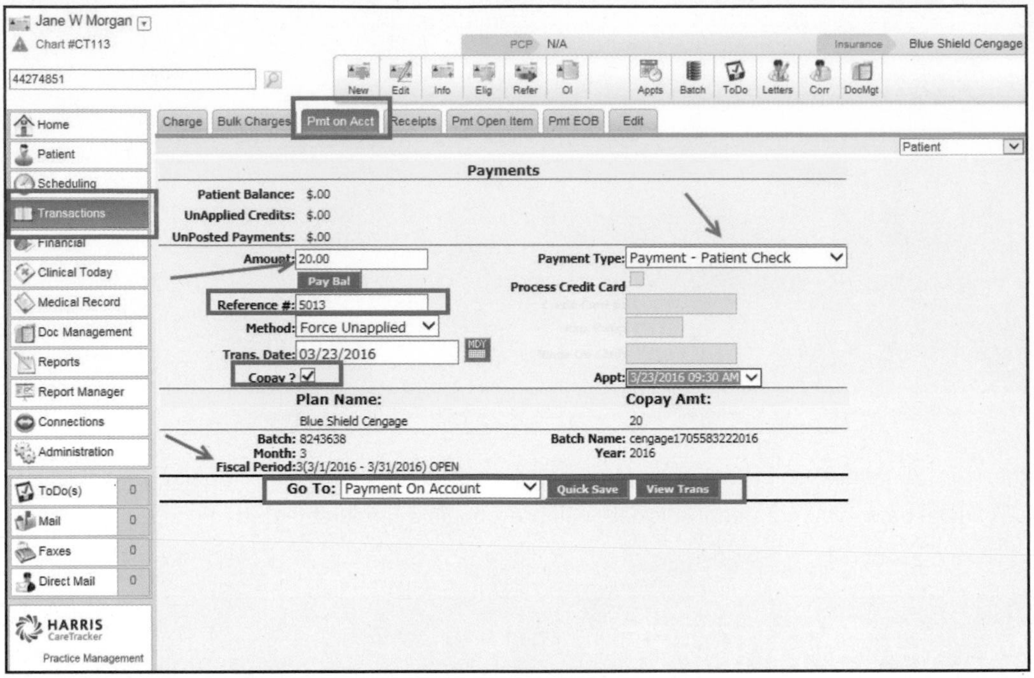

Courtesy of Harris CareTracker PM and EMR

Figure 4-61 Enter Payment on Account

Tip Box

To view a summary of the transaction prior to saving, click *View Trans* (Figure 4-62).

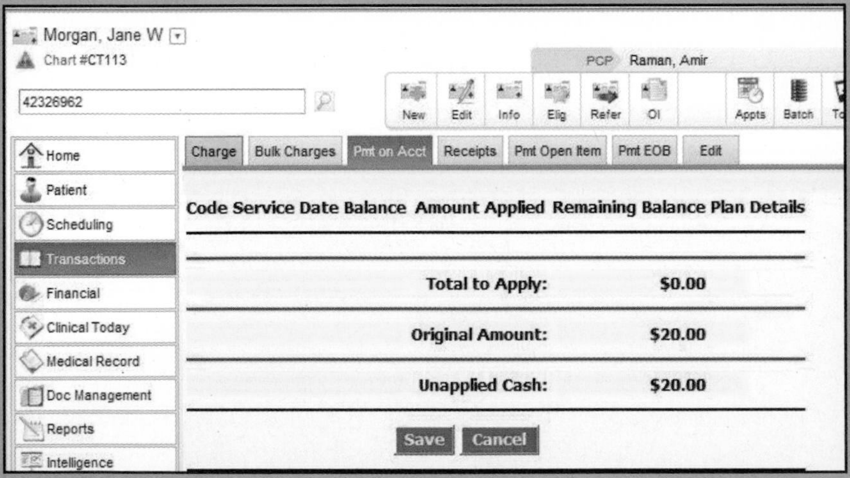

Courtesy of Harris CareTracker PM and EMR

Figure 4-62 View Transaction

11. Click *Quick Save*. Harris CareTracker PM and EMR saves the payment information and launches the application selected in the *Go To* field.

12. You can view the payment in the *Open Batches* field under *Billing* on the *Dashboard* (Figure 4-63).

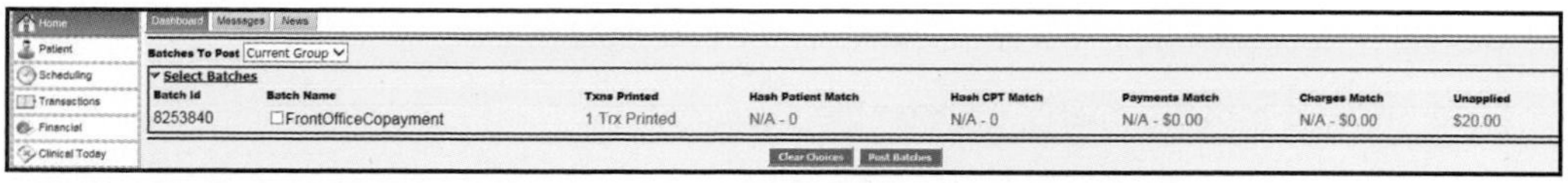

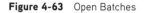

Figure 4-63 Open Batches

FYI

If you are processing a credit card transaction, the live version of Harris CareTracker PM displays the *Process Credit Card* window. If the patient is the cardholder, select the *Same as Patient* checkbox. The application auto-populates the box with the patient's name. To process a credit card transaction:

a. In the *Cardholder Name* box, enter the cardholder's name exactly as it appears on the credit card.
b. In the *Billing Zip Code* box, enter the zip code of the billing address.
c. In the *Card Number* box, enter the credit card number.
d. In the *Expiration Date* field, select the month and year the card expires. In the *CVN* box, enter the 3- or 4-digit number printed on the back of the credit card.
e. Click *Continue*. The application displays the *Payment Confirmation* window.
f. Verify that the information is correct and then click *Make Payment*. The application sends the payment to InstaMed® for processing. The application will display a confirmation message if the transaction was successful.

You will later print a receipt from the *Receipts* tab in the *Transactions* module (Activity 4-18).

Copayment. A copayment is a predetermined (flat) fee that an individual pays for health care services in addition to what the insurance covers. For example, some HMOs require a $10 "copayment" for each office visit, regardless of the type or level of services provided during the visit. Copayments are not usually specified by percentages.

Print Patient Receipts. After entering the payment information in Activity 4-17, print a receipt from the *Receipts* tab in the *Transaction* module. Receipts in Harris CareTracker PM and EMR identify a patient's previous balance, the activity of charges and payments for that date of service, and the new patient balance.

ACTIVITY 4-18: Print Patient Receipts

1. With the patient in context (Jane Morgan), click the *Transactions* module.

2. When the *Transactions* module opens, click on the *Receipts* tab.

3. From the drop-down list at the top of the screen, select who you would like to view the receipt from, *Patient* or *Responsible Party*. (Select "Patient.")

4. Select the date of service for which you need to print a receipt from the *Receipts* list. (Select the date of the payment received, which should also be the same date as your batch.)

5. When a date of service is selected, the receipt displays on the screen.

6. Click on the *Print* button (Figure 4-64), or right-click on the receipt.

   a. When you right-click, a gray pop-up menu appears; select *Print*, and the receipt will print.

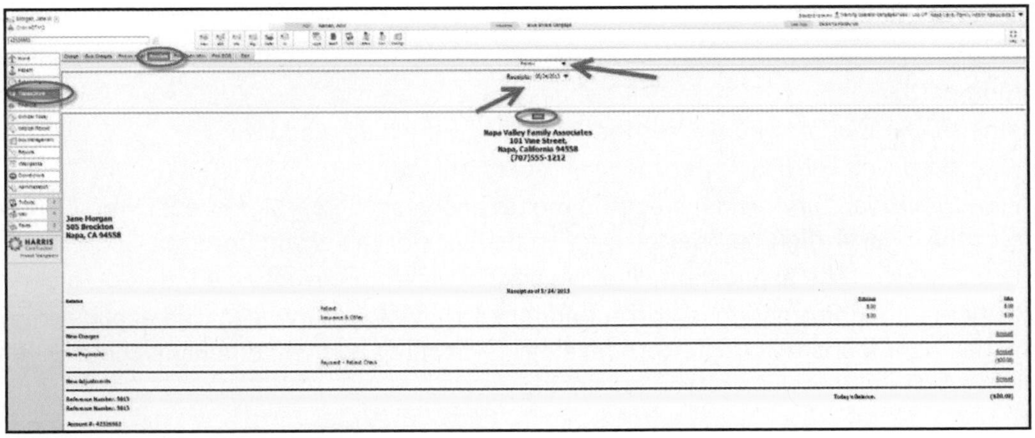

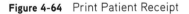

Figure 4-64 Print Patient Receipt

Courtesy of Harris CareTracker PM and EMR

Print the Patient Receipt, label it "Activity 4-18," and place it in your assignment folder.

Now that you have entered copayments, you will complete the process by running a journal and posting your batch as your end-of-day workflow.

Journals

You must run a journal prior to posting your batch to verify that you have entered all the financial transactions correctly in Harris CareTracker PM and EMR. Once you have verified your balance with your journal, post the batch. Journals provide a summary of financial transactions, for example, charges, payments, and adjustments. Typically, each operator who enters financial transactions into Harris CareTracker should run a journal for his or her batch before posting to review and audit only that transactions that he or she entered.

It is important to identify any errors before a batch is posted. Once a batch has been posted, the transactions linked to it are locked in the system and must be reversed to be corrected. Posted errors can only be corrected by reversing the transaction on the patient's account, which occurs in the *Edit* application of the *Transaction* module. It is highly recommended that you run a journal to make sure that your transactions balance for the day is correct before posting your batch.

Harris CareTracker PM and EMR offers multiple drill-down options that allow you to run a journal that fits certain criteria. Open batches are easily chosen from the list of filters. Posted batches are accessible at any time so you can always access an old journal from the *Historical Journals* link (Figure 4-65) under the *Financial Reports* section of the *Reports* application, which alleviates the need to save paper copies of journals.

Courtesy of Harris CareTracker PM and EMR

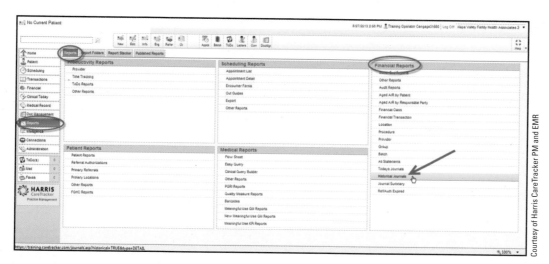

Figure 4-65 Historical Journals Link

Tip Box

For a quick "totals only" view of a batch, the *Open Batches* link on the *Dashboard* displays the total amount of payments, charges, and unapplied money entered into that batch. If the total amount of money collected equals the *Payments Match* or *Unapplied* column, you do not need to run a journal (Figure 4-66).

Courtesy of Harris CareTracker PM and EMR

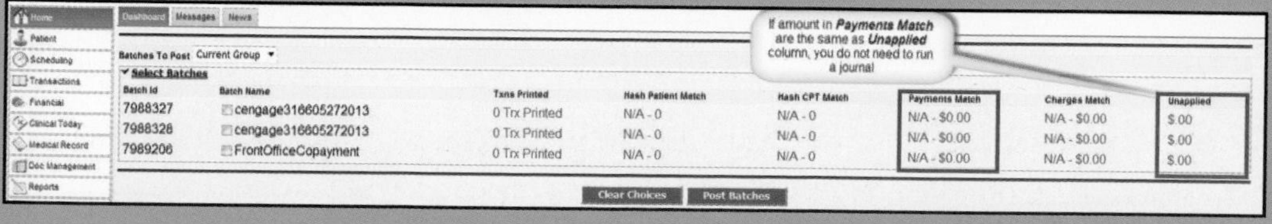

Figure 4-66 Money Collected Equals Payments Match or Unapplied Column

ACTIVITY 4-19: Run a Journal

1. Click the *Reports* module.

2. Click the *Todays Journals* link under the *Financial Reports* section (Figure 4-67). Harris CareTracker PM displays the *Todays Journal Options* screen (Figure 4-68). All of your group's open batches are listed in the *Todays Batches* box.

3. Select a batch to include in the journal either by double-clicking on the batch name or by clicking on the batch and then clicking *Add* (Figure 4-69). Harris CareTracker PM and EMR adds the selected batches to the box on the right. (Add batch "FrontOfficeCopayment.")

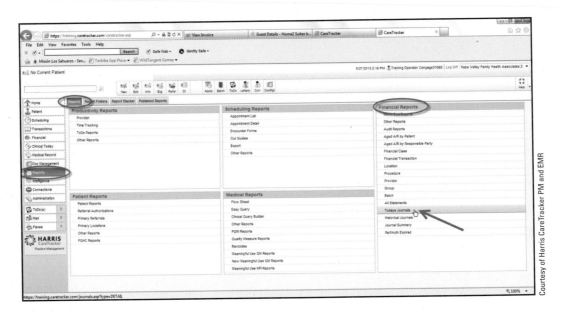

Figure 4-67 Todays Journals Link

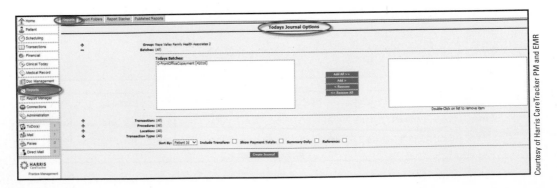

Figure 4-68 Todays Journal Options

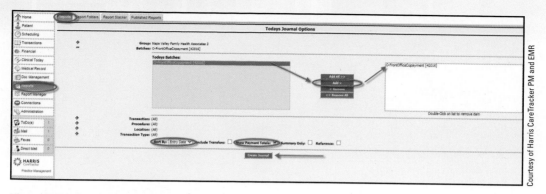

Courtesy of Harris CareTracker PM and EMR

Figure 4-69   Select a Batch for the Journal

4. From the *Sort By* list drop-down, select "Entry Date."

5. Select the *Show Payment Totals* checkbox (Figure 4-69).

6. Click *Create Journal.* Harris CareTracker PM generates the journal (Figure 4-70).

7. To print, right-click on the journal and select *Print* from the shortcut menu.

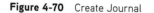

Courtesy of Harris CareTracker PM and EMR

Figure 4-70   Create Journal

Print the Journal screen, label it "Activity 4-19," and place it in your assignment folder.

After balancing the transactions in your journal, you can post your open batch (Activity 4-20). Batches should only be posted after a journal has been generated and you have verified your journal balances. Posting batches locks the transactions permanently in Harris CareTracker. All transactions will show on reports generated in Harris CareTracker, and any corrections to posted transactions must be made via the *Edit* application in the *Transactions* module. *Open Batches* can also be viewed and posted by clicking on the *Open Batches* link under the *Billing* section of the *Dashboard* on the *Home* page.

Tip Box

- As a best practice, you should close out your batch at the end of each day; however, wait until instructed to do so in a particular activity in this text.
- All transactions must be posted before running any *Month End* report in Harris CareTracker, and *Periods* cannot be closed with open batches linked to them.
- A password may be required to post a coworker's batch.

ACTIVITY 4-20: Post a Batch

After generating a journal for the batch(es) you would like to post, review, identify, and correct transactions errors, if any, prior to posting the batch.

To post your batch:

1. Click the *Administration* module. The application opens the *Practice* tab (Figure 4-71).

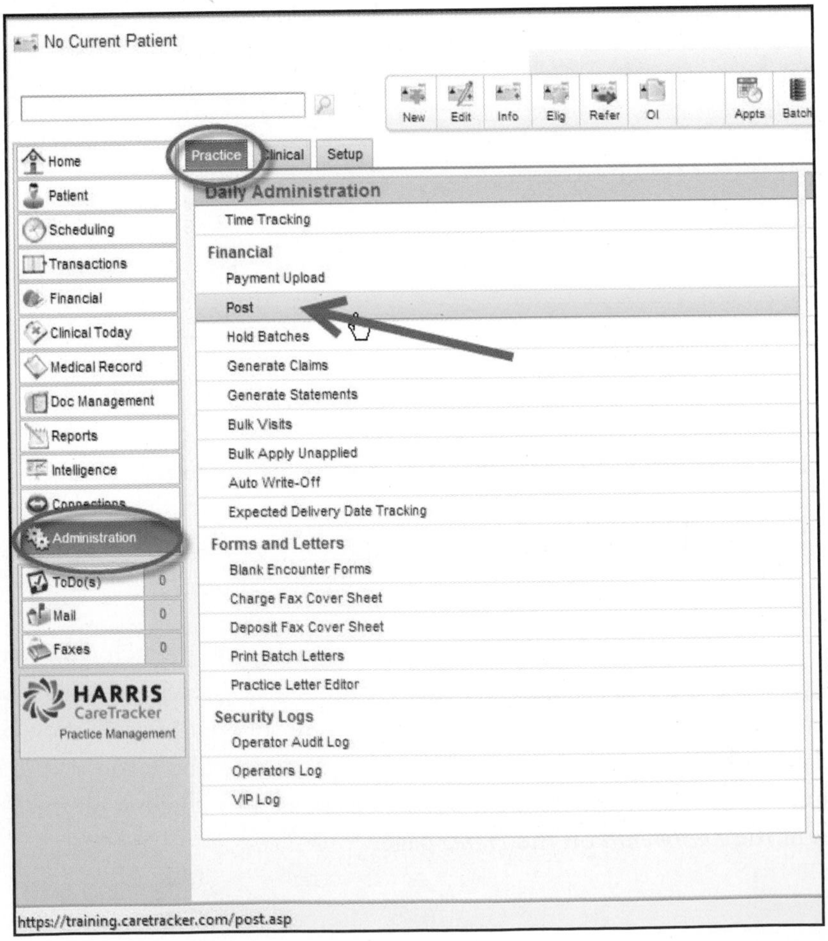

Courtesy of Harris CareTracker PM and EMR

Figure 4-71 Post Link from Admin Practice Tab

Chapter 5
Preliminary Duties in the EMR

Key Terms

American Recovery and
  Reinvestment Act
  (ARRA)
attestation period
Certification
  Commission for
  Health Information
  Technology (CCHIT®)
encounter

Health Information
  Technology for
  Economic and
  Clinical Health
  (HITECH) Act
lot
meaningful use

Learning Objectives

1. Define meaningful use and list its stages.
2. Discuss tools within Harris CareTracker PM and EMR that assist with meaningful use.
3. View and read the meaningful use dashboard in Harris CareTracker PM and EMR.
4. Activate the care management registries in Harris CareTracker PM and EMR.
5. Navigate throughout the Medical Record module.
6. View the patient's encounter information, medications, allergy information, and problem list.
7. State the three types of alerts in Harris CareTracker PM and EMR.
8. View, change, and print a chart summary in Harris CareTracker EMR.
9. Perform routine maintenance functions in Harris CareTracker PM and EMR such as adding a room, editing a room, adding a custom resource, adding favorite labs, removing favorite labs, and managing immunizations.

Certification Connection

1. Discuss the use of electronic medical records (EMRs) and the effects and implications of federal regulation to the health care industry.
2. Adhere to federal, state, and local laws relating to exchange of information and describe elements of meaningful use and reports generated.
3. Communicate in language the patient can understand; demonstrate effective and courteous telephone techniques.
4. Access, edit, and store patient information in the EHR database.
5. Manage data and document accurately in the patient record using the EHR.

Adapted from national standards of the National Healthcareer Association (NHA), Commission on Accreditation and Allied Health Education Program (CAAHEP), and Accrediting Bureau of Health Education Schools (ABHES)

INTRODUCTION

In the first four chapters, you learned a great deal about Harris CareTracker PM—the practice management side of the Harris CareTracker software. This chapter introduces you to Harris CareTracker EMR—a fully integrated, CCHIT®-certified, cloud-based EHR solution guaranteed to help providers meet meaningful use requirements, a term you will learn more about later in the chapter. The abbreviation **CCHIT®** stands for **Certification Commission for Health Information Technology**, an organization appointed by the Department of Health and Human Services (HHS) to certify electronic medical record software. Professionals using Harris CareTracker Physician EMR can access electronic health records seamlessly from any location through a secure and centralized gateway. Combining clinical and business workflows into one comprehensive system helps providers save staff time, enhance practice productivity, and simplify administrative workflows. Harris CareTracker Physician EMR is a web-based system that provides secure, one-click access to patient charts, refill requests, and lab results from any Internet-connected computer and is fully integrated with Harris CareTracker's Practice Management.

Learning to use the robust functionality of Harris CareTracker software will prepare you to use any EMR software on the market. In this chapter, you will learn the basics of electronic medical records and how to navigate throughout the *Medical Record* module within Harris CareTracker EMR.

ELECTRONIC MEDICAL RECORDS

Learning Objective 1: Define meaningful use and list its stages.

In Chapter 1, you learned that electronic medical records (EMRs) are patient records in digital format. EMRs can be found in all health care environments, but this chapter focuses on the utilization of EMRs in ambulatory care settings. For providers to obtain full reimbursement from governmental agencies such as Medicare and Medicaid, they must be in full compliance with specific guidelines set forth by those agencies. EMRs assist providers with meeting those guidelines.

Meaningful Use

EMRs have been in use for the past couple of decades, but their widespread adoption has skyrocketed in the past few years. This is largely due to Medicare and Medicaid financial incentives offered by the federal government for practices that meet meaningful use as well as the penalties that will take place later in the decade for not instituting EMR.

Background of Meaningful Use

The **Health Information Technology for Economic and Clinical Health (HITECH) Act** was signed into law on February 17, 2009, to promote the adoption and meaningful use of health information technology. HITECH was enacted as part of the **American Recovery and Reinvestment Act (ARRA)**, also known as the "stimulus bill." HITECH provides the Department of Health and Human Services (HHS) with the authority to establish programs to improve health care quality through the promotion of health information technology. Components of HITECH are promoted through incentives paid to providers for complying with the act. In future years, providers will face penalties through payment reductions for noncompliance of the bill.

Meaningful use is the way in which EHR technologies must be implemented and used for a provider to be eligible for the EHR Incentive Programs and to qualify for incentive payments. These incentives specify three components of meaningful use:

- The use of a certified EHR in a meaningful manner
- The use of certified EHR technology for electronic exchange of health information to improve quality of health care
- The use of certified EHR technology to submit clinical quality and other measures

The purpose of **meaningful use** is not only to institute the adoption of EMRs, but to ascertain that practices use their EHR software to its fullest. Benefits of meaningful use include complete and accurate medical records, better access to information, and patient empowerment. One of the major goals of meaningful use is to make medical records interoperable so that immediate access can be given to any provider who works with the patient. Three stages are associated with meaningful use.

Stage 1: Data Capture and Sharing Stage.   This stage focuses on the following:

- Electronic capturing of health information in a coded format
- Using electronically captured health information to track key clinical conditions and communicate information for care coordination purposes
- Implementing clinical decision support tools to facilitate disease and medication management
- Reporting information for quality improvement and public health information

Two sets of objectives must be met to prove attestation for this stage: core and menu. All of the core objectives are required; however, eligible providers may choose which menu set objectives to follow. Eligible providers (EPs) must be credentialed with Medicare and may be a doctor of medicine or osteopathy, doctor of dental surgery or medicine, doctor of podiatric medicine, doctor of optometry, or a chiropractor. Medicaid EPs include physicians, dentists, certified nurse-midwives, nurse practitioners, and physician assistants. Providers in the health care setting can only apply for attestation with either Medicare or Medicaid but not both.

Meaningful Use Criteria for Eligible Professionals.   Meaningful use criteria require providers to meet 14 core objectives, 5 out of 10 menu set objectives, and 6 total clinical quality measures. Figures 5-1A and 5-1B illustrate what is included in the core and menu set objectives. (In Figure 5-1A, please note that core objective C-12 was required through 2013, but will not be a requirement moving forward.) Stage 1 was implemented in 2011 and 2012.

Stage 2: Advance Clinical Processes.   This stage focuses on expanding on Stage 1 criteria to encourage the use of health information technology (HIT) for continuous quality improvement at the point of care and the exchange of health information in the most structured format possible. Criteria for Stage 2 include:

- More rigorous health information exchange (HIE)
- Increased requirements for e-prescribing and incorporating lab results
- Electronic transmission of patient care summaries across multiple settings
- More patient-controlled data

The final rule for Stage 2 was released in October 2012 and is expected to be implemented in 2014. In Stage 2, eligible providers must meet 17 core objectives and 3 of 6 menu objectives. Figures 5-2A and 5-2B illustrate the objectives for Stage 2 meaningful use.

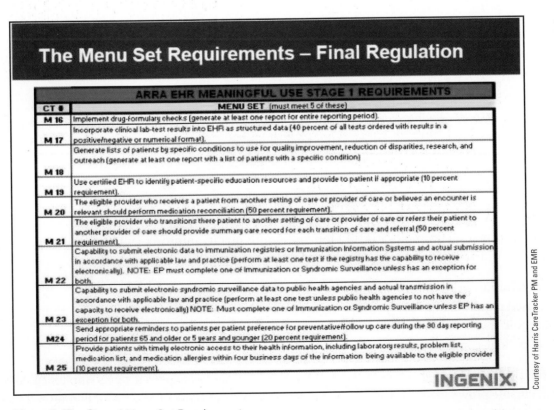

List of Core Requirements – Final Regulation

ARRA EHR MEANINGFUL USE STAGE 1 REQUIREMENTS

CT #	CORE REQUIREMENTS (must meet all of these)
C 1	Record demographics as structured data for preferred language, race, ethnicity, date of birth, and gender (50 percent requirement).
C 2	Record and chart changes in vital signs (BP, height, weight, & display BMI); additionally, plot and display growth charts for children age 2 to 20 including BMI (50 percent requirement).
C 3	Maintain an up-to-date problem list of current and active diagnoses based on ICD-9-CM or SNOMED CT (80 percent of all unique patients admitted have at least one entry or an indication of "no problems are known" recorded as structured data).
C 4	Maintain active medication list with at least one entry or indication of "no currently prescribed medications" as structured data (80 percent requirement).
C 5	Maintain active medication allergy list with at least one entry or indication of "no known medication allergies" as structured data (80 percent requirement).
C 6	Record smoking status for patients 13 years old or older as structured data (50 percent requirement).
C 7	Provide patient with clinical summary for patients for each office visit within 3 business days (more than 50 percent for all office visits).
C 8	Provide patients with electronic copy of their health information (problems, medication, medication allergies, diagnostic test results) upon request (50 percent of patients must receive electronic copy within three days).
C 9	Generate and transmit permissible prescriptions electronically — eRx (40 percent requirement, does not apply to hospitals)
C 10	Use CPOE for medication orders directly entered by any licensed healthcare professional who can enter orders into the medical record per state, local, and professional guidelines. (30 percent for patients with at least one medication ordered through CPOE)
C 11	Implement drug-drug and drug-allergy interaction checks (functionality is enabled for these checks for the entire reporting period)
C 12	Implement capability to electronically exchange key clinical information among providers and patient authorized entities (Perform at least one test of EHR's capacity to exchange information)
C 13	Implement one clinical decision support rule relevant to specialty or high clinical priority along with and ability to track compliance for that rule.
C 14	Protect electronic health information created or maintained by the certified EHR technology through the implementation of appropriate technical capabilities (conduct or review a security risk analysis in accordance with the requirements and implement security updates as necessary)
C 15	Report ambulatory clinical quality measures to CMS or states (For 2011, provide aggregate numerator, denominator, and exclusions through attestation, 2012 submit electronically).

© Ingenix, Inc. 6

INGENIX.

Figure 5-1A   Stage 1 List of Core Requirements

The Menu Set Requirements – Final Regulation

ARRA EHR MEANINGFUL USE STAGE 1 REQUIREMENTS

CT #	MENU SET (must meet 5 of these)
M 16	Implement drug-formulary checks (generate at least one report for entire reporting period).
M 17	Incorporate clinical lab-test results into EHR as structured data (40 percent of all tests ordered with results in a positive/negative or numerical format).
M 18	Generate lists of patients by specific conditions to use for quality improvement, reduction of disparities, research, and outreach (generate at least one report with a list of patients with a specific condition)
M 19	Use certified EHR to identify patient-specific education resources and provide to patient if appropriate (10 percent requirement).
M 20	The eligible provider who receives a patient from another setting of care or provider of care or believes an encounter is relevant should perform medication reconciliation (50 percent requirement).
M 21	The eligible provider who transitions there patient to another setting of care or provider of care or refers their patient to another provider of care should provide summary care record for each transition of care and referral (50 percent requirement).
M 22	Capability to submit electronic data to immunization registries or Immunization Information Systems and actual submission in accordance with applicable law and practice (perform at least one test if the registry has the capability to receive electronically). NOTE: EP must complete one of Immunization or Syndromic Surveillance unless has an exception for both.
M 23	Capability to submit electronic syndromic surveillance data to public health agencies and actual transmission in accordance with applicable law and practice (perform at least one test unless public health agencies to not have the capacity to receive electronically) NOTE: Must complete one of Immunization or Syndromic Surveillance unless EP has an exception for both.
M24	Send appropriate reminders to patients per patient preference for preventative/follow up care during the 90 day reporting period for patients 65 and older or 5 years and younger (20 percent requirement).
M 25	Provide patients with timely electronic access to their health information, including laboratory results, problem list, medication list, and medication allergies within four business days of the information being available to the eligible provider (10 percent requirement).

INGENIX.

Figure 5-1B   Stage 1 Menu Set Requirements

Eligible Professionals

Report on all 17 Core Objectives:
1. Use computerized provider order entry (CPOE) for medication, laboratory and radiology orders
2. Generate and transmit permissible prescriptions electronically (eRx)
3. Record demographic information
4. Record and chart changes in vital signs
5. Record smoking status for patients 13 years old or older
6. Use clinical decision support to improve performance on high-priority health conditions
7. Provide patients the ability to view online, download and transmit their health information
8. Provide clinical summaries for patients for each office visit
9. Protect electronic health information created or maintained by the Certified EHR Technology
10. Incorporate clinical lab-test results into Certified EHR Technology
11. Generate lists of patients by specific conditions to use for quality improvement, reduction of disparities, research, or outreach
12. Use clinically relevant information to identify patients who should receive reminders for preventive/follow-up care
13. Use certified EHR technology to identify patient-specific education resources
14. Perform medication reconciliation
15. Provide summary of care record for each transition of care or referral
16. Submit electronic data to immunization registries
17. Use secure electronic messaging to communicate with patients on relevant health information

Courtesy of CMS.gov

Figure 5-2A Stage 2 List of Core Requirements

Report on 3 of 6 Menu Objectives:
1. Submit electronic syndromic surveillance data to public health agencies
2. Record electronic notes in patient records
3. Imaging results accessible through CEHRT
4. Record patient family health history
5. Identify and report cancer cases to a State cancer registry
6. Identify and report specific cases to a specialized registry (other than a cancer registry)

Courtesy of CMS.gov

Figure 5-2B Stage 2 Menu Set Requirements

Stage 3: Improved Outcomes. This stage focuses on the following:

- Promoting improvements in quality, safety, and efficiency
- Clinical decision support for national high-priority conditions
- Patient access to self-management tools
- Improving population health

This stage is expected to be implemented in 2017.

Tools within Harris CareTracker to Assist Providers with Meaningful Use

Learning Objective 2: Discuss tools within Harris CareTracker PM and EMR that assist with meaningful use.

The *Meaningful Use Dashboard* within Harris CareTracker PM tracks a provider's progress toward meeting the Medicare and Medicaid EHR Incentive Program reporting requirements for the core and menu set items. The dashboard displays a progress bar next to each of the measures that has a reporting requirement. Figure 5-3A illustrates a graphing screen of the core requirements for Dr. Olivia Sherman and Figure 5-3B illustrates the graphing features of the menu set requirements for Dr. Olivia Sherman. (Dr. Sherman is not a provider in our environment.)

The dashboard's default date range is determined by when the provider begins the **attestation period**, or the date that begins the 90-day reporting period of meeting the core and menu measures listed previously. The dashboard calculates these measures over the previous 90 days.

From the dashboard you can

- Customize the requirements displayed on the dashboard for each participating provider
- View a status of a provider's progress for the last 90 days (percentages updated nightly)

Tip Box

Before we start working in the EMR side of Harris CareTracker, we need to review settings within the PM side and make the appropriate adjustments to accommodate each provider's preference.

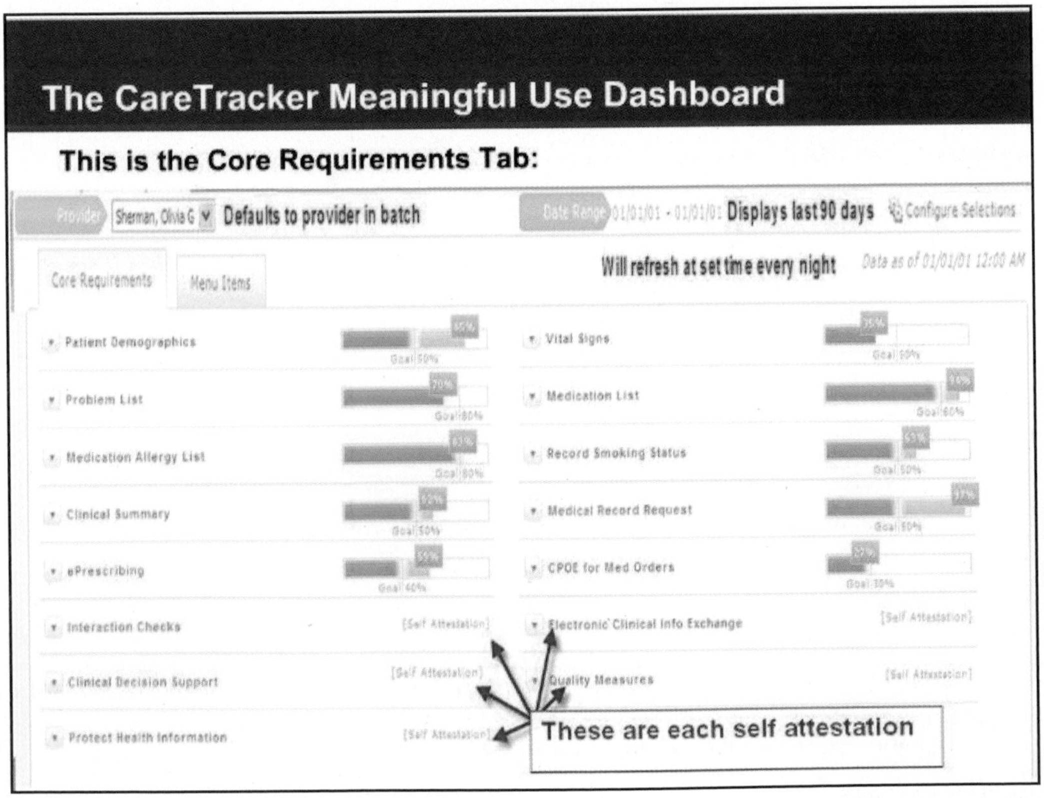

Figure 5-3A   Core Requirements for Dr. Olivia Sherman

Courtesy of Harris CareTracker PM and EMR

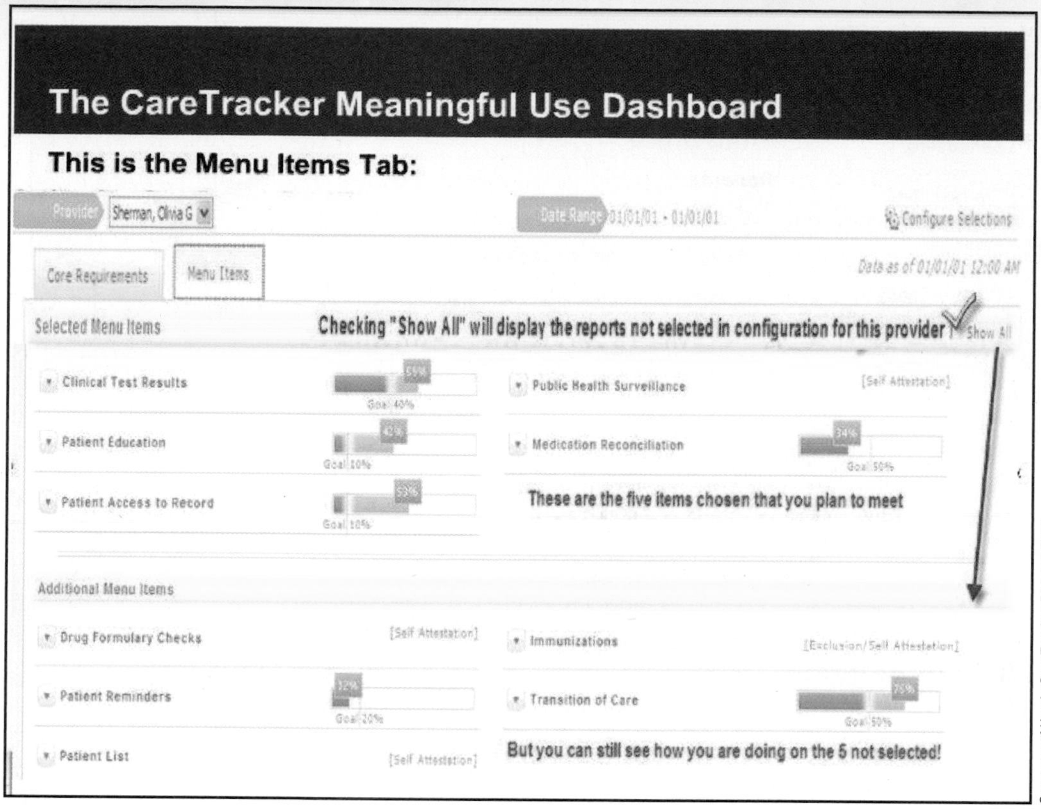

Courtesy of Harris CareTracker PM and EMR

Figure 5-3B Menu Requirements for Dr. Olivia Sherman

- Hover over the percentage bar to review the data used to calculate the provider's percentage
- Click the *Menu Items* tab and then the drop-down arrow to download reference documents or run Key Performance Indicator (KPI) reports

Learning Objective 3: View and read the meaningful use dashboard in Harris CareTracker PM and EMR.

ACTIVITY 5-1: Viewing the *Meaningful Use Dashboard*

Note: Any time you are working in the EMR side of Harris CareTracker, you need to make sure that "Compatibility View" is turned off in your Internet Explorer browser. If you experience any functionality issues, please check your settings.)

1. Click the *Home* module.
2. Click the *Meaningful Use* tab under the *Dashboard* tab (Figure 5-4). Harris CareTracker PM displays *the Meaningful Use Dashboard.*
3. From the *Provider* list, select the name of the provider whose data you want to view. In this case, click on "Dr. Brockton". Harris CareTracker PM displays the provider's percentages on the *Core Requirements* tab (Figure 5-5).

Print the Core Requirements screen, label it "Activity 5-1A," and place it in your assignment folder.

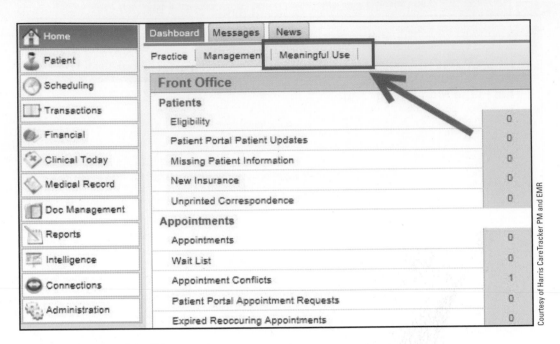

Figure 5-4 Meaningful Use Tab

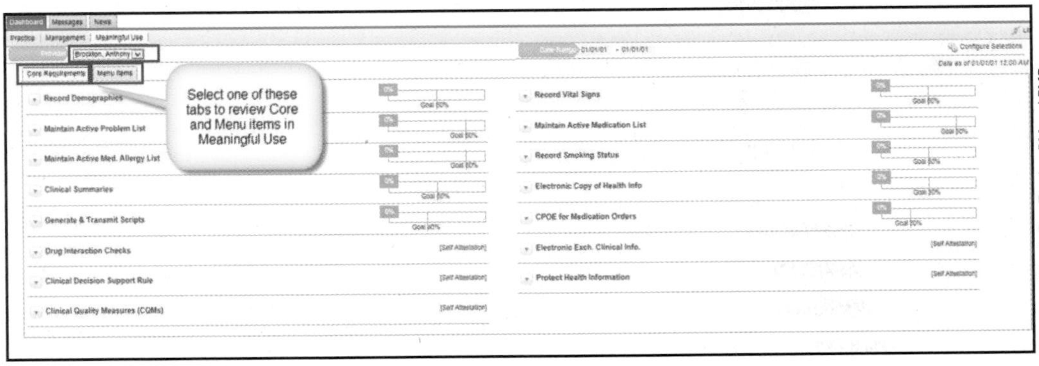

Figure 5-5 Dr. Brockton's Core Requirements

4. Click the *Menu Items* tab to view the *Menu Items* requirements. On the *Menu Items* tab, select the *Show All* checkbox on the right-hand side of the screen to view any excluded requirements.

Print the Menu Items screen, label it "Activity 5-1B," and place it in your assignment folder.

Because this is a training environment, you are only able to see the shell; no meaningful use statistics are available. Figure 5-6 illustrates what a *Core Requirements* tab looks like in a fully functional environment.

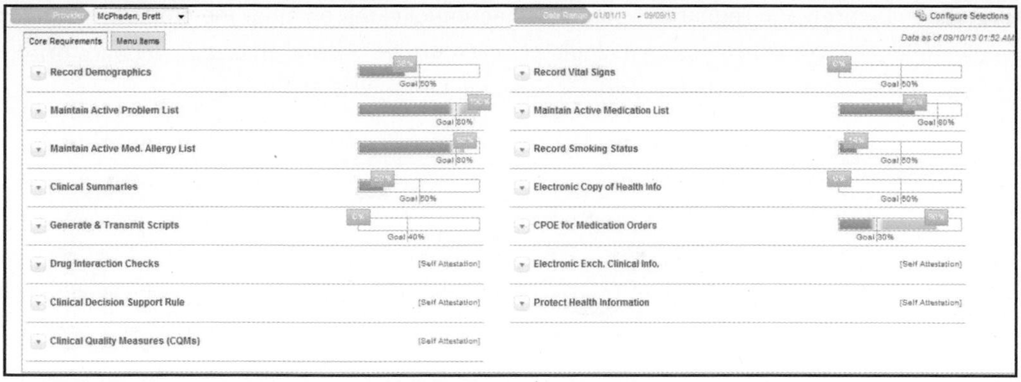

Courtesy of Harris CareTracker PM and EMR

Figure 5-6 Core Requirements in a Fully Functional Environment

Activating Care Management

Learning Objective 4: Activate the care management registries in Harris CareTracker PM and EMR.

The *Care Management* feature in Harris CareTracker PM and EMR allows practices to set clinical measures for health maintenance and disease management registries. The registries will assist with early identification of disease and early treatment. Keeping up to date with immunizations will help to prevent future disease and control costs associated with those diseases. This feature also assists in meeting some of the standards of meaningful use.

By default, clinical measures are turned off in Harris CareTracker PM and EMR. You need to activate the registries and measures you want to make available to the providers in your group. As you will observe, these registries will check to ascertain that the patient is up to date with preventive testing and immunizations. After activation, the registries and measures selected are included in the *Pt Care Management* application of the *Medical Record* module and the *Care Management* application of the *Clinical Today* module. Registries are repopulated with the *Clinical Today/Population Management* tab. Once activation occurs, anytime you open the patient's chart, you can see where he or she falls within the registries and help the patient to come into compliance with testing or procedures.

ACTIVITY 5-2: Activating Care Management Items

1. Click on the *Administration* module and then click the *Clinical* tab.
2. Click the *Care Management Activation* link under the *Maintenances* heading (Figure 5-7A). Harris CareTracker PM and EMR launches the *Care Management Activation* application.

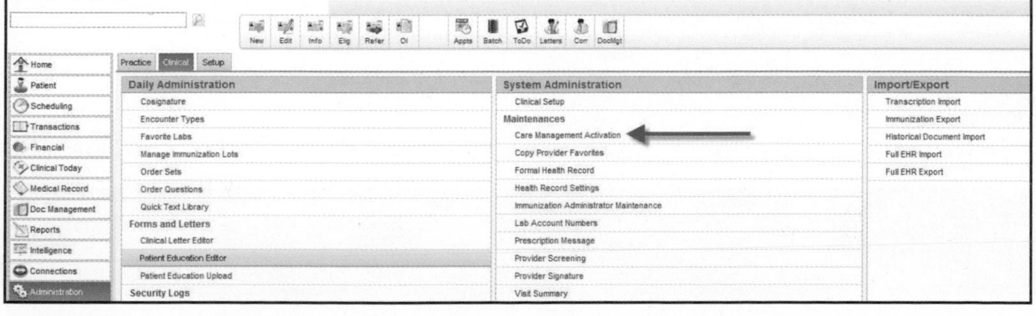

Courtesy of Harris CareTracker PM and EMR

Figure 5-7A Care Management Activation Link

3. Select all of the measures and registries listed by selecting/clicking on all of the boxes. The check boxes are dynamic and will auto-save on a single click. (A green "Saved" message appears briefly when each box is clicked to indicate the settings are saved [Figure 5-7B]).

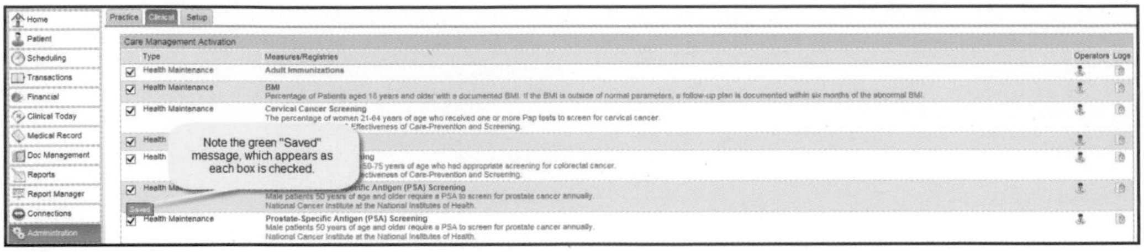

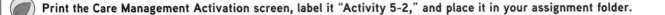

Figure 5-7B Care Activation Measures and Registries

Print the Care Management Activation screen, label it "Activity 5-2," and place it in your assignment folder.

4. Now click back on the *Clinical* tab and the *Care Management Activation* link to view the saved screen with all of the boxes checked.

Critical Thinking

As a clinical medical assistant, it will be your job to help patients stay current with prevention measures and disease management goals. This not only helps the practice stay in compliance with meaningful use, but also promotes improved overall health for the patient. Review Figure 5-8 and identify the patient's overdue test(s).

Outline an action plan to assist the patient in getting back on track with overall health prevention and maintenance. Share the action plan with the patient, and, if possible, schedule any necessary future appointments during the current visit to help the patient reach his or her overall goals. Submit your action plan to your instructor for class discussion.

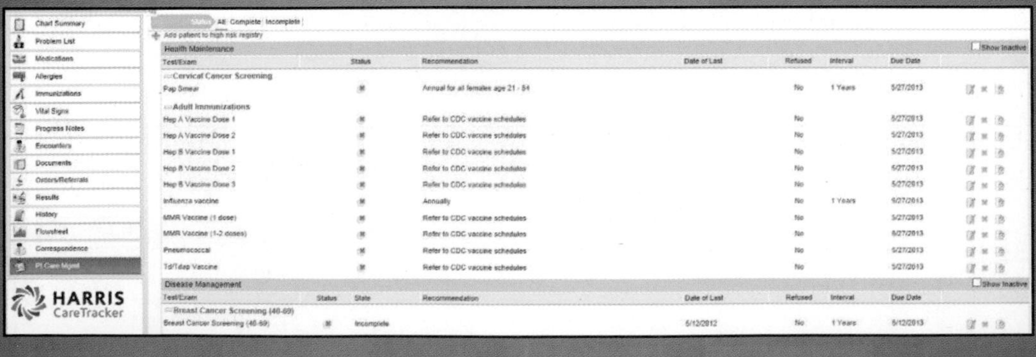

Figure 5-8 Patient Care Management Screen

Tip Box

To access the *Patient Care Management* screen in Harris CareTracker:

- Click on the *Medical Record* pane (you must have a patient in context).
- Click on the *Pt Care Mgmt* pane in the lower-left corner of your screen, and the patient's health maintenance record will display.
- The red "x" in the status column indicates that the patient is overdue for the test/exam recommendations.
- You can also sort the status by clicking on "All," "Complete," or "Incomplete" in the *Status* row at the top of the page.

NAVIGATING THE MEDICAL RECORD MODULE

Learning Objective 5: Navigate throughout the Medical Record module.

The *Medical Record* module is designed to mimic a paper chart and to follow the provider's normal workflow, facilitating effective EHR documentation for a patient. The module is accessed by pulling the patient into context on the *Name Bar* and then clicking the *Medical Record* module. If a patient has an appointment scheduled, you can click the patient name in the *Appointments* application of the *Clinical Today* module to launch the *Medical Record* module. You will learn more about the *Clinical Today* module in Chapter 6. Some of the primary advantages of the *Medical Record* module in Harris CareTracker PM and EMR are as follows:

- Reduces or eliminates chart supply and storage, transcription costs, malpractice premiums, and other costs
- Replaces paper charts and file cabinets with electronic files and minimizes space required to store paper charts
- Maximizes revenue with effective patient services, improves documentation capabilities, improves coding accuracy through use of templates, and enhances charge capturing
- Increases clinical and staff efficiency through reduced data entry, high-quality documentation, patient education, and more
- Includes multitasking capability to work on a number of patient records simultaneously
- Provides a user-friendly interface that helps customize the electronic paper chart to suit user needs

The *Medical Record* module consists of four main components: *Patient Detail Bar, Patient Health History* pane, *Clinical Toolbar*, and *Chart Summary*. Table 5-1 provides a brief description of each component.

TABLE 5-1 Medical Records Module Components

Component	Description
Patient Detail Bar	Provides a summarized view of demographic, appointment, and clinical information pertinent to the patient
Patient Health History Pane	A series of panes reviewing, entering, and editing historical patient information such as allergies, problem list, medications, and more
Clinical Toolbar	A series of tool buttons used as a workflow tool during a patient's appointment to record information such as progress notes, medications, immunizations, *Message Center*, visits, and more
Chart Summary	Provides an overview of a patient's medical record

Courtesy of Harris CareTracker PM and EMR

Patient Detail Bar

The *Patient Detail Bar* (Figure 5-9) can be found at the top of the window once you open the patient's medical record. Table 5-2 describes the components of the *Patient Detail Bar*.

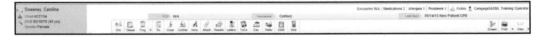

Figure 5-9 Patient Detail Bar

Courtesy of Harris CareTracker PM and EMR

TABLE 5-2 Patient Detail Bar Components

Component	Description
Patient Information	Located just to the left of the patient's name and includes the patient's name, address, telephone numbers, provider's name, and appointment information.
Patient Alert	A box that appears as a red triangle ⚠ below the *Patient Information Bar* and contains three types of alerts: clinical alerts, patient care management alerts, and clinical notes. The red triangle appears both inside and outside of the patient's record once the patient's name is brought into context. If the patient does not have any clinical alerts, a blue check mark appears in the space where the red triangle would normally appear to illustrate that there are no clinical concerns at this time.
Patient's Chart Number	Located beside the *Patient Alert* ⚠ and identifies the chart number assigned to the patient.
Break the Glass	The hammer ⚒ located below the *Patient Alert* icon. It allows users to review VIP patient charts, and patient charts from other groups when the practice has more than one group. Even though the user is not in the specified group, by breaking the glass, the user is able to review the contents of the patient's chart for that session. Users who have "Break the Glass" privileges must provide a reason for breaking the glass.
Patient's DOB and Age	This is located beside the hammer and lists the patient's birth date and age.

TABLE 5-2 (*Continued*)

Component	Description
Sex	Located just below the patient's DOB and states the patient's sex.
PCP	Located just above the clinical tool bar and lists the patient's primary care provider.
Insurance	Located to the right of the PCP and lists the patient's insurance provider.
Next Appointment Date	Located just to the right of the insurance information. Displays the patient's next scheduled appointment.
Last Appointment Date	Located to the right of the next appointment information. Lists when the patient's last appointment took place.
Encounter	Located above and to the right of the next appointment information. This is the area that you click on when you want to review dates of previous encounters or to create a new encounter.
Medications	Located beside encounter information and lists how many medications the patient is taking. By clicking on "Medications," you can see the names of the medications the patient is taking and their doses.
Allergies	Located by the medication information and lists the number of allergies the patient has. By clicking on "Allergies," you can see a listing of the patient's allergies.
Problems	Located beside the allergy information. This lists the number of diagnoses or problems that are considered current. By clicking on "Problems," you can see a list of diagnoses and ICD codes for the patient.
Notes	Located beside the problems. This lists any notes about the patient such as what the patient wants to be called, reminder information, etc.
Training Operator	Should include your sign-in name.

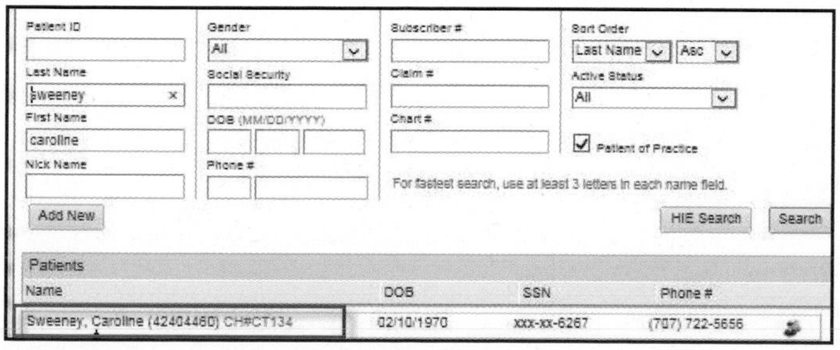

Courtesy of Harris CareTracker PM and EMR

ACTIVITY 5-3: Viewing a Summary of Patient Information

1. In the *ID* search box on the *Name Bar*, enter the last name "Sweeney" and hit [Enter]. The *Patient Search* dialog box displays with a list of patients matching the search criteria you entered.

2. Click on Caroline Sweeney's name to bring her record into context (Figure 5-10).

Figure 5-10 Click on Caroline Sweeney's Name to Bring Up Her Medical Record

3. Click on the *Patient* module, which will open the *Demographics* tab.

4. You will notice that in Caroline's demographics window, no primary care provider (PCP) has been selected. Click on *Edit*, then scroll down to *PCP*, click on the drop-down list, and select "Anthony Brockton" as her PCP. Click *Save*.

5. Click on the *Medical Record* module.

6. A clinical alert comes up alerting you that the patient is allergic to codeine. Click on *Close* to exit the box.

7. To view Caroline's summary information, click the *Patient Information* icon ⬛ to the left of the patient's name. Figure 5-11 illustrates what the summary looks like once you click on the *Patient Information* icon.

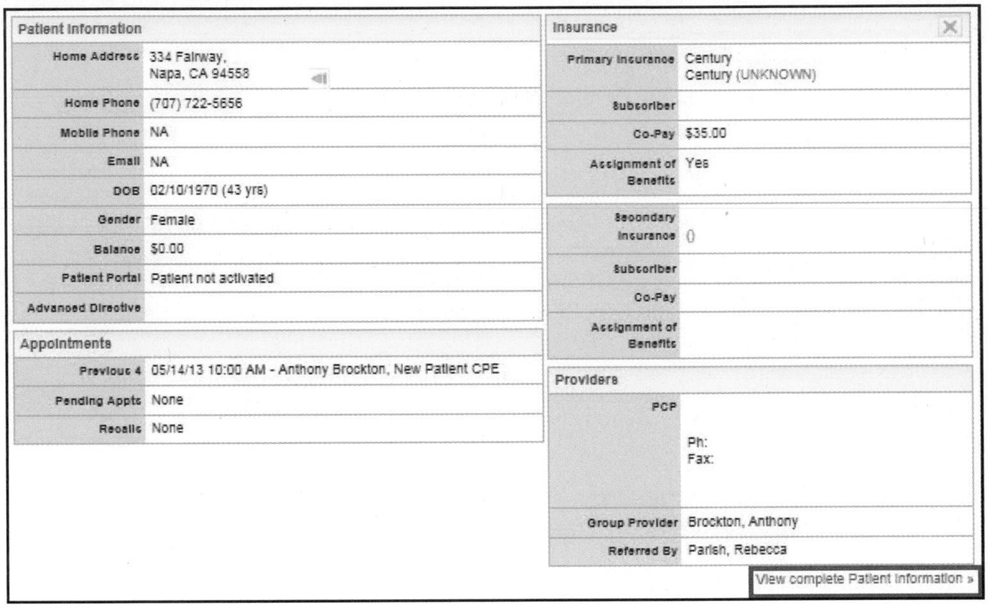

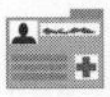

Patient Information		Insurance		✕
Home Address	334 Fairway, Napa, CA 94558 ◀	Primary Insurance	Century Century (UNKNOWN)	
Home Phone	(707) 722-5656	Subscriber		
Mobile Phone	NA	Co-Pay	$35.00	
Email	NA	Assignment of Benefits	Yes	
DOB	02/10/1970 (43 yrs)			
Gender	Female	Secondary Insurance	()	
Balance	$0.00	Subscriber		
Patient Portal	Patient not activated	Co-Pay		
Advanced Directive		Assignment of Benefits		
Appointments		**Providers**		
Previous 4	05/14/13 10:00 AM - Anthony Brockton, New Patient CPE	PCP		
Pending Appts	None		Ph: Fax:	
Recalls	None			
		Group Provider	Brockton, Anthony	
		Referred By	Parish, Rebecca	
			View complete Patient Information »	

Courtesy of Harris CareTracker PM and EMR

Figure 5-11   Patient Information Screen

8. To view additional patient information details, click the *View complete Patient Information* link on the lower right of the window. Figure 5-12 illustrates what the window should like once you click on the *View complete Patient Information* link.

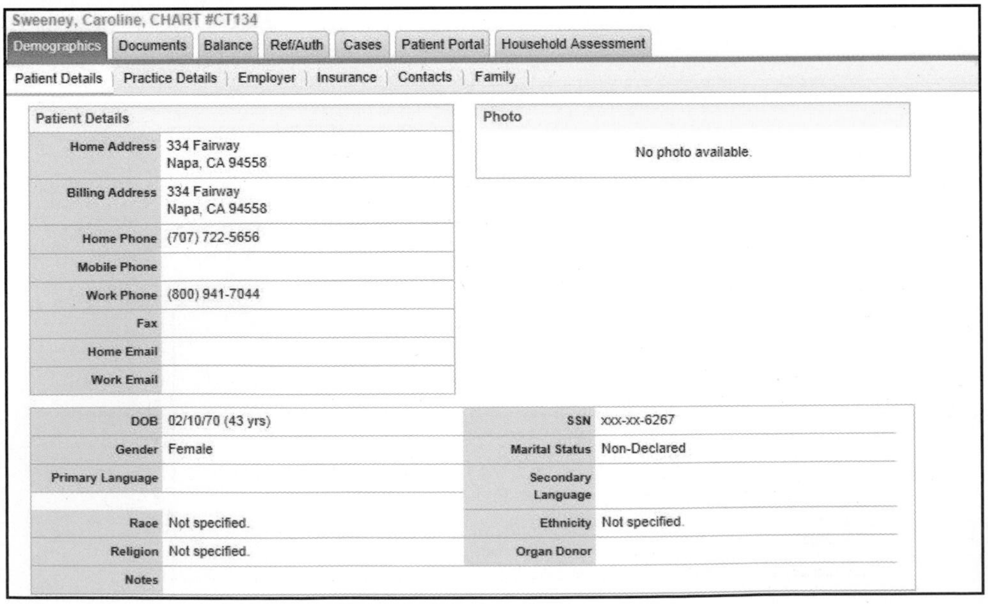

Sweeney, Caroline, CHART #CT134

Demographics | Documents | Balance | Ref/Auth | Cases | Patient Portal | Household Assessment

Patient Details | Practice Details | Employer | Insurance | Contacts | Family

Patient Details		Photo	
Home Address	334 Fairway Napa, CA 94558	No photo available.	
Billing Address	334 Fairway Napa, CA 94558		
Home Phone	(707) 722-5656		
Mobile Phone			
Work Phone	(800) 941-7044		
Fax			
Home Email			
Work Email			
DOB	02/10/70 (43 yrs)	SSN	xxx-xx-6267
Gender	Female	Marital Status	Non-Declared
Primary Language		Secondary Language	
Race	Not specified.	Ethnicity	Not specified.
Religion	Not specified.	Organ Donor	
Notes			

Courtesy of Harris CareTracker PM and EMR

Figure 5-12   View Complete Patient Information Link

Print the View complete Patient Information screen by right-clicking on the screen and selecting the Print function. Label it "Activity 5-3" and place it in your assignment folder.

9. Close out "X" from this screen.

10. Close out of Caroline Sweeney's *Chart Summary* by clicking "X" on the browser window.

Viewing Encounter Information

Learning Objective 6: View the patient's encounter information, medications, allergy information, and problem list.

An **encounter** is an interaction with a patient on a specific date at a specific time and includes visits, phone calls, renewal requests, results, and more. Each patient can have many encounters, each encounter can have many services, and each service can have many CPT® codes associated with it. You must review, capture visit information, transcribe, sign, and bill appointment-based patient "visit"-type encounters, something you will learn more about in subsequent chapters. Additionally, you must capture visit information and bill custom encounters that are flagged as "Billing Required." You must also transcribe and sign notes for encounters that are flagged as "Signed Note Required."

In addition, the *Encounters* application enables you to view the primary diagnosis pertaining to an encounter and sort encounters based on specific diagnoses. This makes it easy to review data for a specific diagnosis when seeing patients for a recurring problem.

ACTIVITY 5-4: Viewing the Encounters Application, Active Medications, Allergies, and Problems

1. Pull patient Caroline Sweeney into context.

2. Click on the *Medical Record* module.

3. To view Caroline Sweeney's encounter information, click on the word *Encounter* (which appears blue) in the detail bar (at the top right of the screen). A box with a listing of the patient's previous encounters will pop up as well as an option to create a new encounter (Figure 5-13). Make a note of the date of the patient's only encounter.

5/14/2013

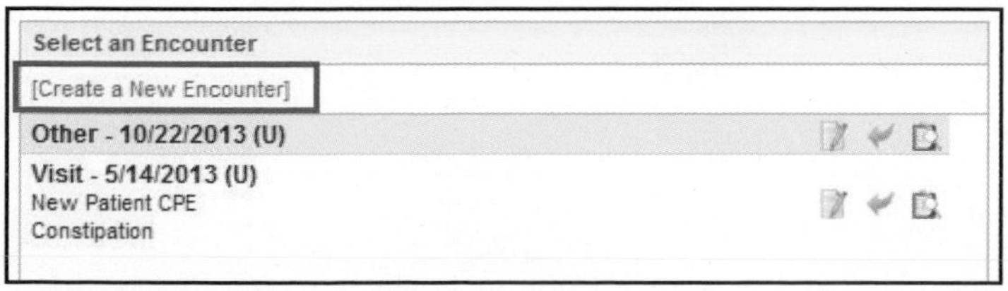

Figure 5-13 Creating a New Encounter

4. Close the encounter window by clicking on the "X" in the top right corner of the window.

5. To view clinical information for the patient, such as the active medications, allergies, and problems, click the corresponding links in the *Patient Detail* bar (located in the upper-right portion of your screen on the same line following *Encounter*).

On a blank sheet of paper write down the date of the patient's only encounter, a listing of the patient's active medications, and any problems listed for the patient. Label the page "Activity 5-4" and place it in your assignment folder.

6. Close out Caroline Sweeney's chart summary by clicking "X" on the browser window.

Learning Objective 7: State the three types of alerts in Harris CareTracker PM and EMR.

Viewing Patient Alerts. In Chapter 3, you learned about patient alerts. This chapter expands on the clinical components of this feature. You can view clinical alert information for a patient by clicking on the *Alert* ⚠ icon next to the chart number in the *Medical Record* module. Harris CareTracker PM and EMR displays the *Clinical Alerts* dialog box with three patient alert types. Table 5-3 describes each alert type.

TABLE 5-3 Alert Types

Alert	Description
Clinical Alerts	Alerts with important information related to the patient's health. The clinical alerts are categorized to display alerts for patient allergies, medications, diagnoses, and more.
	Additionally, for OB/GYN practices, the clinical alerts provide you the ability to view estimated gestational age (EGA) alerts. However, EGA alerts display only if a patient has V22.0-V22.2, V23.0-V23.5, V23.7-V23.9, V23.41, V23.49, V23.81-V23.86, or V23.89 recorded as an active diagnosis.
Patient Care Management Alerts	Alerts for overdue important patient health maintenance and disease management items.
Clinical Notes	Clinical notes entered in the *Demographic* application of the *Patient* module.

Courtesy of Harris CareTracker PM and EMR

ACTIVITY 5-5: Viewing Patient Alerts in the Patient's Medical Record

1. Pull patient Caroline Sweeney into context.

2. Click on *Medical Record*.

3. When you open the *Medical Record*, the alert box automatically pops up. Review the information in the box before closing it out. Close out of the box by clicking on *Close*.

4. Click on the red triangle ⚠ to the left of the chart number. Notice that the information that pops up here is the same clinical alert information that popped up when you opened the medical record.

Tip Box

You might need to scroll down the screen to see all the information.

Write down any alerts listed for Caroline on a piece of paper. Label the page "Activity 5-5" and place it in your assignment folder.

5. Click *Close* on the *Clinical Alerts* box.
6. Close Caroline Sweeney's *Chart Summary* screen.

Patient Medical History Pane

The *Patient Medical History* pane (Figure 5-14) is a series of panes located to the left of the *Chart Summary* in the *Medical Record* module that you can use to access different applications for reviewing, entering, and editing patient information such as diagnoses, medications, and more. The function of each pane is described in Table 5-4.

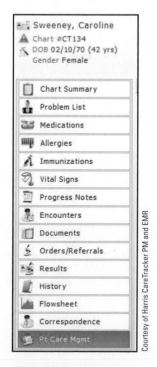

Figure 5-14 Patient Medical History Pane

TABLE 5-4 Patient Medical History Panes

Patient Medical History Pane	Function
Chart Summary	A view-only window displaying a summary of patient medical information. The *Chart Summary* is customizable based on the layout and level of detail you want to see.
Problem List	A list of chronic and ongoing patient problems. The *Problem List* application helps you to add and edit patient diagnoses including conditions managed by other physicians.
Medications	Displays all prescribed medications for the patient. The *Medications* application helps you to add and edit routine and over-the-counter (OTC) medications, medications provided by other providers, and also renew existing prescriptions.
Allergies	A list of patient allergies. The *Allergies* application helps you to add and edit allergies and other types of sensitivities. It is important to keep all allergy information updated, especially medication allergies, for screening purposes.
Immunizations	A list of immunizations given to the patient. The application provides access to child and adult immunization schedules and helps record any immunizations refused by the patient.
Vital Signs	*Vital Signs* displays patient statistics such as height, weight, and blood pressure taken during each office visit or at home. The *Vital Signs* application helps you to record vital signs for each "visit" type encounter. Harris CareTracker PM and EMR supports graphing of vital signs to help identify trends.
Progress Notes	Displays information about patient visits documented via quick text, point and click, dictation, or a combination of methods. It is important to review and sign notes taken during a visit.
Encounters	Displays all patient encounters. These encounters can vary from a telephone conversation to an office visit.
Documents	Displays all scanned or uploaded documents and voice recordings for the patient; for example, clinical documents, insurance cards, or identification cards. You can open the documents in the *Document Viewer* to add annotations, edit, delete, and sign.
Orders/Referrals	Displays test orders and referrals for the patient. The *Orders* application works simultaneously with the *Results* application to provide quick access to test results of completed orders, enabling entering of manual results and linking to lab results received electronically. The *Referrals* application enables you to manage the process of patient movement between primary care providers, specialists, and institutions.
Results	Displays patient test results. Abnormal results display in red to help identify issues needing immediate attention. The *Results* application works simultaneously with the *Orders* application, enabling you to view the order associated with the result.
History	Displays patient information such as the family, past medical and social history. The application enables recording more information for existing and additional family members when necessary.
Flowsheet	Displays clinical measures, allowing you to track several aspects of a patient's health at one time. *Medical Flow Sheets* are most commonly used for tracking vital statistics, diabetic insulin dosages, pain assessment, lab results, blood pressure, medication start and stop dates, physical assessment, and drug frequency. It is also a good solution for pediatric growth charts and prenatal recordings.
Correspondence	Displays all *To Do*(s) for the patient and other communications such as patient education, recall, or collection letters provided or mailed to the patient.
Pt Care Mgmt	Displays a list of overdue preventive or maintenance items such as screening plans that need to be completed for the patient.

CLINICAL SP⬤TLIGHT

To familiarize yourself with these panes, go into Caroline Sweeney's medical record, click out of the alert box, and click on each of the panes in the *Patient Medical History Pane* (e.g., click on *Chart Summary, Problem List, Medications*, etc.). You will learn the specifics of each pane in future activities.

Clinical Toolbar

The *Clinical Toolbar* (Figure 5-15) is a convenient workflow tool you can use to record information during a patient appointment. The toolbar can be found in the *Chart Summary* tab of the *Medical Record* module and contains a series of tool buttons. The function of each button is described in Table 5-5.

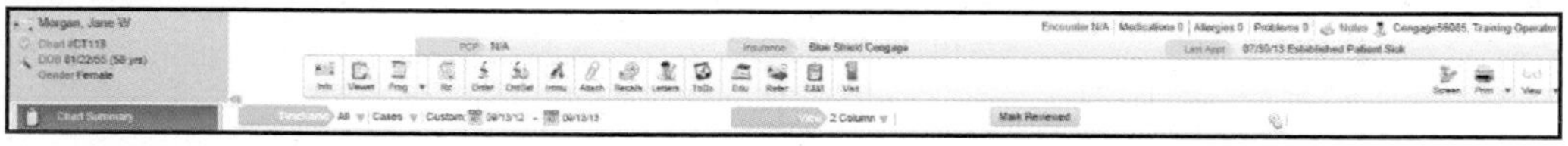

Figure 5-15   Clinical Toolbar
Courtesy of Harris CareTracker PM and EMR

TABLE 5-5   Parts of the Clinical Toolbar

Clinical Tool Button	Function
Patient Information	The *Patient Information* window provides access to a patient's demographic, appointment, and other information. The information is grouped into categories and is accessible by clicking the specific tab. You can also view a picture of the patient, if available. For information on the *Patient Information* window, see *Name Bar > Info* in the *Help* system.
Chart Viewer	The *Chart Viewer* provides a quick and easy way to access other applications when documenting a clinical encounter at the point of care. Each section corresponds to data saved in Harris CareTracker PM and EMR for the patient.
Progress Note	The *New Progress Notes* application helps you document the patient visits in various methods that include diagnosis specific guidelines, provider specific templates, pick list templates, dictation, or a combination of all. Harris CareTracker PM and EMR supports a variety of data entry methods including quick text, pen-tablets with handwriting recognition, voice recognition, or point-and-click mechanism.
Prescriptions (Rx)	The *Rx Writer* application (Surescripts® certified for prescription routing), uses the Surescripts® network to transmit electronic prescriptions directly to a selected pharmacy. A medication is always screened for interactions before it is prescribed. Additionally, the application provides a dosing calculator to view dosage recommendations for medications based on weight and age.

(Continues)

TABLE 5-5   *(Continued)*

Clinical Tool Button	Function
Order	The *Orders* application enables you to enter new orders and process orders by printing and sending to a clinical lab or by sending electronically via the Health Level 7 (HL7) interface. Orders sent electronically provide speed and efficiency for processing and reduces the amount of time spent filling in the lab requisition and related paperwork. **Note:** Electronic orders are currently being implemented in Harris CareTracker and will be available soon. Presently there are some bi-directional interfaces with labs, but the majority are uni-directional, which means a *Results*-only HUB interface has been created (e.g., you write an order, print it, hand it to the patient; the patient goes to the lab, completes the requested tests; the lab sends the results back to the customer through the system [electronically]).
Order Set	The *Order Set* application enables you to group patient orders for a specific diagnosis or condition. This promotes efficiency during the clinical decision-making process, standardizes the patient care processes, expedites the process of order entry, and reduces delays due to inconsistent or incomplete orders. The *Order Set* application helps create, modify, and manage order sets, making it available among all providers.
Immunizations	The *Immunization* application facilitates documenting immunizations administered during a patient visit. Additionally, the application helps administer vaccinations from a "lot" and helps you manage information on immunization lots that pertain to the group. **Lot** is defined by the U.S. Food and Drug Administration as a collection of primary containers or units of the same size, type, and style manufactured or packed under similar conditions and handled as a single unit of trade.
Attachments	The *Document Management Upload* application helps upload or scan documents that include anything from a letter to a medical report for the patient. Examples of documents include lab results, radiology reports, dictations, photographs, and insurance cards. In addition, you can record audio files with information about the patient. For example, you can record a voice mail message that you left for the patient regarding a treatment process.
Recalls	The *Recall* application helps create patient reminders and letters for events such as annual physical exams, follow-up consultations, and lab tests. This feature helps the office to keep track of patients and ensure that proper medical care is provided.
Letters	The *Letters* application helps generate and print anything from a letter to a label for a patient by extracting information from the patient medical record. For example, referral letters, surgery prior consent letters, and appointment letters.
Message Center	The *Messages* application facilitates patient-related communications with patients (if the patient is registered in Harris CareTracker's Patient Portal), office staff, and Harris CareTracker PM and EMR Support Department staff without having to pull or file a chart. For example, a provider can send a *ToDo* to the front office staff to call the patient. There are three components in the Message Center: (1) New ToDo (2) New Fax, and (3) New Mail.
Patient Education	The *Patient Education* application gives you access to a comprehensive library of education material provided by Krames StayWell (the largest provider of interactive, print and mobile patient education solutions, consumer health information, and population health management communications in the country). This is useful to view and print disease-specific educational information you can give to a patient. The application also provides links to clinical websites (such as Medline Plus) and specialty-specific associations.

TABLE 5-5 *(Continued)*	
Clinical Tool Button	**Function**
Referral	The *Referral* application helps manage inbound and outbound referrals and authorizations. This helps manage the process of patient movement between primary care providers, specialists, and institutions.
E&M Evaluator	The *E&M Evaluator* application helps identify the most appropriate E&M procedure (CPT®) code to use when charging for office visits and consultations. The code is calculated based on the information documented during the visit. Additionally, the application helps you apply either the 1995 or the 1997 E&M Documentation Guidelines issued by the American Medical Association (AMA) and the Centers for Medicare and Medicaid Services (CMS) to identify the correct code for the level of service provided.
Visits	The *Visits* application helps capture information such as CPT® and ICD codes about the patient encounter. The electronic format supports a paperless information capturing system and is helpful for submitting claims to the corresponding insurance companies in an expedited manner, helping to increase the practice cash flow.
Screen	The *Screen* feature enables you to check for drug interactions in real time for the patient in context. This complete screening is for informational purposes only and includes interactions based on active diagnoses, medications and allergies, patient's age and weight, duplicate therapy, food interactions, and precaution screening.
Print	The *Print* feature helps export patient data into a PDF format in one- or two-column layout. Additionally, you can print the chart summary, formal medical record, visit summary, and also print reports pertaining to each section in the patient's medical record. For example, you can access the *Medications* application, and click *Print* on the *Clinical* toolbar to print the Medication Summary Report.
View	The *View* feature enables you to view the Clinical Log and the Continuity of Care Document (CCD) of the patient. Additionally, the feature displays interfaces active for your company. However, you can access the interface only if data is available for the patient in context.

Courtesy of Harris CareTracker PM and EMR

You will be using these tools throughout your training activities.

Chart Summary

Learning Objective 8: View, change, and print a Chart Summary in Harris CareTracker EMR.

The *Chart Summary* is a paperless format of a patient's medical record. It is a proprietary display that serves as a medical and legal record of a patient's clinical status, care history, and caregiver involvement.

The information on the *Chart Summary* is taken from various applications within Harris CareTracker PM and EMR. Information available in the *Chart Summary* includes contact and personnel information for providing medical services, problem and medication lists, lab results, patient history, and other information. You can access the *Chart Summary* by clicking on the *Medical Record* module.

ACTIVITY 5-6:   Accessing a Patient Chart Summary Using the Name Bar

1. Pull patient Caroline Sweeney into context.

2. Click the *Medical Record* module.

3. Review the *Clinical Alerts* dialog box and close.

4. By default, the *Chart Summary* tab displays from the *Patient Health History* pane. (Your screen should look like Figure 5-16.) Review all of the categories in the *Chart Summary* by scrolling up and down using the scroll bar.

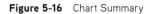

Figure 5-16   Chart Summary

5. To change the look of the *Chart Summary*, find the gray *View* tab in the middle of the page, just below the *Clinical Toolbar* (Figure 5-17). Click on the drop-down arrow next to the *View* tab and change the view to "3 Column."

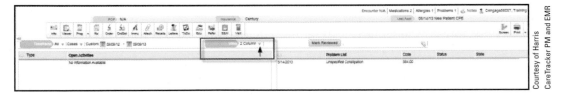

Figure 5-17   View Column Drop-Down Menu

Click on the drop-down arrow next to the Printer 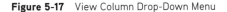 icon and select "Print Chart Summary." Label the printed chart summary "Activity 5-6" and place it in your assignment folder.

6. Close Caroline Sweeney's *Chart Summary* screen.

MAINTENANCE FUNCTIONS THAT AFFECT HARRIS CARETRACKER EMR

Learning Objective 9: Perform routine maintenance functions in Harris CareTracker PM and EMR such as adding a room, editing a room, adding a custom resource, adding favorite labs, removing favorite labs, and managing immunizations.

We have finished our navigation of the *Medical Record* module and are ready to make other adjustments in the PM side of Harris CareTracker. These adjustments will affect available options and other features displayed on the EMR side. There are several maintenance options in Harris CareTracker; however, we only spotlight a few features that impact the EMR.

Room Maintenance

It is important to have an efficient appointment workflow to better serve the patient during an appointment. The *Room Maintenance* feature helps you set up rooms to keep track of a patient appointment by updating a patient's location during his or her stay at your office. Building upon room maintenance activities completed in Chapter 2, continue with Activity 5-7, which illustrates how to add and name rooms within the system.

ACTIVITY 5-7: Adding a Room

1. Click the *Administration* module and then click the *Setup* tab.
2. Click the *Room Maintenance* link at the bottom of the *Scheduling* section (Figure 5-18).

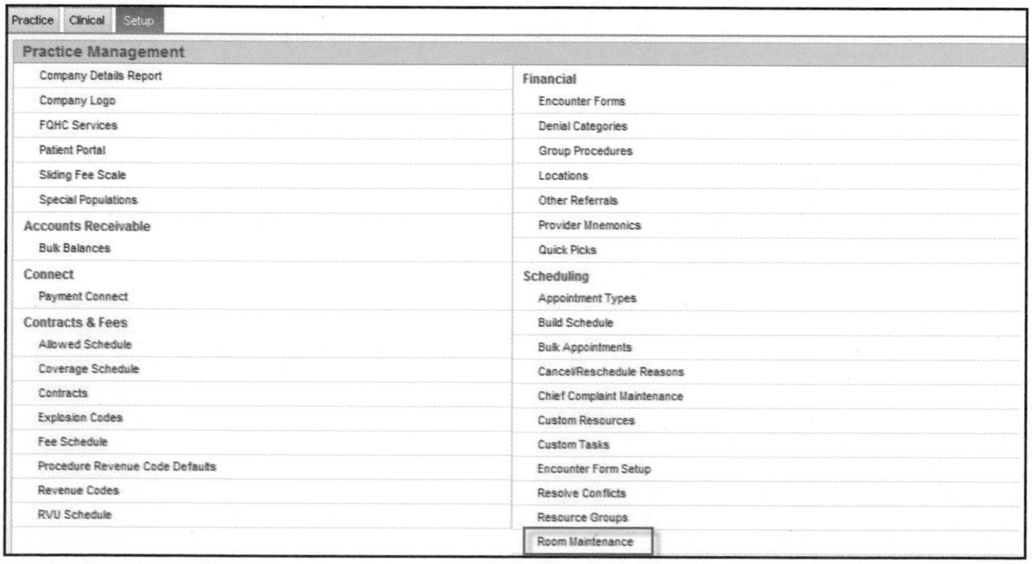

Figure 5-18   Room Maintenance Link

3. Click the drop-down menu beside (*Select*) to see what rooms are already in the system. (You will notice that there are two rooms listed for our environment—"Exam Room #1" and "Exam Room 2.")
4. Click *Add* beside the (*Select*) drop-down menu.
5. Enter "Exam Room #3" in the *Room Name* box (Figure 5-19).

FYI

A "Room Short Name" field is available, which is not necessary to complete unless a short version or acronym of the room name is often used.

6. Select "Napa Valley Family Health Associates 2" from the *Group* list.
7. Select "Napa Valley Family Associates" from the *Location* list. (These lists are useful for multi-location practices.)
8. By default, the *Active* field is set to "Y". This means the room is active (Figure 5-19).

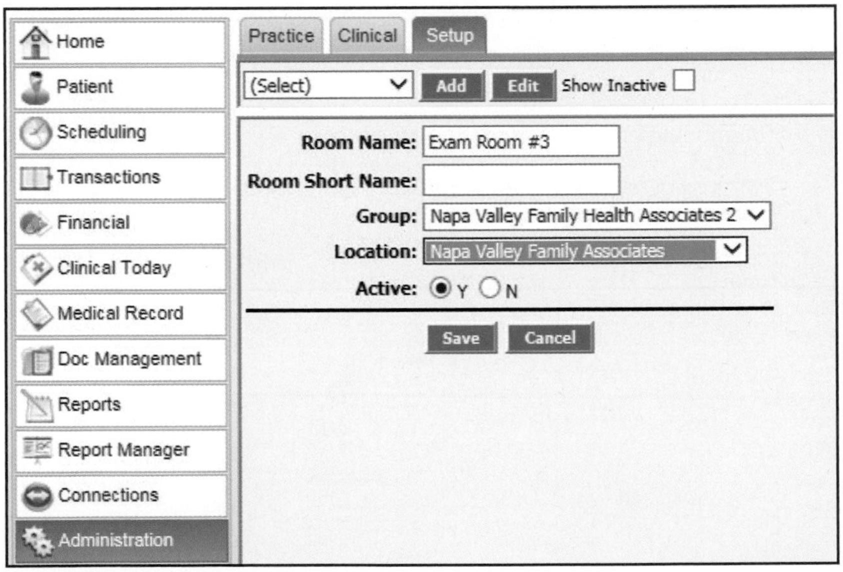

Courtesy of Harris CareTracker PM and EMR

Figure 5-19 Add Exam Room #3

9. Click *Save*. The application adds the room.
10. Click on the drop-down menu. "Exam Room #1", "Exam Room 2", and "Exam Room #3" should appear in the drop-down list.
11. Now repeat the same procedure, adding the following rooms: "Triage Room" and "Cardiac Bay" with the same *Group* and *Location* as in Steps 6–7.

12. Click on the (*Select*) drop-down menu. All the rooms you added should appear in the drop-down list.
13. Click on the "Cardiac Bay" room listing.

If you have a screen shot application with a "10-second delay" feature, you will be able to capture the drop-down list. If not, print the information from the Cardiac Bay field to illustrate that it was added to the list. Label it "Activity 5-7" and place it in your assignment folder.

After a room is created you can edit the room's name, group, or location. You can also activate or deactivate a room.

ACTIVITY 5-8: Editing a Room

1. Click the *Administration* module and then click the *Setup* tab.
2. Click the *Room Maintenance* link at the bottom of the *Scheduling* section.
3. (Optional) If you want to view all rooms created in Harris CareTracker PM and EMR including inactive rooms, select the *Show Inactive* checkbox. (All of our rooms are active.)
4. Select "Exam Room #3" from the drop-down menu and then click *Edit* (Figure 5-20).

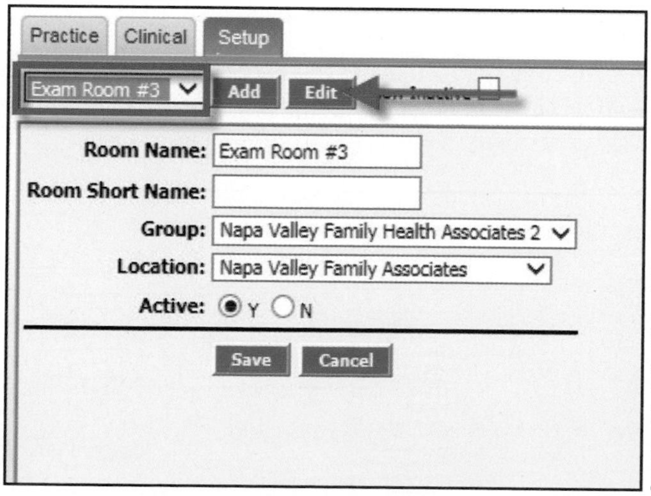

Courtesy of Harris CareTracker PM and EMR

Figure 5-20 Edit an Exam Room

5. Change the name of the room to "Procedure Room" and click *Save*.

Print a copy of the window that illustrates you changed the name of the room to Procedure Room. Label it "Activity 5-8" and place it in your assignment folder.

6. Click back on the *Administration* module.

7. Click on the *Setup* tab and then select the *Room Maintenance* link at the bottom of the *Scheduling* section.

8. Click the drop-down menu beside (*Select*). Make certain that "Exam Room 3" is no longer an option and that "Procedure Room" is now an option. (If your changes did not go through, start again from Step 2.)

Custom Resources

There may be times where you will need to add *Resources* to the system. Resources can be people, places, or things. Providers are always considered a resource, but an exam room or a piece of equipment can also be considered a resource. Something that requires a schedule is considered a resource because it has specific availability with days and times it can provide certain services. If the resource does not need a set schedule then it is not considered a "resource" in Harris CareTracker PM and EMR.

After a resource is entered in the system, you can customize the resource, assign it to resource classes, and assign it to a resource group for scheduling purposes. Building upon the activities you completed in Chapter 2, add a custom resource (Activity 5-9).

ACTIVITY 5-9: Adding Custom Resources

1. Click the *Administration* module and then click the *Setup* tab.

2. Click the *Custom Resources* link (Figure 5-21) under the *Scheduling* section. Harris CareTracker PM displays the *Schedule Resource* page. All providers in the practice are listed as *Available Resources*.

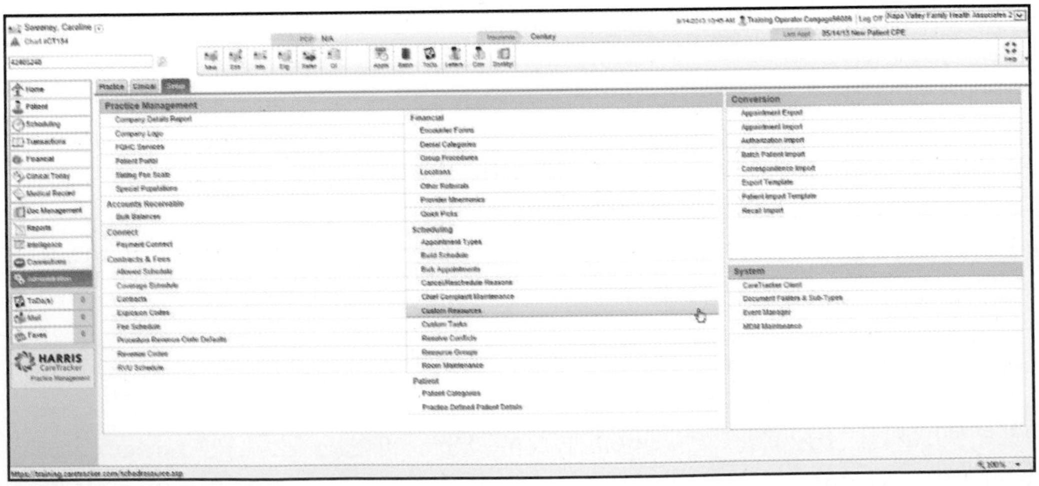

Figure 5-21 Custom Resources Link

3. Click *New* to the right of the *Available Resources* list. Harris CareTracker PM displays a dialog box, prompting you to enter a name for the resource.

4. In the dialog box, enter "Accent Laser Machine" (Figure 5-22).

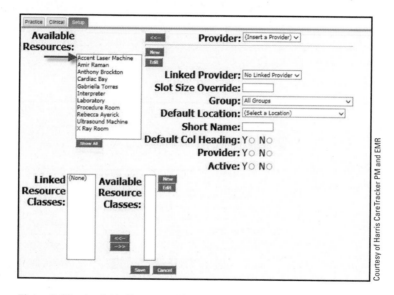

Figure 5-22 Add an Available Resource

5. Click *OK.* The application adds the resource to the *Available Resources* list (Figure 5-23).

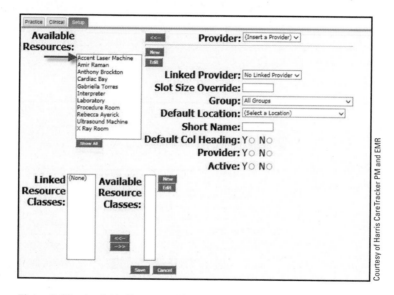

Figure 5-23 Available Resources List

> Print a copy of the Available Resources screen, indicating that the Accent Laser Machine is now in the Available Resources box. Label it "Activity 5-9" and place it in your assignment folder.

Favorite Lab Maintenance

Every office has a few select labs they work with. Napa Valley Family Health Associates has its own lab, but some insurance companies require patients to go to a lab that they contract with. This is known as an "In Network" lab. The lab agrees to do testing for a fraction of the usual charge in exchange for the increased volume of patients. This results in a win for both the insurance company and the lab. Another lab may also be used when a test is requested that is not available through the Napa Valley lab.

As you learned in Chapter 2, the *Favorite Labs* link is where you create a list of commonly used labs for the practice. In Activity 2-10 you selected a lab from the drop-down list available in the global database. In Activity 5-10 you will add new labs that are not in the database. This expedites the ordering process by avoiding the need to go through a long list of facilities supported by Harris CareTracker PM and EMR each time you create an order.

ACTIVITY 5-10: Adding Favorite Labs

1. Click the *Administration* module and then click the *Clinical* tab.
2. Click the *Favorite Labs* link under the *Daily Administration* heading. This launches the *Favorite Lab Maintenance* application (Figure 5-24).

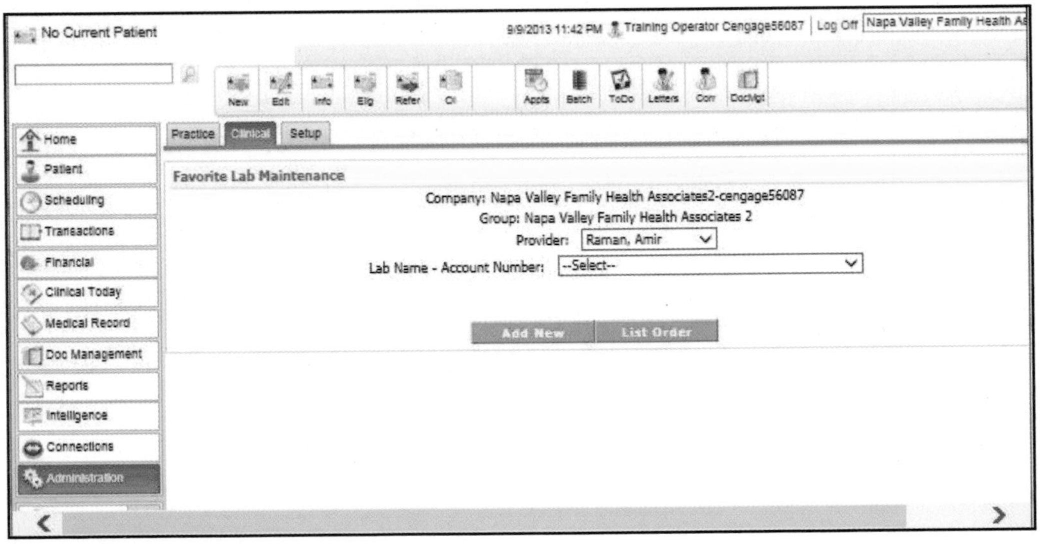

Courtesy of Harris CareTracker PM and EMR

Figure 5-24 Favorite Lab Maintenance Application

3. In the *Provider* box, click on the drop-down menu and select "Rebecca Ayerick." (**Note:** Even though you are selecting Dr. Ayerick, all providers will have access to the lab once you successfully add it to your favorites.)
4. Click *Add New*. (**Note:** This may take a few moments to populate.)

Tip Box

In some cases you are able to select the lab name from the *All Labs* box by clicking on the drop-down menu, and then selecting the lab you want to add to your favorites list (the application will automatically populate the lab address fields) as you did in Activity 2-10; however, the needed labs are not available in the drop-down list so you will need to add the requested information. In this activity, you will be adding two separate labs.

5. Add the two labs listed in Table 5-6, starting with the Napa Valley Lab information first.

TABLE 5-6 Favorite Lab Information

Napa Valley Family Health Associates Laboratory		CareTracker Inc. Health Labs of America	
Lab Address	101 Vine Street	Lab Address	6584 Elm Street
Lab City	Napa	Lab City	Napa
Lab State	CA	Lab State	CA
Lab Zip	69875	Lab Zip	69875
Lab Account #	785698	Lab Account #	986547
Lab Fax	707-555-1217	Lab Fax	707-986-6985

6. Click *Save.* You should receive a message that Napa Valley Family Health Associates Lab has been successfully added to the database. (**Note:** This may take a few moments to save. Wait for the message before moving on.) Now repeat the steps to add CareTracker Inc. Health Labs of America.

7. After both labs have been successfully added to the database, click *Done.*

8. Click on the drop-down arrow beside *Lab Name-Account Number.*

9. Scroll down and click on "Napa Valley Family Health Associates Laboratory" in the drop-down box. (**Note:** You will see there are numerous labs with the same name. This is because every time an operator adds a lab, it is added to the entire database.)

Once the NVFHA Lab is in context, print the screen and label it "Activity 5-10A." Do the same with CareTracker Inc. Health Labs of America, and label it "Activity 5-10B." Place both activities in your assignment folder.

Removing a Favorite Lab.   To remove labs from your favorites, follow the instructions in Activity 5-11.

ACTIVITY 5-11: Remove a Favorite Lab

1. Click the *Administration* module and then click the *Clinical* tab.

2. Click the *Favorite Labs* link under the *Daily Administration* header. This launches the *Favorite Lab Maintenance* application.

3. Click the lab you want removed from the *Lab Name-Account Number* drop-down list. (Select "Test Facility" lab, the one you created in Activity 2-10. If you do not see "Test Facility" on your list, complete Activity 2-10 before moving forward with this activity.)

4. Click *Delete*. A message prompts to confirm the delete action.

Print the Favorite Labs screen with the Delete message, label it "Activity 5-11," and place it in your assignment folder.

5. Click *OK*.

6. When the record has been successfully deleted from the database, click *Done*. The facility is removed from the list of favorite labs.

Manage Immunization Lots

The *Manage Immunization Lots* application enables you to manage immunization lots that pertain to groups. When immunizations are received, you can add the lot information for the immunizations to the system. After an immunization lot is added, the system keeps track of the inventory and deducts administered immunization from the quantity in the lot. Tracking inventory ensures that required immunizations can be reordered in a timely manner.

The *Manage Immunization Lots* application also enables you to modify lots, make lots inactive, and delete lots as necessary.

Tip Box

You can also add and manage immunization lots via the *Add Immunization Lot* and *Edit Immunization Lot* dialog boxes accessed via the *Immunization* application in the *Clinical Toolbar*.

ACTIVITY 5-12: Adding an Immunization Lot

1. Click the *Administration* module, and then click the *Clinical* tab.
2. Click the *Manage Immunization Lots* link under the *Daily Administration* header. Harris CareTracker PM and EMR displays the *Immunization Lots* application, which displays existing immunization lots that have not yet been exhausted.

> **Tip Box**
>
> Immunization lots are practice specific and not determined by the provider selected in the *Admin Provider* list. Therefore, lot details recorded display in the *Lots* list for all providers.

3. Click *+ Add Immunization Lot* (Figure 5-25) located to the far right of your screen. Harris CareTracker displays the *Add Immunization Lot* dialog box (Figure 5-26).

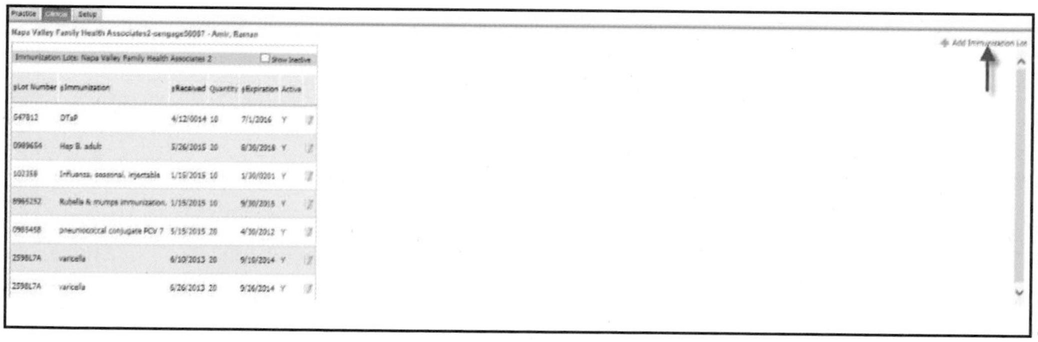

Courtesy of Harris CareTracker PM and EMR

Figure 5-25 Adding an Immunization Lot

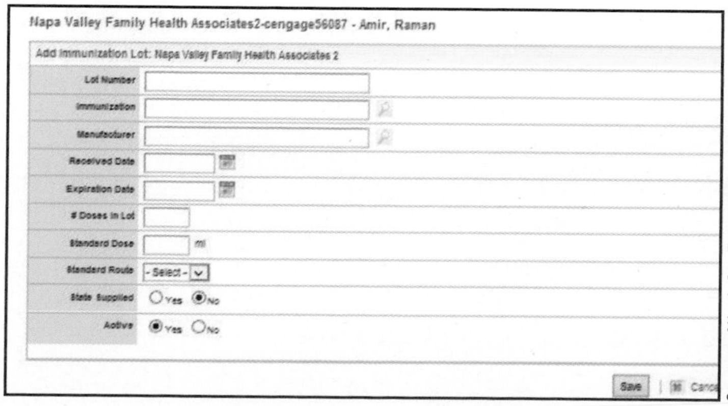

Courtesy of Harris CareTracker PM and EMR

Figure 5-26 Add Immunization Lot Dialog Box

4. In the *Lot Number* box, enter "MMR" followed by your operator number. (For example, if your operator number is "Cengage59290" you would enter the lot number "MMR59290".)
5. In the *Immunization* box, type "MMR" and then click the *Search* icon.
6. Click on the word "MMR" under *Search Results* (Figure 5-27).

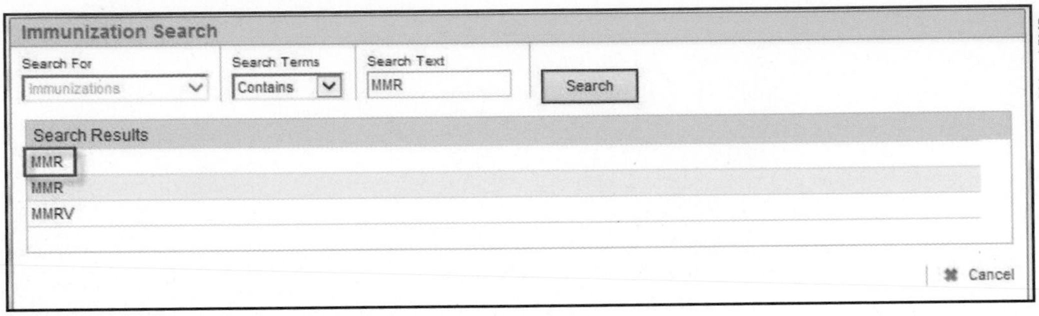

Courtesy of Harris CareTracker PM and EMR

Figure 5-27 Select MMR in the Immunization Search Box

7. In the *Manufacturer* box, type the word "MedImmune" and then click the *Search* icon. Select the radio dial (Figure 5-28) next to "MedImmune" under *Search Results*.

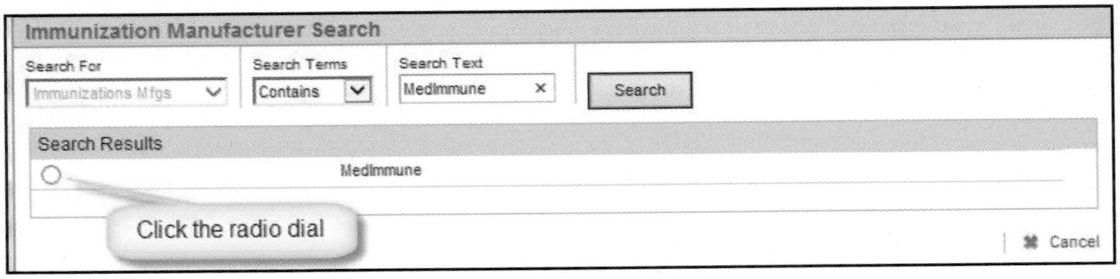

Courtesy of Harris CareTracker PM and EMR

Figure 5-28 Radio Button

8. In the *Received Date* box, click on the calendar and select today's date.
9. In the *Expiration Date* box, type in a date that is 15 months from today's date.
10. In the *# Doses in Lot* box, type "10".
11. In the *Standard Dose* box, type "0.5".
12. In the *Standard Route* box, click the drop-down menu and select "SC" for "subcutaneous."
13. In the *State Supplied* category, click "No".
14. In the *Active* category, select "Yes".
15. Your dialog box should look like Figure 5-29. Click on *Save*.

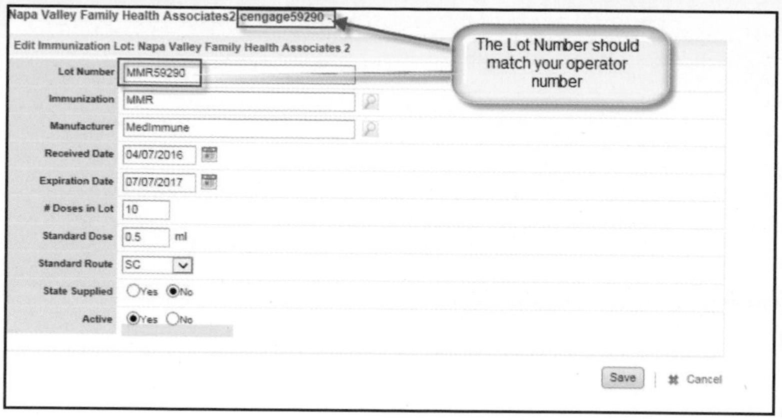

Courtesy of Harris CareTracker PM and EMR

Figure 5-29 Completed Add Immunization Lot Box

Print the screen listing the Immunization Lots for NVFA to illustrate that the vaccine has been added to the list. Label it "Activity 5-12" and place in your assignment folder. (In order to find the lot you entered, it may help to sort the list by Received Date.)

ACTIVITY 5-13: Modify an Immunization Lot

1. Click the *Administration* module, and then click the *Clinical* tab.
2. Click the *Manage Immunization Lots* link under the *Daily Administration* header. Harris CareTracker PM and EMR displays the *Immunization Lots* application with active lots.
3. Scroll down and click the *Edit* icon (Figure 5-30) next to the Varicella lot received on 06/10/2013.

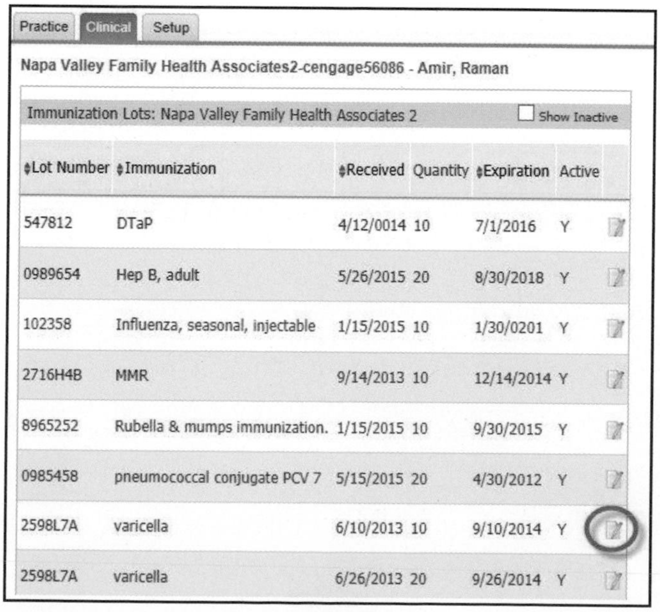

Courtesy of Harris CareTracker PM and EMR

Figure 5-30 Edit an Immunization Lot

4. You realize that you double counted a box in the last shipment of Varicella received on 06/10/2013 with the lot number of #2598L7A. Instead of having 10 doses in the lot you have 20 doses. Make the change and then click *Save*.

Scroll down and print the screen listing the Immunization Lots for NVFA to illustrate that the vaccine has been modified. Label it "Activity 5-13" and place in your assignment folder.

SUMMARY

The electronic medical record consists of a wide range of capabilities. In this chapter you learned some of the basic functions of Harris CareTracker EMR. The concept of meaningful use was introduced, and the stages of meaningful use were discussed. For providers to collect the financial incentives associated with Stage 1 meaningful use, they must go through a rigorous 90-day attestation period where they demonstrate that they have met the core and menu requirements. The provider must demonstrate attestation for a full year during the second year of the program. Meaningful Use Stage 2 requires two full years of attestation in order to receive financial incentives.

Meaningful use standards and the financial incentives created by the federal government for EMR implementation will have a substantial impact on the breadth and scope of EMR use in the near future. As the use of electronic medical records becomes more widespread, the need for medical professionals to be familiar with them and to be proficient in their use will become more critical.

Most of the activities in this chapter were designed to assist you in getting ready to work in the electronic medical record and learn how to navigate Harris CareTracker EMR. As you begin your career in health care, this basic knowledge of electronic medical records will be essential to your success.

Chapter 6

Patient Work-Up

Key Terms

advance directive
anthropometric
contraindication
encounter
family history
flowsheet template
growth chart
iteration
open encounter

open order
patient history
progress note
sensitive information
SIG
Surescripts®
ToDo
transfer
unsigned note

Learning Objectives

1. List major applications of the Clinical Today module.
2. View daily appointments in Clinical Today.
3. Perform check-in duties and track patients throughout their visits.
4. Describe basic tasks of the medical assistant when working in Clinical Today.
5. View prescription renewals and new prescriptions within Clinical Today.
6. Retrieve the patient's EMR and update sections within the patient medical history panes.
7. Record vital signs and document the patient's chief complaint.
8. View and create Flow Sheets within Harris CareTracker EMR.
9. Create and print a growth chart.
10. Update the Patient Care Management application.
11. Create and print a Progress Note.

Certification Connection

1. Perform routine practice management and clinical EHR tasks within a health care environment according to appropriate protocols.
2. Enter live data into an EHR and assist clinicians with charting.
3. Execute clinical workflows within a health care facility per protocol.
4. Coordinate patient flow within the back office clinical setting (e.g., check-in, transfer to a room, record vital signs and patient history, create outgoing referrals, and check out patients).
5. Execute data management using electronic health care records such as the EMR.
6. Locate requested information in the chart and complete tasks (orders) called out in the progress note.
7. Verify eligibility.

Adapted from national standards of the National Healthcareer Association (NHA), Commission on Accreditation and Allied Health Education Program (CAAHEP), and Accrediting Bureau of Health Education Schools (ABHES)

INTRODUCTION

As a medical assistant working in a clinical capacity, you will be responsible for completing the patient's work-up and documenting your findings; however, this is only a small portion of your responsibilities. You will also be responsible for screening patient phone calls, handling prescription requests, tracking lab results, and responding to messages from providers and other staff members within the practice. The *Clinical Today* module within Harris CareTracker PM and EMR helps to categorize and organize these tasks, improving quality and efficiency throughout the day. As a result, providers and staff members are continuously in sync with one another, enhancing communications, and, ultimately, patient care. This chapter introduces you to the *Clinical Today* module and provides activities representative of those you will perform in the industry.

This chapter also focuses on how to build the patient's electronic health record. As a student medical assistant working in the Harris CareTracker system, you will learn how to track patients throughout the visit, record vital signs and chief complaints, enter medication and history information, and transcribe physical and diagnostic findings for the provider. These activities comprise the front end of the clinical portion of the visit; the back end of the patient visit is discussed in Chapter 7.

SETTING OPERATOR PREFERENCES IN THE BATCH APPLICATION

The *Batch* application in Harris CareTracker PM and EMR enables you to set up your operator preferences based on the workflow for your role. This reduces the number of clicks required to get from one application to the other, making navigation through Harris CareTracker easy. As a medical assistant working in a clinical capacity, you will want your screen to open in the *Clinical Today* module each time you log in to Harris CareTracker. Selecting the appropriate setting from the *Login Application* in your *Batch* preferences will take you directly to the *Clinical Today* module after logging in. Activity 6-1 will assist you in making the appropriate changes to your preferences.

ACTIVITY 6-1: Setting Operator Preferences in Your Batch Application

1. To set up operator preferences click *Batch* on the *Name Bar*. Harris CareTracker PM and EMR displays the *Operator Encounter Batch Control* dialog box.

2. Click on the *Edit* button.

3. Click on the drop-down arrow beside *Provider* and select "Dr. Raman," if he has not already been selected.

4. Click on the drop-down arrow beside *Resource* and select "Dr. Raman," if he has not already been selected.

5. Click on the drop-down arrow beside *Show Alerts* and select "Yes".

6. In the *Login Application* box, click on the drop-down arrow and select "Clinical".

7. Click on *Save*. Now every time you log in to Harris CareTracker, you will be taken directly to the *Clinical Today* module.

8. Click "X" in the right-hand corner to close the dialog box.

OVERVIEW OF THE CLINICAL TODAY MODULE

Learning Objective 1: List major applications of the Clinical Today module.

Within Harris CareTracker EMR the *Clinical Today* module is the area where most medical assistants working in a clinical capacity spend their time. The *Clinical Today* module works as an electronic desk. It organizes and helps manage tasks by displaying items to be worked on daily. It also automates a large number of routine tasks, thereby increasing productivity. In addition, the module helps track patient workflow efficiently by displaying information about scheduled appointments and patient movements within the clinic. The application helps track the care of one or more patients in the practice and provides instant access to a patient's medical record that includes test results, clinical information, and more. The *Clinical Today* module consists of three main applications: *Appointments*, *Tasks*, and *Population Management*. This chapter focuses on the *Appointments* and *Tasks* applications.

Appointments

Learning Objective 2: View daily appointments in Clinical Today.

The *Appointments* application (Figure 6-1) consists of patient and non-patient appointments scheduled via the *Book* application in the *Scheduling* module. The application mimics most features in the *Scheduling* module, enabling you to manage appointments and the appointment workflow. You can use the application to update, confirm and cancel appointments, update the appointment status, access the patient's medical record, view the patient's open activities, capture visit information, and more.

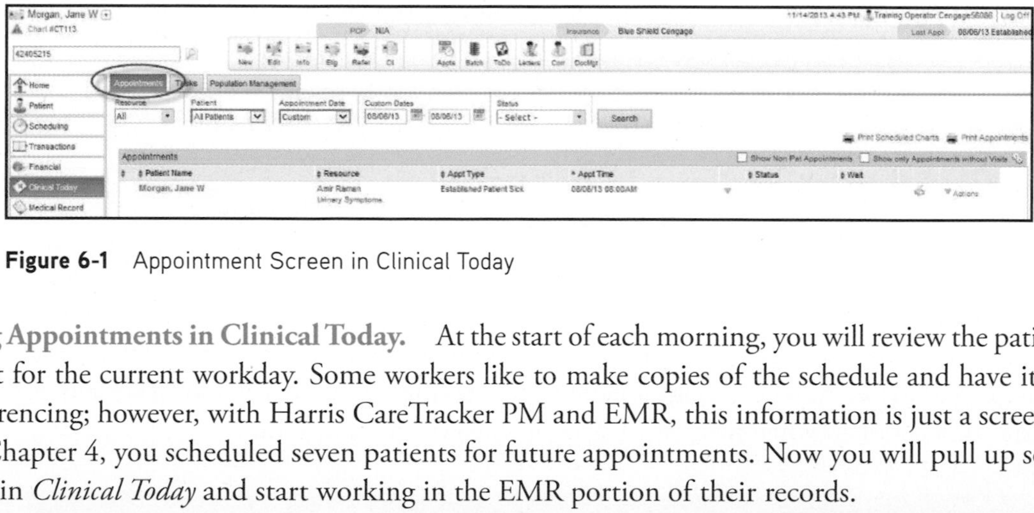

Figure 6-1   Appointment Screen in Clinical Today

Viewing Appointments in Clinical Today.   At the start of each morning, you will review the patient appointment list for the current workday. Some workers like to make copies of the schedule and have it close by for easy referencing; however, with Harris CareTracker PM and EMR, this information is just a screenshot away.

In Chapter 4, you scheduled seven patients for future appointments. Now you will pull up some of these patients in *Clinical Today* and start working in the EMR portion of their records.

> ⚠️ **Alert**
>
> When you click on *Clinical Today*, the screen automatically defaults to the patients scheduled for the current date. For Activity 6-2, you will need the dates of the appointments you scheduled for patients in Chapter 4.

ACTIVITY 6-2: Viewing Appointments

1. Click on *Clinical Today*.

2. Click on the drop-down arrow under *Resource* and select "All".

3. Click on the drop-down arrow under *Patient* and select "All Patients".

4. Click on the drop-down arrow under *Appointment Date* and select "Custom".

5. Click on the calendar beside the first box under *Custom Dates* and select the date you scheduled your patient appointments in Chapter 4. (If you scheduled your patients on different dates, select the date that you scheduled Jane Morgan.)

6. Click in the second box to the right of the calendar under *Custom Dates*. The date that you inserted in the first box should automatically populate in this box.

7. In the status box, click on the drop-down arrow and select "All" (Figure 6-2).

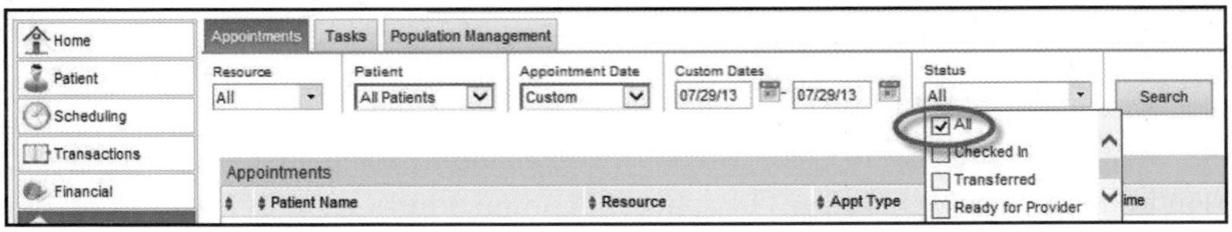

Figure 6-2 Select All

8. Click on *Search*. (The appointment screen with Ms. Morgan's appointment should now appear.)

🖉 **Print a screenshot of your Appointment screen from Clinical Today. Label it "Activity 6-2" and place it in your assignment folder.**

Learning Objective 3: Perform check-in duties and track patients throughout their visits.

Checking In and Transferring Patients.   In Chapter 4 you practiced checking in patients. Patients are typically checked in upon arrival. This cues the clinical staff that the patient is ready to be taken back to the exam room. Once the patient has been transferred to the exam room, you will alert the staff of the patient's current status. Activity 6-3 describes how to change a patient's status from "Checked In" to "Transferred." **Transfer** refers to the status of a patient when he or she has been taken to an exam room.

ACTIVITY 6-3: Transferring a Patient

1. Click on *Clinical Today*.

2. Match the search parameters to those set in Activity 6-2. Click *Search*.

3. Jane Morgan's appointment should be listed in the *Appointments* window. Her current status is green, which means that she has already been checked in. Change her status by clicking on the drop-down arrow in her *Status* column and selecting "Transfer."

4. The *Patient Location* box will pop up. Select the radio button next to "Exam Room # 1." Click *Select* (Figure 6-3). (**Note:** If the there is nothing listed in the *Patient Location* box, make sure that the Compatibility View setting is turned off, and try again.)

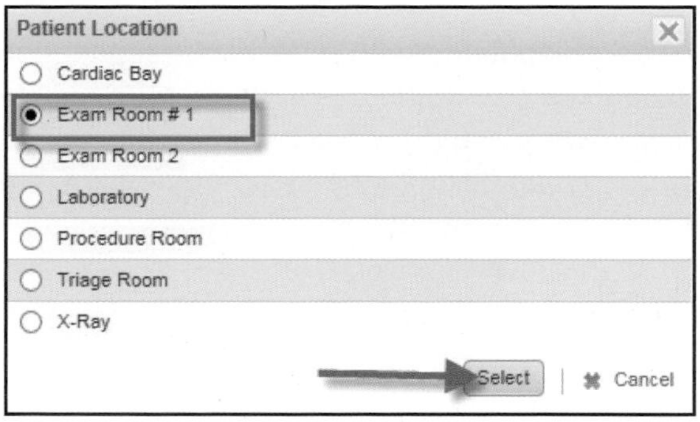

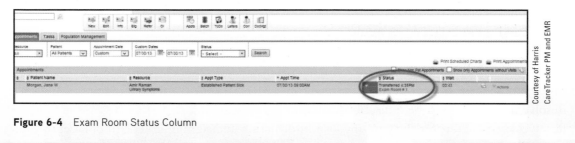

Figure 6-3　Patient Location Box

5. Ms. Morgan's entry line should now be blue, indicating that she has been transferred to the exam room. The appropriate exam room number will now appear in the *Status* column (Figure 6-4).

Figure 6-4　Exam Room Status Column

Tasks Menu

Learning Objective 4: Describe basic tasks of the medical assistant when working in Clinical Today.

The *Tasks* menu (Figure 6-5) displays an up-to-date number of any outstanding activities, such as lab results pending review, incomplete encounters, documents pending review, and more. Clicking on a specific task category will direct you to the list of items that requires attention. An **encounter** is an interaction with a patient on a specific date and time. Encounter types include visits, phone calls, referrals, results of a test, and more.

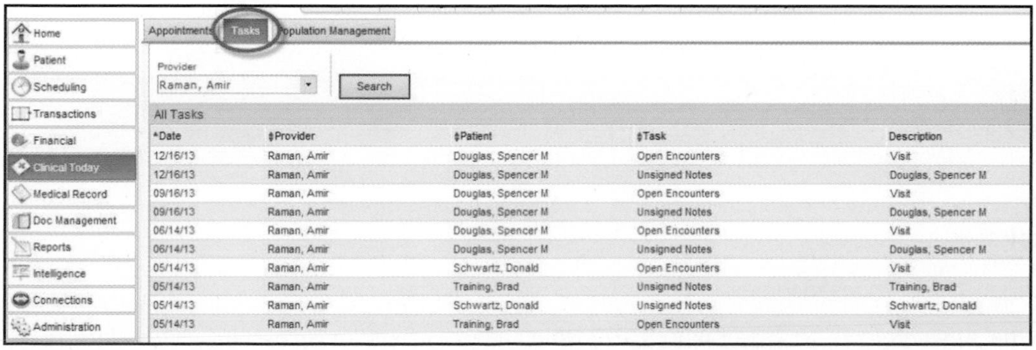

Figure 6-5　Tasks Menu

The *Tasks* application provides an integrated view of all open and active tasks that require attention. The tasks list helps you to efficiently manage routine tasks occurring throughout the practice and provide improved patient services. The tasks list provides the capability to manage the following:

- Complete all daily tasks in a timely manner.
- Create, reply, and transfer *ToDo*(s), mail, and fax messages. A **ToDo** is Harris CareTracker's internal messaging system.
- Review and sign unsigned test results.
- Review **open orders** (diagnostic tests that have been ordered but have no results).
- Efficiently manage prescription renewal requests.
- Efficiently manage patient documents.
- Resolve notes that must be transcribed.
- Resolve **open encounters** by entering visit information and signing notes. An open encounter is documentation of a patient visit that took place that was never completed.
- Resolve unmatched attachments.

ACTIVITY 6-4: Viewing Tasks

To View Tasks:

1. Click on the *Clinical Today* module.
2. Click on the *Appointments* tab (see Figure 6-1). (**Note:** You may need to reset the *Custom Date* to Ms. Morgan's appointment [see Activity 6-2]).

3. Find the *Quick Tasks* heading all the way over on the right side of the window. Click on the drop-down menu beside *Open Encounters*. (**Note:** You may need to scroll down in the tab to view all the *Open Encounters* [Figure 6-6].) *Quick Tasks* will populate as you work in Harris CareTracker entering patient data.

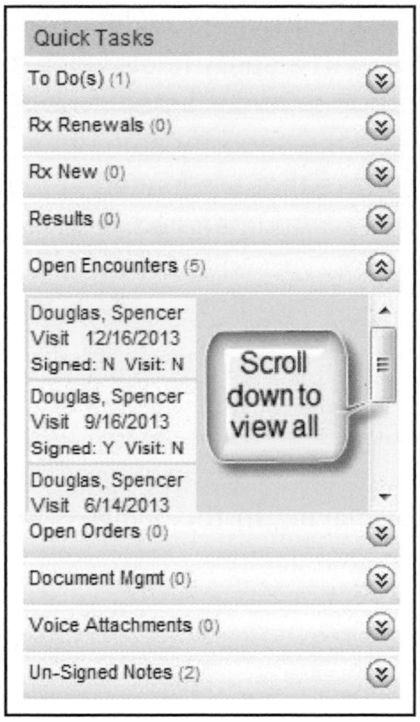
Quick Tasks
To Do(s) (1)
Rx Renewals (0)
Rx New (0)
Results (0)
Open Encounters (5)
Douglas, Spencer
Visit 12/16/2013
Signed: N Visit: N
Douglas, Spencer
Visit 9/16/2013
Signed: Y Visit: N
Douglas, Spencer
Visit 6/14/2013
Scroll down to view all
Open Orders (0)
Document Mgmt (0)
Voice Attachments (0)
Un-Signed Notes (2)

Courtesy of Harris CareTracker PM and EMR

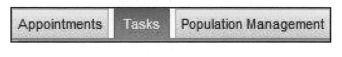

Figure 6-6 Open Encounters

4. (FYI) Information related only to the provider selected in your batch will appear in the *Quick Tasks* pane. To display all tasks for every provider, you will need to access the *Tasks* tab. (See the FYI box on the following page.)

5. All open tasks can be reviewed by selecting the *Tasks* tab in *Clinical Today* (Figure 6-7). In the *Provider* box, click on the drop-down arrow and select "All". Click the *Search* button. The screen will populate with a list of all open and active tasks pertaining to patients for all providers (Figure 6-8).

Appointments
Tasks
Population Management

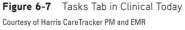

Figure 6-7 Tasks Tab in Clinical Today

Courtesy of Harris CareTracker PM and EMR

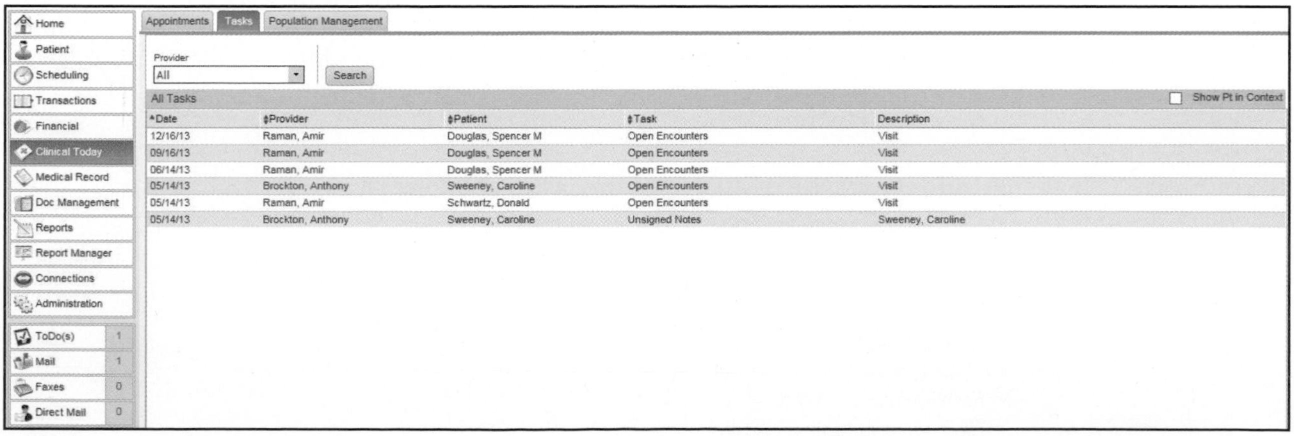
Home
Patient
Scheduling
Transactions
Financial
Clinical Today
Medical Record
Doc Management
Reports
Report Manager
Connections
Administration
ToDo(s) 1
Mail 1
Faxes 0
Direct Mail 0
Appointments
Tasks
Population Management
Provider
All
Search
All Tasks
Show Pt in Context
Date Provider Patient Task Description
12/16/13 Raman, Amir Douglas, Spencer M Open Encounters Visit
09/16/13 Raman, Amir Douglas, Spencer M Open Encounters Visit
06/14/13 Raman, Amir Douglas, Spencer M Open Encounters Visit
05/14/13 Brockton, Anthony Sweeney, Caroline Open Encounters Visit
05/14/13 Raman, Amir Schwartz, Donald Open Encounters Visit
05/14/13 Brockton, Anthony Sweeney, Caroline Unsigned Notes Sweeney, Caroline

Courtesy of Harris CareTracker PM and EMR

Figure 6-8 Open and Active Tasks

FYI

Tasks that display in the *Tasks* tab pertain to the provider associated with the operator. If you are not a provider, or not associated with a specific provider, the *All Tasks* list in the center of the screen displays tasks only for the provider listed in your batch. However, the tasks you can view and access are based on the security settings assigned to your role in Harris CareTracker PM and EMR. The only tasks that are loaded in the training environment thus far are *Open Encounters* and *Unsigned Notes*. An **unsigned note** is a progress note that was never signed. As you complete more activities, you will see more tasks populate in this window.

Table 6-1 describes the information displaying in the columns of the *All Tasks* section of the *Tasks* tab. Refer back to Figure 6-8 as you review this table.

TABLE 6-1 All Tasks Columns

Column	Description
Date	**Note:** The date that displays is based on the type of task on the line item. • *Document Management* tasks – Document date • *Fax* tasks – Date the fax was received • *Lab Results* tasks – Reported date • *Mail* tasks – Date the mail was received • *Open Encounters* tasks – Encounter date • *Open Orders* tasks – Due date for the order • *Rx New* tasks – Original date of the prescription • *Rx Renewals* tasks – Written date of the Rx • *ToDo* tasks – Last modified date • *Unsigned Notes* tasks – Encounter date • *Untranscribed Notes* – Encounter date • *Voice Attachments* – Document date
Provider	Displays the provider associated with the task
Patient	Displays the patient associated with the task
Task	Displays the task name
Description	**Note:** The description is based on the type of task on the line item. • *Document Management* tasks – Document name • *Fax* tasks – Where the fax was sent from • *Lab Results* tasks – Report status and test name • *Mail* tasks – Where the mail message was received from • *Open Encounters* tasks – Note (signed or not signed) • *Open Orders* tasks – Test description • *Rx New* tasks – Medication name • *Rx Renewals* tasks – Medication name

TABLE 6-1 *(Continued)*

Column	Description
	• *ToDo* tasks – Subject line on the *ToDo* • *Unsigned Notes* tasks – Patient name • *Untranscribed Notes* tasks – File name (.wav) • *Voice Attachments* tasks – File name (.wav)

Courtesy of Harris CareTracker PM and EMR

FYI

To review a particular task, click on the line item that corresponds with the task you want to review. Harris CareTracker PM and EMR opens the task in a new window. The window that opens is determined by the type of the task. Figure 6-9 illustrates an unsigned note that needs to be completed by the provider, and Figure 6-10 illustrates the open order screen (no orders have yet been entered).

Courtesy of Harris CareTracker PM and EMR

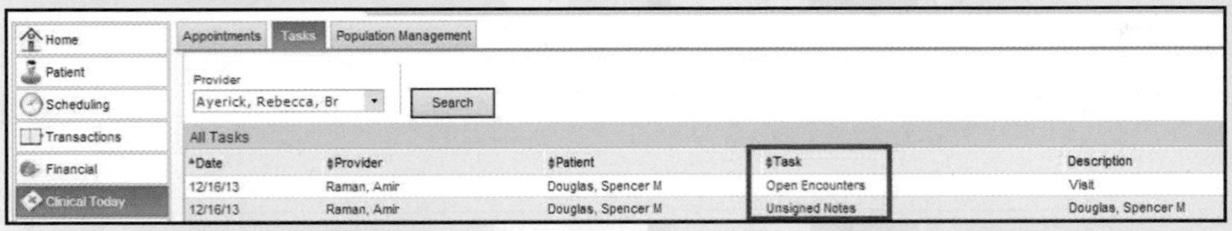

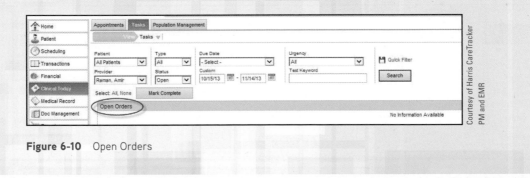

Figure 6-9 Unsigned Note That Needs Completion

Courtesy of Harris CareTracker PM and EMR

Figure 6-10 Open Orders

Critical Thinking

One of your patients called early this morning for a prescription request. She stated that she is completely out of her blood pressure medication. The task is showing up in the prescription renewal column, but it does not appear that the physician has addressed it yet. It is now closing time and the physician has already left the office. Is there anything that can be done to assist the patient? Is there any patient education that can be given to this patient so that this scenario does not occur again?

Learning Objective 5: View prescription renewals and new prescriptions within Clinical Today.

Viewing Prescription Renewals.   The *Rx Renewals* application displays a list of renewal requests sent electronically by the pharmacy and patient to the provider set up in your batch. The *Rx Renewal* application can be accessed via the *Tasks* tab in the *Clinical Today* module. If you were working for a provider using Harris CareTracker EMR, your practice would need to first enroll in the **Surescripts®** network—a network used by thousands of physicians nationwide to prescribe medications without the use of paper, pens, or fax. Surescripts® is the largest network of its kind and provides electronic connectivity between pharmacies and physician offices. Once enrolled in the Surescripts® network, the practice would be required to send five new prescriptions to receive renewal requests, and accept or deny the request within 48 hours. Surescripts® monitors and requires at least a 90% response rate. If the response rate falls below 90% for more than four weeks, Surescripts® terminates the ability to electronically receive renewal requests. As a clinical medical assistant, you will need to work with the provider to keep the response rate above 90%.

To receive prescription renewal requests (Figure 6-11) from a patient, the practice must enroll the patient in the Harris CareTracker *Patient Portal* application supported by Harris CareTracker PM and EMR. All requests made by a patient using the Harris CareTracker *Patient Portal* application are saved in the *Rx Renewals* application (*Tasks* tab in *Clinical Today*) for the medical assistant to review. The *Patient Portal* is not active in your student version of Harris CareTracker (Figure 6-12).

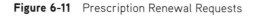

Figure 6-11   Prescription Renewal Requests

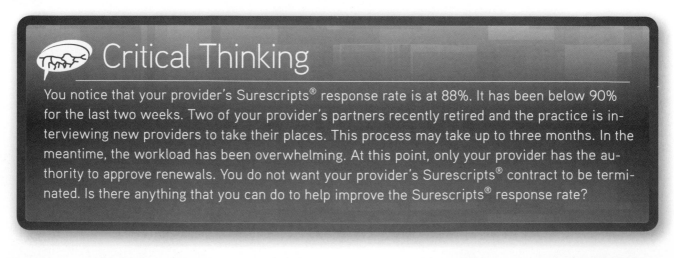

Figure 6-12   Patient Portal

Critical Thinking

You notice that your provider's Surescripts® response rate is at 88%. It has been below 90% for the last two weeks. Two of your provider's partners recently retired and the practice is interviewing new providers to take their places. This process may take up to three months. In the meantime, the workload has been overwhelming. At this point, only your provider has the authority to approve renewals. You do not want your provider's Surescripts® contract to be terminated. Is there anything that you can do to help improve the Surescripts® response rate?

Table 6-2 describes the information displaying in the *Rx Renewals* application. Refer back to Figure 6-11 as you review this table.

TABLE 6-2   Rx Renewal Columns

Column	Description
Type	Where the renewal request initiated from. Renewal requests can be initiated by a patient or a pharmacy.
Patient Name	The name of the patient associated with the renewal request.
Drug	The name of the medication that requires a refill.
Provider	The name of the provider who originally issued the prescription.
Phone/Fax	The pharmacy phone and fax numbers.
Pharmacy	The name of the pharmacy where the prescription was filled previously. You can click on the line item to view the pharmacy address information.
Active Dates	The date and time Harris CareTracker EMR received the renewal request.
Notes	Notes entered by the pharmacy or patient when creating the renewal request.

Courtesy of Harris CareTracker PM and EMR

ACTIVITY 6-5:   Viewing Rx Renewals

1. Click on the *Clinical Today* module.
2. Select the *Tasks* tab.
3. View the *Tasks* panes on the right side of the window.
4. Click on the *Rx Renewals* link (Figure 6-13) in the *Tasks* pane.

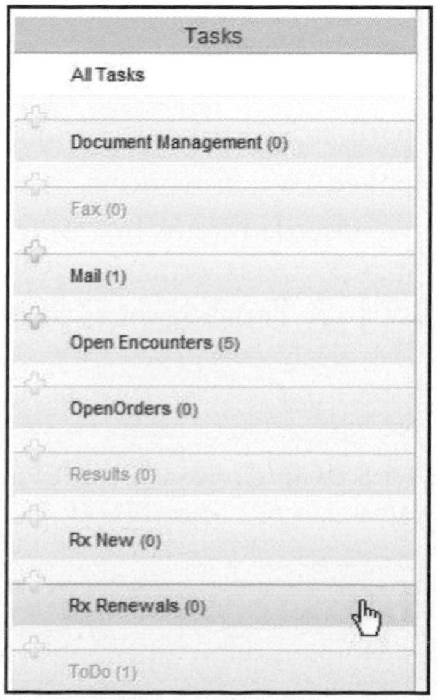

Figure 6-13   Rx Renewals Link in Tasks Pane

Courtesy of Harris CareTracker PM and EMR

5. To set your parameters, click on the word "All" beside *Provider*.

6. Click on the word "All" for *Request Type*.

7. For *Status*, click on "Active".

8. Click on "All" beside the *Dates* tab (Figure 6-14).

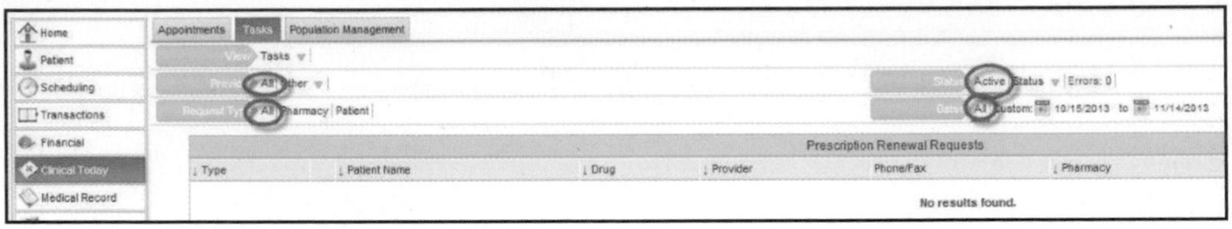

Figure 6-14 Viewing Rx Renewals Tab

FYI

Setting the parameters to "All" in the *Rx Renewals* application allows you to review all active prescription renewals for all providers in the practice.

Print this screen, even though it does not show any prescription renewals. Label it "Activity 6-5" and place it in your assignment folder.

Viewing New Prescriptions. The *Rx New* application displays a list of prescriptions that are not transmitted electronically, printed, or failed transmission that you must review and resolve on a daily basis. Additionally, you can view details for each prescription listed and reorder a prescription, eliminating the need to reenter redundant information, view interactions, and more. Along with prescription renewals, new prescriptions can be viewed from the *Tasks* tab in *Clinical Today*. Instead of clicking on the *Rx Renewal* link, click on *Rx New* on the right-hand side of the screen and follow the prompts.

This chapter has just briefly touched on a few of the available functions in the *Clinical Today* module. Harris CareTracker PM and EMR provides users with an assortment of tools to streamline and organize information so that important tasks are never overlooked. When working in the industry, you should review electronic tasks throughout the workday and resolve unsettled items in a timely manner.

RETRIEVING AND UPDATING THE PATIENT'S ELECTRONIC MEDICAL RECORD

Learning Objective 6: Retrieve the patient's EMR and update sections within the patient medical history panes.

Once the patient has been checked in and transferred to an exam room, you are ready to bring up his or her electronic medical record (EMR). In the case of Jane Morgan, she is an established patient; however, Napa Valley Family Health Associates is in the middle of transitioning from paper records to Harris CareTracker PM and Physician EMR. Because Ms. Morgan's chart has not yet been converted, you will need to build her chart from scratch.

ACTIVITY 6-6: Bringing Up the Patient's Chart

1. Click on *Clinical Today*.

2. In the appointment screen within *Clinical Today*, bring up the date of Jane Morgan's appointment.

3. Click on Ms. Morgan's name. The patient's *Chart Summary* will open in a new window (Figure 6-15).

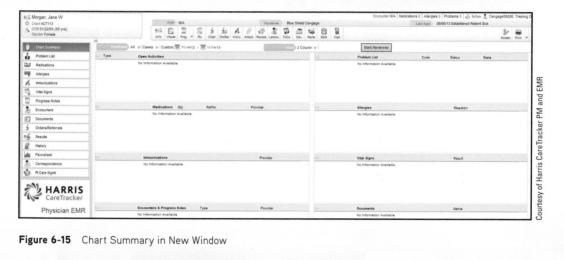

Figure 6-15   Chart Summary in New Window

The order in which you complete activities in the patient's chart is purely subjective. Some medical assistants start by entering the vital signs and chief complaint, and then adding new medications, allergies, and history information. The order really does not matter as long as you complete the process. We are going to start the process by creating the patient's current medication list.

Updating the Patient's Medication List

In the patient's *Chart Summary*, the *Medications* application allows you to manually update the patient's medication list. New prescriptions can also be added here; however, you will only enter the patient's current medications at this time. Table 6-3 describes all medication status categories within the *Medications* application. It is important to ensure that all active medications are recorded to screen for interactions when prescribing new medications.

TABLE 6-3	Medication Status Categories
Status	**Description**
Active	A medication the patient is currently taking.
Inactive	A medication the patient is not taking at the present time.
Discontinued	A medication discontinued for the patient.

(Continues)

Status	Description
Erroneous	A medication entered in error for the patient.
Completed	A medication the patient has completed by taking the full recommended dosage.
Medication Refused	A medication the provider recommended, but the patient refused to take. **Note:** All patients with a Medication Refused status and an active diagnosis of asthma are excluded from the Asthma Pharmacologic Therapy (NQF 0047) quality measure report.
Failed	A medication that the patient did not respond well to.

TABLE 6-3 (*Continued*)

Courtesy of Harris CareTracker PM and EMR

ACTIVITY 6-7: Adding a Medication to a Patient's Chart

1. Following the steps used in Activity 6-6, bring up Jane Morgan's patient chart using the *Clinical Today* module.

2. In the *Patient Medical History* pane, click on the *Medications* link (Figure 6-16). The *Medications* window displays.

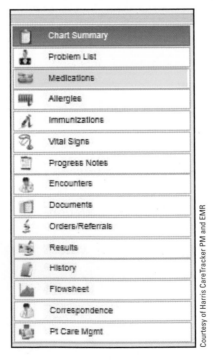

Figure 6-16 Medications Link

Courtesy of Harris CareTracker PM and EMR

3. Click + *Patient Med*, which is located at the top right side of the screen (Figure 6-17). The *Medication* dialog box will display (Figure 6-18).

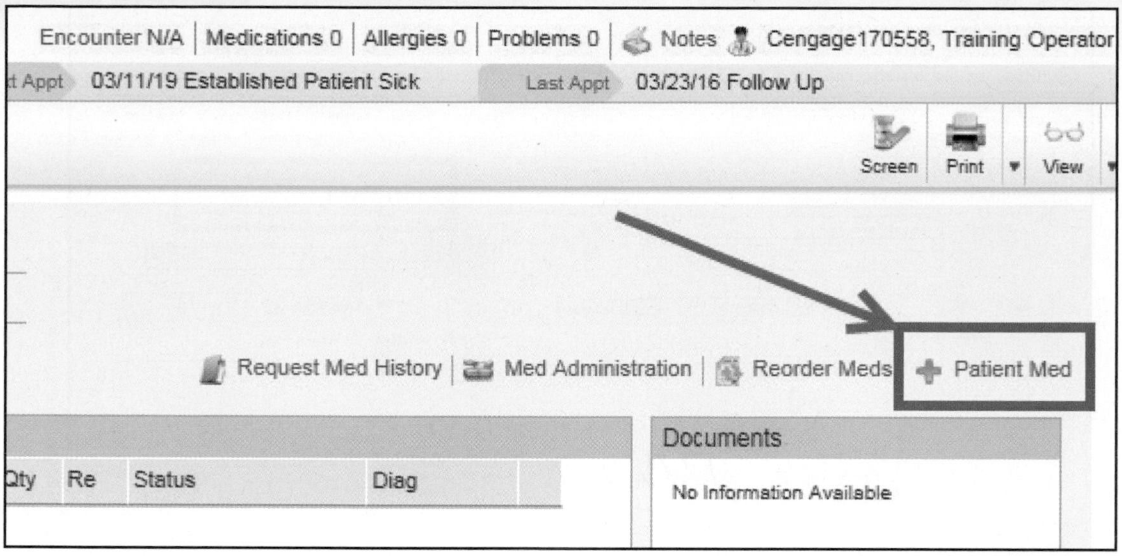

Figure 6-17   Add a Patient Medication

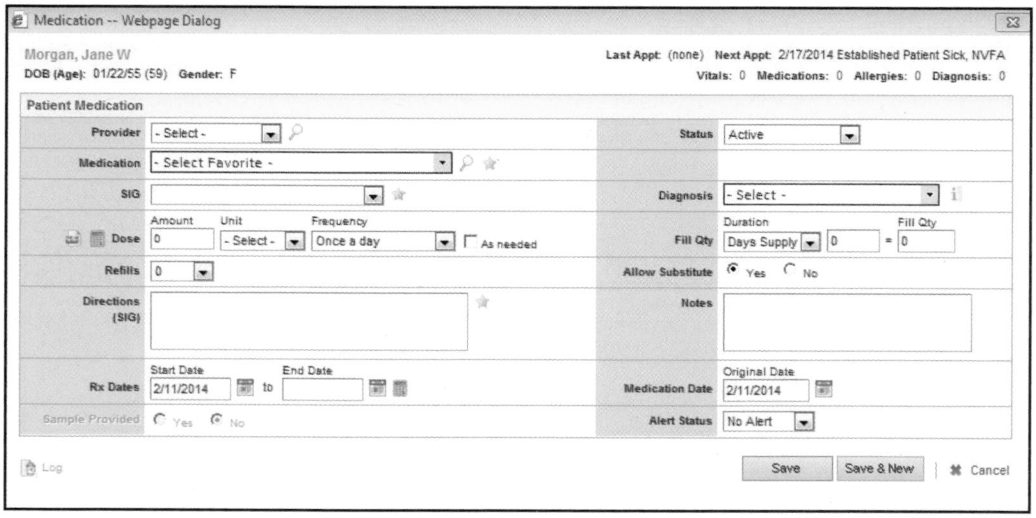

Figure 6-18   Medication Dialog Box

4. In the *Provider* drop-down list, select "Amir Raman".

FYI

The *Provider* list displays the group providers first, followed by the referring providers.

5. By default, the *Status* list is set to "Active" (Figure 6-19), but you can change to another applicable status if necessary. Refer to Table 6-3 for a complete listing of medication statuses. (Leave the *Status* as "Active.")

6. In the *Medication* field, click on the drop-down arrow (Figure 6-20). Ms. Morgan is currently taking Boniva to help slow down her osteoporosis. Click on "Boniva Oral Tablet 150 mg". An *Interaction Screening* box will pop up (Figure 6-21).

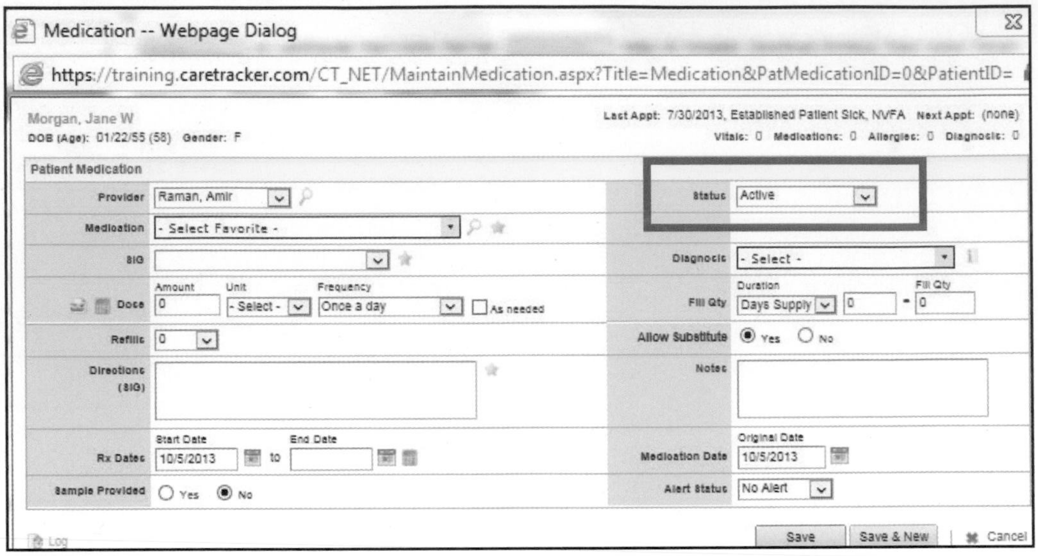

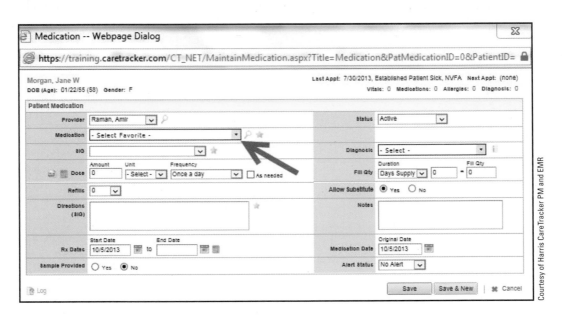

Figure 6-19   Status List Set to Active

Figure 6-20   Medication Field Drop-Down Arrow

> ⚠️ **Alert**
>
> Selected medications are screened for possible **contraindications** in regard to the patient's active medications, allergies, and problems. A contraindiciation is something (a symptom or condition) that makes a particular treatment or procedure inadvisable. The *Interaction Screening* box alerts you if the interaction is higher than the severity level set in your configurations. If the screening triggers an interaction that is higher than the severity settings set for the provider in the batch, the *Interaction Screening* dialog box displays.

7. Acknowledge the screening by selecting one or more *Override Reasons* and entering notes. Select "Benefit outweighs risk" (see Figure 6-21). **Note:** If you click *Cancel* in the *Interaction Screening* dialog box before accepting an override reason you may receive an error message.

8. Click *Accept* (see Figure 6-21).

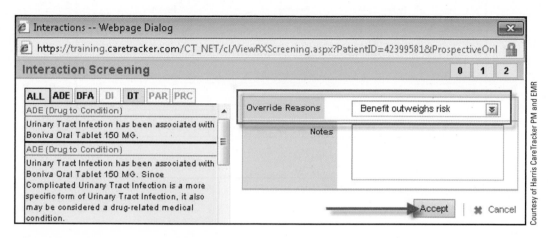

Figure 6-21   Interaction Screening Dialog Box

9. You will skip over the SIG box for now. Refer to the FYI box below. Once a SIG is saved as a favorite, you will be able to select it from the manage favorites icon. **SIG** is an abbreviation for *signa* in Latin (meaning "label" or "sign"). SIG codes are specific dosage instructions that are given when prescribing medications.

FYI

The drop-down selections only display if a SIG is associated as a favorite to the medication selected and auto-populates in the specific fields. Because nothing has been loaded to the system prior to this exercise, you will need to enter the SIG information manually.

10. Enter the dosage information in the *Dose* boxes. Enter "1" in the *Amount* box, "Tablet" in the *Unit* box, and "Once every month" in the *Frequency* box (Figure 6-22).

11. Tab down to the *Rx Dates* field. Because the medication is not being renewed, remove any dates that appear in the *Start Date* box. Leave the *End Date* box blank as well.

12. The patient states that she started taking the medication on October 1 of last year. Insert this information in the box titled *Original Date* on the right side of the screen (Figure 6-23).

13. Because you are not creating a new prescription, no other information needs to be entered. Click *Save*.

14. "Boniva Oral Tablet 150 MG" should now appear in the *Medications* box of the *Patient Medical History* Pane (Figure 6-24).

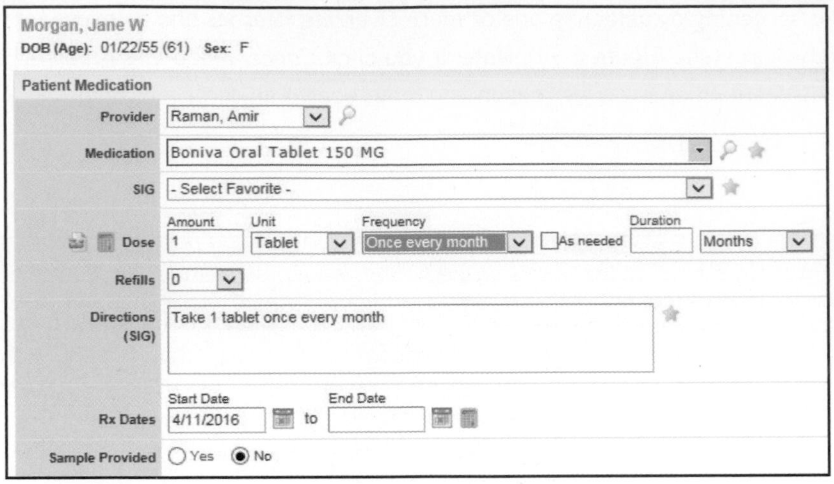

Morgan, Jane W
DOB (Age): 01/22/55 (61)   Sex: F

Patient Medication

Provider	Raman, Amir
Medication	Boniva Oral Tablet 150 MG
SIG	- Select Favorite -

Dose
Amount	Unit	Frequency		Duration	
1	Tablet	Once every month	☐ As needed		Months

Refills   0

Directions (SIG)   Take 1 tablet once every month ★

Rx Dates
Start Date   4/11/2016   to   End Date

Sample Provided   ○ Yes   ● No

Figure 6-22   Dose - Amount, Unit, Frequency

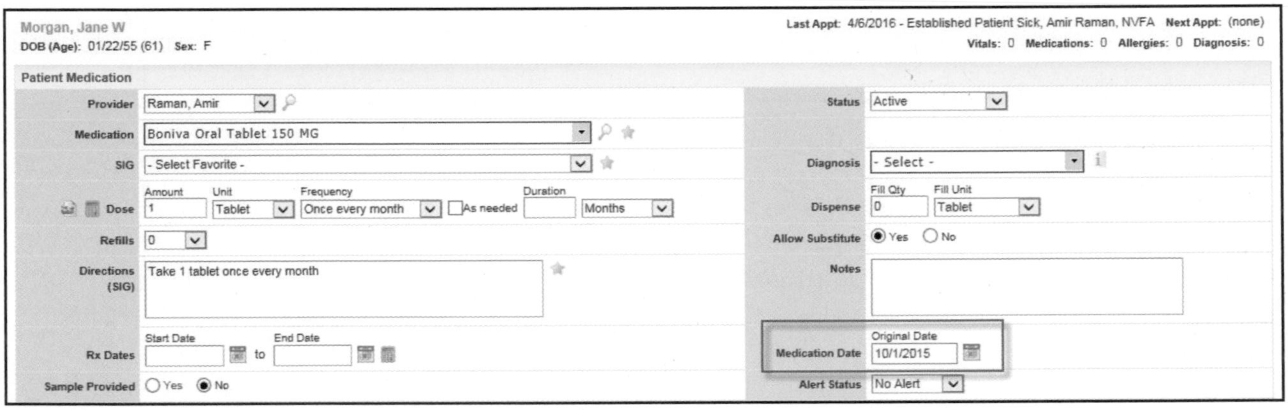

Morgan, Jane W
DOB (Age): 01/22/55 (61)   Sex: F

Last Appt: 4/6/2016 - Established Patient Sick, Amir Raman, NVFA   Next Appt: (none)
Vitals: 0   Medications: 0   Allergies: 0   Diagnosis: 0

Patient Medication

Provider	Raman, Amir		Status	Active
Medication	Boniva Oral Tablet 150 MG		Diagnosis	- Select -
SIG	- Select Favorite -			

Dose
Amount	Unit	Frequency	Duration		Dispense	Fill Qty	Fill Unit
1	Tablet	Once every month ☐ As needed	Months			0	Tablet

Refills   0

Allow Substitute   ● Yes   ○ No

Directions (SIG)   Take 1 tablet once every month ★   Notes

Rx Dates
Start Date   to   End Date

Medication Date   Original Date   10/1/2015

Sample Provided   ○ Yes   ● No

Alert Status   No Alert

Figure 6-23   Original Date

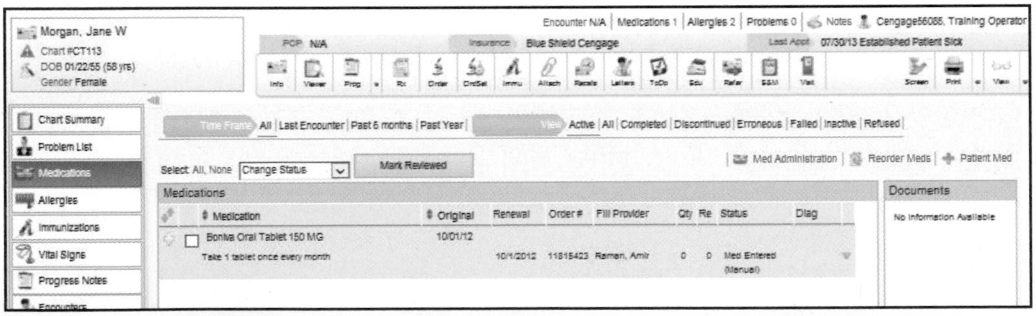

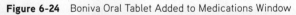

Morgan, Jane W
Chart #CT113
DOB 01/22/55 (58 yrs)
Gender Female

Encounter N/A   Medications 1   Allergies 2   Problems 0   Notes   Cengage56086, Training Operator
PCP N/A   Insurance Blue Shield Cengage   Last Appt 07/30/13 Established Patient Sick

Info Viewer Prog Rx Order OrdSet Immu Attach Recalls Letters ToDo Edu Refer E&M Visit   Screen Print View

- Chart Summary
- Problem List
- Medications
- Allergies
- Immunizations
- Vital Signs
- Progress Notes
- Encounters

Time Frame All | Last Encounter | Past 6 months | Past Year   View Active | All | Completed | Discontinued | Erroneous | Failed | Inactive | Refused

Select: All, None   Change Status   Mark Reviewed
Med Administration   Reorder Meds   Patient Med

Medications

	‡ Medication	‡ Original	Renewal	Order #	Fill Provider	Qty	Re	Status	Diag
☐	Boniva Oral Tablet 150 MG	10/01/12							
	Take 1 tablet once every month		10/1/2012	11815423	Raman, Amir	0	0	Med Entered (Manual)	

Documents
No information Available

Figure 6-24   Boniva Oral Tablet Added to Medications Window

Updating the Patient's Allergy Information

The *Allergies* application helps add new and existing allergies to a patient's medical record. It is important to ensure that all active allergies are recorded for accurate drug–allergy contraindication checks when prescribing medications and ordering immunizations.

ACTIVITY 6-8: Adding an Allergy to a Patient's Chart

1. If you are not in Jane Morgan's medical record, access it following the steps used in Activity 6-6.
2. In the *Patient Medical History* pane, click on *Allergies*. Harris CareTracker EMR displays the *Allergies* window.
3. Click + *Add Allergy* (Figure 6-25). Harris CareTracker EMR displays the *Patient Allergy* dialog box (Figure 6-26).

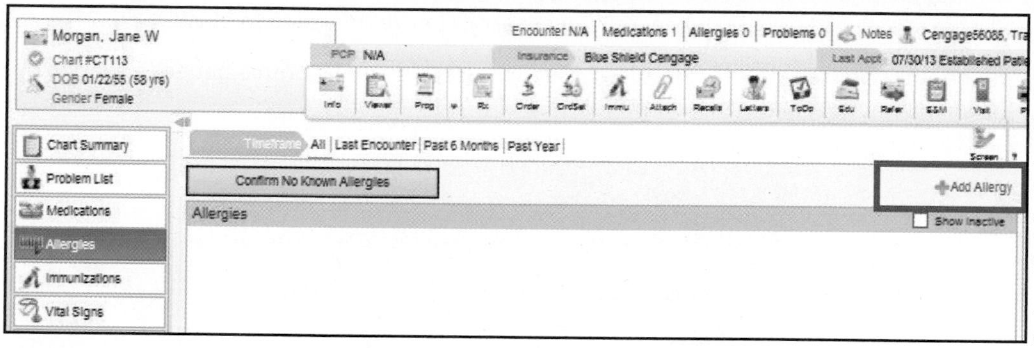

Courtesy of Harris CareTracker PM and EMR

Figure 6-25 Add Allergy

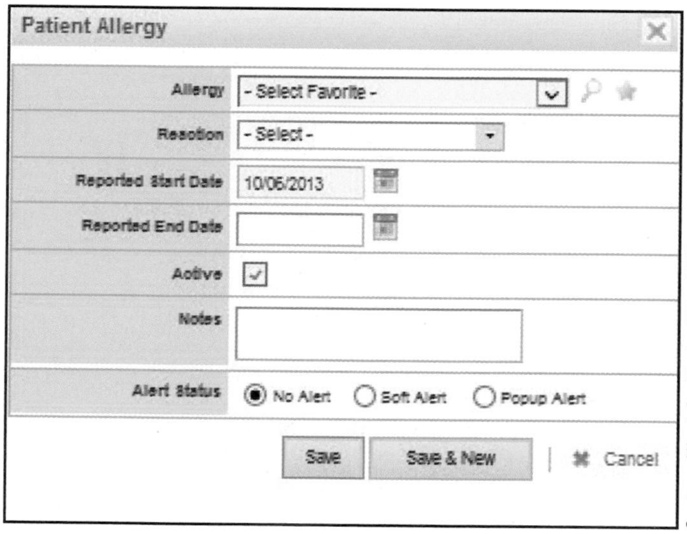

Courtesy of Harris CareTracker PM and EMR

Figure 6-26 Patient Allergy Dialog Box

4. Ms. Morgan is allergic to codeine, so this information will need to be entered in her electronic chart. Search for codeine by clicking on the *Search* icon next to the *Allergy* field. (**Note:** If codeine has been previously entered as a favorite in the system it will appear in the drop-down *Allergy* list. We will mimic searching for it as though it were not saved as a favorite.)
5. In the *Search Text* box, type "Codeine." Click the *Search* button.
6. A list of several medications will pop up that include the word "codeine." If "Codeine" is already on the favorites list, it will be indicated by the *On Favorites* icon.
7. Click on the search result, "Codeine Phosphate." The *Patient Allergy* window will reappear with "Codeine Phosphate" listed beside *Allergy*.

8. In the *Reaction* box, click on the drop-down arrow and select "Anaphylaxis". (**Note:** Click on the drop-down arrow again to remove the drop-down list. "Anaphylaxis" is now selected.)

9. In the *Reported Start Date* box, enter the date of onset for the allergy in MM/DD/YYYY format or click the *Calendar* ⊞ icon to select the date. Enter a start date of April 1 of last year.

10. Leave the *Reported End Date* blank.

11. By default, the *Status* is set to *Active* to indicate that the allergy is an active allergy. (**Note:** The active checkbox is read only and is updated based on *Reported End Date* status.)

12. In the *Notes* box, enter additional comments, if necessary. (Leave this section blank.)

13. By default, the *Alert Status* is set to "No Alert". Due to the seriousness of this patient's allergy, click on "Popup Alert" (Figure 6-27).

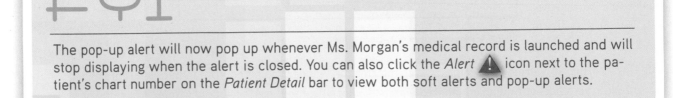

Figure 6-27   Popup Alert

FYI

The pop-up alert will now pop up whenever Ms. Morgan's medical record is launched and will stop displaying when the alert is closed. You can also click the *Alert* ⚠ icon next to the patient's chart number on the *Patient Detail* bar to view both soft alerts and pop-up alerts.

14. Click *Save & New* to save and add another allergy without exiting the *Patient Allergy* dialog box.

15. Add "Peanuts [NS]" as a new allergy for Ms. Morgan and save it as a favorite.

    a. In the *Reaction* box, scroll down the list and select both "Diarrhea" and "Vomiting".

    b. In the *Reported Start Date* box, enter a date that is 10 years prior to the date of the appointment.

    c. Leave the *Reported End Date* box blank.

d. In the *Notes* section, type the following: "The reported start date is just an estimate. Patient doesn't know the actual day or year she had the reaction."

e. Select "Soft Alert" in the *Alert Status* category.

16. Click *Save.* "Peanuts" and "Codeine" will now be listed in the *Allergies* pane (Figure 6-28).

Courtesy of Harris CareTracker PM and EMR

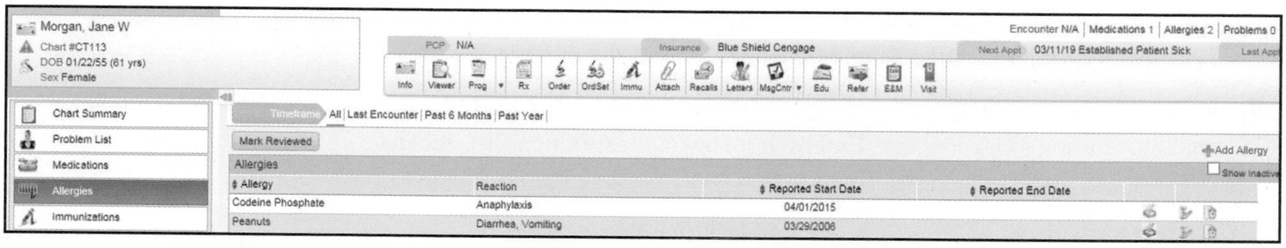

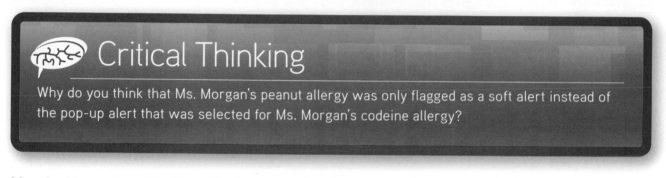

Figure 6-28 Allergies Pane

Critical Thinking

Why do you think that Ms. Morgan's peanut allergy was only flagged as a soft alert instead of the pop-up alert that was selected for Ms. Morgan's codeine allergy?

Updating the Patient's Immunization Status

The *Immunizations* module allows you to enter history information regarding the patient. It also allows you to enter immunizations you administer in your office. Activity 6-9 describes how to enter a patient's past immunizations.

ACTIVITY 6-9: Entering Past Immunizations in a Patient's Chart

1. If you are not in Jane Morgan's medical record, access it following the steps used in Activity 6-6.

2. In the *Patient Medical History* pane, click on *Immunizations.* Harris CareTracker EMR displays the *Immunizations* window.

3. Click on the + *Add Past/Refused Immunization* link (Figure 6-29).

Courtesy of Harris CareTracker PM and EMR

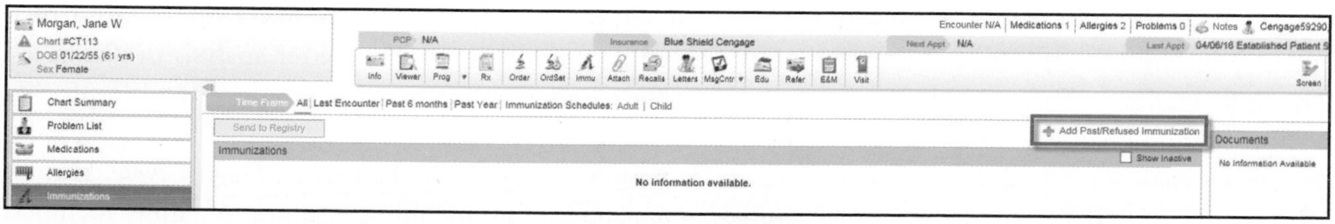

Figure 6-29 Add Past/Refused Immunization Link

4. Type in the word "Tetanus" in the *Immunization* field and then click on the *Search* 🔍 icon.

5. An *Immunization Search* dialog box will pop up. Click on "tetanus toxoid, absorbed" under *Search Results*. The selected immunization will now appear in the *Immunization* field.

6. Because Ms. Morgan's tetanus immunization was not administered at Napa Valley Family Health Associates, the only other information that can be entered is when she received the shot and where she received it. Ms. Morgan stated that she received the shot on March 3 of last year. Type this information in the *Admin Date* box.

7. Enter a description in the *Administration Notes* field. Ms. Morgan stated that she received the tetanus shot at America's Urgent Care. Enter the following description: "Pt. received Tetanus shot at America's Urgent Care after stepping on a nail."

8. Click *Save*. Your *Immunizations* pane should match Figure 6-30.

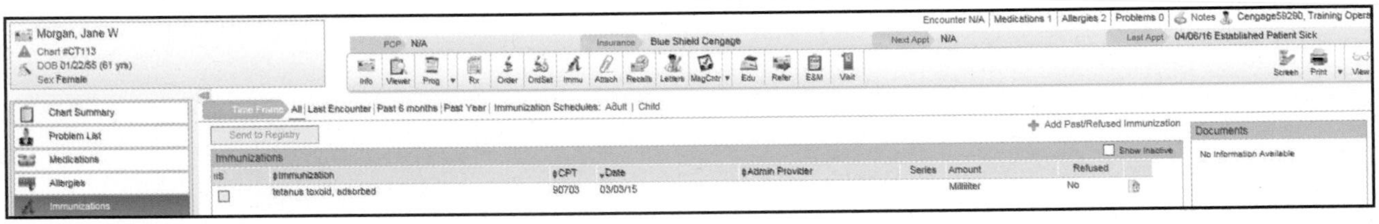

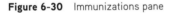

Figure 6-30   Immunizations pane

Courtesy of Harris CareTracker PM and EMR

🔴 **Print your chart summary using the following instructions, which will illustrate the work you did in the last three activities.**

- Click on *Chart Summary* in the *Patient Health History Pane*.

- Click on the drop-down arrow beside the printer 🖨 icon in the upper-right corner of the screen.

- Click on *Print Chart Summary*. A new window will pop up.

- Click the *Print* button. Label this "Activities 6-7, 6-8, and 6-9" and place it in your assignment folder.

Accessing the History Application

The *History* application helps capture and review a patient's past medical, family, and social history information from one central location using different data entry methods. It is important to record and review history data because they enable the provider to form a diagnosis and treatment plan together with the clinical examination. The *History* application provides quick and easy data entry methods, such as checkboxes, drop-down lists, text boxes, and more, to record information. In addition, you can also click *Mark Reviewed* for each category to ensure that historical information presented is reviewed to provide better analysis in diagnoses. This information is automatically made available in the *History* section of each progress note, improving documentation quality and patient care.

An alternative method to document history information is directly via the patient *Progress Note*. History information recorded here is also recorded in the *History* application, including addition of family members to the *Family History* section.

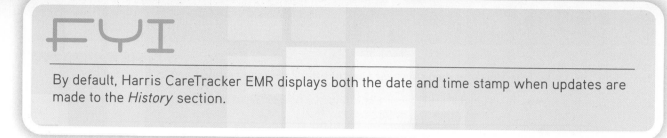

FYI

By default, Harris CareTracker EMR displays both the date and time stamp when updates are made to the *History* section.

Table 6-4 describes information found in the *History* application.

Type	Description
TABLE 6-4 History Application Descriptions	
Patient History	By default, the *History* window displays the **patient history**, which consists of past medical and social history information. Past medical history includes details such as any operations, illnesses, and accidents. Social history includes information on tobacco and alcohol usage.
Sensitive Info	This displays **sensitive information** such as a patient's human immunodeficiency virus (HIV) or sexually transmitted disease (STD) statuses and information on overuse of alcohol and/or chemicals.
Family History	**Family history** displays part of a patient's medical history in which questions are asked in an attempt to find out whether the patient has hereditary tendencies toward particular diseases. Family history is to be present in all members' charts, including children.
Advance Directives	**Advance directives** are the legal documents, such as the living will, durable power of attorney, and health care proxy, that allow people to convey their decisions about end-of-life care ahead of time. Advance directives provide a way for patients to communicate their wishes to family, friends, and health care professionals and to avoid confusion later on, should they become unable to do so. Ideally, the process of discussing and writing advance directives should be ongoing, rather than a single event. Advance directives can be modified as a patient's situation changes. Even after advance directives have been signed, patients can change their mind at any time.
Attachments	In addition to capturing health history information electronically, you can scan or attach health history forms filled by a patient via the *Document Management Upload* application. All history forms assigned as type "Clinical" and subtype "History" display under this tab. You can edit, delete, or annotate documents if necessary.
Log	The log displays a history of all activities performed in the *History* section of the patient's medical record.
Preview	Preview displays a summary view of all history information recorded for the patient. In addition, the preview displays the specific date an item is recorded or updated in the patient's medical record.

ACTIVITY 6-10: Entering a Patient's Medical History

1. If you are not in Jane Morgan's medical record, access it following the steps used in Activity 6-6.
2. Click on the *History* tab. Harris CareTracker EMR displays the *History* window (Figure 6-31).

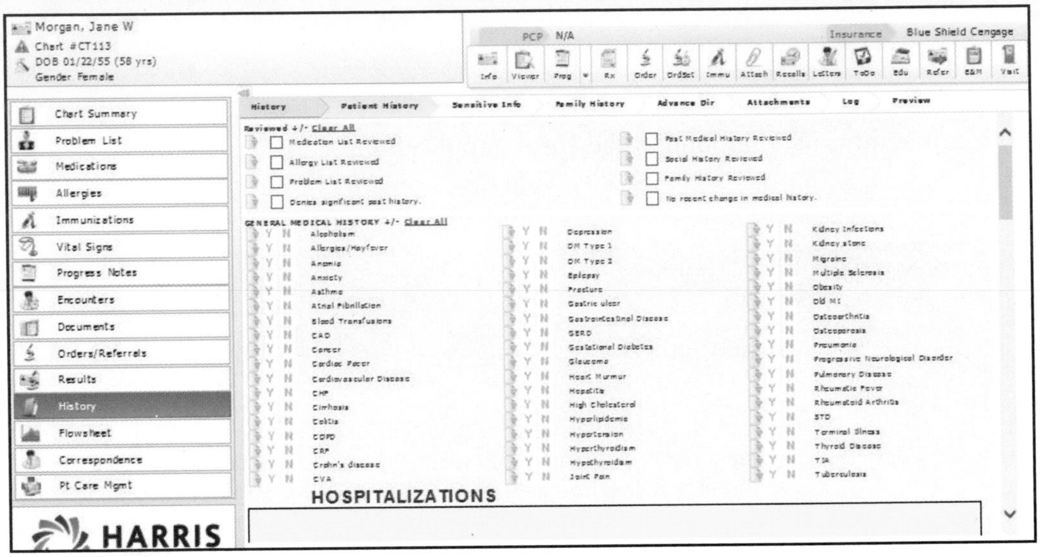

Courtesy of Harris CareTracker PM and EMR

Figure 6-31 History Window

3. In the *General Medical History* section of the *Patient History* screen, click "Yes" on the conditions listed in Table 6-5. Click on the *Finding Details* icon to the left of the "Y" boxes and follow the instructions in Table 6-5 regarding information to insert in the *Comments* box (Figure 6-32). Click the *X* on the top right of the *Comments* box to close and save each comment. (**Note:** It may take a few moments for the dialog box to activate to enter text.)
4. Enter the following information in the *Hospitalizations* box:
   a. Tonsillectomy at age 3. Doesn't know which hospital.

TABLE 6-5 General Medical History Information for Jane Morgan

Condition	Details
Allergies/Hay Fever	*Comment:* Usually occurs in the spring of each year. Onset: During childhood. Doesn't know the year. Takes OTC allergy relief medication during flare-ups. (Refer to Figure 6-32.)
Asthma	Under *Severity*, click the box beside "mild." *Comment*: Diagnosed 10 years ago. Has had 2–3 attacks in the past 10 years. Last attack approximately five years ago. Not taking any meds for this condition.
Depression	*Comment:* Has not been formally diagnosed. Has periods of sadness and crying. Doesn't want to do anything during these bouts. Onset: About one year. Occurs a couple of times a month and lasts for a few days.
Joint Pain	*Comment:* Intermittent pain (flare-ups approx 2–3 times per year). Never been formally diagnosed. Mainly in fingers and toes. Onset date approx three years ago.

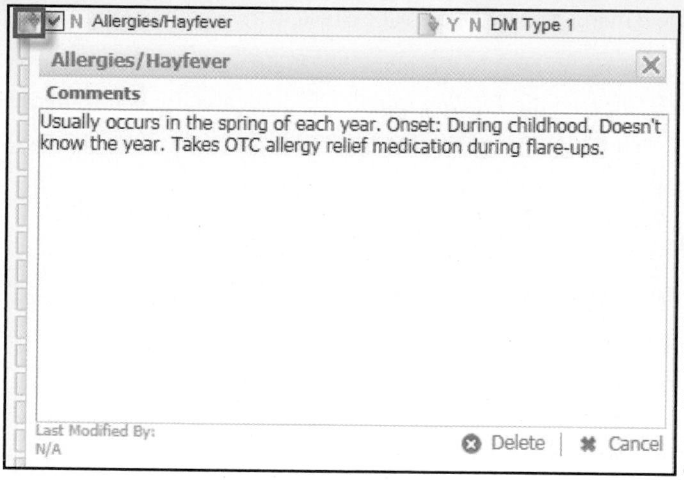

Figure 6-32   Allergies/Hay Fever Comments Box

   b. Hospitalized for the birth of her three children at County General. No complications.

   c. No other hospitalizations.

5. Enter the following information in the *Other Medical History* box: "Five-year history of UTIs. Approximately 1–2 episodes/year. Treatment: Antibiotics."

6. In the *Tobacco Assessment* section, click on the drop-down menu next to the blank box/field to the right of *Smoking Status* and select "Never Smoker". Beside *Tobacco User* click on the "N" for No. Leave everything else in this section blank. (Note that the *Tobacco Assessment* section supports Stage 1 Meaningful Use.)

7. Enter the following information in the *Social History* section:

   a. Click on the drop-down menu next to the blank box/field to the right of *Alcohol Use* and select "Non-Drinker".

   b. Click on the drop-down menu next to the blank box/field to the right of *Caffeine Use* and select "2 servings per Day". Click on the *Finding Details* icon next to *Caffeine Use* and put a check mark beside "coffee" and "tea." In the *Comments* box state the following: "Drinks 1 cup of coffee and 1 glass of iced tea daily." Click the *X* to close out of the box.

   c. *Drug Use*: Click on the "N" for No.

   d. *Sun Protection*: Click on the "Y" for Yes. Click on the *Finding Details* icon. Place a check mark in the "sunglasses" and "sunscreen" boxes. Click on *SPF* and select the "30" box. Click the *X* to close out of the *Sun Protection* box.

   e. *Tattoos*: Click on the "N" for No.

   f. *Sexually Active*: Click on the "Y" for Yes. Click on the *Finding Details* icon and enter the following in the *Comments* box: "In a monogamous relationship with husband. No concerns." Click the *X* to close out of the box.

   g. Click on the drop-down menu next to the blank box/field to the right of *Race* and select "Caucasian".

   h. Click on the drop-down menu next to the blank box/field to the right of *Native language* and select "English".

   i. *Physical Abuse*: Click on the "N" for No.

   j. *Domestic Violence*: Click on the "N" for No.

   k. Click on the drop-down menu next to the blank box/field to the right of *Education Level* and select "Bachelors Degree".

l. Click on the drop-down menu next to the blank box/field to the right of *Marital Status* and select "Married".

m. Click on the drop-down menu next to the blank box/field to the right of *Exercise Habits* and select "moderate >3 x/wk". Click on the *Finding Details* icon and enter the following in the *Comments* section: "Walks 1–2 miles twice a week with husband." Click the *X* to close out of the box.

n. *Seatbelts*: Click on the "Y" for Yes.

o. *Body Piercings*: Click on the "N" for No.

p. *Birth Control Method*: Leave all boxes blank in this section.

q. Click on the drop-down menu next to the blank box/field to the right of *Religion* and select "Christian".

r. *Occupation*: Enter "Nurse".

s. *Other Social History* box: Leave blank.

8. In the *Depression Screening* section, click on the drop-down box next to the blank box/field beside *Little interest or pleasure in doing things* and select "Occasionally". Click on the drop-down box next to the blank box/field beside *Feeling down, depressed, or hopeless* and select "Occasionally". Leave the *Date of Last Depression Screening* field blank.

9. Enter the following information in the *OB/GYN History* section:

a. *LMP:* Leave blank.

b. *Menopause has occurred*: Click on the "Y" for Yes. Click on the *Finding Details* icon and enter the following in the *Comments* box: "Age of Onset: 48, + night sweats, + hot flashes, and problems with concentration." Click the *X* to close out of the box.

c. *History of abnormal pap smears*: Click on the "N" for No.

d. *Sexually Active*: This information should have been pulled in from information you entered during the social history. If not, click on the "Y" for Yes, and click on the *Finding Details* icon. Enter the following in the *Comments* box: "In a monogamous relationship with husband. No concerns." Click the *X* to close out of the box.

e. *Ectopic Pregnancy*: Click on the "N" for No.

f. *Menarche Age*: Enter "13".

g. *Birth Control:* Leave these boxes blank.

10. Enter the following information in the *Pregnancy Summary* section:

a. *Gravida*: Select "4" from the drop-down menu next to the blank box/field.

b. *Term:* Select "2" from the drop-down menu next to the blank box/field.

c. *Preterm*: Select "1" from the drop-down menu next to the blank box/field.

d. *AB:* Skip over this category.

e. *Live Children*: Select "3" from the drop-down menu next to the blank box/field.

f. *Miscarriage*: Select "1" from the drop-down menu next to the blank box/field.

11. Leave the *Other OB-GYN History* box blank.

12. In the *Surgical/Procedural* section, select the box for *Breast Lumpectomy* and click on the associated *Finding Details* icon. In the *Breast Lumpectomy* box, select "left" for the *Location*. In the *Comments* section, enter: "Had lumpectomy in May of 2010. Biopsy negative for cancer cells." Click the *X* to close out of the box. Leave all other boxes in this section blank.

13. Leave the *Other Surgical History* box blank.

14. Enter the following information in the *Preventive Care* section (for all dates, use the previous year unless otherwise indicated):

a. *Colonoscopy:* Enter 03/12/20XX

b. *Dilated Eye Exam*: Enter 01/04/20XX

c. *Flu Vaccine*: Enter 10/12/20XX

d. *Mammography*: 05/12/20XX

e. *Pap Smear*: 05/15/20XX (3 years ago)

15. In the *Self-Management Goal* box, enter: "Lose 10 pounds this year and start exercising 3x/week."

16. Click *Save*.

Go to the top right of the History pane. Click on the drop-down arrow beside the Print icon. Click on Print Patient History. When the box opens, you should see the patient's history form. Print this form, label it "Activity 6-10A" and place it in your assignment folder.

CLINICAL SPOTLIGHT

There are times a patient will refuse to answer questions outlined on the template. If so, leave the field blank. Do not check "Y" or "N." There is no option of "patient refused" but you could free text a comment in the notes box by clicking the *Finding Details* icon.

17. Click on the *Sensitive Info* tab. Your screen should match Figure 6-33 (though no selections will have been made yet).

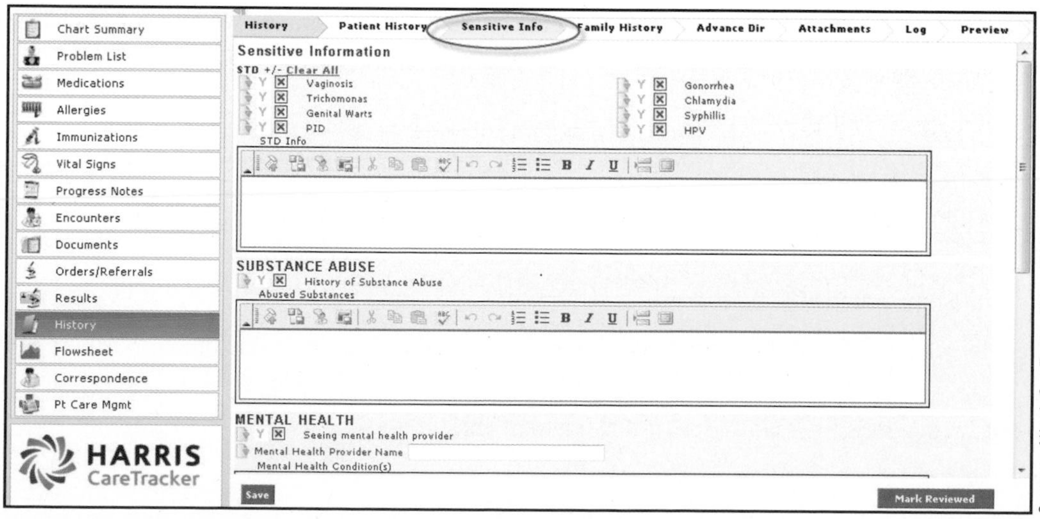

Courtesy of Harris CareTracker PM and EMR

Figure 6-33 Sensitive Info Tab

18. In the *STD* section, click "N" for each disease listed. (**Note:** An easy way to mark all categories with the same response is to click on the [+/-] sign between *STD* and *Clear All*. For this scenario, click on the [-] sign. All diseases should now have a red "X" [indicating 'No'] beside their names.)

19. Ms. Morgan has no history of substance abuse so click on the "N" beside *History of Substance Abuse*.

20. Ms. Morgan is not seeing any mental health providers so click on the "N" beside *Seeing mental health provider*.

21. Ms. Morgan has never had an HIV test. Enter the following comment in the text box below *HIV Status*: "Patient has never had an HIV test but states that she has been in a monogamous relationship with her husband over the past 25 years."

22. Leave the *Medicare High Risk Criteria* section blank because Ms. Morgan is not enrolled in Medicare.

FYI

Normally, Medicare pays for a Pap test every three years for females who are asymptomatic. However, Medicare may pay for annual Pap tests when the patient is considered high risk for cervical and vaginal cancers. Those conditions include the following:

- Early onset of sexual activity (under 16 years of age)
- Multiple sexual partners (five or more in a lifetime)
- History of a sexually transmitted infection (STI) (including human immunodeficiency virus [HIV] infection)
- Fewer than three negative Pap tests or no Pap tests within the previous seven years
- DES (diethylstilbestrol) exposed daughters of women who took DES during pregnancy

These guidelines may or may not have changed with the implementation of the Affordable Care Act and it is important that the practice continually review updates on current rules and regulations.

---

23. Click *Save*.

Click on the drop-down arrow beside the Print icon. Select Print Sensitive Information. When the box opens, you should see the Sensitive Information Form. Print this form and label it "Activity 6-10B." Place it in your assignment folder.

24. Click on the *Family History* tab.

25. Select the *Mother* tab (Figure 6-34). Enter the following information in this section:

   a. Ms. Morgan's mother is still alive. Click on the drop-down menu next to the blank box/field to the right of *Status* and select "Alive".

   b. In the *Age* box, enter "78".

   c. Select the checkbox next to *In good health* to indicate the general health status of Ms. Morgan's mother.

   d. Ms. Morgan's mother suffers from GERD and hypertension. Click on the "Y" for Yes next to these two diseases.

   e. Click *Save*.

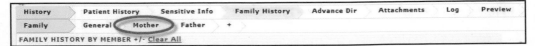

Figure 6-34   Mother Tab
Courtesy of Harris CareTracker PM and EMR

26. Select the *Father* tab. Enter the following information in this section:

    a. Ms. Morgan's father died in a car accident at age 30. Click on the drop-down menu next to the blank box/field to the right of *Status* and select "Deceased".

    b. In the *Other conditions* text box at the bottom of the screen, enter the following comment: "Ms. Morgan's father died in a car accident at the age of 30."

    c. Click *Save*.

Click on the drop-down arrow beside the Print icon. Select Print Family History. When the box opens, you should see the **Family History By Family Member form. Print this form, label it "Activity 6-10C" and place it in your assignment folder.**

Recording Patient's Vital Signs and Chief Complaint

Learning Objective 7: Record vital signs and document the patient's chief complaint.

The *Vital Signs* application allows you to record the patient's vital data at every encounter in the office and includes the patient's blood pressure, temperature, pulse respiration, height, weight, oxygen saturation reading, and pain level. This helps to guide clinical decisions about treatment and to identify the need for additional diagnostic measures. Activity 6-11 describes how to record a patient's vital signs.

ACTIVITY 6-11:   Recording a Patient's Vital Signs

1. If you are not in Jane Morgan's medical record, access it following the steps used in Activity 6-6.

2. In the *Patient Health History* pane, click on *Vital Signs*. Harris CareTracker EMR displays the *Vital Signs* window with vital data taken during the current and past encounters at the office or at home. Because this is Ms. Morgan's first visit since the EMR was instituted, no vital signs have been entered yet.

3. Click on *Record Vital Signs* in the lower-left pane of the screen (Figure 6-35).

4. Using the information in Table 6-6, enter the appropriate values in the *Record Vital Signs* dialog box (Figure 6-37).

5. In the *Chief Complaint* box, type the following: "Patient complains of urinary symptoms over the last three days."

6. Click *Save*. The vital data automatically update the vital grid with the measurements and the date the vitals are recorded. (**Note:** The vital data automatically update the progress note for the same encounter and display the data in the corresponding narrative.)

7. In Activity 6-12 you are going to be working with flow sheets, which graph a variety of different measurements. Because we can add multiple iterations in one visit for vital signs, click back on *Record Vital Signs* at the bottom left corner of the window pane.

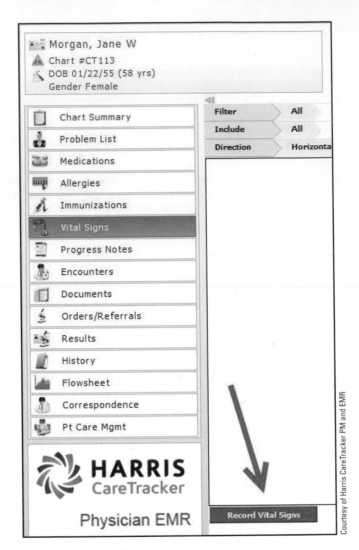

Figure 6-35   Record Vital Signs

FYI

If an encounter is in context, the *Record Vital Signs* dialog box will display. If an encounter is not in context, the *Select Encounter* dialog box displays (Figure 6-36) and you must create an encounter. An encounter already exists for this patient because you went in through the *Appointment* application in *Clinical Today*; however, if the patient was not coming in for an appointment, but rather just stopping by to have his or her vital signs monitored, you would need to create an encounter to record your measurements.

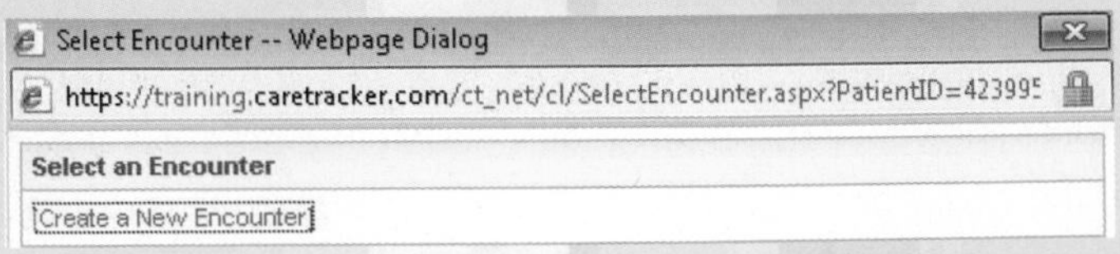

Select Encounter -- Webpage Dialog

https://training.caretracker.com/ct_net/cl/SelectEncounter.aspx?PatientID=423995

Select an Encounter

Create a New Encounter

Figure 6-36   Select Encounter Dialog Box

Courtesy of Harris CareTracker PM and EMR

TABLE 6-6   Vital Signs for Jane Morgan

Measurement Category	Reading
Height	5 ft 6 in
Weight	160 lb
Body Mass Index	This will automatically populate.
Blood Pressure	146/90
Pulse Rate	84 bpm
Temperature	98.4 °F
Respiratory Rate	16
Pulse Oximetry	97%
Pain Level	7/10

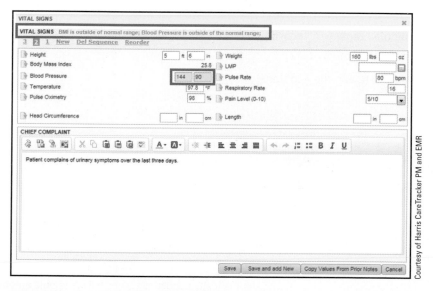

Figure 6-37   Record Vital Signs Dialog Box

Critical Thinking

Did you notice how the blood pressure field turned orange and the note "BMI is outside of normal range; Blood Pressure is outside of the normal range" appeared in orange next to Vital Signs after the measurements were saved (see Figure 6-37)? This is because the patient is out of the normal ranges for those two categories. What should the medical assistant do when the patient's vital signs are elevated?

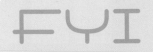

You can record vital data such as height, weight, temperature, head circumference, and length using metric and standard measurements. By default, the vital data are converted from one unit of measure to another.

FYI

You can record multiple **iterations** (the act of repeating) of vital data by clicking *Save and Add New*. When you record multiple iterations, the *Chart Summary* and *Progress Note* display the date and the iteration number for each instance. When vital data are recorded via the progress note, the *Vital Signs* application automatically updates with the same data.

8. Using the information in Table 6-7, record two more sets of readings so that you can graph your results in the flow sheet activity (Activity 6-12).

9. Click *Save and add New* to add the additional readings.

TABLE 6-7 Additional Vital Sign Readings for Jane Morgan

Measurement Category	Second Reading	Third Reading
Height	5 ft 6 in	5 ft 6 in
Weight	160 lb	160 lb
Body Mass Index	This should automatically populate.	This should automatically populate.
Blood Pressure	148/92	144/90
Pulse Rate	84 bpm	80 bpm
Temperature	98.8 °F	97.8 °F
Respiratory Rate	16	16
Pulse Oximetry	99%	98%
Pain Level	6/10	5/10

10. Once you are finished, click on *Save*. Now all three measurements should appear.

Click on the drop-down arrow beside the Print icon. Select Print Vital Signs Form. When the box opens you should see the Vital Signs form. Print this form, label it "Activity 6-11" and place it in your assignment folder.

FYI

Filtering Vital Data

The *Vital Signs* application enables you to filter vital data based on the location the vitals are monitored and the date the vitals are recorded. Additionally, you can filter to view vitals pertaining to a specific case.

To filter vital data:

- Access the *Medical Record* module using one of the following methods:
  - Pull the patient into context, and click the *Medical Record* module.
  - If the patient has an appointment, click the patient's name in the *Appointments* tab of the *Clinical Today* module.
- In the *Patient Health History* pane, click *Vital Signs*. Harris CareTracker EMR displays the *Vital Signs* window with vital data taken during the current and past encounters at the office or at home.
- Do one of the following:
  - To filter vitals based on the location recorded, click either the *Recorded at Home* or the *Recorded in the Office* tabs.
  - To filter vitals based on the date the vitals are recorded, click on the *Last Encounter*, *Past 6 months*, or *Past Year* tabs (Figure 6-38).

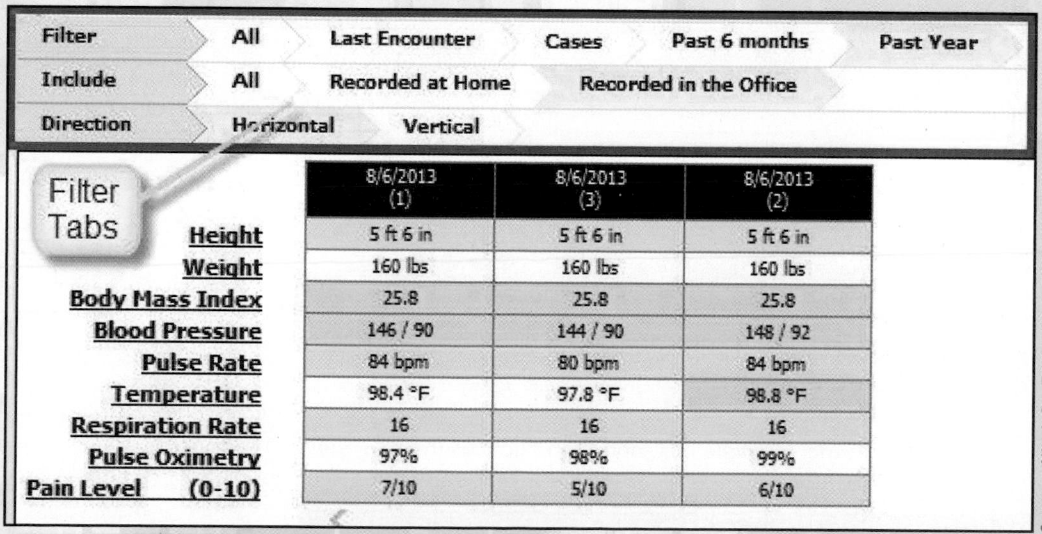

	8/6/2013 (1)	8/6/2013 (3)	8/6/2013 (2)
Height	5 ft 6 in	5 ft 6 in	5 ft 6 in
Weight	160 lbs	160 lbs	160 lbs
Body Mass Index	25.8	25.8	25.8
Blood Pressure	146 / 90	144 / 90	148 / 92
Pulse Rate	84 bpm	80 bpm	84 bpm
Temperature	98.4 °F	97.8 °F	98.8 °F
Respiration Rate	16	16	16
Pulse Oximetry	97%	98%	99%
Pain Level (0-10)	7/10	5/10	6/10

Courtesy of Harris CareTracker PM and EMR

Figure 6-38 Filtering Vital Data-Horizontal View

- To filter vitals pertaining to a specific case, click the *Cases* tab. In the *Select Cases* dialog box, select the checkbox for the case you want and click *Select*.

Viewing Flow Sheets

Learning Objective 8: View and create FlowSheets within Harris CareTracker EMR.

The *Flowsheet* application provides electronic management of clinical data entry and review of patient progress over time using different flowsheet templates. A **flowsheet template** is a profile with selected items. Data in a patient medical record can be pulled into a flow sheet, eliminating the need for double entry. It accommodates multidisciplinary documentation requirements and is linked to *Progress Notes, Vital Signs*, and the *Results* applications. The application displays patient information that includes lab results, medications, vitals, and other medical data in a table or graph view.

The table view includes two formats: vertical grid (Figure 6-39) and horizontal grid. In a vertical grid, the columns represent vitals taken, and rows represent an interval of time. The horizontal grid represents the data in the reverse layout. The different formats enable you to analyze data over time from a variety of viewpoints on a single display screen.

Filter	All	Last Encounter	Cases	Past 6 months	Past Year					
Include	All	Recorded at Home	Recorded in the Office							
Direction	Horizontal	Vertical								

	Height	Weight	Body Mass Index	Blood Pressure	Pulse Rate	Temperature	Respiration Rate	Pulse Oximetry	Pain Level (0-10)
8/6/2013 (1)	5 ft 6 in / 167.6 cm	160 lbs/72.57 kg	25.8	146/90	84 bpm	98.4 °F/36.9 °C	16	97%	7/10
8/6/2013 (3)	5 ft 6 in / 167.6 cm	160 lbs/72.57 kg	25.8	144/90	80 bpm	97.8 °F/36.6 °C	16	98%	5/10
8/6/2013 (2)	5 ft 6 in / 167.6 cm	160 lbs/72.57 kg	25.8	148/92	84 bpm	98.8 °F/37.1 °C	16	99%	6/10

Courtesy of Harris CareTracker PM and EMR

Figure 6-39 Vital Signs Vertical Grid

ACTIVITY 6-12: Viewing a Flow Sheet

1. If you are not in Jane Morgan's medical record, access it following the steps used in Activity 6-6.

2. In the *Patient Health History* pane, click on *Flowsheet*. Harris CareTracker EMR displays the *Flowsheet* window.

3. Generally, you can select a template from the *Saved Views* drop-down list, but the template you will need for this activity has not been saved yet. Click the *Search* 🔍 icon to the right of *Saved Views* (Figure 6-40). Harris CareTracker EMR displays the *Manage Flowsheet Templates* dialog box.

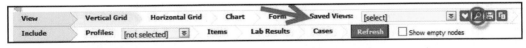

View	Vertical Grid	Horizontal Grid	Chart	Form	Saved Views:	[select]			
Include	Profiles:	[not selected]	Items	Lab Results	Cases	Refresh	☐ Show empty nodes		

Figure 6-40 Saved Views

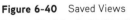
Courtesy of Harris CareTracker PM and EMR

4. Enter "Vital Signs" in the *Template* box, and then click on the plus sign (Figure 6-41).

🔍 **Templates**   ❤ **Favorites**

Template: [vital signs]   [×]   🔍 **Search**
          +
Warning! Select Provider when searching for Provider Flowsheet!

⊞ 👤 FAMILY - PSYCHOLOGIST [+]
⊞ 👤 GENERAL PRACTICE [+]
⊞ 👤 OBSTETRICS - OBSTETRICS AND GYNECOLOGY [+]

Courtesy of Harris CareTracker PM and EMR

Figure 6-41 Enter Vital Signs in Template Box

5. The *Flowsheet Template* dialog box will appear. In the *Name* box, type "Vital Signs."

6. In the *Specialty* box, click on the drop-down arrow and select "FAMILY MEDICINE".

7. In the *View* box, click on the drop-down arrow and select "Chart".

8. Next to the *Scope* box, click on the drop-down arrow and select "COMPANY".

9. Click on the checkbox next to *In Favorites* to make this a favorite you can select for further activities.

10. Click on the drop-down arrow in the *Flowsheet Profile* box, scroll down, and select "Vital Signs".

11. A list of flow sheet items comes up that you can select for your profile (Figure 6-42). Click on the checkboxes next to *Blood Pressure, Body Mass Index, Height, Pain Level, Pulse Oximetry, Pulse Rate, Respiration Rate,* and *Weight.* **Note:** You will need to scroll down the screen to view all options of the Flowsheet Profile.

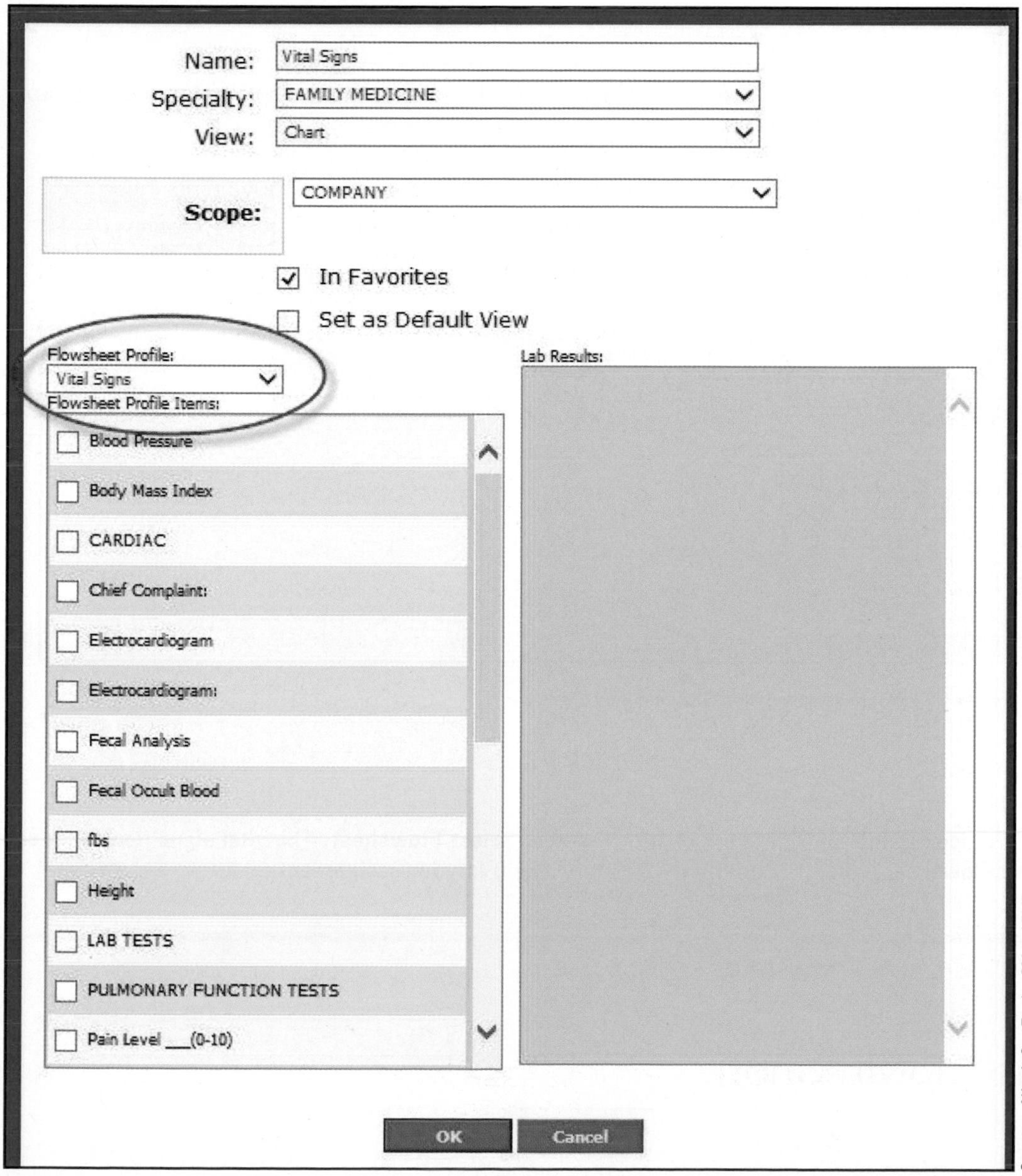

Figure 6-42 Flowsheet Profiles

12. Click *OK*.

13. The *Manage Flowsheet Template*s application will pop up with the new specialty heading *Family Medicine*. (**Note:** You may need to click the *Search* button for your screen to refresh with the new template.)

14. Click on the [+] sign beside *Family Medicine*. You should now see the *Vital Signs* heading (Figure 6-43).

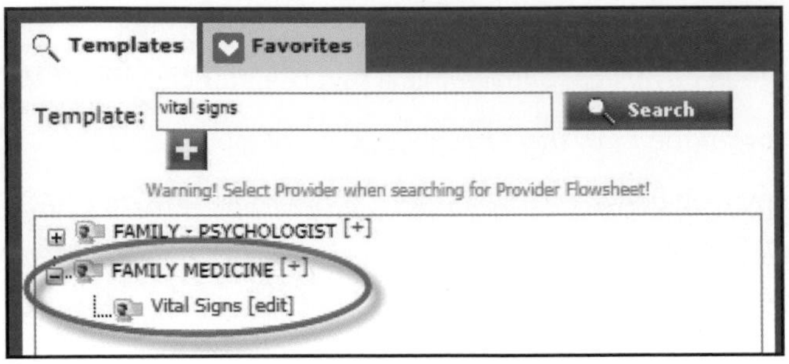

Figure 6-43   Vital Signs Heading

15. Click on the *Vital Signs* heading, which will take you back to the original *Flowsheet* application box (Figure 6-44).

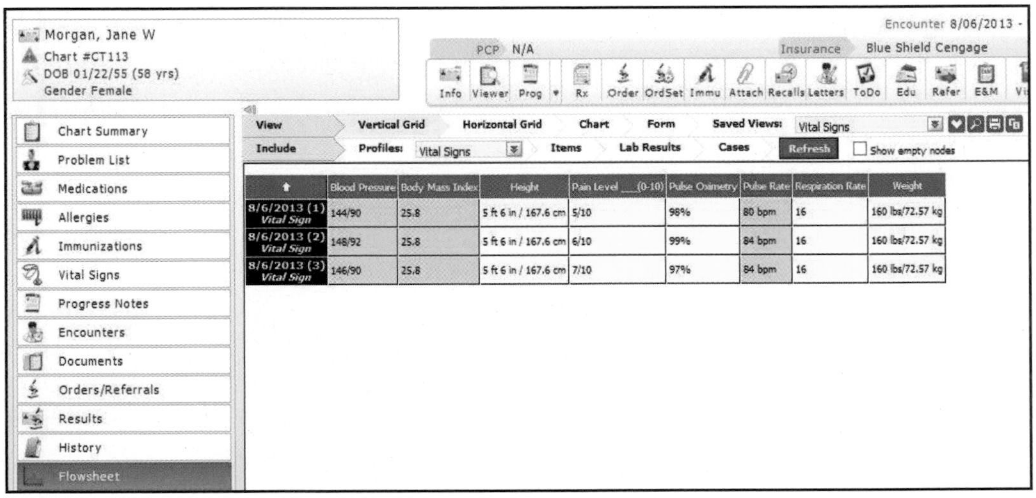

Figure 6-44   Flowsheet Application Showing Vital Signs

16. Change the view by clicking on the *Horizontal Grid* tab.

Click on the Print icon in the top right corner of the screen. Select Flowsheet. The vital signs flowsheet should open. Print this flowsheet, label it "Activity 6-12," and place it in your assignment folder.

Pediatric Growth Chart

Learning Objective 9: Create and print a growth chart.

According to the U.S. Department of Health and Human Services, **growth charts** provide a graphical method to compare a child's achieved growth with that of children of the same age and sex from a suitable reference population. For clinical use, such charts show selected percentiles of **anthropometric** variables such as weight, height, or body mass index (BMI) plotted against age or weight plotted against height. Anthropometric refers to a measurement or description of the physical dimensions and properties of the body, especially on a comparative basis; typically, it is used on upper and lower limbs, neck, and trunk.

Harris CareTracker EMR allows users to create, view, and print pediatric growth charts from the *Flowsheet* application in the patient's EMR. Table 6-8 illustrates the units of measure for specific age groups.

TABLE 6-8   Pediatric Growth Chart Units of Measure for Age

Age	Units of Measure
Birth to 6 days	Age is measured in days and is indicated with a "d."
7 days to 1 month	Age is measured in weeks and days and is indicated by "wks" or "wk/d."
1 month to 36 months	Age is measured in months and weeks and is indicated by "mos," "mo/wks," or "wk."
3 years to 21 years	Age is measured in years and months and is indicated by "yrs," "yr/mos," or "mo."

Harris CareTracker PM and EMR houses the standard growth charts available from the Centers for Disease Control and Prevention (CDC) and World Health Organization (WHO). Table 6-9 highlights the different growth charts available in Harris CareTracker EMR.

TABLE 6-9   Types of Growth Charts in Harris CareTracker EMR

Growth Charts for Boys	Growth Charts for Girls
Boys HC/WT for Length 0–36 mos	Girls HC/WT for Length 0–36 mos
Boys Length/Weight for Age 0–36 mos	Girls Length/Weight for Age 0–36 mos
Boys BMI for Age 2–20 years	Girls BMI for Age 2–20 years
Boys Stature/Weight for Age 2–20 yrs	Girls Stature/Weight for Age 2–20 yrs

ACTIVITY 6-13:   Creating a Growth Chart

1. Pull patient Spencer Douglas into context.
2. Click on the *Medical Record* module.

3. Click on the *Flowsheet* tab in the *Patient Health History* pane.

4. Click on the drop-down arrow beside *Profiles* and select "Boys Length/Weight for Age 0–36 months" (Figure 6-45).

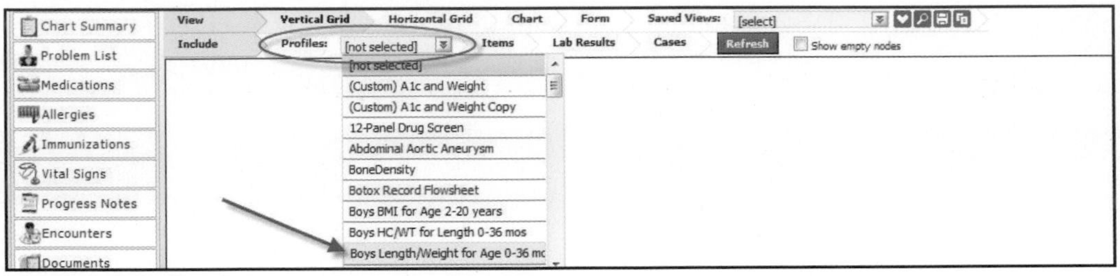

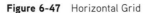

Figure 6-45 Flowsheet Profiles - Boys

5. Click on the *Items* tab (Figure 6-46).

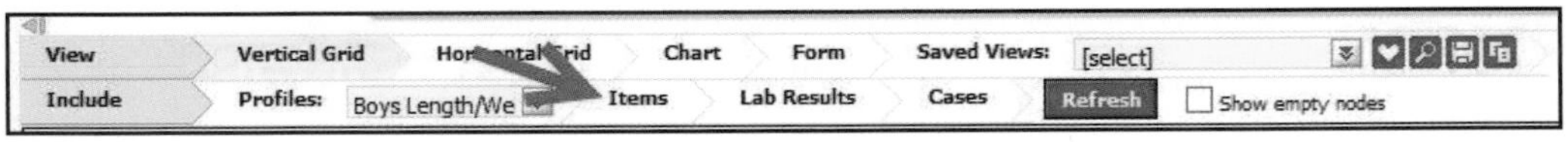

Figure 6-46 Flowsheet Items Tab
Courtesy of Harris CareTracker PM and EMR

6. The *Select Flowsheet Items* box displays. Check the boxes for "Weight" and "Length" and then click on *Select*.

7. Notice that three different weights and lengths are already entered for Spencer at different age intervals. The current view is set on *Vertical Grid*. Click on *Horizontal Grid* (Figure 6-47).

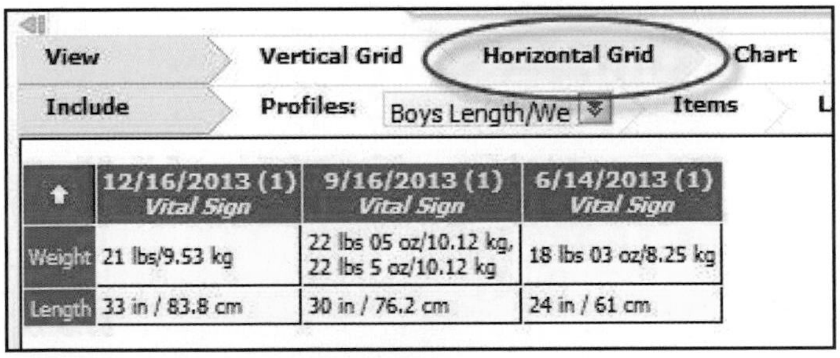

	12/16/2013 (1) Vital Sign	9/16/2013 (1) Vital Sign	6/14/2013 (1) Vital Sign
Weight	21 lbs/9.53 kg	22 lbs 05 oz/10.12 kg, 22 lbs 5 oz/10.12 kg	18 lbs 03 oz/8.25 kg
Length	33 in / 83.8 cm	30 in / 76.2 cm	24 in / 61 cm

Figure 6-47 Horizontal Grid

8. To bring up Spencer's growth chart, click on the *Chart* tab in the *View* row.

Click on Print in the View row. Label the growth chart "Activity 6-13" and place it in your assignment folder.

Critical Thinking

Where was Spencer on the growth chart for all three visits? Is there cause for concern about Spencer? Why or why not? See Figure 6-48.

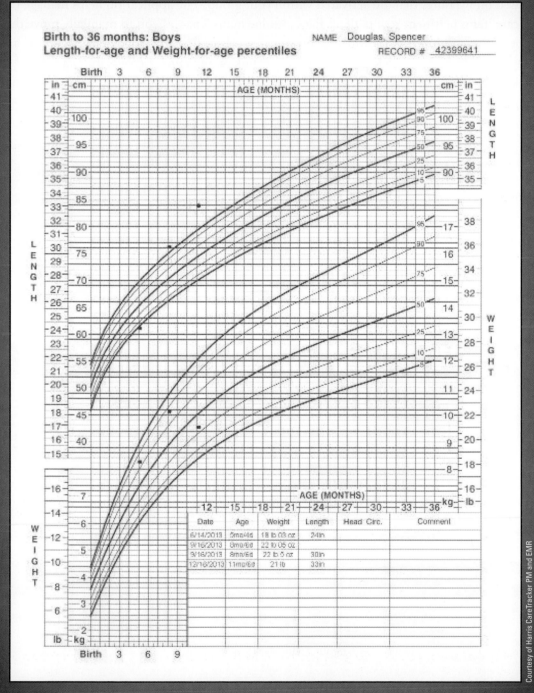

Figure 6-48 Spencer Douglas Growth Chart

Accessing the Patient Care Management Application

Learning Objective 10: Update the Patient Care Management application.

The *Patient Care Management* application is used as a proactive reminder tool to improve the care management process. The patient is evaluated and moved to specific health maintenance and disease management registries based on measures that are activated within your group. The application helps manage the recurring preventive care items pertinent to a patient, flags overdue items, enables you to manually move the patient to a high-risk registry, and more. Additionally, you can view a list of care management items that are complete and pending for the patient by clicking the *Pt Care Mgt* link on the *Patient Health History* pane of the *Medical Record* module.

> # FYI
>
> The care recommendations in the *Health Maintenance* and *Disease Management* registries are based on CDC and National Committee for Quality Assurance/Healthcare Effectiveness Data and Information Set (NCQA/HEDIS) guidelines.

Table 6-10 provides a description of each section within the *Patient Care Management* application. Table 6-11 provides a further description of each column within the application.

TABLE 6-10   Sections within the Patient Care Management Application

Section	Description
Health Maintenance	This section displays all tests/exams that a patient is due for that are part of *Health Maintenance* registries.
Disease Management	This section displays all tests/exams that a patient is due for OR is required to have according to disease management measures. Click the *Expand* ➕ icon in the *Disease Management* section to view all items that are part of the disease management measure.

Courtesy of Harris CareTracker PM and EMR

TABLE 6-11   Columns within the Patient Care Management Application

Column	Description
Test/Exam	The test or exam for which the patient qualifies.
Status	Indicates the status of the test or exam. • Indicates that the test or exam is complete. • Indicates that the test or exam is missing or overdue. • Indicates that the patient refused the test or exam.

TABLE 6-11   *(Continued)*

Column	Description
State	Indicates how well a disease management item is controlled. (**Note:** This is available only in the *Disease Management* section.)
Recommendation	The recommendation for having the specific test or exam performed.
Date of Last	The last date the test or exam was done.
Refused	The date the patient refused the test or exam. However, if the test or exam belongs to a series, the due date for the next test or exam will display under the *Due Date* column based on the interval set for the test or exam.
Interval	The duration between the last and next test or exam.
Due Date	The date the patient is due for the specific test or exam.
OS (Order Set)	If a *Patient Care Management* (PCM) item is associated with an order set, you can click on the *Order Set* icon to open the order set in a new window. If the PCM items is associated with multiple order sets, you can point to the *Order Set* icon to view the list of order sets. The order sets are grouped under provider, group, and company categories allowing you to click and open in a new window.
Actions (Edit, Activate/ Deactivate/Log)	Provides you the ability to edit, activate and deactivate, and view the log pertaining to the care management item.

The *Patient Care Management* application enables you to update information, such as the due date or interval for a test/exam, and flag a test or exam that is refused by a patient. Additionally, you can remove a care management item that is due for a patient or move the patient to a high-risk registry if necessary. In Activity 6-14, you will access and update the *Patient Care Management* screen.

ACTIVITY 6-14: Accessing and Updating Patient Care Management Items

1. If you are not in Jane Morgan's medical record, access it following the steps used in Activity 6-6.

2. In the *Patient Health History* pane, click on the *Pt Care Mgmt* tab. Harris CareTracker EMR displays the *Patient Care Management* window with all health maintenance and disease management items for the patient (Figure 6-49). The list includes both pending and completed items.

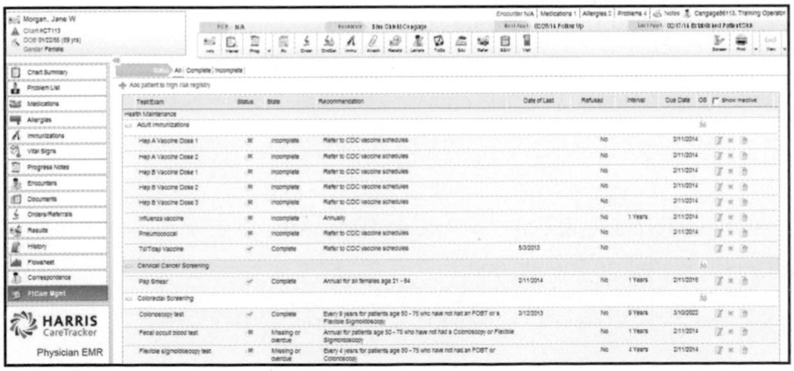

Figure 6-49   Patient Care Management Window

3. As you are reviewing the registry, note that the information collected during the history phase automatically populated in this section, such as the dates of the patient's last colonoscopy and Pap test. While reviewing the registry information with Ms. Morgan, she states that she just remembered she received an influenza vaccine on October 12 of last year. The patient received the immunization at America's Urgent Care. Click the *Edit* ![icon] icon in the row in which Influenza appears. Harris CareTracker EMR displays the *Edit Test/Exam* dialog box (Figure 6-50).

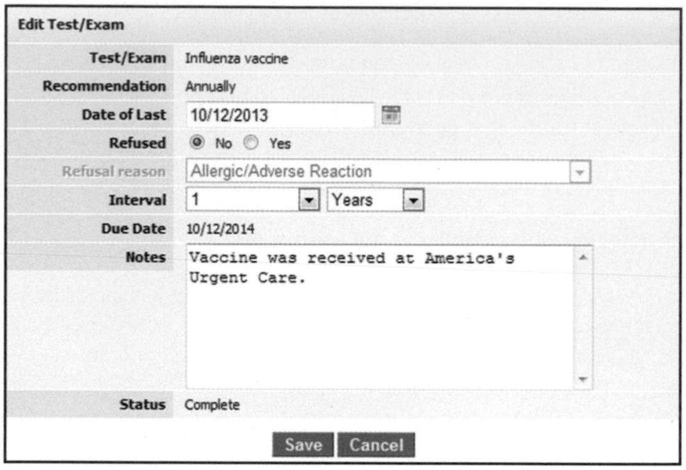

Figure 6-50 Edit Test/Exam Dialog Box

4. In the *Edit Test/Exam* box, enter October 12 of last year in the *Date of Last* field.

5. Leave the other fields blank because the vaccine was not administered at the Napa Valley Family Health Associates facility. Type the following in the *Notes* box: "Vaccine was received at America's Urgent Care."

FYI

By default, the date is auto filled in the *Date of Last* box based on the information available in Harris CareTracker EMR. However, you can change the date if necessary. Additionally, you can update the interval between the last and the next, mark a test that a patient has refused with the refusal reason, and enter additional notes. The due date and the status of the test or exam are automatically calculated based on the last date the exam was performed and the interval.

6. Click *Save*. (**Note:** You may have to close out of the *Patient Care Management* window and re-open it before the influenza entry is updated on the screen.)

FYI

You can remove a patient care management item from the list by clicking the *Deactivate* ✖ icon. The inactive item appears dimmed and you can select the *Show Inactive* checkbox to view the item.

Print the updated Patient Care Management list, label it "Activity 6-14," and place it in your assignment folder.

CLINICAL SP⬤TLIGHT

Many of the new "Pay for Performance" health care models require the medical assistant to review patient Health and Disease Management registries prior to the scheduled appointment. Following review, the medical assistant writes a plan, establishing steps that will be taken to bring the patient into compliance. The provider reviews the plan and makes necessary adjustments. Electronic orders are placed in the EMR prior to the appointment so that the "Catching Up" process can be performed throughout the visit. If the patient refuses any of the items listed in the plan, the medical assistant will click on the *Edit* [ ] icon and signify that the patient refused the item. The reason for refusal is then entered in the *Notes* section of the dialog box. Sharing this information with the provider prior to patient examination gives the provider an opportunity to encourage those prevention or maintenance items that the patient refused.

Critical Thinking

Review the items that Ms. Morgan is behind on and write a plan listing the following:

- Immunizations that may be given today
- Screenings that should be scheduled prior to patient departure

What are some reasons the patient may refuse these items? What can you do as a health care advocate to assist patients who are refusing due to financial constraints?

CREATING PROGRESS NOTES

Learning Objective 11: Create and print a Progress Note.

Progress notes are the heart of the patient record. They serve as a chronological listing of the patient's overall health status. Data pertaining to the findings from the visit are entered into the progress note. Most EMR software programs, including Harris CareTracker EMR, have progress note templates, copy and paste features, and automatic population tools, which make creating progress notes simplistic and efficient. The software also assists in promoting consistency from one provider to the next.

The *Progress Notes* application displays a list of notes recorded during each patient appointment and is required for medical, legal, and billing purposes. The note includes information such as the patient's history, medications, and allergies as well as a complete record of all that occurred during the visit. The application provides a quick and easy way to review and sign notes and helps identify notes that must be signed by a co-signer.

Progress Note Templates

Each predefined specialty and condition specific template available in Harris CareTracker EMR simplifies the process of documenting a patient encounter at the point of care. Harris CareTracker EMR provides several template types, each offering a specific layout and custom options. These options allow providers to select the template that best suits their documenting needs. Staff members can also pull in sections of a prior note and insert documents and images into templates if necessary. Standard templates can be broken down by specialty and template styles. Table 6-12 describes the standard templates available in Harris CareTracker EMR.

TABLE 6-12 Progress Note Templates	
Template	**Description**
Option 1	This template consists of two tabs and is recommended for providers who prefer using a simple version of a template with quick text or dictation. One tab consists of text boxes for Chief Complaint and History of Present Illness (CC/HPI), History (HX), Review Of Systems (ROS), Physical Exam (PE), Tests, Procedures (Proc), and Assessment and Plan (A&P). The second tab consists of structured data elements that link to the Quality Measure reports in Harris CareTracker PM and EMR.
Option 2	This template consists of eight tabs and is recommended for providers who prefer using a simple version of a template with quick text or dictation. Seven tabs consist of text boxes to document the Chief Complaint and History of Present Illness (CC/HPI), History (HX), Review Of Systems (ROS), Physical Exam (PE), Tests, Procedures (Proc), and Assessment and Plan (A&P) in each tab. The last tab consists of structured data elements that link to the Quality Measure reports in Harris CareTracker PM and EMR.
Option 3	This template consists of eight tabs and is recommended for providers who are using the structured option or combination of structure and quick text to document a note. The template provides data elements in one screen and additional elements in a pop-up window to be used as necessary. This option allows for no scrolling within the template.
Option 4	This is recommended for providers who are using the structured option or combination of structure and quick text to document a note. All data elements are organized in one screen, enabling you to scroll through to document patient information.

ACTIVITY 6-15: Accessing and Updating the Progress Notes Application

1. If you are not in Jane Morgan's medical record, access it following the steps used in Activity 6-6.
2. In the *Clinical Toolbar*, click the *Progress Notes* tab. If an encounter is in context, which in this case it is, Harris CareTracker EMR displays the *Progress Notes* template window (Figure 6-51). (**Note:** If documenting a progress note that is not based on an appointment, the *Encounter* dialog box displays, enabling you to create a new encounter. If you are getting an *Encounter* dialog box, it means that you did not have an encounter in context. Repeat step 1 if necessary.)

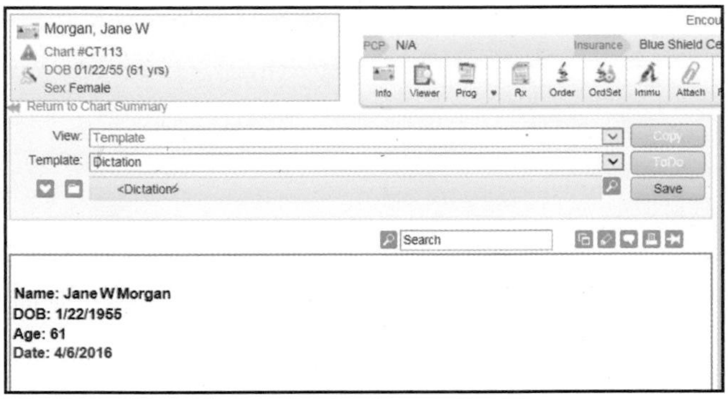

Courtesy of Harris CareTracker PM and EMR

Figure 6-51 Progress Notes Template Window

3. By default, the *View* field displays "Template." (Skip this box at this time.)
4. In the *Template* field, click on the drop-down arrow and select "IM OV Option 4 (v4) w/A&P" (Figure 6-52). Complete the note by navigating through each tab. (The provider would ordinarily work in the progress note, but because the provider is not available you will be entering the information for the provider.)

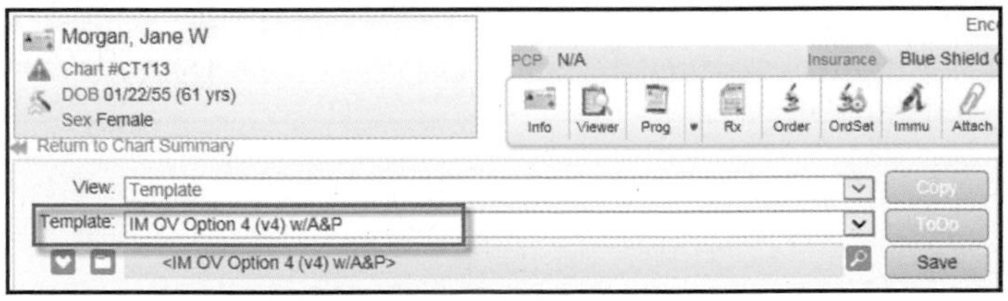

Courtesy of Harris CareTracker PM and EMR

Figure 6-52 IM OV Option 4 Template

5. All the information you entered regarding Ms. Morgan's medical history, allergy information, medication list, vital signs, and preventive care are now populated within the progress note. The *CC/HPI* tab will be showing on the right side of the screen (Figure 6-53). Review the note you wrote regarding the patient's chief complaint. The provider will expand a bit on the complaint by developing the History of Present Illness (HPI). Scroll down to the *History of Present Illness* box and type the following:

   "Patient has a five-year history of UTIs (1-2 infections/year). Current episode includes frequency, urgency, and pain upon urination (7/10). Pt. denies fever, blood, or pus in urine, or the presence of vaginal symptoms. No back or abdominal pain. Patient drinks very little water and has at least two beverages per day which include caffeine. Last UTI was approximately three months ago. Treatment included a ten-day treatment of Bactrim DS. Patient states she completed the treatment and was free of urinary symptoms. Patient did not follow up for a post check." Your documentation should match Figure 6-53.

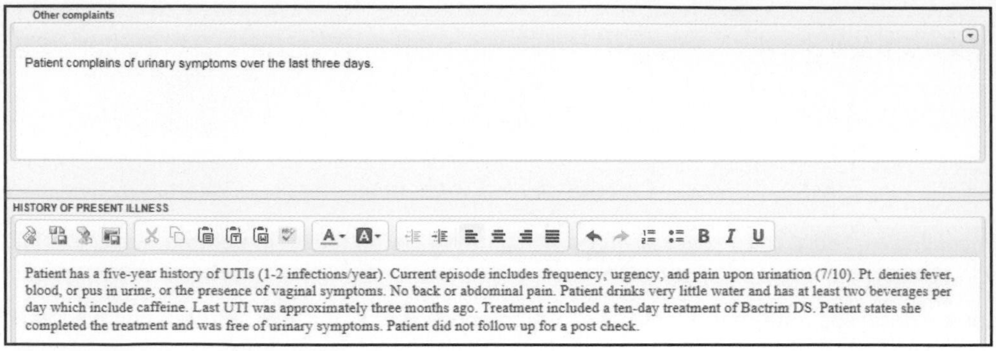

Other complaints

Patient complains of urinary symptoms over the last three days.

HISTORY OF PRESENT ILLNESS

A· A·   B I U

Patient has a five-year history of UTIs (1-2 infections/year). Current episode includes frequency, urgency, and pain upon urination (7/10). Pt. denies fever, blood, or pus in urine, or the presence of vaginal symptoms. No back or abdominal pain. Patient drinks very little water and has at least two beverages per day which include caffeine. Last UTI was approximately three months ago. Treatment included a ten-day treatment of Bactrim DS. Patient states she completed the treatment and was free of urinary symptoms. Patient did not follow up for a post check.

Courtesy of Harris CareTracker PM and EMR

Figure 6-53   Jane Morgan HPI

6. Click on *Save*, located in the template box in the middle of the screen (Figure 6-54).

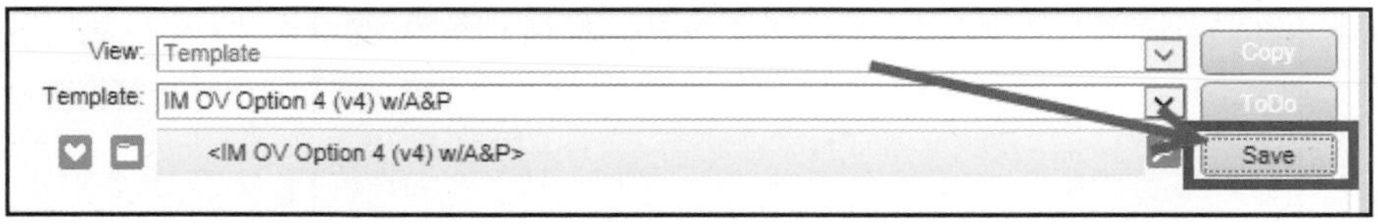

View: Template   Copy
Template: IM OV Option 4 (v4) w/A&P   ToDo
      <IM OV Option 4 (v4) w/A&P>   Save

Figure 6-54   Save Button for Template Screen
Courtesy of Harris CareTracker PM and EMR

7. Click on the *HX* tab on the right side of the progress note (center of screen). Review the information that you entered while collecting the patient history. Because you are acting as the provider in this section, indicate that you reviewed each section of the history by clicking on the plus sign next to *Reviewed* at the top of the screen. Check marks will now appear next to each box in the *Reviewed* section (Figure 6-55).

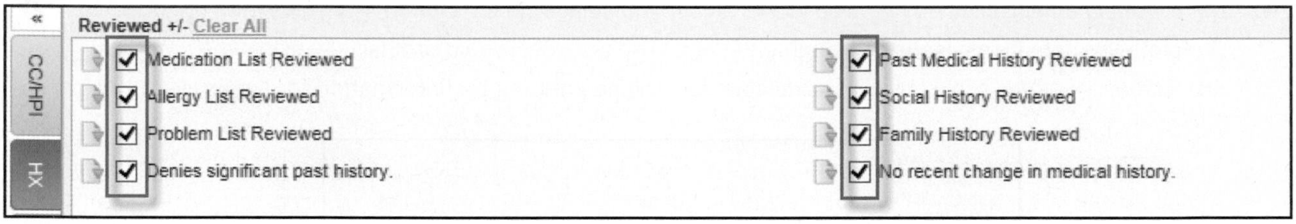

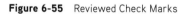

Reviewed +/- Clear All

CC/HPI   ☑ Medication List Reviewed   ☑ Past Medical History Reviewed
      ☑ Allergy List Reviewed   ☑ Social History Reviewed
      ☑ Problem List Reviewed   ☑ Family History Reviewed
HX   ☑ Denies significant past history.   ☑ No recent change in medical history.

Courtesy of Harris CareTracker PM and EMR

Figure 6-55   Reviewed Check Marks

8. Click on *Save* to update the note.

9. Click on the *ROS* tab. Refer to Table 6-13 to complete this section of the progress note.

10. Click *Save* to update the progress note with the ROS findings.

11. Click on the *PE* tab. Use Table 6-14 to complete this portion of the note.

12. Click *Save* to update the progress note with the PE findings.

13. Skip the *TESTS* and *PROC* tabs.

14. Click on the *ASSESS* tab.

15. It was discovered during the exam that the patient has hypertension. The provider also diagnosed the patient with a urinary tract infection (UTI) and dysuria. Although a list of ICD-9 codes is shown in the *Diagnoses* section of the *ASSESS* tab, you will be selecting ICD-10 codes associated with the provider's diagnoses. Click on the *Search* icon to the right of the *-Select-* drop-down menu at the top of the screen. In the *Diagnosis Search* window that pops up, enter "hypertension" in the *Search Text* field and click the *Search* button. Click

TABLE 6-13   Completing the ROS Tab

Section	Entry
Constitutional	Check the box beside *No constitutional symptoms.*
Eyes	Check the box beside *No eye symptoms.*
ENMT	No entry.
Neck	Check the box beside *No neck symptoms.*
Breasts	No entry.
Respiratory	Check the box beside *No respiratory symptoms.*
Cardiovascular	Click on the minus symbol so that *N* for No is selected for each box. Now click on the *Y* beside "cold hands or feet."
Gastrointestinal	Check the box beside *No GI symptoms.*
Genitourinary	Select *Y* for Yes for the following categories: "dysuria," "burning on urination," "urgency," and "frequency." Select *N* for No for all other genitourinary (GU) symptoms.
Skin	No entry.
Musculoskeletal	No entry.
Neurological	No entry.
Psychiatric	Select *Y* for Yes for depression, and *N* for No for all other symptoms.
Hematologic	No entry.
Endocrine	No entry.

TABLE 6-14   Completing the PE Tab

Section	Entry
General	Click the plus sign beside *General* so that a check mark is placed beside each box in the section.
HEENT	*Head*: Check the box beside *Negative head exam.* *Eyes*: Click on the *Y* for Yes next to "PERRL." Click on the *N* for No next to "EOMI" and "scleral icterus." *ENT*: No entry.
Neck	Check the box beside *Negative neck exam.*

(Continues)

TABLE 6-14 *(Continued)*

Section	Entry
Lymphatics	No entry.
Chest	*Chest:* Check the box beside *Negative chest exam.* *Breasts*: No entry. *Lungs*: Check the box beside *Negative lung exam.*
Heart	Check the box beside *Negative heart exam.*
Abdomen	Click on the minus sign beside *Abdomen* so that a red "X" is placed beside each box in the section. Click the *Y* for Yes beside "soft" and "tenderness." Click on the *Finding Details* icon beside "tenderness" and enter the following in the *Comments* section: "The abdomen was soft with minimal tenderness to palpation in the left periumbilical and left lower quadrant. There was no guarding or rebound." Click on the *X* to close out of the box.
Genitourinary	Check the box beside *Negative genitourinary exam.*
Musculoskeletal	No entry.
Neurologic	No entry.
Mental Status Exam	No entry.
Skin	No entry.

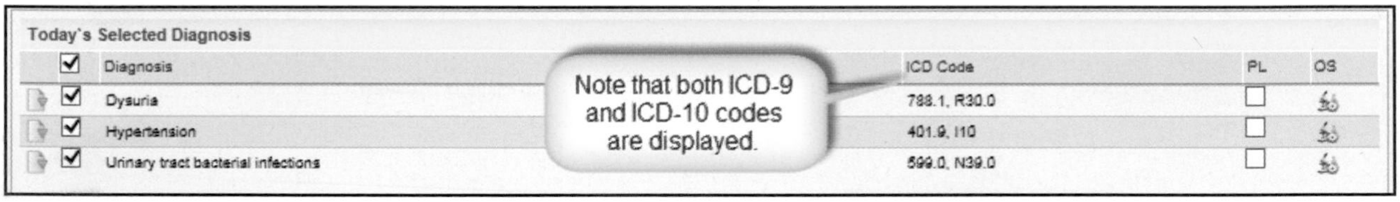

Courtesy of Harris CareTracker PM and EMR

Figure 6-56 Record ICD Code in Assessment Box

on "Hypertension" in the results section of the *Diagnosis Search* window (note that it has already been marked as a favorite diagnosis.) Search for and select "urinary tract infection" and "dysuria" as well. After selecting each diagnosis, scroll down to the bottom of the *ASSESS* tab, and see all selected codes listed under *Today's Selected Diagnosis.* Both the ICD-9 and ICD-10 versions of the code are listed (Figure 6-56).

16. Click *Save* to update the progress note with the *Assessment* information.

17. Click on the *PLAN* tab to record the provider's plans. Document the following in the *Additional Plan Details* box (Figure 6-57):

a. Stat lab test - "Urinalysis dipstick panel by Automated test strip"

b. Send Urine out for lab test "Urinalysis microscopic panel [#volume] in urine by automated count"

c. Give patient educational handouts for UTI and Hypertension

d. Bactrim DS Oral Tabs (80-160 mg), Sig 1 tab bid for 5 days, No refills

e. Patient to return in 10 days for a Follow-Up UA and BP check

f. Set patient up for a referral with a urologist

Prevention Goals

g. Patient to have her first Hepatitis B shot today

h. Set patient up for a mammogram

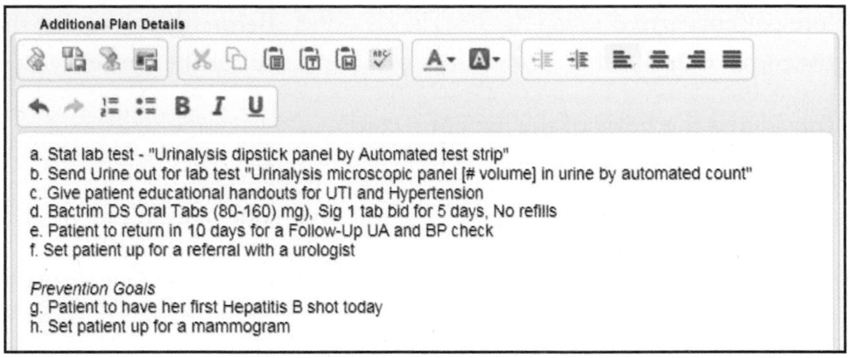

Figure 6-57   Additional Plan Details Box

18. Click *Save*.

Click the orange Print 🖪 icon in the middle of the screen. The Clinical Note dialog box will open. Click the Print button to print a copy of the progress note. Label it "Activity 6-15" and place it in your assignment folder.

19. Click on the *Return to Chart Summary* link at the top left of the screen to return to the patient's medical record.

There are many different things you can do with the progress note including changing the template, filtering the progress note, editing a progress note, deleting a progress note, and adding an addendum. Instructions for these functions can be found in the *Help Documents* section of Harris CareTracker PM and EMR. The progress note that you created in this chapter is not yet complete. You will complete the note in Chapter 7.

SUMMARY

In this chapter you learned all about the patient's EMR. Electronic medical records help to organize the chart and keep the office running efficiently. Harris CareTracker PM and EMR provides users with lots of tools to keep up with clinical documentation and tasks.

It is your job to work on electronic tasks throughout the day and to help your provider stay on task as well. It is important to remember that even though Harris CareTracker EMR provides all this robust technology, the patient is always your first priority. Do not get trapped behind the technology during the visit. Always remember to look up from the computer so that you can study the patient's face and body language. Treat your patient the way that you would want to be treated.

Check Your Knowledge

Select the best response.

_____ 1. Electronic tasks should be checked:

    a. Before patients arrive
    c. Before departing for the day
    b. Between patients
    d. All of the above

_____ 2. What is considered the heart of the patient record?

    a. The patient's medication list
    c. The allergy list
    b. Progress notes
    d. The patient's medical history

_____ 3. What application in Harris CareTracker EMR features information regarding prevention and disease management measures?

    a. *Task* menu
    c. *Patient Care Management* application
    b. *Clinical Toolbar*
    d. None of the above

_____ 4. An unsigned note in Harris CareTracker EMR refers to which of the following?

    a. A prescription that has not been signed
    c. A message that has not been signed
    b. A fax that has not been signed
    d. A progress note that has not been signed

_____ 5. Once enrolled in Surescripts®, the practice is required to send a minimum of how many prescriptions within 48 hours to receive renewal requests and to accept or deny requests?

    a. 1
    c. 10
    b. 5
    d. 15

_____ 6. Manual and electronic results are saved in which of the following locations?

    a. *Dashboard* tab (*Results* link)
    b. *Tasks* tab within *Clinical Today* (in the *Results* section)
    c. Both a and b
    d. None of the above

_____ 7. An encounter is an interaction with a patient and includes all of the following except:

    a. Visits
    c. ICD codes
    b. Payments
    d. CPT® codes

_____ 8. Transfer status means that a patient has been transferred to:

    a. The examination room
    c. Radiology
    b. Checkout
    d. Another provider

_____ 9. Selected medications are screened for possible contraindications in regard to:

    a. The patient's active medications
    c. The patient's problems
    b. The patient's allergies
    d. All of the above

_____10.   When a patient is allergic to a medication, what type of alert would be most appropriate?

    a. Pop-up alert

    b. Soft alert

    c. No alert

    d. There is no set standard

mini-case studies

Note: Case studies must be completed in every chapter since future chapter activities build upon them.

For Case Studies 6-2 through 6-6, you will need to refer to the appointment dates for Adam Thompson, Barbara Watson, Craig X. Smith, Ellen Ristino, and Jordyn Lyndsey that you scheduled in Chapter 4. You will also be referencing the appropriate source documents found in Appendix A.

Case Study 6-1

Using the steps in Activity 6-4, recheck the quick tasks list for Dr. Raman. (Make sure that Dr. Raman is selected as the provider in your clinical batch.):

1. How many open encounters do you have?
2. How many unsigned notes do you have?
3. How many open orders do you have?

 Write the answers down on a separate sheet of paper. Label this "Case Study 6-1" and place it in your assignment folder.

Case Study 6-2

Using the steps you learned throughout this chapter and the information packet for Adam Thompson found on page 624 of Appendix A, update Mr. Thompson's medical record and create a progress note.

 After entering all of the information provided in the packet, print a chart summary (label it "Case Study 6-2A") and progress note (label it "Case Study 6-2B") and place them in your assignment folder.

Case Study 6-3

Using the steps you learned throughout this chapter and the information packet for Barbara Watson found on page 630 of Appendix A, update Ms. Watson's medical record and create a progress note.

 After entering all of the information provided in the packet, print a chart summary (label it "Case Study 6-3A") and progress note (label it "Case Study 6-3B") and place them in your assignment folder.

Case Study 6-4

Using the steps you learned throughout this chapter and the information packet for Craig X. Smith found on page 635 of Appendix A, update Mr. Smith's medical record and create a progress note.

 After entering all of the information provided in the packet, print a chart summary (label it "Case Study 6-4A") and progress note (label it "Case Study 6-4B") and place them in your assignment folder.

Case Study 6-5

Using the steps you learned throughout this chapter and the information packet for Ellen Ristino found on page 637 of Appendix A, update Ms. Ristino's medical record and create a progress note.

 After entering all of the information provided in the packet, print a chart summary (label it "Case Study 6-5A") and progress note (label it "Case Study 6-5B") and place them in your assignment folder.

Case Study 6-6

Using the steps you learned throughout this chapter and the information packet for Jordyn Lyndsey found on page 642 of Appendix A, update Ms. Lyndsey's medical record and create a progress note.

 After entering all of the information provided in the packet, print a chart summary (label it "Case Study 6-6A") and progress note (label it "Case Study 6-6B") and place them in your assignment folder.

Resources

The Harris CareTracker PM and EMR Help homepage represents a wealth of information for the electronic health record (https://training.caretracker.com/help/CareTracker_Help.htm).

Department of Health and Human Services (DHHS) Centers for Medicare and Medicaid Services (CMS). (2003, June 6). *Medicare hospital manual.* Retrieved from http://www.cms.gov/Regulations-and-Guidance/Guidance/Transmittals/downloads/R804HO.pdf

U.S. Department of Health and Human Services. (2013, February 11). *Construction of LMS Parameters for the Centers for Disease Control and Prevention 2000 Growth Charts,* by Katherine M. Flegal, Ph.D., Office of the Director, National Center for Health Statistics; and Tim J. Cole, Ph.D., MRC Centre of Epidemiology for Child Health, Institute of Child Health, University College London, UK. National Health Statistics Report (No. 63). Retrieved from http://www.cdc.gov/nchs/data/nhsr/nhsr063.pdf

Chapter 7

Completing the Visit

Key Terms

accession
adjudication
advance beneficiary
 notice (ABN)
Ask at Order Entry
 (AOE)
compendium
contraindication
dispensable (drug)

formulary
order
Real Time Adjudication
 (RTA)
routed (drug)
Rx Norm
SIG
stat
"Tall Man" lettering

Learning Objectives

1. Complete requisitions for diagnostic orders: specialists, labs, and radiology.

2. Search for pharmacies, manage a list of favorites, and create and print prescriptions.

3. View, add, and create immunization records.

4. Search for, customize, and provide patient education materials for patients.

5. Access the Correspondence application to add, filter, customize, and print patient correspondence.

6. Create outgoing and incoming patient referrals.

7. View and resolve open encounters and unsigned notes by completing the visit and signing the Progress Note.

Certification Connection

1. Utilize EMR and practice management (PM) systems.

2. Perform routine PM and clinical EHR tasks within a health care environment according to appropriate protocols.

3. Coordinate patient flow within the back office clinical setting (e.g., check-in, transfer to a room, record vital signs and patient history, create outgoing referrals, and check out patients).

4. Access, edit, and store patient information in the EHR database.

5. Enter live data into an EHR and assist clinicians with charting.

6. Acquire external patient data (labs, radiology reports, patient visit summaries, and more); edit the patient medical record in the EHR within your scope of practice.

7. Locate requested information in the chart and complete tasks (orders) called out in the progress note.

8. Adhere to federal, state, and local laws relating to exchange and transmission of patient information for external use.

9. Describe how to use and find the most current ICD, CPT®, and HCPCS codes in an EMR.

10. Identify the impact of HIPAA for the medical assistant; adhere to rules pertaining to the confidentiality and release of PHI.

Adapted from national standards of the National Healthcareer Association (NHA), Commission on Accreditation and Allied Health Education Program (CAAHEP), and Accrediting Bureau of Health Education Schools (ABHES)

INTRODUCTION

Now that you have completed the EMR activities in Chapter 6, you will move forward and complete tasks from the *Assessment* and *Plan* (A&P) tabs located in the patient's progress note. These activities are often referred to as "completing the visit." To generate claims, charges must be captured for the patient's appointment. The *Visit* application allows you to capture charges and enter CPT®, NDC, and ICD codes for a patient's appointment. The *Visit Summary* application enables you to define patient, provider, visit, and chart information to include in the *Visit Summary* reports generated by your group.

You will place orders and prescriptions, provide educational material for patients, create referrals, document immunizations you administer, sign the progress note, and schedule follow-up appointments as indicated. To complete activities in this chapter, you will refer back to the patient's progress note *Assessment and Plan* (Figure 7-1). Many of the advanced features of Harris CareTracker EMR's applications are introduced in this chapter, but you will also be directed to the *Help* section where appropriate for more details.

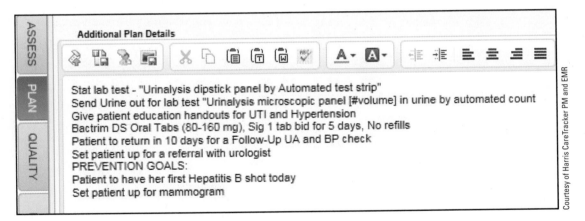

Figure 7-1   Assessment and Plan for Jane Morgan

COMPLETING REQUISITIONS FOR DIAGNOSTIC ORDERS

Learning Objective 1: Complete requisitions for diagnostic orders: specialists, labs, and radiology.

The *Orders* application in Harris CareTracker EMR enables you to manage and track orders such as laboratory, radiology, pathology, and physical therapy directly from the patient's medical record. This ensures that all orders placed are followed up on by the office for patient compliancy. The *Orders* application works simultaneously with the *Results* application by providing quick access to test results of completed orders and enables entering manual results and linking to results received electronically.

Tip Box

If you find that when you access a patient's medical record you receive a pop-up alert indicating some missing information (e.g., consent, PCP, NPP, etc.), it is best practice to update the patient's record in the demographics screen.

ACTIVITY 7-1: Access the Orders Application

1. Access patient Jane Morgan's *Medical Record* module using one of the following methods:

   a. Pull patient Jane Morgan into context and click the *Medical Record* module.

   b. If the patient has an appointment, click the patient's name in the *Appointments* application of the *Clinical Today* module. (To find an appointment date with the patient in context, click on the *History* tab of the *Scheduling* module. It displays the most current appointment for the patient in context in either the *Pending Appointments* or *Rescheduled Appointments* sections in the center of the screen.)

2. In the *Patient Health History* pane, click *Orders/Referrals* (Figure 7-2). The *Orders* window displays with outstanding orders for the patient. You will see that there are no outstanding orders at this time; however, to view more details about an open order, you would do the following:

   a. Click the order number.

   b. To sort orders in the required sequence, click the column heading.

   c. Use the *Expand* ✛ icon to view the orders for the patient.

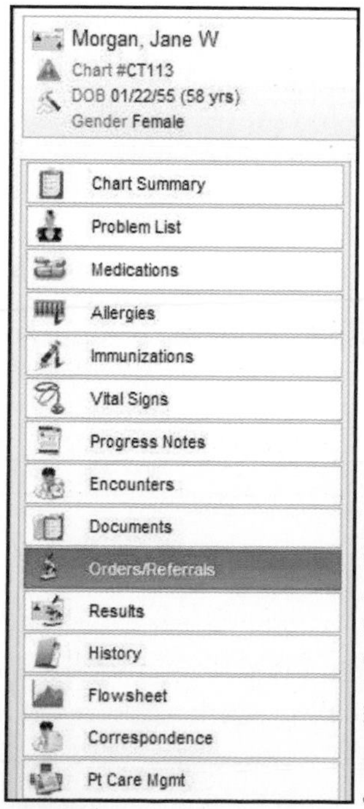

Figure 7-2 Orders/Referrals Application

Courtesy of Harris CareTracker PM and EMR

Tip Box

The *Expand* ➕ icon next to an order indicates that the order includes multiple tests (Figure 7-3). You can click on the *Expand* ➕ icon to view tests included in the order. You can move the pointer over the document to view additional details and click to view scanned and attached orders by clicking the specific document under the *Documents* section.

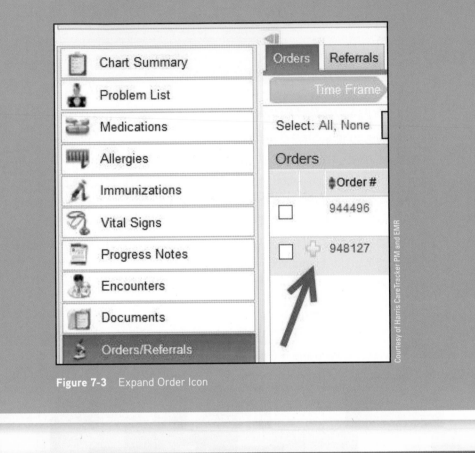

Figure 7-3 Expand Order Icon

Table 7-1 describes the information displaying in the columns of the *Orders* window (Figure 7-4).

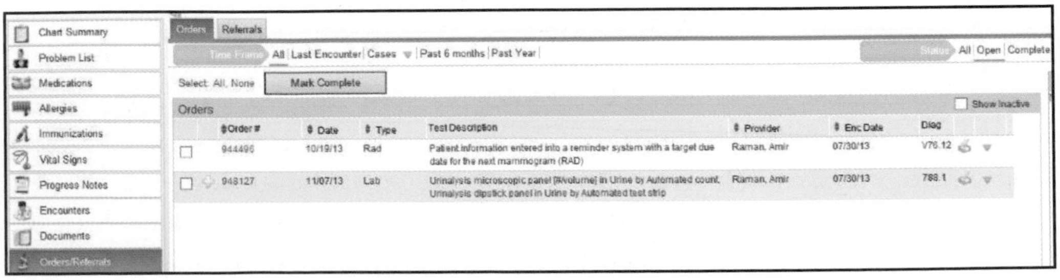

Figure 7-4 Orders Window

TABLE 7-1	Orders Columns
Column	**Description**
Order #	Indicates a unique, system-assigned identifier to track the order. This identifier is often referred to as an accession.
Date	Displays the date the order must be completed. (**Note:** The *Due Date* column is updated to display Stat if you set the urgency to Stat when creating the order. **Stat** refers to "immediately" or "without delay.")
Type	Displays the type of the order. Order types include lab, diagnostic imaging, and procedure.
Test Description	Displays a description about the order.
Provider	Displays the provider who created the order.
Enc Date	Displays the encounter date associated with the order.
Diag	Displays the diagnoses associated with the order.

Courtesy of Harris CareTracker PM and EMR

Tip Box

You can view notes entered by moving the pointer over the *Note* icon. However, the *Note* icon is dimmed if notes are not available for the order.

Enter New Lab Orders

The *Orders* application, accessed by clicking *Orders* on the *Clinical Toolbar*, allows you to order tests directly from the *Medical Record* module.

An **order** consists of a list of tests to perform on one or more patient specimens; for example, blood or urine. In many cases, each order is tracked with a unique, system-assigned identifier. This identifier (which is usually a number) is often referred to as an **accession**. When an order is created, the application enables you to preview, print, fax, or send electronically to the facility that will be completing the order. The order is saved as an open order in the *Orders* application and *Open* activities sections of the patient's medical record, enabling you to track outstanding orders for the patient. Additionally, the order is saved to the *Practice* tab of the *Home* module under the *Clinical* header, as well as the *Open Orders* application of the *Clinical Today* module.

The *Open Orders* application provides a quick and efficient way to track the progress of and resolve open orders to expedite patient treatment. This process replaces the manual log books that were used to keep track of labs and other diagnostic tests.

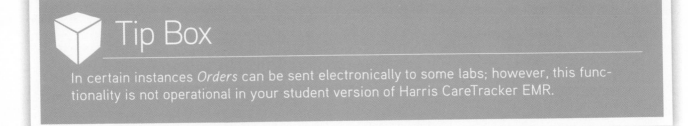

Tip Box

In certain instances *Orders* can be sent electronically to some labs; however, this functionality is not operational in your student version of Harris CareTracker EMR.

The *Orders* application enables you to answer *Ask at Order Entry (AOE)* or custom questions, provide physician instructions, produce Medicare waivers for tests that may not be covered, and more. You can also manage a list of favorite facilities, tests, and test notes. Using patient Jane Morgan, complete the *Assessment and Plan* (A&P) *Orders* as outlined in the progress note from her encounter that you created in Chapter 6 (see Figure 7-1). You will refer back to her A&P throughout this chapter's activities. The first activity will be to add a new lab order (Activity 7-2).

ACTIVITY 7-2: Add a New Lab Order

1. Pull patient Jane Morgan into context, and then click the *Medical Record* module.

2. In the *Clinical Toolbar*, click *Order* 🔬.

3. If an encounter is in context, Harris CareTracker EMR displays the *New Order* dialog box. If an encounter is not in context, Harris CareTracker EMR displays the *Select Encounter* dialog box. Click on the encounter you created in Chapter 6, and the *Order* screen (Figure 7-5) will appear.

Figure 7-5 Order Screen

4. Verify that patient information such as medications, allergies, and diagnoses are up to date in the medical record by hovering over each category in the upper-right corner of the *Order* dialog box (Figure 7-5). Add and update the information as necessary. (For example, hover over the *Medications* category, and click *+ New Medication* from the list. This launches the *Medication* dialog box to add the medication information your provider ordered in the *Plan* section of the note. Close the *Medication* box and continue with placing your lab order.)

5. By default, the *Status* is set to "Open" in the *Order* dialog box (Figure 7-5).

6. By default, the *Order Type* is set to "Lab". Leave this setting as is.

FYI

The *Order Type* defaults to the option selected in the *Default Order Type* list in the *Set Chart Summary Defaults* dialog box. You can change the order type by selecting *Lab, Diag. Imaging,* or *Procedure*.

Tip Box

You can only select one order type per order and you must select the correct type to view pertinent tests.

7. By default, the *Ordering Physician* list displays the provider associated with the encounter. Confirm that the provider listed is Dr. Raman.

8. The *Facility* list displays the default facility set for the order type. If a default facility has not been set but has been saved as a favorite, click the drop-down list. A list of favorites will appear. Select *Napa Valley Family Health Associates Laboratory*. (**Note**: If the required facility were not on the list, you would click the *Search* 🔍 icon to search for the required facility.)

9. *(Optional)* If you want to copy the result to another provider, in the *Copy Result To* list click other providers to whom you wish to route results. If the provider is not on the list, click the *Search* 🔍 icon to search for the provider.

Tip Box

To search for the required facility:

- Enter the name of the facility, phone number, city, state, or zip code in the specific boxes. (**Note:** If you are searching for a facility by name, you must enter at least two characters for the name.)
- Click *Search*. A list of facilities displays, matching the search criteria.
- Click the facility you want. The selected facility auto populates in the *Facility* list.

Note: You can add a facility from the search results to the favorites list by clicking the *Add as Favorites* ⭐ icon. When a facility is added to the favorites list, Harris CareTracker PM and EMR displays the *On Favorites* ⭐ icon, indicating that the facility is in the favorites list. You can also click the *Manage Favorites* ⭐ icon next to the *Facility* list to add or remove facilities from the provider's favorites list. Each facility location is associated with a **compendium** supported by Harris CareTracker PM and EMR. A compendium is a summary or abstract containing the essential information in a concise, but brief, form. If a default facility for the order type is set, the *Manage Favorites* ⭐ icon displays next to the facility. You can point to the icon to view the default *Order Type* for the facility.

Tip Box

To search for the provider:

- Enter the last name, UPIN, or NPI in the specific boxes.
- Enter other information such as name, city, state, or zip code, if known.
- Click *Search*. Harris CareTracker PM and EMR displays a list of providers matching the search criteria.
- Click the provider you want. The selected provider autopopulates in the *Copy Result To* list.

Note: The *Copy Result To* list includes all providers in the group, the patient's active providers, and providers listed in the *Refer Provider From* and *Refer Provider To* lists in the *Quick Picks* application of the *Administration* module. If you select a provider from the search results, the provider name displays under the *Current Encounter* section in the *Copy Result To* list.

10. In the *Diagnosis* list, click the diagnosis from the drop-down list that is associated with the order (select Dx code "R30.0"). If the diagnosis is not in the list, search for the required diagnosis. (**Note:** The *Diagnosis* list is separated into two sections. The *Current Encounter* section contains

any ICD codes that are selected within the progress note or selected from the search result list and displays at the top of the list. The *Favorites* section contains all diagnoses saved to the *Favorites* list.)

Tip Box

To search for a diagnosis:

- Click the *Search* 🔍 icon next to the *Diagnosis* list. Harris CareTracker EMR displays the *Diagnosis Search* dialog box.
- In the *Search Text* box, enter the name, partial name, or diagnosis code.

Note: If a partial name search does not return the result expected, enter the full name of the diagnosis or the code.

- Click *Search*. Harris CareTracker EMR displays a list of diagnoses that match the search criteria.
- Click the diagnosis you want.

11. In the *ABN given to Pt* field, choose "Yes" or "No" to indicate if an advance beneficiary notice was given to the patient. This notifies the patient that Medicare can deny payment for that specific service and that the patient is responsible for payment if denied. Select "No" because the patient does not have Medicare as her insurance.

12. In the *Due Date* box, enter the date the order is due in MM/DD/YYYY format. (Select the date of the patient's encounter and collection.) If you were to select the time period from the list, Harris CareTracker

ADMINISTRATIVE SPOTLIGHT

The **advance beneficiary notice (ABN)** is a written notice (the standard government form CMS-R-131) that a patient receives from physicians, providers, or suppliers before they furnish a service or item to the patient, notifying them that Medicare will probably deny payment for that specific service or item; the reason the physician, provider, or supplier expects Medicare to deny payment; and that the patient will be personally and fully responsible for payment if Medicare denies payment. ABNs alert beneficiaries that Medicare might not reimburse for certain services even though physicians have ordered them, ask for patients' consent regarding financial liability when Medicare denies coverage, and notify patients with Medicare insurance that either a service or services rendered will be the patient's financial responsibility to the physician/facility (lab) for payment.

For information regarding ABNs and for a current form, access the CMS website (http://www.cms.gov).

EMR would automatically calculate the due date. Because you are working in the EMR on a date other than the current date, you will need to use the MM/DD/YYYY format for consistency; however, Harris CareTracker EMR will automatically date stamp your work with the day you perform the activity.

13. In the *Coll. Date & Time* box, enter the date and time for collecting the specimen. Use the date of the encounter and a time of 30 minutes past the patient's set appointment time (for example, if Jane Morgan's visit was on July 30, 2013, at 9:00 a.m., the UA collection time would be 9:30 a.m.).
14. In the *Time of Day* list, click the time of the day for completing the order, "Morning," "Afternoon," or "Evening."
15. In the *Frequency* field, select "Single Order" or "Repeat" to indicate if the order is a single order or must be repeated (select "Single Order"). (**Note**: If the *Frequency* is set to "Repeat," you can click the *Repeat* link to display the *Test Frequency* dialog box (Figure 7-6), enabling you to record additional details about the tests that must be repeated.)

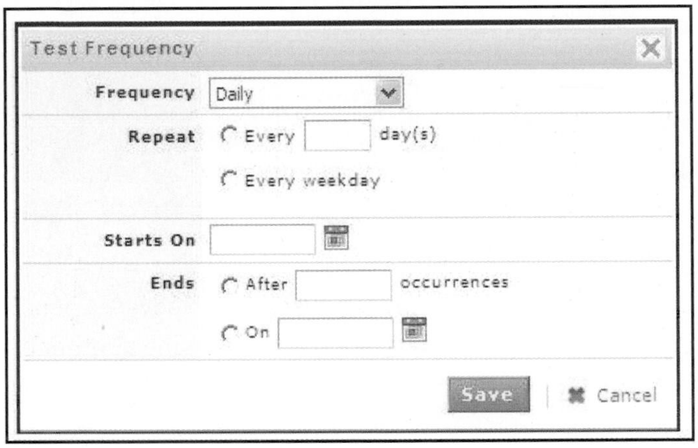

Courtesy of Harris CareTracker PM and EMR

Figure 7-6 Test Frequency Dialog Box

Tip Box

The fields in the *Test Frequency* dialog box are based on the *Frequency* selected. You can select Daily, Weekly, Monthly, or Yearly from the *Frequency* list.

16. *(Optional)* In the *Patient Notes* box, enter any notes about the order you want to display on the order form.
17. The *New Test* section displays favorite tests for the order type, provider, and facility selected. (**Note**: To add a test to your favorites, you would click the *Search* icon to search for the required test.)

Tip Box

To search for the test:

- The *Search For* list defaults to the order type selected.
- By default, the *Search Field* list displays "Description."

Note: The options in the *Search Field* list are based on the order type you select. If you are searching for a lab type order test, you can search by "Logical Observation Identifiers Names and Codes (LOINC) Code" and Order Code. If you are searching for a procedure type order test, you can search by "CPT® Code."

- By default, the *Search Terms* list displays "Contains." However, you can change the option to "Begins with" if necessary.
- In the *Search Text* box, enter the keyword (for example, "Urinalysis").
- Click *Search*. Harris CareTracker EMR displays a list of tests that match the selected order type and the compendium associated with the facility.
- Find the test you want and add the test from the search results to the favorite list by clicking the *Add as Favorites* ⭐ icon. When a test is added to the favorites list, Harris CareTracker EMR displays the *On Favorites* ☆ icon, indicating that the test is on the *Favorites* list.

Note: If a facility is not selected and the order type is set to "Lab," Harris CareTracker EMR searches the default master compendium. You can also click the *Manage Favorites* ⭐ icon in the *New Test* section to add or remove tests from the provider's *Favorite* list. You must always have an order type selected to view tests for the order type.

18. Select the tests indicated in the patient's A&P. Start by selecting the radio dial button next to "Urinalysis dipstick panel in Urine by Automated test strip" in the *New Test* section. (**Note:** You may see multiple entries in the *New Test* field. That is because each time an operator selects a test as a favorite, it populates in the favorites field.)

19. (*Optional*) Click the *Custom Order Questions* link to enter additional information for the test. Only fields with information display in the *Order* form.

Tip Box

The *Custom Order Questions* link is unavailable if the facility selected has an associated lab-specific compendium such as LabCorp. However, if the facility does not have a lab-specific compendium associated but has additional fields defined via the *Order Questions* application, Harris CareTracker EMR activates the *Custom Order Questions* link.

FYI

- *Ask at Order Entry (AOE)* represents questions you must provide to the lab when sending an order electronically or submitting a printed order. The AOE questions are based on the compendium associated with the facility and the test selected. If you do not select a facility when you create an order, Harris CareTracker EMR displays tests and associated AOE questions from the Harris CareTracker PM and EMR master compendium.
- If the practice had created *Order Sets*, when you click the *AOE* 🔬 icon, the required questions display with a red background. If the AOEs are required and you do not answer the questions, a message alerts you that the required AOEs are missing for the tests. You can choose to answer the questions in the *Order Set* window or answer the questions in the *Orders* dialog box before saving the order. You would answer the AOE questions, if required.

Tip Box

By default, a test that is a part of the Harris CareTracker PM and EMR compendium includes the fasting information as part of the AOE questions.

20. In the *Urgency* field, select "Routine" or "Stat" based on the urgency level of the order.

    Select "Routine" for standard orders and "Stat" if results must be processed immediately. (Select "Stat" for this order.)

21. In the *Fasting* field, select the option based on the fasting requirements for the test. (Select "None.")

22. In the *Test Note* box, enter notes specific to the test to display on the order form. (No notes are required.)

Tip Box

You can also click the *Manage Favorites* icon ⭐ next to the *Test Note* box to add or remove notes from the provider's favorite list.

23. Click *Add Test.* The test is added to the *Tests Summary* section. You can add multiple tests that are of the same order type, if necessary. You can also edit, view notes pertaining to the test, or remove a test from the *Test Summary* section.

24. Using the same settings, add an additional test: "Urinalysis microscopic panel [#/volume] in Urine by Automated count."

Tip Box

If creating an order that includes two or more tests with different settings, a message prompts, indicating that there is a conflict with the setting and provides you the ability to assign common settings for all tests. However, if you want each test to have different settings, you must create separate orders for each test.

25. At the bottom of the screen, select the appropriate option to process the order (select *Print*). Each option is described in the *Order Actions* listed in Table 7-2.

TABLE 7-2 Order Actions

Action	Description
Send	Saves the order to the patient's medical record and the *Open Orders* application of the *Home* and *Clinical Today* modules. The order is also electronically transmitted via the Health Level (HL7) interface to the selected facility. (**Note**: The *Send* option is enabled only if an order interface is set up for the selected facility and your practice. This functionality is not available in your student version of Harris CareTracker PM and EMR.)
Print	Saves the order to the patient's medical record and the *Open Orders* application of the *Home* and *Clinical Today* modules. The order also displays in PDF format, enabling you to print. If an order has multiple tests, Harris CareTracker PM and EMR prints all tests at once. If the ABN given to Pt is set to "Yes" at the time the order is created, the ABN also displays after the order form to print. (**Note**: If your group is not activated to send orders electronically, Harris CareTracker PM and EMR defaults to the *Print* option.)
Fax	Saves the order to the patient's medical record and the *Open Orders* application of the *Home* and *Clinical Today* modules and faxes the order to the facility. (**Note**: Only the order form is sent to the facility. Additionally, a default fax number displays if the fax number is entered in the *Favorite Labs* application of the *Administration* module. If a fax number is not available for the lab, you must select the fax number from your address book.)
ToDo	Enables you to create a *ToDo*, referencing the order. For example, the provider may send a message asking the finance department to call the insurance to approve the charge for the order.
Record	Saves the order to the patient's medical record and the *Open Orders* application of the *Home* and *Clinical Today* modules to send or print at a later time.
Mark Complete	Marks the selected tests or the entire order as complete. (**Note**: By default, selecting the *Mark Complete* checkbox selects checkboxes pertaining to all tests included in the order.)

26. Your screen of Ms. Morgan's *Order* should look like Figure 7-7. Click *Save* to generate the order number and save the order. A copy of the order(s) is saved in the *Open Activities* section at the top of the patient's *Chart Summary*. Additionally, the open order displays in the *Today's Open Activities* dialog box when you access the patient's medical record from the *Clinical Today* module.

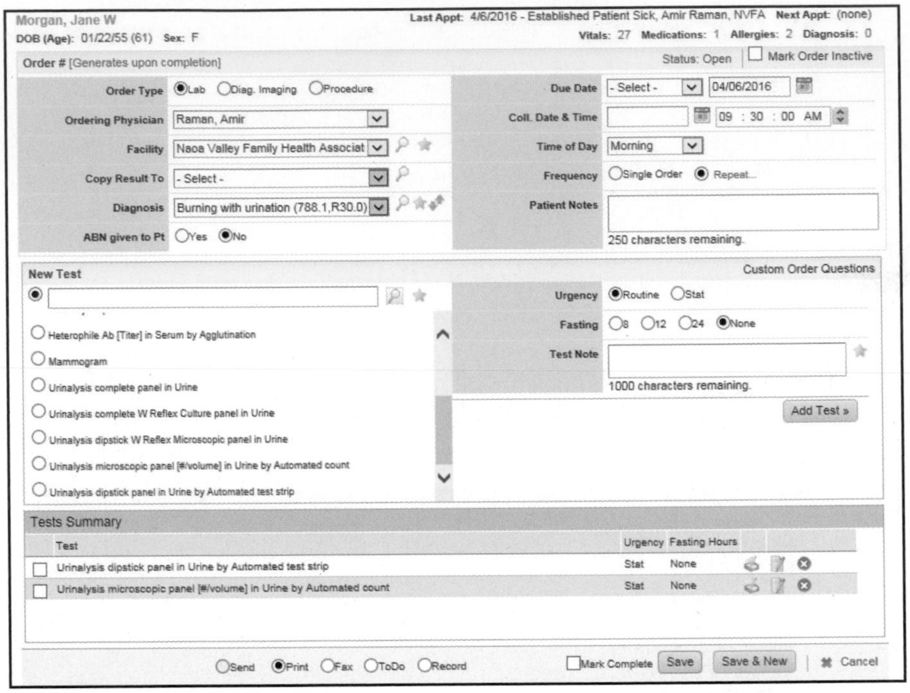

Courtesy of Harris CareTracker PM and EMR

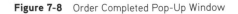

Figure 7-7 Jane Morgan Lab Order

27. Once the order is saved, a pop-up box (Figure 7-8) will display the completed order. (It may take a few moments for the completed order to display.) Print or save the order.

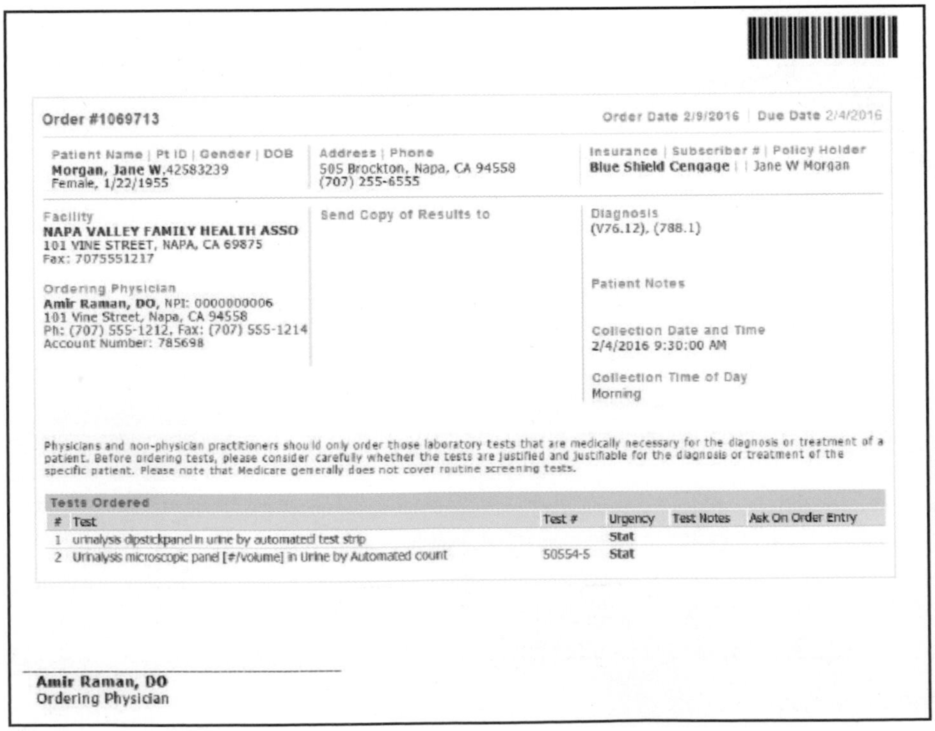
Order #1069713

Order Date 2/9/2016 | Due Date 2/4/2016

Patient Name | Pt ID | Gender | DOB
Morgan, Jane W,42583239
Female, 1/22/1955

Address | Phone
505 Brockton, Napa, CA 94558
(707) 255-6555

Insurance | Subscriber # | Policy Holder
Blue Shield Cengage | | Jane W Morgan

Facility
NAPA VALLEY FAMILY HEALTH ASSO
101 VINE STREET, NAPA, CA 69875
Fax: 7075551217

Send Copy of Results to

Diagnosis
(V76.12), (788.1)

Ordering Physician
Amir Raman, DO, NPI: 0000000006
101 Vine Street, Napa, CA 94558
Ph: (707) 555-1212, Fax: (707) 555-1214
Account Number: 785698

Patient Notes

Collection Date and Time
2/4/2016 9:30:00 AM

Collection Time of Day
Morning

Physicians and non-physician practitioners should only order those laboratory tests that are medically necessary for the diagnosis or treatment of a patient. Before ordering tests, please consider carefully whether the tests are justified and justifiable for the diagnosis or treatment of the specific patient. Please note that Medicare generally does not cover routine screening tests.

Tests Ordered

#	Test	Test #	Urgency	Test Notes	Ask On Order Entry
1	urinalysis dipstickpanel in urine by automated test strip		Stat		
2	Urinalysis microscopic panel [#/volume] in Urine by Automated count	50554-5	Stat		

Amir Raman, DO
Ordering Physician

Courtesy of Harris CareTracker PM and EMR

Figure 7-8 Order Completed Pop-Up Window

Tip Box

The *Open Activities* section in the *Chart Summary* displays open orders that are overdue. Overdue tests display "Due" and the due date in red. An order with an urgency of "Stat" displays a bold "S" in parenthesis (**S**) in the test description. For example: "Due 07/30/2013 - Urinalysis microscopic panel [#volume] in Urine by Automated count; Urinalysis dipstick panel in Urine by Automated test strip (Figure 7-9)."

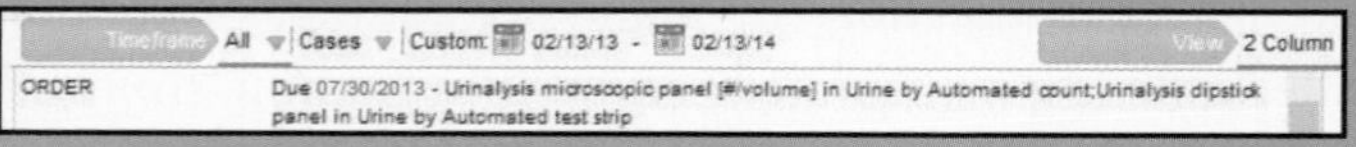

Figure 7-9 Open Activities for Jane Morgan

Courtesy of Harris CareTracker PM and EMR

🌱 **Print the lab order. Label it "Activity 7-2" and place it in your assignment folder.**

The *Orders* application has a number of advanced features that improve workflow in the medical practice. These include the ability to filter the list of orders on the status, the date of the order, the case associated with the order, or the tests included in the order. In addition, the *Orders* application consists of both open and complete orders for a patient. When you create an order for a patient, the order is saved in the patient's medical record, enabling you to track the progress of the order. When results are received, through mail, fax, or electronically, you can enter the results manually, or link to the electronic result, and update the status of the order in the *Open Orders* application of the *Quick Tasks* menu in *Clinical Today* and the *Practice* tab in the *Home* module. When results are entered for an outstanding order and marked as "complete," the order is removed from the *Open Activities* section of the patient's medical record. Additionally, the order is removed from the *Open Orders* application. Furthermore, you can print a copy of the order created for the patient or create a copy of the order when you want to order the same tests again. You will practice recording lab results in Chapter 8 activities.

To print patient test orders to share with other health care professionals treating the patient, click on the drop-down arrow next to the order entry and select *Print* (Figure 7-10). This helps review the history of tests, enabling you to prevent unnecessary duplication of tests and increase the efficiency of patient care by ordering the required tests.

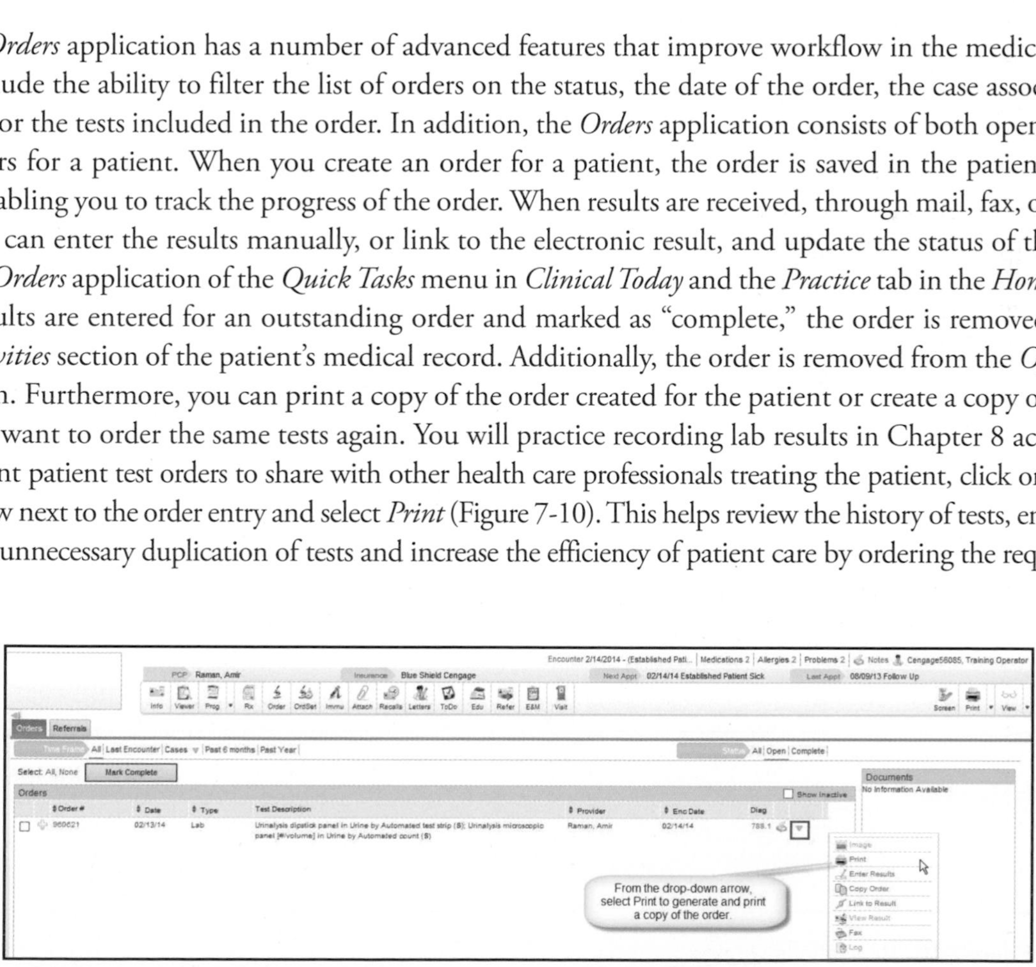

Figure 7-10 Print Lab Order

Courtesy of Harris CareTracker PM and EMR

CREATING AND PRINTING PRESCRIPTIONS

Learning Objective 2: Search for pharmacies, manage a list of favorites, and create and print prescriptions.

In Chapter 6 you were introduced to the *Medications* application in Harris CareTracker EMR. This chapter focuses on managing favorite medications, searching for pharmacies, and creating and printing prescriptions.

The *Medications* application consists of the past and current medications the patient is taking. The list also includes medications prescribed, medications administered, and samples given to the patient. You can maintain the complete list of medications by manually adding, prescribing, uploading via the *Document Management* module, and importing medication information from a Continuity of Care Document (CCD).

You can manage the list by reviewing the medication history, updating medication details, flagging medications that need attention, renewing, and electronically transmitting prescribed medications, and more. All the active medications recorded for the patient display in various locations in Harris CareTracker PM and EMR.

FYI

Access the *Medical Record* module using one of the following methods:

1. Pull the patient into context, and click the *Medical Record* module.
2. If the patient has an appointment, click the patient's name in the *Appointments* application of the *Clinical Today* module.

   a. In the *Patient Health History* pane, click *Medications*. Harris CareTracker EMR displays the *Medications* window.

Table 7-3 describes the columns of the *Medications* window. Refer to Figure 7-11 when reviewing Table 7-3.

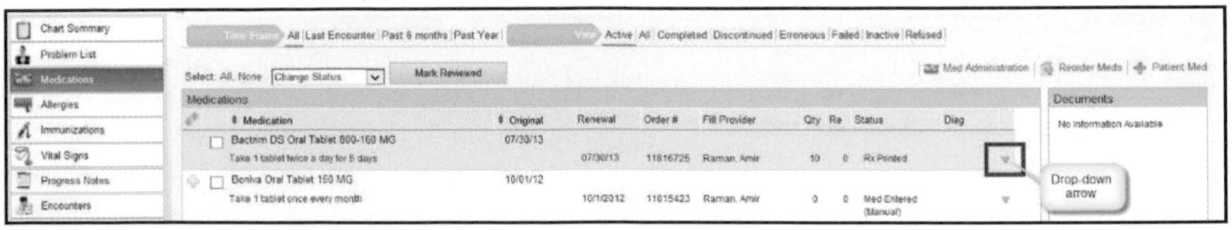

Figure 7-11 Medications Window

Courtesy of Harris CareTracker PM and EMR

TABLE 7-3	Medications Columns
Column	**Description**
Medication	The name of the medication dosage (SIG) information. The dosage is the information entered in the *Directions* (SIG) box when adding a medication or creating a prescription. For inactive medications, the *Medication* column displays the reason and the end date recorded in the *End Date* box when deactivating the medication. Example: Flomax Oral Capsule 0.4 MG (Inactive; Discontinued as of 05/17/2009).
Original	The original date for taking the medication. This is the date entered in the *Medication Date* box when adding a medication or creating a prescription.
Renewal	The original date or the dates the medication was reordered. This is the date entered in the *Start Date* box when adding a medication or creating a prescription.
Order #	A unique, system-assigned identification number for medications added or prescriptions ordered.
Fill Provider	The provider who ordered the medication.
Qty	The total quantity of the medication ordered. This is the quantity that is calculated in the *Fill Qty* box when adding a medication or creating a prescription.
Re	The number of refills allowed for the medication. The information is the option selected from the *Refills* list when adding a medication or creating a prescription.
Status	Indicates if the medication was added manually or imported from a CCD. Additionally, the column displays the status for prescriptions based on the action option selected when creating the prescription.
Diag	The diagnoses treated with the medication. These are the diagnoses you selected from the *Diagnosis* list when adding a medication or creating a prescription.
Actions	• Interactions: Displays interactions that were returned when the medication was added to the patient's medical record. If no interactions were returned, the *Interactions* 🔲 icon appears dimmed. • Reorder: Displays the original order for review and edit as necessary to reorder the medication. • Print: Displays the confirmation dialog box to enter information required to reprint the prescription. • Fax: Displays the *New Fax* dialog box to enter information required to fax the prescription. • Send Electronically: Displays the confirmation dialog box to enter information required to resend the prescription. • Log: Displays activity related to the medication.
Documents	Displays medications that are uploaded or scanned via the *Document Management* module. The list is sorted based on the document date entered when you upload or scan the document. You can move the pointer over the document to view a summary of the medications and click the document to open in the *Document Viewer*.

In Chapter 6 you reviewed the *Rx Writer* application, Surescripts®, and the requirements prior to creating and transmitting prescriptions electronically to a pharmacy. Additional features of the *Rx Writer* application are outlined in Table 7-4.

TABLE 7-4 Rx Writer Application Features
The application is *RxHub* certified and electronically routes up-to-date patient medication history and pharmacy benefit information at every point of care. This helps improve patient safety and saves the time required to create and renew prescriptions.
Allows you to verify and update information, such as the patient's last vital signs, medications, allergies, and diagnoses, to identify possible adverse effects during screening. To verify, add, or update information, hover over each category on the upper-right-hand corner of the *Rx Writer* application.
Displays easy-to-read formulary specific messages and generic cost-effective suggestions when writing a prescription.
Allows you to calculate dosage recommendations for the medication based on weight and age.
Allows you to create provider preferences such as favorite medications, SIGs, and pharmacy notes to simplify the prescription writing process.
Supports an extensive national drug database, interaction screening, and medication education information in different languages.
In addition to sending prescriptions electronically, allows you to print and fax prescriptions.

Courtesy of Harris CareTracker PM and EMR

CLINICAL SPOTLIGHT

If a prescription includes a controlled (scheduled) drug, you can only print the prescription to provide to the patient and cannot transmit it electronically.

Create Prescriptions

The *Rx* application allows you to create prescriptions for both controlled (scheduled) and noncontrolled drugs. All prescriptions created through the *Rx Writer* application are recorded in the *Medications* application with the name, Rx Norm code, dosage, and other pertinent data. **Rx Norm** is a standardized nomenclature for clinical drugs and drug delivery devices produced by the National Library of Medicine (NLM). The Rx Norm code supports interoperability between EHR systems.

ADMINISTRATIVE SP⬤TLIGHT

Prerequisites for creating a prescription

As best practice, you can set up the following prior to using the *Rx* application to create a prescription. This will also make the process for creating a prescription quick and easy.

- To see a patient's frequently used pharmacies in the list (Figure 7-12), set up the patient's favorite pharmacies via the *Relationships* application in the *Patient Demographics* module. For more information on adding patient pharmacies, see *Patient* module > *Relationships* > *Adding a Patient Pharmacy* in the *Help* system.

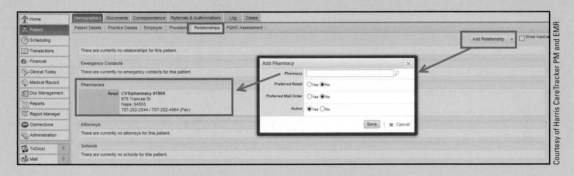

Figure 7-12   Frequently Used Pharmacies

- To see pharmacies frequently used by the practice, set the list of practice pharmacies via the *Quick Picks* application in the *Administration* module. For more information on the *Quick Picks* application, see *Administration Module* > *Setup* > *Financial* > *Quick Pick Setup* in the *Help* system.
- To check the selected medication for contraindications with the patient's active medications, problems, and allergies, set provider level screening preferences for the provider via the *Provider Screening* application. A **contraindication** is a symptom or condition that makes a particular treatment or procedure inadvisable. For more information on the *Provider Screening* application, search for "Provider Screening" in the *Search* tab in the *Help* system.
- To display a custom message on the prescription, set up a prescription message via the *Prescription Message* application. For more information on setting up prescription messages, search for "Provider Screening" in the *Search* tab in the *Help* system.
- To include a signature in the printed prescription, upload the digital signature of the provider. For more information on provider signature maintenance, see *Administration Module* > *Clinical Administration* > *System Administration* > *Provider Signature* in the *Help* system.
- To send the prescription as a fax, set up an account with *MyFax*®, and a *Fax* queue. For information on setting up an account with *MyFax*®, search for "Faxing Setup" in the *Search* tab in the *Help* system.

Manage a List of Favorites.   The *Rx Writer* application helps save favorite or most commonly prescribed medications, commonly used SIGs, and pharmacy notes to your list of favorites. This avoids having to search for medications, create SIGs, or enter pharmacy notes when creating future prescriptions. **SIG** is an abbreviation for the Latin word *signa* (meaning "label" or "sign"). SIG codes are specific dosage instructions that are given when prescribing medications.

You will now add a medication as a function of managing your list of favorites (Activity 7-3). It is important to know that you will need to click in the boxes of the dialog box versus using the [Tab] key when adding medications/prescriptions. In addition, when you fill in the number of days in the quantity box, the SIG will pull the information into the screen.

ACTIVITY 7-3:   Add a Medication as a Function of Managing the List of Favorites

1. Access the *Chart Summary* of Jane Morgan by clicking on her appointment in the *Clinical Today* module to add the medication noted in her progress note *A&P* (see Figure 7-1).

2. In the *Clinical Toolbar*, click the *Rx* icon. (This will launch the *Prescription* dialog box.)

3. By default, the *Filling Provider* list displays the provider set in your batch. However, you can click another provider to add to your favorites. Confirm that the *Filling Provider* displays Dr. Raman.

4. If you had previously entered *Favorite Medications*, you could click the *Manage Favorites* ⭐ icon next to the *Medication* box. If you notice that the *Favorites* ⭐ icon is grayed out, this means no medications have been saved to *Favorites*. When you have *Favorites*, the *Manage Favorites* dialog box (Figure 7-13) displays a list of favorites or commonly prescribed medications. You would also be able to view favorite pharmacy notes and SIGs by clicking the specific pane under the *Favorites* section.

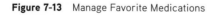

Manage Favorites: Amir Raman		Favorites
FavoriteMedications		
Add Medication [_____] 🔍 [Add]		Allergies
Boniva Oral Tablet 150 MG	⊗	
Atenolol Oral Tablet 100 MG	⊗	Facilities
Doryx Oral Tablet Delayed Release 150 MG	⊗	
Avapro Oral Tablet 150 MG	⊗	Lab Tests
Avapro Oral Tablet 75 MG	⊗	
Pepcid Oral Tablet 20 MG	⊗	Medications
Bactrim DS Oral Tablet 800-160 MG	⊗	
Cipro Oral Tablet 750 MG	⊗	Pharmacy Notes
Oxycodone-Acetaminophen Oral Tablet 5-325 MG	⊗	
Lipisorb Oral Liquid	⊗	SIG
Lipitor Oral Tablet 10 MG	⊗	Test Notes

Courtesy of Harris CareTracker PM and EMR

Figure 7-13   Manage Favorite Medications

5. First, check the *Medication* drop-down list to see if the prescribed medication is listed (Bactrim DS Oral Tablet 800-160 MG). If it is listed, select it and skip to step 11. If not, click the *Search* 🔍 icon. The *Medication Search* dialog box displays to search for a medication. By default, the *Search For* field displays "Medications". By default, the *Drug Type* list is set to "Dispensable". **Dispensable** (capable of being dispensed, administered, or distributed) includes the medication name and dosage information.

FYI

In your student environment, the *Drug Type* list is grayed out and automatically set to "Dispensable." In the real-world version of Harris CareTracker EMR you can also select "Routed Drug" to record the medication without any dosage information. **Routed** refers to the way that a drug is introduced into the body, such as oral, enteral, mucosal, parenteral, or percutaneous.

6. By default, the *Search Terms* list is set to "Contains"; however, you can change the option to "Begins with" if necessary.

7. Enter a keyword in the *Search Text* box. (Enter "Bactrim.")

8. Select the *Include Generics* checkbox to include generic versions of the medication in the search results. The generic version displays in *italics* for easy identification.

9. Click *Search*. Harris CareTracker EMR displays a list of medications matching the search criteria. (**Note:** By default, the search results do not show obsolete medications. To view medications that are obsolete, select the *Show Obsolete Drugs* checkbox. The obsolete medications appear dimmed in the search results. You cannot save obsolete medications.)

10. Scroll down to select the medication noted in the *A&P*: Bactrim DS Oral Tablet 800-160 MG (Figure 7-14). First, if not already saved as a *Favorite*, click the *Add as Favorite* ⭐ icon to add to your medication favorites. Then click the medication selected. (**Note:** If an *Interaction Screening* dialog box appears, select "Benefit outweighs risk" as the *Override Reason* and then click *Accept*.)

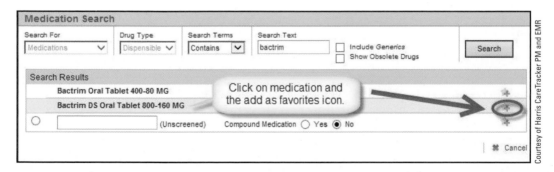

Figure 7-14   Bactrim Search Results

Tip Box

When you are searching for medications, you can click on the *Add as Favorite* ⭐ icon on as many medications as you want to include in your favorites. This will save time in the future when entering medications. In addition, you can click on the *Add as Favorite* ⭐ icon for the SIG once entered, which will make your workflows more efficient.

(*Continues*)

(Continued)

If the required medication is not in the list, scroll to the bottom of the list and select the radio dial button next to *Unscreened* and then type the medication name. Medications that are not a part of the drug database are not screened against the patient's active allergies, problems, and other medications. You can add a medication including a free text medication to the provider's favorite list by clicking the *Add as Favorite* ⭐ icon next to the medication name. The free text medication you add to the favorite list pertains to the provider selected when searching for the medication. Additionally, you can enter favorite SIG information for the free text medication.

11. Continue completing the prescription by adding the SIG, as noted in the *Progress Note* ("SIG: 1 tab bid for 5 days, No refills") in the *Dose* line of the *New Prescription* section. You can also click the *Dosing Calculator* 🖩 icon, and the calculator will display the advised SIG. If the *Dosing Calculator* returned the SIG noted in the A&P, click on the radio dial, then scroll down and click *Select*. The SIG will populate in the *Prescription* dialog box. If the SIG returned by the *Dosing Calculator* is not the same as noted in the *Progress Note*, enter the SIG manually. In this case, the SIG will need to be entered manually.

   a. For *Amount*, enter "1."

   b. For *Unit*, select "Tablet."

   c. For *Frequency*, select "Twice a day."

   d. Enter a *Duration* of "5 Days."

FYI

The *Rx Writer* application includes the dosing calculator that provides dosing recommendations for the medication the provider is prescribing based on the weight and age of the patient. You must enter the patient's weight to provide weight-based decision support. Additionally, the calculator takes into consideration other factors, such as the reason for prescribing the medication, type of the dose, route, and other special conditions, enabling you to customize recommendations to suit your preference. However, the ability and the options available to customize dosage recommendations are based on the medication the provider is prescribing.

12. In your student environment, you will need to change the *Start Date* and *Original Date* to reflect the date of the patient's encounter. However, the date stamp for audit purposes will reflect the actual date and time you recorded the information.

FYI

When you click the *More Information* link next to the *Med Formulary* field, Harris CareTracker EMR displays the *Formulary-Additional Information* dialog box (Figure 7-15) with formulary, co-pay, coverage, and alternatives. **Formulary** is defined by the Centers for Medicare & Medicaid Services (CMS) as a list of prescription drugs covered by a prescription drug plan or another insurance plan offering prescription drug benefits (also called a drug list) (see Table 7-5).

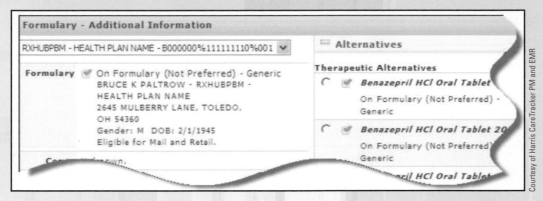

Figure 7-15 Formulary Information Dialog Box

You can select the original or an alternative medication and click *Select*. (**Note:** The selected medication is screened against the patient's active diagnoses, medications, and allergies. If the screening triggers an interaction that is higher than the severity settings set for the provider in the batch, the *Interaction Screening* dialog box displays for you to acknowledge the screening.)

13. Click *Add Rx* (Figure 7-16) and the prescription summary will display the newly added medication (Figure 7-17).

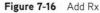

Figure 7-16 Add Rx

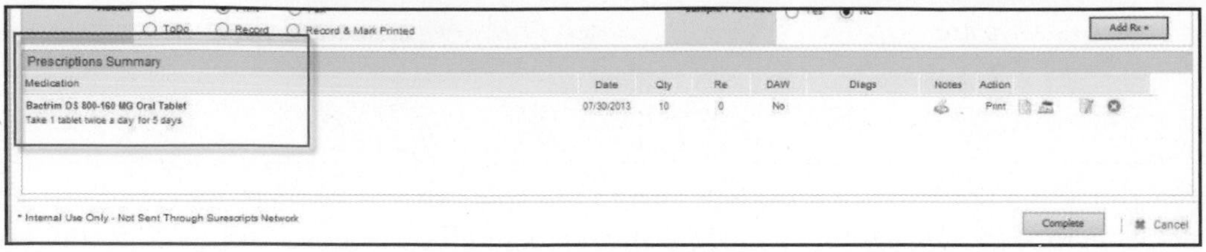

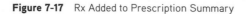

Figure 7-17 Rx Added to Prescription Summary

14. Click *Complete* to finish the prescription. The prescription will open in a new window (Figure 7-18).

15. If your prescription did not print, follow the instructions in Activity 7-4 to reprint the prescription. Use reprint reason of "printer out of paper."

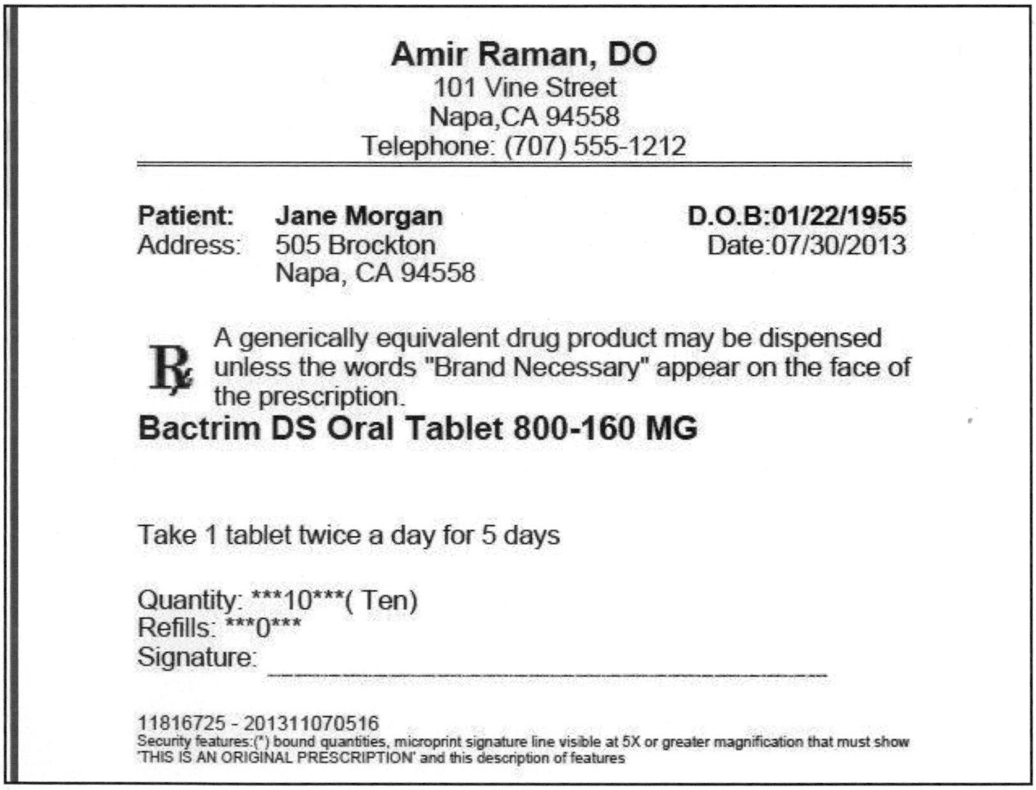

Amir Raman, DO
101 Vine Street
Napa,CA 94558
Telephone: (707) 555-1212

Patient: **Jane Morgan**	**D.O.B:01/22/1955**
Address: 505 Brockton	Date:07/30/2013
Napa, CA 94558	

℞ A generically equivalent drug product may be dispensed unless the words "Brand Necessary" appear on the face of the prescription.

Bactrim DS Oral Tablet 800-160 MG

Take 1 tablet twice a day for 5 days

Quantity: ***10***(Ten)
Refills: ***0***
Signature: _____

11816725 - 201311070516
Security features:(*) bound quantities, microprint signature line visible at 5X or greater magnification that must show
'THIS IS AN ORIGINAL PRESCRIPTION' and this description of features

Figure 7-18 Print Bactrim Rx

 Print the Bactrim prescription ordered for Jane Morgan. Label it "Activity 7-3" and place it in your assignment folder.

The tiered formularies are displayed with color-coded symbols, as described in Table 7-5.

TABLE 7-5 Formulary Symbols

Symbol	Description
☆	The medication is formulary compliant and is preferred.
📋✓	The medication is formulary compliant but not preferred.
✖	The medication is not formulary compliant and the payment is the patient's responsibility if prescribed.

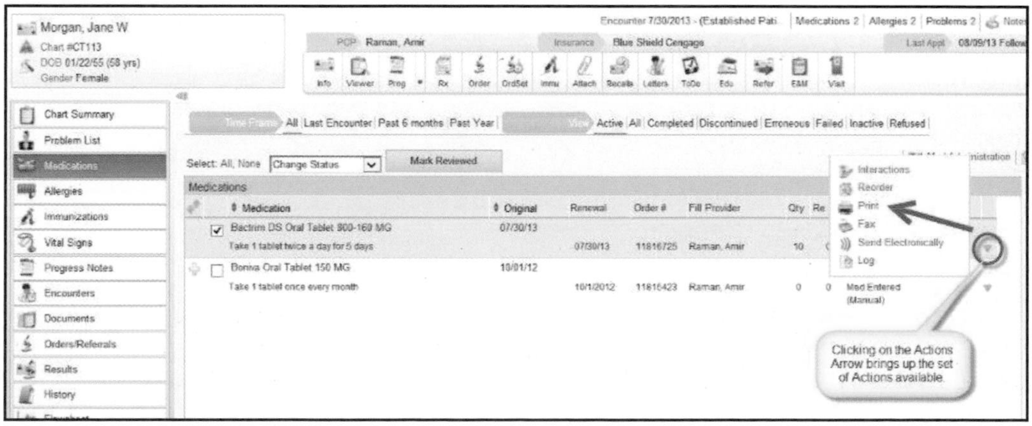

Courtesy of Harris CareTracker PM and EMR

Print Prescriptions

The *Medications* application helps review and print prescription information to give to a patient or fax to a pharmacy.

ACTIVITY 7-4: Reprint a Prescription

1. With patient Jane Morgan in context, click the *Medical Record* module.

2. In the *Patient Health History* pane, click *Medications*. Harris CareTracker EMR displays the *Medications* window.

3. Click on the checkbox next to the prescription you want to reprint. (Select *Bactrim*.)

4. In the *Actions* menu, click the *Arrow* ▼ icon for the prescription and click *Print* (Figure 7-19).

Figure 7-19 Actions Menu - Print

5. A *Reprint Prescription* dialog box will pop up. Select "Printer Out of Paper" as your *Reprint Reason* and click *Print.* The prescription displays in PDF format, enabling you to print.

6. If you had uploaded a digital signature, Harris CareTracker EMR would display the *Provider Signature* dialog box. Because no digital signature has been uploaded, print the prescription as is. In the *Medication* window, the *Status* of the medication changes to "Rx Printed."

Tip Box

By default, the prescription is set up to print on 4" × 6" paper. If you want to print a prescription in one-quarter of the page, click to clear the *Auto-Rotate and Center* checkbox in the *Page* handling section of the *Print* dialog box (Figure 7-20).

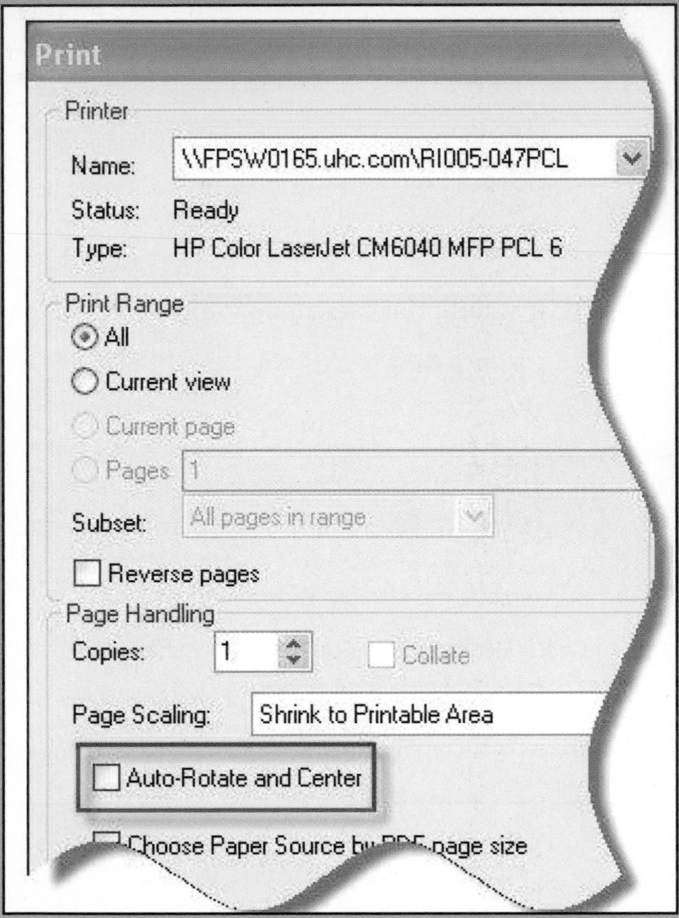

Figure 7-20   Auto Rotate and Center Rx

Print a copy of the prescription. Label it "Activity 7-4" and place it in your assignment folder.

Search for a Pharmacy.   The *Rx Writer* application includes a *Pharmacy* list that includes the following two categories:

- Patient Pharmacies: Displays patient pharmacies listed under the *Relationships* application in the *Patient* module. By default, the *Pharmacy* list displays the patient's preferred pharmacy recorded for the patient in the *Relationships* application of the *Patient* module.

- Favorite Pharmacies: Displays pharmacies your practice most frequently uses. The favorite pharmacy list is set via the *Quick Picks* application of the *Administration* module. To access the application, click the *Administration* module, *Setup* tab, and then click the *Quick Picks* link under the *Financial* section. Click *Pharmacies* from the list to search and add favorite pharmacies for your practice. For more information on the *Quick Pick Setup* application, see *Administration Module > Setup > Financial > Quick Pick Setup* in the *Help* system.

Additionally, the *Rx Writer* application includes a pharmacy search feature, enabling you to search for pharmacies that are not in the patient's active pharmacy list or the practice's favorite pharmacy list. When you write a prescription for a pharmacy that is not in the list, Harris CareTracker EMR adds the pharmacy to the *Other* application in the *Patient* module.

Tip Box

If CVS pharmacy is not in the patient's active pharmacy list, writing a prescription to the pharmacy automatically adds it under the *Active Patient Pharmacies* section in the *Other* application of the *Patient* module.

You need to include the pharmacy information when sending a prescription electronically. Because you cannot send electronic prescriptions in your student version of Harris CareTracker EMR, you can only complete this activity up to the point of searching for a pharmacy. Follow the instructions in Activity 7-5 to familiarize yourself with this task.

ACTIVITY 7-5:   Search for a Pharmacy

1. With patient Jane Morgan in context, click the *Medical Record* module.
2. In the *Clinical Toolbar*, click the *Rx* icon.
3. If an encounter is in context, Harris CareTracker EMR displays the *Prescription* dialog box. (**Note:** If an encounter is not in context, the *Select Encounter* dialog box displays for you to select or create a new encounter. Click on the encounter you already created for this patient. The *Prescription* dialog box will display.)
4. If Ms. Morgan does not have any favorite pharmacies saved yet, you will need to click the *Search* icon next to the *Pharmacy* list. Harris CareTracker EMR displays the *Search Pharmacies* dialog box.
5. Enter search criteria such as name, city, state, zip code, and phone number in the specific boxes to search for the pharmacy you want. In the *Pharmacy Type* list, select the appropriate type of pharmacy. For example, if you want to search for pharmacies that can mail the medication to the patient, select "Mail Order." Enter the following criteria in the *Search Pharmacies* dialog box:
   a. *Name:* CVS
   b. *City:* Napa
   c. *State:* CA
   d. *Pharmacy Type:* Retail

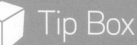

Tip Box

The *State* list defaults to the patient's home address state and is a required field. In the *Name* box, enter the first few characters of the pharmacy name to display more results and prevent from eliminating results based on the way the name is spelled.
Example: Entering *wal* will display all results with walmart, wal mart, and wal-mart.

6. Click *Search*. Harris CareTracker EMR will return all pharmacies matching your criteria. Select "CVS # 1804" (Figure 7-21). (**Note**: If you get an error message, close the dialog box and begin the search over.)

Name	Type	Address	City⬦	ST⬦	ZIP⬦	Phone	Fax
CVS/pharmacy #1804 (eRx)	Retail	675 Trancas St	Napa	CA	94558	707-252-2844	707-252-4864
CVS/pharmacy #7141 (eRx)	Retail	291 S. COOMBS STREET	NAPA	CA	94559	707-252-0101	707-252-0137
CVS/pharmacy #9214 (eRx)	Retail	1558 Trancas St	Napa	CA	94558	707-253-7918	707-253-8719

Courtesy of Harris CareTracker PM and EMR

Figure 7-21 Search Pharmacy Criteria Results

7. Do not add in the medication name or SIG at this time because this activity is only to learn to use the *Search* feature for pharmacies.

8. Click *Cancel* in the bottom right corner of the *Prescription* dialog box.

9. Click *OK* in the *Cancel Prescription* box.

Critical Thinking

State requirements for prescriptions may vary and it is your responsibility to be sure your practice is in compliance. Because you are a medical assistant at Napa Valley Family Health Associates in Napa, California, log in to the *Help* system and click on *State Print Instructions* (*Medical Record Module > Prescriptions > Printing Prescriptions*). Print each of the *State Print Instructions* sheets at the bottom of the screen (California, New Jersey, and New York). Compare and contrast the differences of each state. Write a one-page paper on why you think individual states would have different requirements. Submit the forms and your paper to your instructor for class discussion.

Other Prescription Highlights.   Some medication names may have mixed case lettering in the description name. This is known as **"Tall Man" lettering;** for example, NEXium. This is a standard used to comply with the patient safety initiative endorsed by the Food and Drug Administration (FDA) and Institute for Safe Medication Practices (ISMP). This helps reduce errors between medication names that either look or sound alike.

Interaction Screenings.   The *Rx Writer* application checks for interactions when prescribing a medication to a patient. The screening checks for possible contraindications with the patient's active medications, allergies, and problems and alerts you if the interaction is higher than the severity level you set.

 If an interaction exists for a medication added or prescribed, you can click *Cancel* or "X" in the *Interactions Screening* dialog box and take necessary action to avoid adverse reactions. You can also choose to acknowledge the screening by selecting one or more override reasons and entering notes before clicking *Accept.* The *Interactions Screening* dialog box is color and numerically coded to highlight the severity levels of an interaction (Figure 7-22). It also summarizes the effects and the level of risk of the prescribed medication.

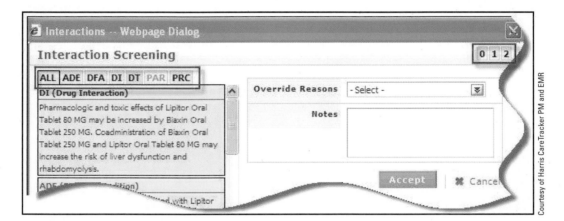

Figure 7-22 Interactions Screening

Tip Box

If a medication, a diagnosis, or an allergy triggered an interaction, you can click the *Interaction* icon for the item in the associated application to display a read-only dialog box with the interactions and override reasons available. The *Interaction* icon appears dimmed if interactions are unavailable.

 The *Levels of Severity* (Numeric and Color Codes) listed in Table 7-6 are the numeric severity indications. The *Levels of Interaction* are described in Table 7-7.

TABLE 7-6 Levels of Severity

Level of Severity	Description
Gray (0)	Indicates minor severity (bothersome or little effect)
Yellow (1)	Indicates moderate severity (deterioration for patient's status)
Green (2)	Indicates major severity (life-threatening or permanent damage)

TABLE 7-7 Levels of Interaction (Tab View)

Level of Interaction	Description	Example
ADE (Drug-to-Condition Interaction)	The prescribed medication has a negative interaction with the patient's existing diagnosis.	The patient suffers from high blood pressure and the prescribed medication has an effect on blood pressure.
DFA (Drug-to-Food Interaction)	The prescribed medication taken with certain food interacts in ways that diminish the effectiveness of the ingested medication or reduce the absorption of food nutrients.	Vitamin and herbal supplements taken with prescribed medications can result in adverse reactions.
DI (Drug-to-Drug Interaction)	The prescribed medication has an effect with the patient's active medications that may cause new and dangerous reactions or may reduce or increase the effects of the prescribed medication.	Mixing antidiabetic medication (e.g., oral hypoglycemics) and beta blockers (e.g., Inderal) can result in decreased response of the antidiabetic drug and increase the frequency and severity of low blood sugar episodes.
DT (Duplicate Therapy)	The prescribed medication is the same as a medication the patient is currently on and is treating the same diagnosis. If a provider prescribes a brand name medication and allows substitution, a duplicate medication message displays when approving a refill request for the generic version of the medication. If the refill request is approved for the generic version, the previously prescribed brand name medication is made inactive on the same date the refill request is received. Additionally, a record is also saved for the generic medication in the patient's active medication list. You can view the brand name medication that was originally ordered by hovering over the generic medication name.	Two sleep medication types are prescribed for the patient.
PAR (Drug to Allergy)	The prescribed medication has allergic reactions and cross sensitivities with the patient allergies.	
PRC (Precaution Screening)	The prescribed medication has precautionary warnings based on factors such as age (pediatric and geriatric) and medical conditions.	

The *Complete Screening* icon in the *Patient Detail* bar enables you to check for interactions in real time for the patient in context. This complete screening is for informational purposes only and includes interactions based on active diagnoses, medications and allergies, patient's age and weight, duplicate therapy, food interactions, and precaution screening.

Fax Prescriptions.   The *Medications* application enables you to fax prescriptions to a pharmacy using the *Message Center* application. You must have an account with *MyFax®* to use the faxing features in Harris Care-Tracker PM and EMR and have a *Fax* queue set up to send the prescription as a fax. Your student version of Harris CareTracker EMR does not have the *MyFax®* feature. For information and instructions on faxing prescriptions, log in to the *Help* system *Contents* tab and select *Faxing Prescriptions (Medical Records* module > *Prescriptions* > *Faxing Prescriptions*).

Submit Prescriptions Electronically.   The *Medications* application helps transmit a saved prescription electronically to a selected pharmacy. This feature is useful to transmit a prescription that failed electronic transmission or is saved to send later. Because your student environment will not electronically transmit prescriptions, you will receive the error message noted in Figure 7-23.

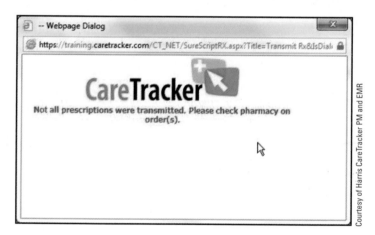

Figure 7-23   Electronic Rx Error Message

In a live environment, the steps to send an electronic prescription are noted in the FYI box.

FYI

Submit a Saved Prescription Electronically

1. Access the patient's *Medical Record* module.
2. In the *Patient Health History* pane, click *Medications*. The *Medications* window displays.
3. In the *Actions* menu, click the *Arrow* icon for the prescription you want and click *Send Electronically* to electronically send the prescription to the pharmacy.

(Continues)

(Continued)

Tip Box

If the prescription was previously sent, faxed, or printed, the *Transmit Rx* dialog box displays.

- In the *Resend Reason* list, click a reason for sending the prescription again. If the reason is not in the list, click "Other (See Comments)." You must select a reason for tracking purposes. The reason and comments are saved in the activity log of the prescription.
- In the *Comments* box, enter the reason or additional comments if necessary.

4. Click *Send*. In the *Medication* window, the *Status* of the medication changes to "Rx Queued" (for Electronic Transmit) or "Rx Sent" (Electronically).

ACCESSING THE IMMUNIZATION APPLICATION

Learning Objective 3: View, add, and create immunization records.

In Chapter 5 you learned how to manage immunization lots in Harris CareTracker EMR. In this chapter you will view, add, and create immunization records. In Chapter 8 you will perform advanced features such as running an immunization lot number report.

The *Immunizations* application consists of a list of newly administered immunizations, immunizations administered in the past, and immunizations the patient refused to have administered. You can maintain the complete list of immunizations by manually recording immunizations, uploading via the *Document Management* module, or importing immunization information from a CCD. You can manage the list of immunizations by reviewing the immunization history, updating, sorting, and printing. All active immunizations recorded for the patient display in various locations in Harris CareTracker PM and EMR.

Additionally, the *Immunizations* application provides access to the Centers for Disease Control and Prevention (CDC) website. The website provides quick reference for recommended child and adolescent immunization schedules and a catch-up schedule for children who missed a scheduled immunization. You can review and print the immunization schedules from the CDC site.

ACTIVITY 7-6: Access the Immunizations Application

1. Pull patient Jane Morgan into context and click the *Medical Record* module.

2. In the *Patient Health History* pane, click *Immunizations*. Harris CareTracker EMR displays the *Immunizations* window with a list of patient immunizations (Figure 7-24).

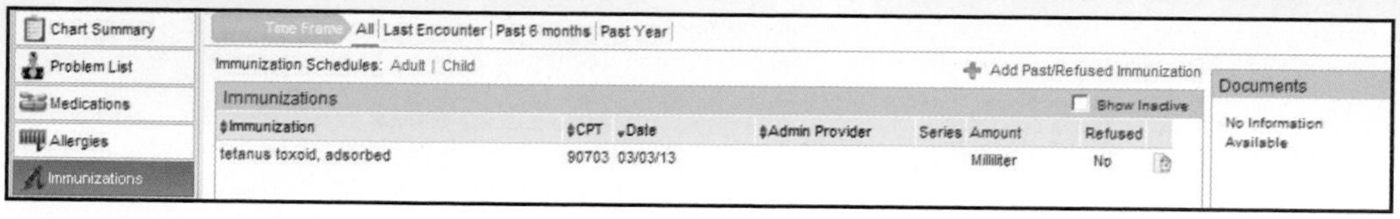

Figure 7-24 . Immunizations Window
Courtesy of Harris CareTracker PM and EMR

Print a screen shot of the Immunizations window. Label it "Activity 7-6" and place it in your assignment folder.

Table 7-8 describes the columns in the *Immunizations* window, as displayed in Figure 7-24.

TABLE 7-8 Immunizations Columns	
Column	**Description**
IIS	Allows you to select the immunization to send to the Immunization registry.
Immunization	The name of the immunization.
CPT®	The CPT® code associated with the immunization.
Date	The date the immunization was administered. By default, the immunization list is sorted by the immunization administered date.
Admin Provider	The provider who administered the immunization.
Series	The series associated with the immunization.
Amount	The dosage amount of the administered immunization.
Refused	Displays if the immunization was refused by the patient. If the immunization was refused, you can move the pointer over *Yes* to view the reason for refusing the immunization.
Log	Displays all activities pertaining to the immunization.
Documents	Displays immunizations that are uploaded or scanned via the *Document Management* module. The list is sorted based on the document date entered when you upload or scan the document.

Courtesy of Harris CareTracker PM and EMR

Add Immunizations

The *Immunizations* application helps maintain a complete record of a patient's immunizations by adding past immunizations administered and immunizations the patient refused to have administered in addition to new immunizations recorded. This helps store an up-to-date record of a patient's immunization history in one location and provides the ability to track immunizations that are due.

The *Immunization Writer* application, accessed by clicking the *Immunizations* ↗ icon on the *Clinical Toolbar,* allows you to maintain an up-to-date record of immunizations by recording information about immunizations administered. This helps your practice report accurate and complete patient immunization records to other entities, track inventory of immunizations, improve patient safety, and more.

ACTIVITY 7-7: Add a New Immunization

Prior to adding a new immunization, you must set your *Administered By* list, which is defined through the *Immunization Administrator Maintenance* application accessed via the *Administration* module (Figure 7-25).

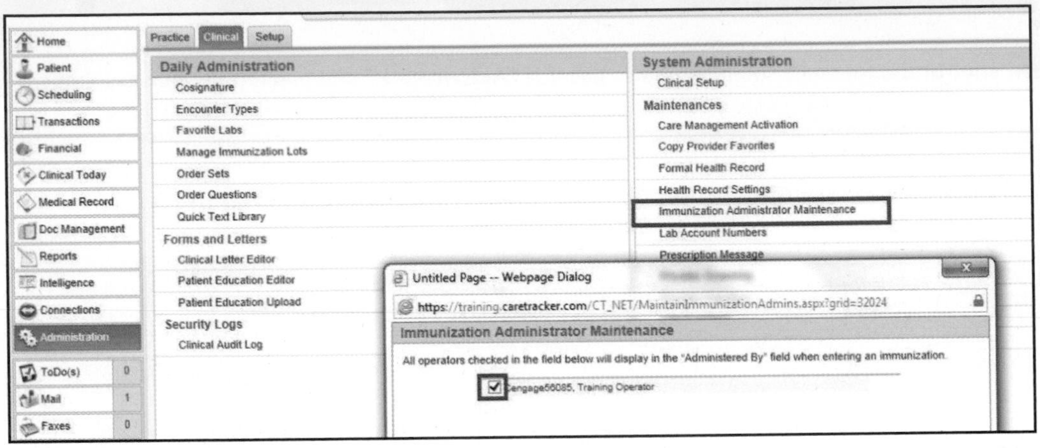

Figure 7-25 Immunization Administrator Maintenance

1. Go to the *Administration* module > *Clinical* tab and select the *Immunization Administrator Maintenance* link. Place a check mark next to your "Training Operator" number, and then click *Save*. You are now ready to add immunizations. (**Note:** You may receive an error message that the web page is trying to close; if so, click *Yes*. You can close out of the *Immunization Administrator Maintenance* dialog box by clicking the "X" in the upper-right corner. You have been added as an administrator to *Immunization Maintenance*.)

2. Pull patient Jane Morgan into context, and then click the *Medical Record* module.

3. In the *Clinical Toolbar*, click the *Immunizations* ⚕ icon.

4. If an encounter is in context, Harris CareTracker EMR displays the *Immunization Writer* dialog box. If there was no encounter in context, the *Select Encounter* dialog box would display for you to select an encounter. Select the encounter you created for this patient in Chapter 6, which will launch the *Immunization Writer* dialog box.

5. Verify that patient information such as diagnoses, medications, and allergies are up to date in the medical record by hovering over each category in the upper-right corner of the *Immunization Writer* application (Figure 7-26).

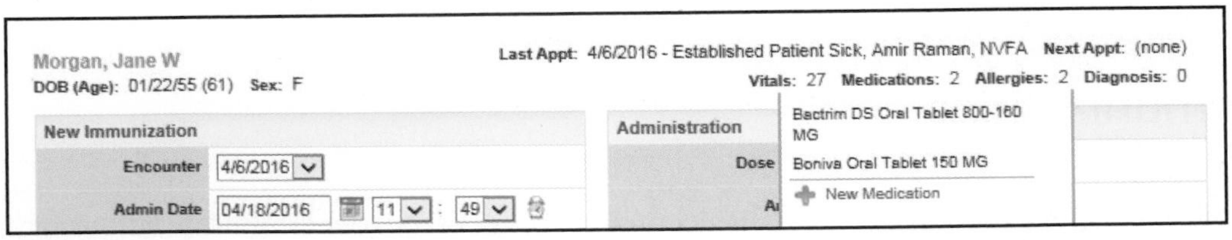

Figure 7-26 Patient Information in Immunization Writer

6. The *Encounter* list defaults to the encounter date selected or created. (Leave as is.)

7. The *Admin Date* defaults to today's date. To change the date of administration, enter the date or click the *Calendar* ⊞ icon to select the date. (Change the *Admin Date* so that it matches the encounter date.) Select the time the immunization is administered. (Enter a time that is 15 minutes past the patient's appointment time).

Tip Box

You can also click the *Reset* 🔄 icon to reset to the current date and time.

8. In the *Administered By* list, click the provider who administered the immunization. The screen should populate with your operator number. (Leave as is.)

9. In the *Ord Provider* list, click the provider who ordered the immunization. (Select "Dr. Raman.")

10. Using the details in Figure 7-27, add immunization lot information by clicking the *Add Lot* ➕ icon. Enter the following information in the *Lot Management* dialog box. (**Note:** Adjust the years in the *Received Date* and *Expiration Date* fields depending on the date of the encounter. For example, if your encounter takes place in 2016, the *Received Date* should occur in 2016, and the *Expiration Date* should be in 2017.)

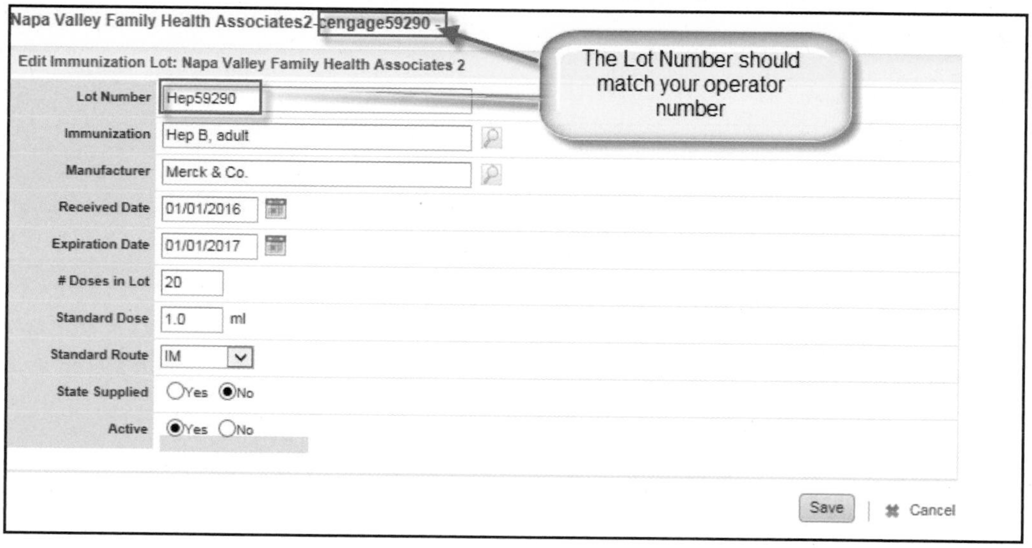

Figure 7-27   Add Immunization Lot

a. Enter the *Lot Number* (enter "Hep" followed by your operator number as the lot number).

b. Click the *Search* 🔍 icon next to *Immunization*.

   i. Enter "Hep B" in the *Search Text* field. Click *Search*.

   ii. Select "Hep B, adult" from the *Search Results* list.

c. Click the *Search* 🔍 icon next to *Manufacturer*.

   i. Enter "me" in the *Search Text* field. Click *Search*.

   ii. Select the radio dial button next to "Merck & Co" under *Search Results*.

d. Enter *Received Date* of January 1, 20XX. (See prior note on the *Received Date*.)

e. Enter *Expiration Date* of January 1, 20XX. (See prior note on the *Expiration Date*.)

f. Enter "20" in the *# Doses in Lot* field.

g. Enter *Standard Dose* of "1.0" mL.

h. Select *Standard Route* of "IM."

i. *State Supplied* defaults to "No."

j. *Active* defaults to "Yes."

k. Click *Save*.

11. Select the lot you just created from the *Lot Number* drop-down list.

CLINICAL SPOTLIGHT

Important!! If the lot number is not selected, a warning message displays, prompting you to select a lot number.

CLINICAL SPOTLIGHT

All state departments of health require reporting the amount of an immunization administered in milliliters (mL).

12. By default, the *Dose Route* list displays the standard route information selected in the *Lot Management* dialog box. However, you can change the method by which the immunization is administered by making another selection from the *Dose Route* list. (Leave the *Dose Route* as "IM.")

13. By default, the *Amount* field displays the amount entered in the *Lot Management* dialog box. You can change this by manually entering another amount. (Leave the *Amount* as "1.0" mL.)

14. In the *Series* list, select the appropriate sequence when the immunization administered is from a series of several shots (i.e., initial challenge and boosters). For example, if administering the patient with a series of hepatitis immunizations and it is the first immunization in the series, select "1" in the *Series* list. (Select "1".)

CLINICAL SPOTLIGHT

Three doses are generally required to complete the hepatitis B vaccine series for adults.

- First injection – given at any time
- Second injection – at least one month after the first dose
- Third injection – six months after the first dose

> ### Tip Box
>
> When documenting a patient encounter, the series information displays in the narrative.

15. In the *Site* list, click the area of the patient's body where the immunization or drug is administered. (Select "Left Deltoid.")

16. In the *VIS Date* box, Harris CareTracker EMR automatically fills in the date from the *Support* database. If the date does not display, enter the date on the *Vaccine Information Statements* (VIS) handed out to the patient when the immunization was administered. (Enter date of the first day of the current year you are working in. For instance, if you are working in 2016, you would enter "01/01/2016.")

17. In the *Date VIS given to Pt* box, enter the date the VIS was given to the patient. (Enter the date of the patient encounter.)

18. By default, the *Adverse Reactions* list is set to "Pt Tolerated Well." However, you can select one or more other reactions the patient had as a result of the immunization administered. (Leave the selection as is.)

19. In the *Administration Notes* box, enter additional comments about the immunization if necessary. (Enter: "Patient to return in 4–5 weeks for second injection, and return 6 months after the 1st dose for 3rd injection.") Your screen should look like Figure 7-28.

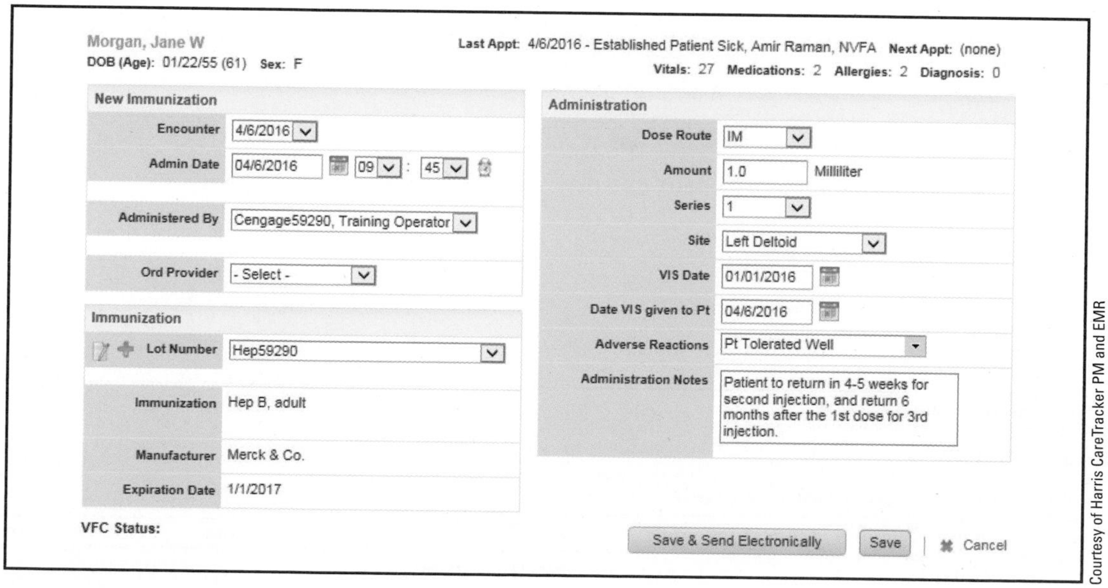

Courtesy of Harris CareTracker PM and EMR

Figure 7-28   Immunization Writer

20. Click *Save* to save the administered immunization to the patient's medical record, *Chart Viewer*, and the narrative of the *Progress Note* template. (**Note:** To save and send the immunization information to the Department of Health in your state, you would click *Save & Send Electronically*.)

21. Refresh your *Immunizations* screen, and you will see the newly added Hep B immunization (Figure 7-29).

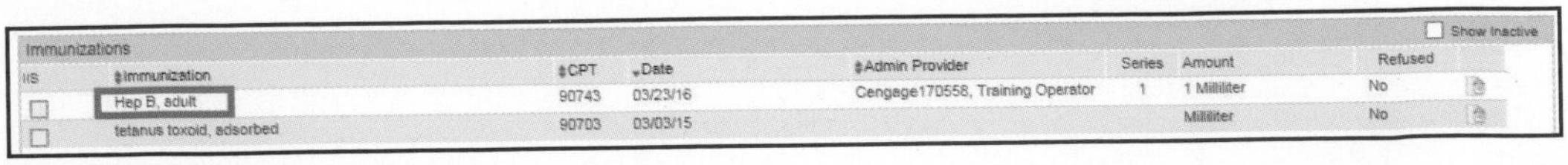

Figure 7-29   Refreshed Immunization Screen
Courtesy of Harris CareTracker PM and EMR

🖊 **Print the updated Immunizations window. Label it "Activity 7-7" and place it in your assignment folder.**

Print Immunization Records

The *Immunizations* application allows you to print immunization records to give to patients. This printed record helps to review the immunization history, provides the ability to know when an immunization is due, and prevents over-immunization. It also helps to share the patient immunization history with other entities such as clinics, schools, and camps, enabling compliance with safety and health regulations.

ACTIVITY 7-8:   Print Immunization Records

1. Pull patient Jane Morgan into context, and then click the *Medical Record* module.

2. In the *Patient Health History* pane, click *Immunizations*. Harris CareTracker EMR displays the *Immunizations* window with a list of immunizations administered to the patient.

3. Click the drop-down arrow next to *Print* 🖨 on the *Patient Detail* bar, and click *Print Immunization*.

4. The patient immunization record opens in a new window (Figure 7-30).

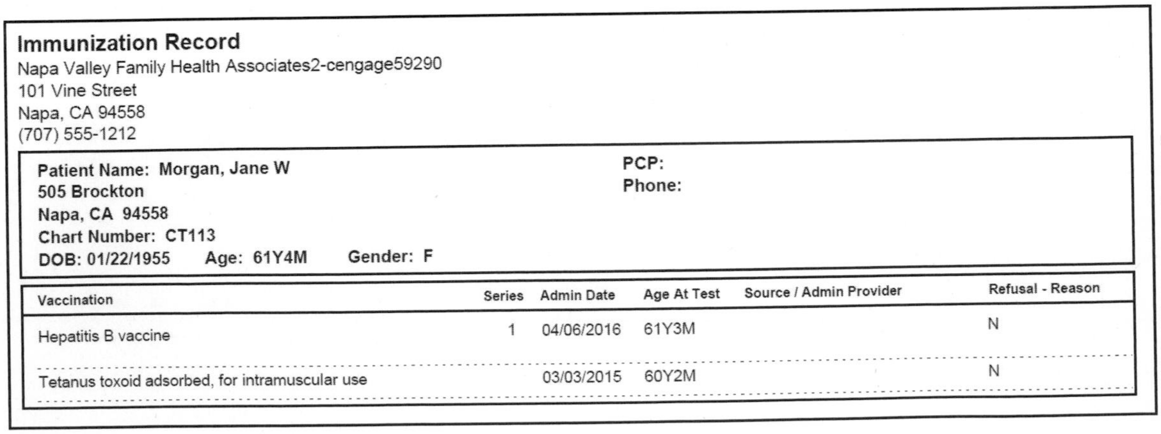

Figure 7-30   Print Immunizations Record

Tip Box

The Immunization Record displays a detailed list of active immunizations for the patient. Immunizations marked as inactive do not display in the report.

Print the Immunization Record. Label it "Activity 7-8" and place it in your assignment folder.

View the Activity Log of an Immunization

The *Activity Log* tracks all activity related to immunizations recorded in the patient's medical record. It is a helpful reference for audit purposes and displays information such as date, user responsible for the action, the action performed, and comments associated with an action.

ACTIVITY 7-9: View the Activity Log of an Immunization

1. With patient Jane Morgan in context, click the *Medical Record* module.

2. In the *Patient Health History* pane, click *Immunizations*. Harris CareTracker EMR displays the *Immunizations* window with a list of immunizations administered to the patient.

3. Click the *Log* icon next to the selected immunization record to view all activity details for that immunization. (Select the log for "Hep B, adult".) The *View Log* dialog box displays. (**Note**: You may need to adjust the date in the *From Date* [select "01/01/2016"] and *To Date* [use current date] boxes to include previously administered immunizations [Figure 7-31]. The activity log displays the information listed in Table 7-9, based on the type of action performed.)

4. In the *Operator* drop-down list, select your operator number.

5. Click *Show Log*.

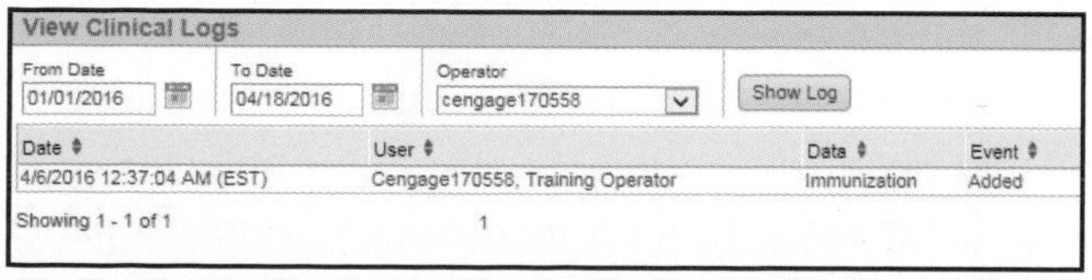

Figure 7-31 View Clinical Logs
Courtesy of Harris CareTracker PM and EMR

Tip Box

You can also click the immunization to view the operator, date, and time the last updates were made. Click the *Log* icon to view all activities associated with the immunization.

Print the Immunization Log. Label it "Activity 7-9" and place it in your assignment folder.

TABLE 7-9 Immunizations Activity Log

Entry	Description
Immunization Added	Displays when the immunization is added to the patient's medical record.
Immunization Accessed	Displays when immunization information is viewed.
Immunization Modified	Displays when information about the immunization is updated. However, this does not include updates to the status of the immunization.
Immunization Removed	Displays when the immunization is changed to an inactive status.

Note: You can filter the activity log by selecting a date range and an operator and then clicking *Show Log*.

PULLING UP AND RECORDING PATIENT EDUCATION

Learning Objective 4: Search for, customize, and provide patient education materials for patients.

The *Patient Education* application provides a comprehensive library of patient education material available through Krames StayWell that covers the most common conditions. You can search for education material using keywords, ICD-9 or CPT® codes, or search for material by navigating the tree structure. The content in this site is updated quarterly based on material received from Krames StayWell. You can also browse a list of favorite education materials via the *Favorites* tab. The material includes access to a database of health care advisories and clinical education handouts in different languages. You can give these materials to a patient based on the patient's condition and treatment options. The application enables searching through hundreds of education material to give a patient, save common material given out to patients as favorites, or link to other online sites with professionally written material. Education handouts given to a patient are recorded in the *Correspondence* and the *Progress Notes* sections of the patient's medical record.

ACTIVITY 7-10:   Access and Search for Patient Education

1. With patient Jane Morgan in context, click on the *Medical Record* module.

2. In the *Clinical Toolbar*, click the *Patient Education* icon.

3. If an encounter is in context, the *Patient Education* dialog box displays and defaults to the tab set in the *Patient Education Default* list in the *Set Chart Summary Defaults* dialog box. If an encounter is not in context, Harris CareTracker EMR displays the *Select Encounter* dialog box. Select the encounter you created for the patient in Chapter 6. This will launch the *Patient Education* dialog box.

4. By default, the *Search By* option is set to "Keywords." However, you can change the search option to CPT® ICD-9, or ICD-10 code if necessary. (Leave as is.)

5. By default, the age and gender criteria default to the information saved for the patient in context. However, you can change the age and gender selections if necessary. (Change the *Age* selection to "All.")

6. In the *Language* list, click the language of the education material you want. (Select "English.")

7. In the blank box above *Language* type in the keywords "Urinary Tract Infection."

8. Click *Search*.

9. Under *Search Results* scroll down and select "Urinary Tract Infections in Women." Click on the *Favorite* icon in the *Search Results* bar to save in your list of *Favorites*.

10. Now enter "High Blood Pressure" in the text box above *Language*.

11. Click *Search*.

12. Scroll down and select "Controlling High Blood Pressure". Click on the *Favorite* icon to save in your list of *Favorites*.

13. Print the handouts for "Urinary Tract Infections in Women" and "Controlling High Blood Pressure." To print the handouts:

    a. Click on the *Favorites* tab at the top of the *Patient Education* dialog box (Figure 7-32).

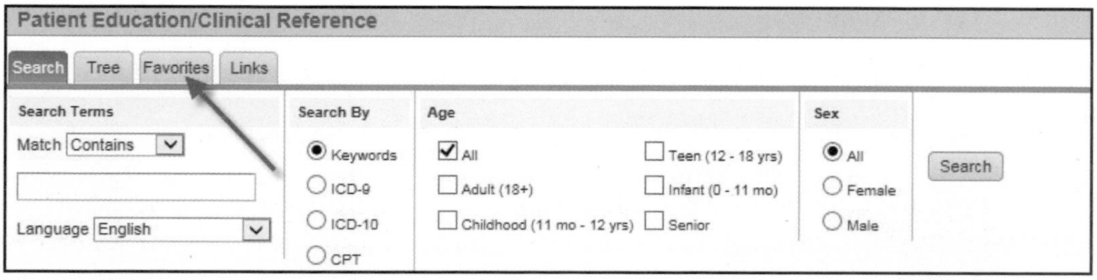

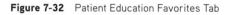

Figure 7-32   Patient Education Favorites Tab

    b. Select the required handout(s) from the *Favorites* list. The handout displays in the *Preview* section of the window.

    c. Click *Print* on the top right of the window to print the handout.

14. *(Optional)* To print multiple handouts from the *Search* tab:

    a. Select the checkboxes pertaining to the handouts you want to print.

    b. Click *Print Checked* located at the bottom of the *Search Results* pane.

Label the printed Patient Education Sheet(s) "Activity 7-10a and 7-10b" and place them in your assignment folder.

You can also search for handouts via the *Tree* tab (Figure 7-33) and via the *Favorites* tab. For more information on these alternative search methods, log in to *Help*, click on the *Contents* tab, and select *Searching for Handouts* (Go to *Medical Record Module > Patient Education > Searching for Handouts*).

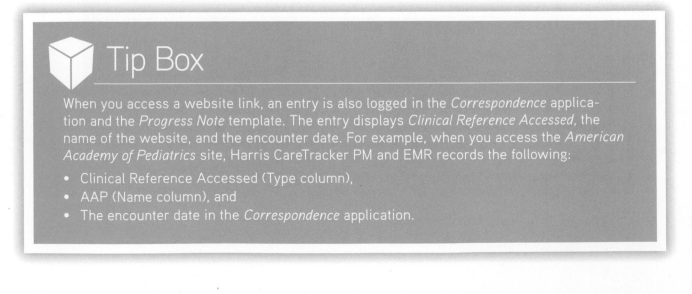

Figure 7-33 Patient Education Tabs

Advanced Features for Patient Education

The *Patient Education* application enables you to customize the content of patient education material based on your requirements. However, the changes you make are only valid for the current encounter and the customized handout cannot be saved as a favorite. If you print the customized handout, the *Patient Education Printed* entry, and a copy of the customized handout are recorded in the *Correspondence* application of the patient's medical record.

The *Patient Education* application enables you to search other online sites for professionally written material as well. Refer to instructions in *Help* for accessing websites for handouts.

Tip Box

When you access a website link, an entry is also logged in the *Correspondence* application and the *Progress Note* template. The entry displays *Clinical Reference Accessed*, the name of the website, and the encounter date. For example, when you access the *American Academy of Pediatrics* site, Harris CareTracker PM and EMR records the following:

- Clinical Reference Accessed (Type column),
- AAP (Name column), and
- The encounter date in the *Correspondence* application.

CREATING CLINICAL LETTERS

Learning Objective 5: Access the Correspondence application to add, filter, customize, and print patient correspondence.

The *Letters* application provides the ability to use letter templates to create letters for patients. You can include the company logo; patient information, such as progress note data; lab reports; and more, in the letter. You can utilize the editor that is similar to other desktop editors like MS Word® to format and edit each letter. After creating the letter, you can save, print, or attach the letter to a *ToDo*, mail, or fax.

FYI

If your practice would like to include a company-specific logo on any letters printed from the *Clinical Letter Editor*, you would complete the following steps to define and set up letter templates via the *Clinical Letter Editor* application:

- To access the *Clinical Letter Editor* application, click on the *Administration* module, select the *Clinical* tab, and then click on the *Clinical Letter Editor* link under the *Forms and Letters* heading.
- You can include the company logo in a letter by uploading the logo via the *Company Logo* application. To access the *Company Logo* application, click on the *Administration* module, and then select the *Setup* tab and *Company Logo* link.

ACTIVITY 7-11: Create Clinical Letters

1. Pull patient Jane Morgan into context, and then click the *Medical Record* module.

2. In the *Clinical Toolbar*, click the *Letters* icon.

3. If an encounter is in context, Harris CareTracker EMR displays the *Letter Manager* dialog box. (**Note:** If an encounter is not in context, Harris CareTracker EMR displays the *Select Encounter* dialog box. Select the encounter you created for the patient in Chapter 6. This will launch the *Letter Manager* dialog box.) To select the *Letter Template* you want to use ("NVFHA Consult Letter Copy"), use one of the following methods:

    a. If the letter is saved as a favorite, select the letter template from the *Letter* list.

    b. If the letter is not in the *Letter* list, click the *Manage Favorites* ☆ icon to search for the required letter.

       i. In the *Manage Letter Favorites* dialog box, select "NVFHA Consult Letter COPY" under *ClinicalNote* (Figure 7-34). The selected letter template will now appear in the *Letter Manager* dialog box.

4. The Harris CareTracker EMR *Letters* application pulls in the referring provider (Dr. Richard Shinaman) and information from the patient encounter, creating the *Consult Letter* to send to Dr. Shinaman (Figure 7-35).

5. In the bottom right corner of the screen, select *Print* to print a copy of the consult letter. (All letter actions are described in Table 7-10.)

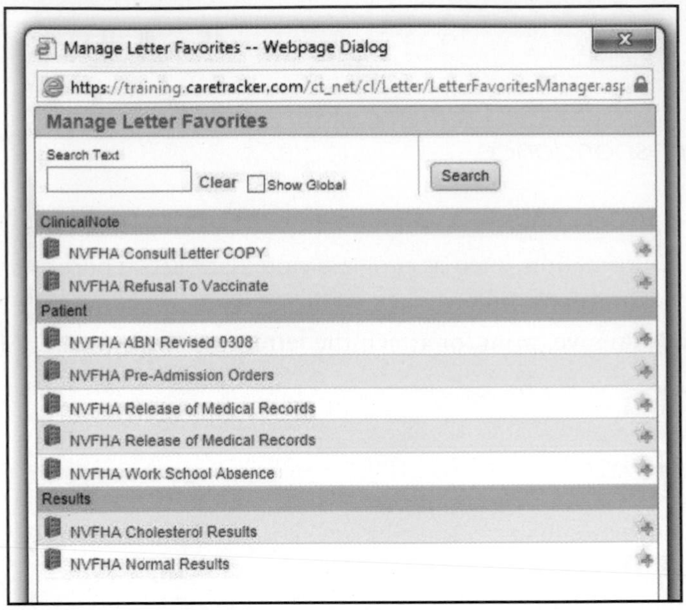

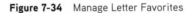

Figure 7-34 Manage Letter Favorites

Tip Box

To save a letter as a favorite and add it to the *Letter* list, click the *Add as Favorite* ⭐ icon to the right of the letter name in the *Manage Letter Favorites* dialog box.

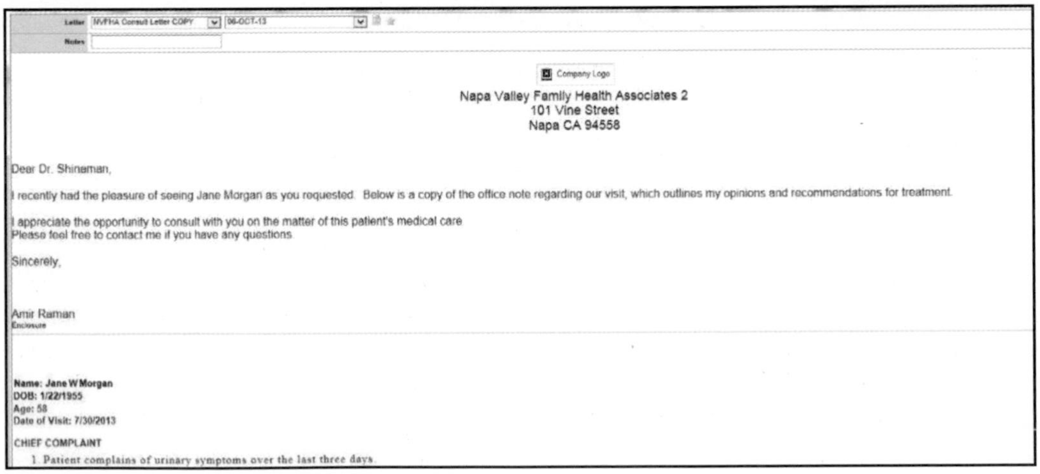

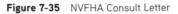

Figure 7-35 NVFHA Consult Letter

Label the printed consult letter "Activity 7-11" and place it in your assignment folder.

Tip Box

If printing a *Clinical Note* type letter, you must select the encounter. This allows you to generate a letter with information and progress note data from the encounter. If printing a *Results* letter type, you must select the specific result to include in the letter.

All letter actions are described in Table 7-10. When a letter is saved, printed, or attached to a *ToDo*, an entry is recorded in the clinical log.

TABLE 7-10 Letter Actions

Action	Description
Save	Click to save and print the letter at a later date. The letter is saved in the *Correspondence* application and displays the *Letter Generated* entry. The name of the letter displays under the *Name* column and notes display under the *Document* column of the *Correspondence* application.
Print	Click to print the letter. When a letter is printed, an entry is recorded with the date and time in the *Correspondence* application.
Msg Center	Point to the *Arrow* ▼ icon next to *Msg Center*, and click the required option to attach the letter as a PDF to a *ToDo* or fax or mail the letter.

Courtesy of Harris CareTracker PM and EMR

Access the Correspondence Application

The *Correspondence* application displays any correspondence your practice has had with the patient in context and with another physician regarding the patient. This includes items such as *ToDo*(s), e-mails, phone calls, letters pertaining to the patient, patient education material given to the patient, and more. This helps keep track of all communications associated with the patient in a central location. The *Correspondence* application is accessible from the following locations:

- *Name Bar* > *Corr* icon
- *Patient Info* icon on the *Name Bar* > *Documents* tab > *Correspondence* tab (Figure 7-36)
- *Home* module > *Practice* tab > *Unprinted Correspondence* link (*Front Office* section)
- *Financial* module > *Correspondence* tab
- *Medical Record* module > *Correspondence* pane

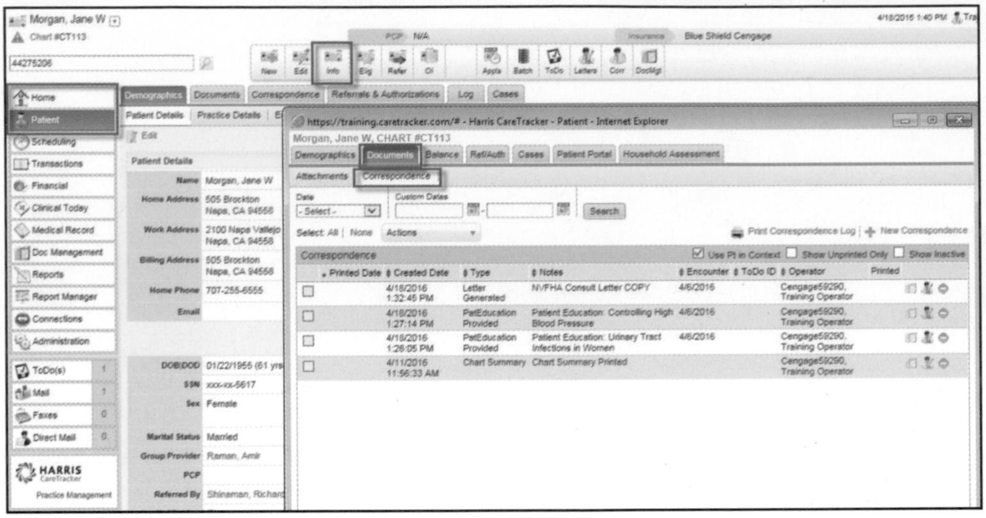

Courtesy of Harris CareTracker PM and EMR

Figure 7-36 Patient Info - Correspondence Tab

Add Patient Correspondence

The *Correspondence* application allows you to add any correspondence, including medical record disclosures associated with a patient. When recording a medical record disclosure, a dialog box displays to enter additional details such as date and information disclosed. Additionally, you can link a correspondence to a specific encounter or to a document uploaded to the patient's medical record.

ACTIVITY 7-12: Add a Patient Correspondence

Patient Jane Morgan requested that a copy of her medical records be mailed to her home address because she is considering relocating to Colorado and wants to have all her records in her possession. She has completed the required authorization form.

1. Pull patient Jane Morgan into context, and then click the *Medical Record* module.
2. In the *Patient Health History* pane, click *Correspondence.* Harris CareTracker EMR displays the *Correspondence* window.
3. Click + *New Correspondence* (Figure 7-37). Harris CareTracker EMR displays the *Add Correspondence* dialog box. The *Printed Date* box is grayed out, so no dates can be entered here.

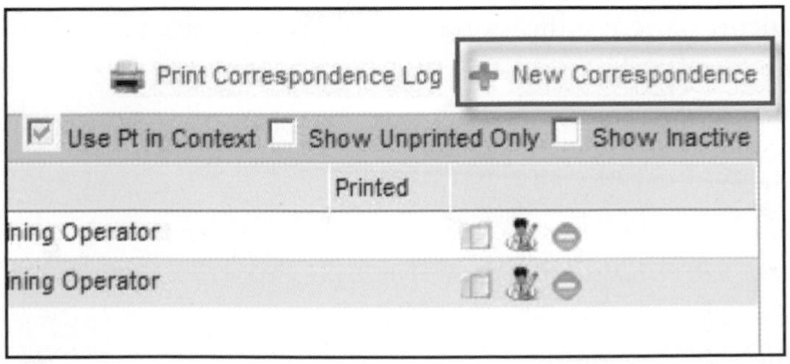

Courtesy of Harris CareTracker PM and EMR

Figure 7-37 Add New Correspondence

4. In the *Type* list, scroll down to "Medical Record Disclosure" and select it.

5. In the pop-up *Correspondence Type* dialog box, enter the following details (Figure 7-38):

   a. *Date of Disclosure*: Enter today's date

   b. *Operator Name*: Enter your operator number

   c. *Reported to*: Enter "Patient, Jane Morgan"

   d. *Recipient's Address*: Leave blank

   e. *Information Disclosed*: Enter "Medical Record"

   f. *Purpose of Disclosure*: Enter "Pt requested copy of medical record"

   g. Click *Save.*

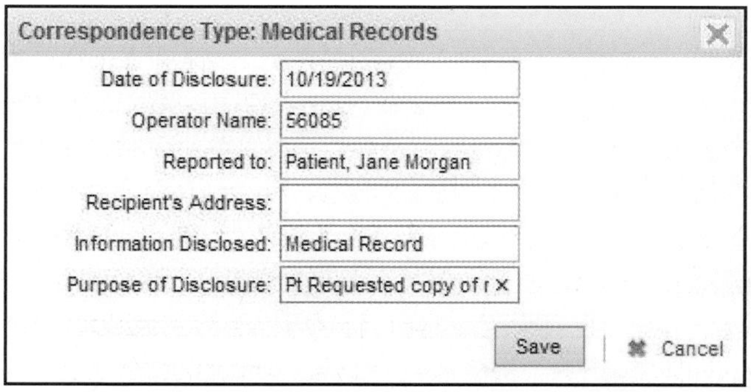

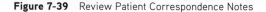

Figure 7-38 Correspondence Type – Medical Records

6. You will be taken back to the *Add Correspondence* dialog box. In the *Encounter ID* list, select the encounter to link to the correspondence. Use the last encounter you created for the patient.

7. In the *Document* list, you would click the attachment given to the patient. No document appears in the list, but your correspondence indicates having mailed a copy of the patient's medical record to her home address.

8. By default, *Active* is set to "Yes." (Leave as is.)

9. In the *Notes* box, you can enter additional comments about the patient correspondence. Verify that the information entered in the *Correspondence Type* dialog box appears here (Figure 7-39).

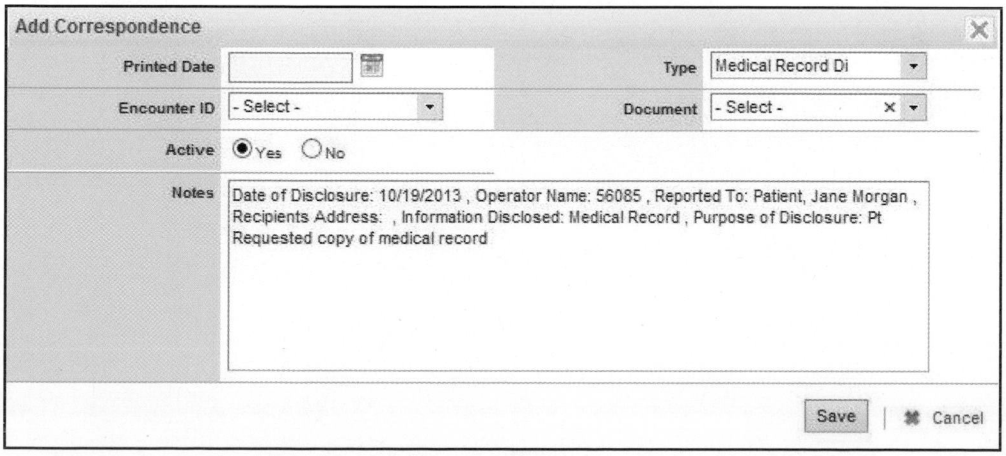

Figure 7-39 Review Patient Correspondence Notes

10. Click *Save*. The correspondence is saved in the *Correspondence* window (Figure 7-40).

Courtesy of Harris CareTracker PM and EMR

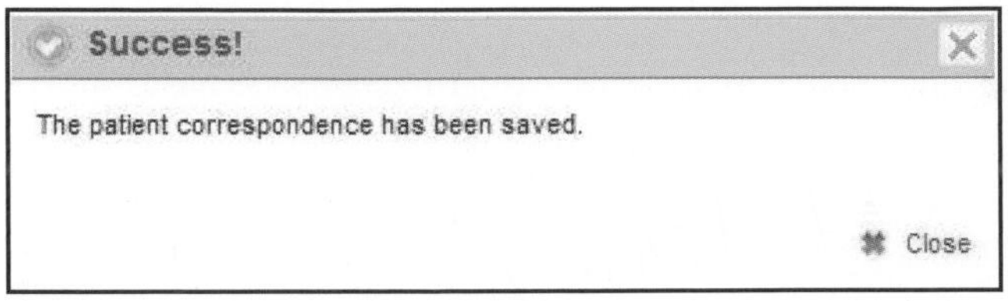

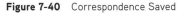

Figure 7-40 Correspondence Saved

Print a screenshot of the Patient Correspondence window. Label it "Activity 7-12" and place it in your assignment folder.

Table 7-11 describes the information that displays in the columns of the *Correspondence* window. You can click a column heading to sort the items on the window.

TABLE 7-11 Correspondence Columns

Column	Description
Printed Date	The original date the correspondence is printed or marked as printed. (**Note**: You can click the *Mark Printed* action in the *Correspondence* application to mark a correspondence as printed.)
Created Date	Displays the date the correspondence is created in MM/DD/YY, HH:MM:SS format.
Type	The correspondence type. For example, Patient Education Provided, Patient Portal, and Patient Visit Summary.
Notes	Displays notes entered in the *Note* field when manually entering the correspondence or creating a *ToDo* or *Fax*. Additionally, the columns display titles of patient education given to a patient or attached to a *ToDo*, names of letters created, approval status of amendment requests made via the *Patient Portal*, and more.
Encounter	Displays the encounter date associated with the correspondence.
ToDo ID	Displays the *ToDo* number associated with *ToDo*-type correspondence.
Operator	Displays the operator who created the correspondence.
Printed	Indicates if practice management letters are generated.
Documents	Allows viewing documents attached to the correspondence.
Letters	Allows viewing letters attached to the correspondence.
Activate/Deactivate	Allows activating and deactivating a correspondence.

Courtesy of Harris CareTracker PM and EMR

Work with Patient Correspondence

The *Correspondence* application allows you to view correspondences and any attachments. You can view any documents or letters attached to patient correspondences in the *Correspondence* window.

ACTIVITY 7-13:   View and Print Correspondence Attachments

1. With patient Jane Morgan in context, click the *Medical Record* module.

2. In the *Patient Health History* pane, click *Correspondence*. Harris CareTracker EMR displays the *Correspondence* window.

3. To view a letter, click the *Letters* icon on the right-hand side of your screen. For example, click the *Letters* icon next to "Patient Education: Controlling High Blood Pressure" to open the letter in a new window. It may take a few moments for the *Letter* to pull up. If the *Letters* icon is grayed out, you cannot view the correspondence in this tab. You can click the *Print* box in the lower-left-hand screen of the letter to print (Figure 7-41).

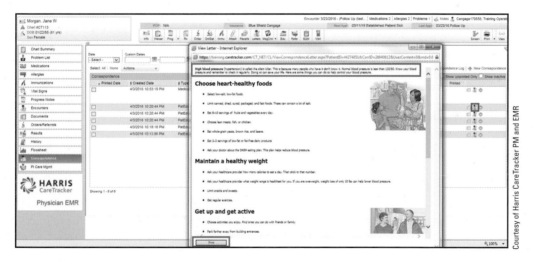

Figure 7-41   Print Patient Education Letter

4. Click *Print* to print the selected letter(s).

🖊 **Print the Patient Correspondence letter. Label it "Activity 7-13" and place it in your assignment folder.**

Activate and Deactivate Correspondence

You can set items as inactive in the *Correspondence* window. Inactive items display the *Set Active* 🔵 icon. You can also change the status of an inactive item to active.

ACTIVITY 7-14: Set an Item as Inactive or Active

1. With patient Jane Morgan in context, click the *Medical Record* module.

2. In the *Patient Health History* pane, click *Correspondence*. Harris CareTracker EMR displays the *Correspondence* window.

3. First, mark the "Patient Education: Controlling High Blood Pressure" document as inactive. Click the *Set Inactive* ⬯ icon pertaining to this correspondence and then click *OK* to confirm the change (Figure 7-42).

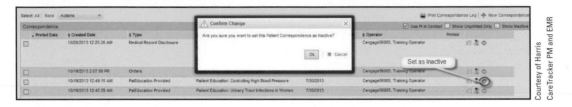

Figure 7-42 Set as Inactive Confirmation Box

4. Check the box in the upper-right-hand corner of your screen to "show inactive" (Figure 7-43).

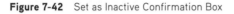

Figure 7-43 Show Inactive Box
Courtesy of Harris CareTracker PM and EMR

🖐 **Print the screen of the Inactive Patient Correspondence, label it "Activity 7-14a," and place it in your assignment folder.**

5. Now, mark the inactive document "Patient Education: Controlling High Blood Pressure" as active by clicking the *Set Active* ⬯ icon pertaining to the inactive correspondence. Click *OK* to confirm the change.

🖐 **Print the screen of the Activated Patient Correspondence, label it "Activity 7-14b," and place it in your assignment folder.**

Print the Correspondence Log

The *Correspondence Log* is a summary of all patient correspondences.

ACTIVITY 7-15: Print the Correspondence Log

1. Pull patient Jane Morgan into context, and then click the *Medical Record* module.

2. In the *Patient Health History* pane, click *Correspondence*. Harris CareTracker EMR displays the *Correspondence* window.

3. Click the *Print Correspondence Log* (Figure 7-44A) link at the top right of the screen. The application displays the log in a new window (Figure 7-45). (**Note:** If the log does not appear within a few seconds, follow the steps in the *Tip Box* below to access the log.)

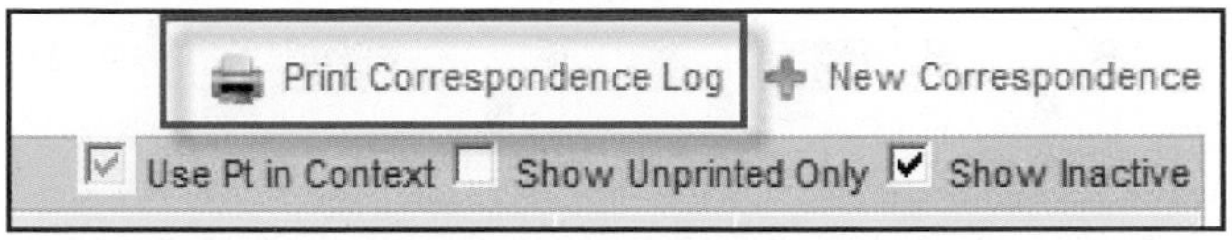

Figure 7-44A Print Correspondence Log

Courtesy of Harris CareTracker PM and EMR

Tip Box

Depending on the version of Internet Explorer you are working in, you may have some difficulty loading the *Correspondence Log*. If you are experiencing difficulty, you can try to troubleshoot using one of the two following methods:

1. Click back on the home screen, where you will see a message at the top of the screen indicating that Internet Explorer has blocked the correspondence file from downloading. Click on the message and select "Download file" from the drop-down menu (Figure 7-44B). The home page will reload.
   a. Go back into the patient's medical record, and in the *Correspondence* module click on the *Print Correspondence Log* link.
   b. A *Generating Report* window will pop up, telling you that the log is processing. (**Note:** If the correspondence log is taking too long to load, you can close out of the *Generating Report* window and the patient's medical record. Go back to the home screen and click the *Medical Record* module. Click the *Correspondence* tab and select the *Print Correspondence Log* link again. The correspondence log PDF should now load quickly.)

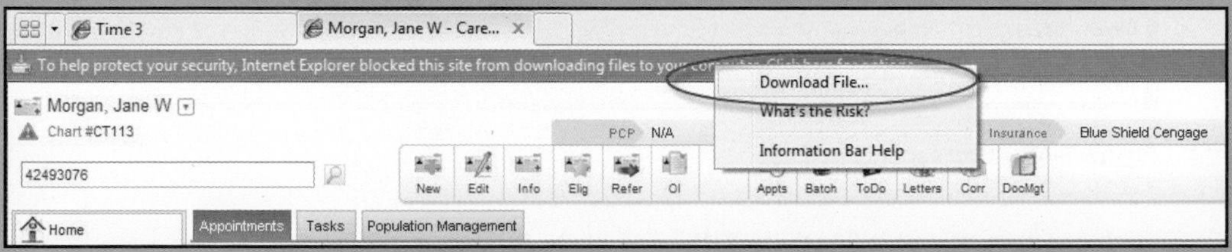

Courtesy of Harris CareTracker PM and EMR

Figure 7-44B Select Download File

2. Click back on the home screen, where you will see the PDF report on the lower part of your screen (Figure 7-44C). You will be asked if you want to *Open* or *Save* the PDF. Click *Open* and then *Print* by right-clicking your mouse in the screen and selecting *Print* from the *Menu*.

(*Continues*)

(Continued)

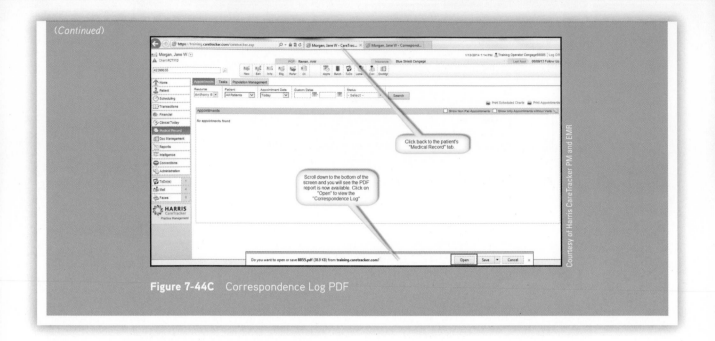

Figure 7-44C Correspondence Log PDF

| Patient Name: | Jane W Morgan | | Print Date: 10/20/2013 |

Account #: 42399638

Napa Valley Family Health Associates2-cengage56085

Type: Medical Record Disclosure Encounter:
Letter: No Letter   Attachment: No Attachment
Date: 12:25:20 am
Notes:
Date of Disclosure: 10/18/2013 , Operator Name: 56086 , Reported To: Patient, Jane Morgan , Recipients Address: , Information Disclosed: Medical Record , Purpose of Disclosure: Pt Requested copy of medical record

Type: Orders   Encounter: 55457779
Letter: No Letter   Attachment: No Attachment
Date: 2:07:56 pm
Notes:
Resend letter regarding mammogram

Type: PatEducation Provided Encounter: 55457779
Letter: No Letter   Attachment: No Attachment
Date: 2:02:07 pm
Notes:

Type: PatEducation Provided Encounter: 55457779
Letter: No Letter   Attachment: No Attachment
Date: 10/19/2013 12:45:29 am
Notes:
Patient Education: Urinary Tract Infections in Women

Figure 7-45 Correspondence Log

Print the Correspondence Log. Label it "Activity 7-15" and place it in your assignment folder.

CREATING REFERRALS

Learning Objective 6: Create outgoing and incoming patient referrals.

The *Referrals and Authorizations* application enables providers to create inbound and outbound referrals and associated authorizations directly via the patient's medical record. You can provide data about the patient's condition and needs, referring and referred-to provider details, treatment authorization data, and referral dates and ranges. Referrals enable you to track patient compliance with the referral instructions, eliminating the need for paperwork.

Tip Box

You can set the *Referrals and Authorizations* application to default to a referral type in the *Referral Default* field (Referral-Incoming, Referral-Outgoing, or Referral-Outgoing New) when creating a batch.

ADMINISTRATIVE SPOTLIGHT

Referrals and authorizations in "pending" status do not display in the *Authorization* list of the *Additional Claim Information* dialog box. This prevents you from linking an incomplete referral or authorization to a claim.

All referrals added via the *Referrals and Authorizations* application display in the patient medical record as well as the *Ref/Auth* application of the *Patient* module, and vice versa.

Access the Referrals and Authorizations Application

There are several ways to access the *Referrals and Authorizations* application:

- Click the *Patient* module and then click the *Referrals & Authorizations* tab.
- Click the *Refer* icon on the *Name Bar*.
- Click the *Medical Record* module and then click the *Refer* icon on the *Clinical Toolbar*.

Create Outgoing Referrals

Outgoing referrals are requests made by the physician to specialists, ancillary providers, or clinics. Most primary care physicians (PCPs) create outgoing referrals; however, many specialists refer out for ancillary services and/or for consults with other specialties.

Tip Box

If a PCP sends a patient to a dermatologist to treat a psoriasis condition, the PCP gives the patient a referral, which is referred to as the outgoing referral.
(**Note:** The authorization number, provider information, from and to dates, and number of authorized visits are mandatory information required to link a referral to a charge.)

ACTIVITY 7-16:   Create an Outgoing Referral

1. To access the *Chart Summary* for patient Christina Stoned, with the patient in context, click on the *Medical Record* module. Christina had been seen by Dr. Brockton on May 14, 2013, and complained of hip and back pain. She was to follow up with Dr. Brockton in one month. However, Christina called the office on June 5, 2013, complaining that the pain had increased and requested a referral to an orthopedic specialist.

2. In the *Clinical Toolbar*, click the *Referrals* 🔳 icon. A *Select Encounter* dialog box will pop up. Select the encounter dated May 14, 2013. Harris CareTracker EMR displays the *Referrals and Authorizations* dialog box.

3. If the default selection is set to *Outgoing Referral* in your batch, leave as is. If not, change the field to *Outgoing Referral* for this activity.

4. If the *Default Referral to Billing Provider* list is set to "Yes" in your batch, then the *Referral From* list defaults to the billing provider set in the batch. However, you can select a different provider if needed. Confirm that Dr. Brockton is listed as the referring provider.

5. From the *Referral To* list, select the provider to whom you want to refer the patient. Click the *Search* 🔍 icon to search for a provider.

   a. In the *Provider Search* dialog box, enter the *Name* and *State* information for Dr. Robert Rovner in San Ramon, California. Click *Search*.

   b. Click on Robert Rovner's name under the *Provider Name* heading and Harris CareTracker EMR will pull his information into the referral dialog box.

📦 Tip Box

The *Referral To* list displays the providers in your *Refer Provider To* quick pick list. The *Referral From* list displays the providers in your *Refer Provider From* quick pick list. The quick pick list is set up via the *Quick Picks* application. The *Quick Picks* application is accessible by clicking the *Administration* module, *Setup* tab, and then clicking the *Quick Picks* link under the *Financial* section.

---

6. If the provider you are referring to is within the same practice as the referring from provider (internal), Harris CareTracker EMR automatically populates the information in the *Group* and *Specialty* lists. If the provider is outside the practice (external), you must select the provider's group and specialty. (Select "Orthopaedic Surgery" in the *Specialty* field.)

7. By default, the *Transition of Care* list is set to "Yes" to indicate that the outgoing referral is a transition of care to another provider. However, you can change the option if necessary. (Select "No.")

8. Change the *Auth. Date* to June 5, 2013 (the date Christina called, requesting a referral).

9. *(Optional – Authorization)* Christina's insurance does not require an authorization.

FYI

Authorizations:

- If you need to enter an authorization for the referral in the *Authorization* section:
  - Enter the authorization date in the *Auth. Date* box or click the *Calendar* 📅 icon to select the date from the calendar.
- Enter the authorization number in the *Authorization #* box. Do not use symbols.

📦 Tip Box

If you need to send the referral number instead of an authorization number, select *Referral #* as the qualifier (Figure 7-46). The authorization number prints in box 23 of the Health Care Financing Administration (HCFA) claim form.

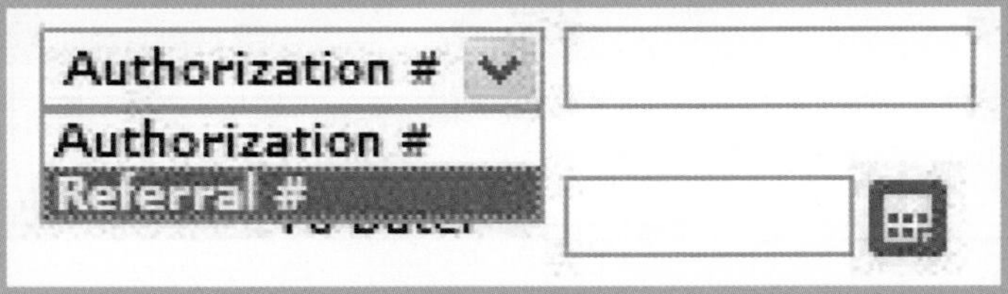

Figure 7-46   Referral #

Courtesy of Harris CareTracker PM and EMR

- Enter the dates for which the authorization is valid in the *From Date* and *To Date* boxes.
- Select the authorization type:
  - *Visits*: Authorizes a set number of visits. When a charge for a visit is entered into the system, Harris CareTracker EMR automatically deducts a visit from the remaining visits that are authorized.
  - *Amount*: Authorizes a set monetary amount. Harris CareTracker EMR does not calculate and deduct a dollar amount when charges are saved for the patient.
  - *Hours*: Authorizes a set number of hours. Harris CareTracker EMR does not calculate and deduct the time when charges are saved for the patient.
- Enter the authorized amount in the *Visits, Amount,* or *Hours* box. (The box displayed is linked to the authorization type selected.) Example: Six (6) *Visits* authorized (such as in a Physical Therapy *Authorization*).
  - *(Optional)* Click *+ Notes* to enter comments related to the authorization.

10. Click *Save & Print* (Figure 7-47). Harris CareTracker EMR saves the referral (Figure 7-48). (**Note:** Once you have saved the referral, you may have to close out of the *Referrals and Authorizations* dialog box to see the *Referral Print* screen.)

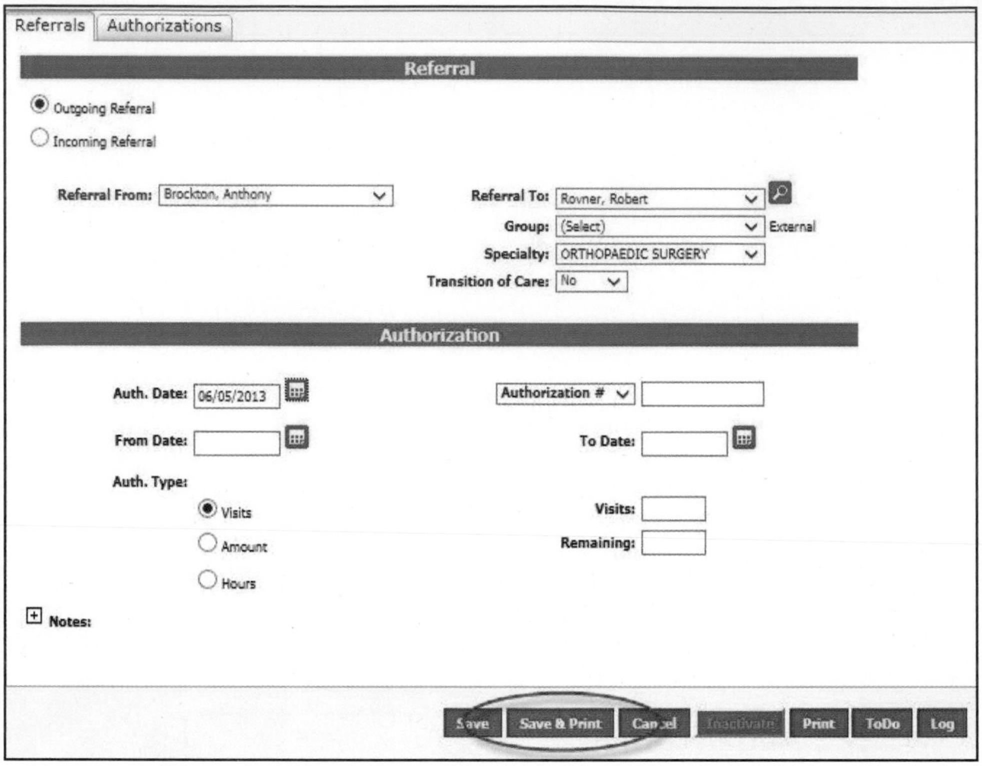

Figure 7-47 Referral to Dr. Rovner

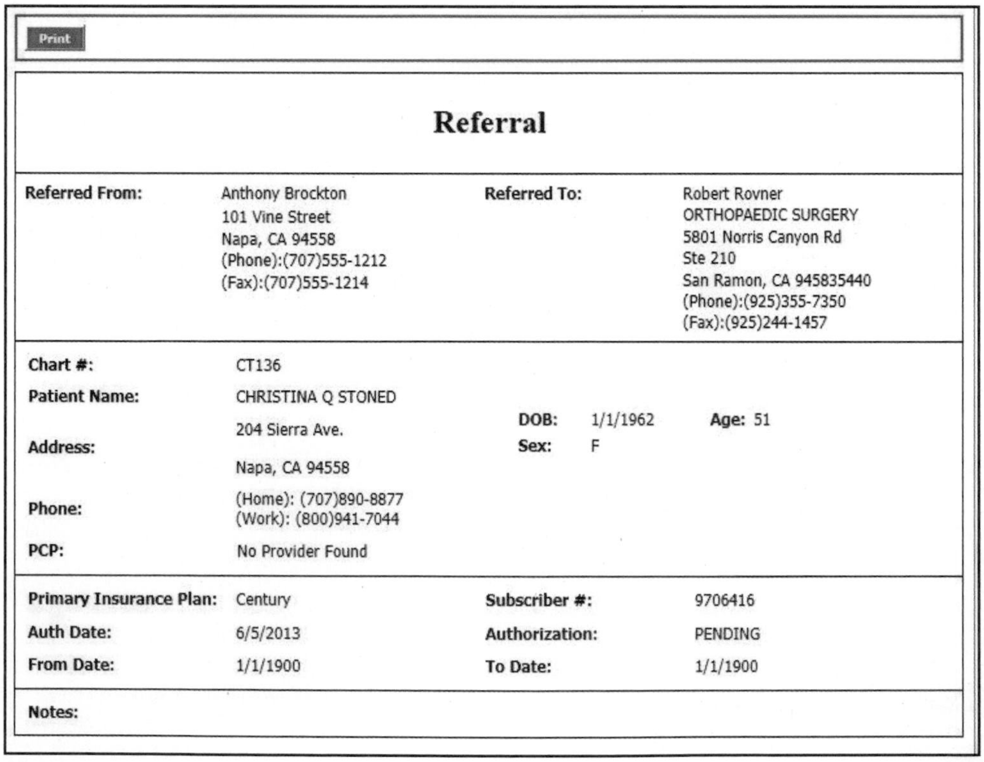

Print

Referral

Referred From:	Anthony Brockton 101 Vine Street Napa, CA 94558 (Phone):(707)555-1212 (Fax):(707)555-1214	**Referred To:**	Robert Rovner ORTHOPAEDIC SURGERY 5801 Norris Canyon Rd Ste 210 San Ramon, CA 945835440 (Phone):(925)355-7350 (Fax):(925)244-1457
Chart #:	CT136		
Patient Name:	CHRISTINA Q STONED		
Address:	204 Sierra Ave. Napa, CA 94558	**DOB:** 1/1/1962 **Sex:** F	**Age:** 51
Phone:	(Home): (707)890-8877 (Work): (800)941-7044		
PCP:	No Provider Found		
Primary Insurance Plan:	Century	**Subscriber #:**	9706416
Auth Date:	6/5/2013	**Authorization:**	PENDING
From Date:	1/1/1900	**To Date:**	1/1/1900
Notes:			

Figure 7-48 Referral Form for Christina Stoned

Print the Outgoing Referral by clicking on the Print button, or by right-clicking your mouse and selecting Print from the menu. Label it "Activity 7-16" and place it in your assignment folder.

Create Incoming Referrals

Incoming referrals are generally received by specialty physicians and must be processed during check-in or on a pre-visit basis. The referral is necessary for the specialty provider to receive appropriate payment.

> **Tip Box**
>
> If a women's health care specialist receives a referral from an outside practice to treat a patient for polycystic ovarian syndrome, the referral is referred to as an incoming referral.

Prior to creating incoming *Referrals*, you must set up your providers in the "Refer Provider To" list via the *Quick Picks* link. In previous chapters you learned how to create *Quick Picks*. Follow the steps in Activity 7-17 to add your providers to the *Quick Picks* list.

ACTIVITY 7-17: Add Your Providers to the Quick Picks List

1. Click on the *Administration* module > *Setup* tab > *Financial* header > *Quick Picks* link.
2. In the *Screen Type* drop-down, scroll down and select *Refer Provider To*.
3. Your screen will display "There are no quick picks."
4. Click the *Search* icon and enter the providers of NVFHA (Rebecca Ayerick, Anthony Brockton, Gabriella Torres, and Amir Raman). Enter the provider's last name and state (California) to narrow your search (Figure 7-49). Click *Search*.

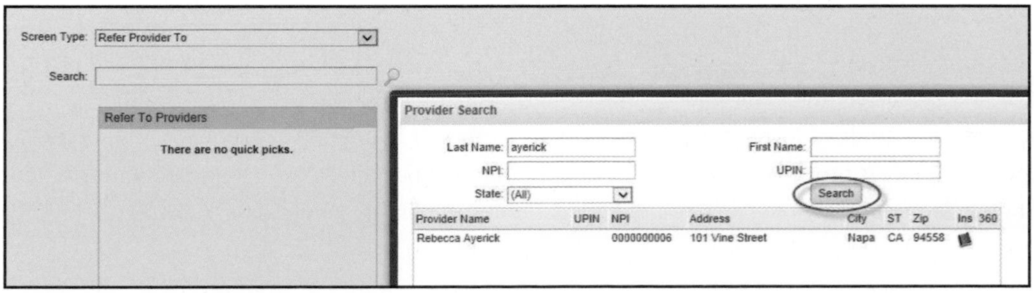

Courtesy of Harris CareTracker PM and EMR

Figure 7-49 Quick Pick – Refer Providers To

5. Click on each NVFHA provider's name and the provider will be added to your "Refer Provider To" *Quick Pick* list.
6. Click *Close* to exit out of the *Success* box after each provider has been added. When you have completed each entry, your screen should look like Figure 7-50.

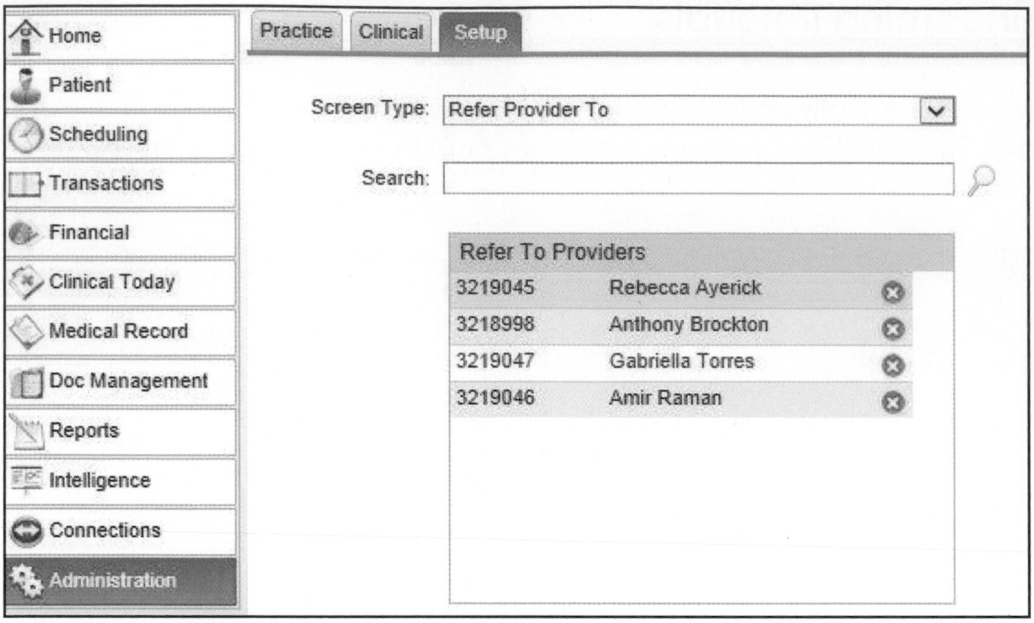

Courtesy of Harris CareTracker PM and EMR

Figure 7-50 Refer Provider To Quick Pick List

Now that your referring provider *Quick Picks* have been set up, you will be able to create an incoming referral (Activity 7-18).

ACTIVITY 7-18: Create an Incoming Referral

1. Pull patient James Smith into context and then click on the *Medical Record* module. Mr. Smith was referred to Dr. Ayerick of NVFHA as his new PCP by orthopaedic specialist Dr. David Dodgin.

2. In the *Clinical Toolbar*, click the *Referrals* 🔖 icon. The *Referral and Authorization* dialog box displays. If the patient has an encounter in the system, you will be taken directly to the *Referrals* dialog box. If there is no previous encounter for the patient, you will be prompted to select (or create) an encounter. Select the most recent encounter for the patient. If the patient does not have a previous encounter listed, select the *Create a New Encounter* link and enter the following information in the *Create a New Encounter* dialog box:

   a. *Type*: Select "Other"

   b. *Service Date*: Enter the date of the appointment you scheduled for Mr. Smith in Chapter 4.

   c. *Responsible Provider*: Select "Dr. Ayerick"

   d. *Patient Case*: Leave as "Default"

 e. *Location*: Leave as "NVFA"

 f. *Transition of Care*: Leave as "No"

 g. Click *Ok*.

3. In the *Referrals and Authorizations* dialog box, select *Incoming Referral* if not already selected (Figure 7-51). (The default selection for this field is set in your batch.)

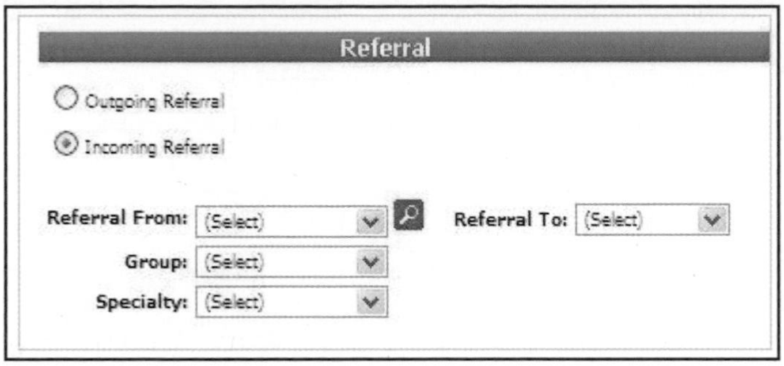

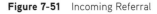

Referral

 ○ Outgoing Referral

 ◉ Incoming Referral

 Referral From: (Select)   🔍   **Referral To:** (Select)

   Group: (Select)

  Specialty: (Select)

Courtesy of Harris CareTracker PM and EMR

Figure 7-51   Incoming Referral

4. Click *New*. Harris CareTracker PM and EMR displays the incoming referral fields. (**Note:** If the patient did not have a previous encounter, the *New* button will not display until you save this incoming referral, allowing you to create another. Skip this instruction and continue with the rest of the activity if the *New* button is not displayed.)

5. In the *Referral From* list, select the provider referring the patient. (Select "David Dodgin.")

 a. Alternatively, click the *Search* 🔍 icon to search for a provider. If you use the search feature to select a provider, Harris CareTracker EMR automatically adds the provider to the *Active Patient Providers* section in the *Other* application of the *Patient* module.

6. In the *Specialty* field, select "Orthopaedic Surgery" from the drop-down list.

7. The *Referral To* list defaults to the billing provider set in your batch (if the batch setting of *Default Referral* to Billing provider is listed as "Yes"), but you can select a different provider if needed. (Select "Dr. Ayerick.")

8. No authorization is required; however, change the date to your encounter date (the first appointment date the patient has/had with Dr. Ayerick) in the *Auth. Date* field.

9. *(Optional)* If you need to enter an authorization for the referral, follow the instructions noted in the *Outgoing Referral* "FYI" box in Activity 7-16.

10. Click *+ Notes* to enter comments related to the authorization. Enter notes: "James Smith is a patient of Dr. Dodgin and has recently moved to Napa and would like to establish with Dr. Ayerick as his PCP" (Figure 7-52).

11. Click *Save & Print*. Harris CareTracker EMR saves the referral and the *Print* dialog box will appear (Figure 7-53). (**Note:** You may need to close out of the *Referrals and Authorizations* dialog box to see the *Referral Print* box.)

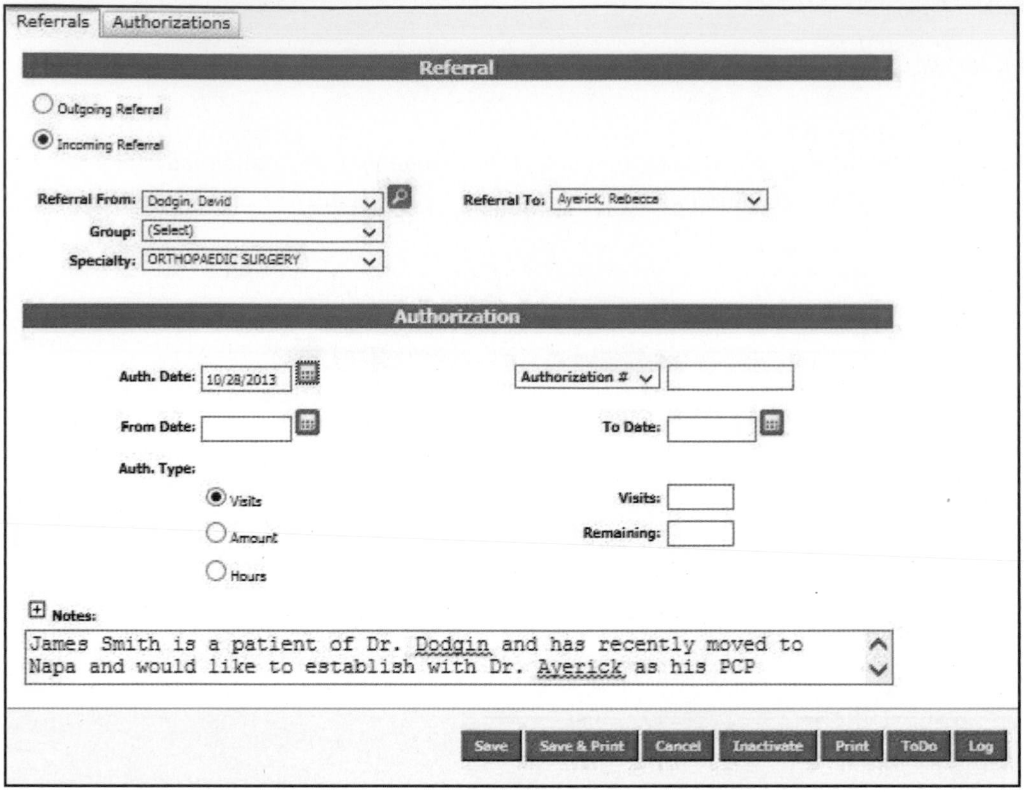

Figure 7-52   Incoming Referral for James Smith

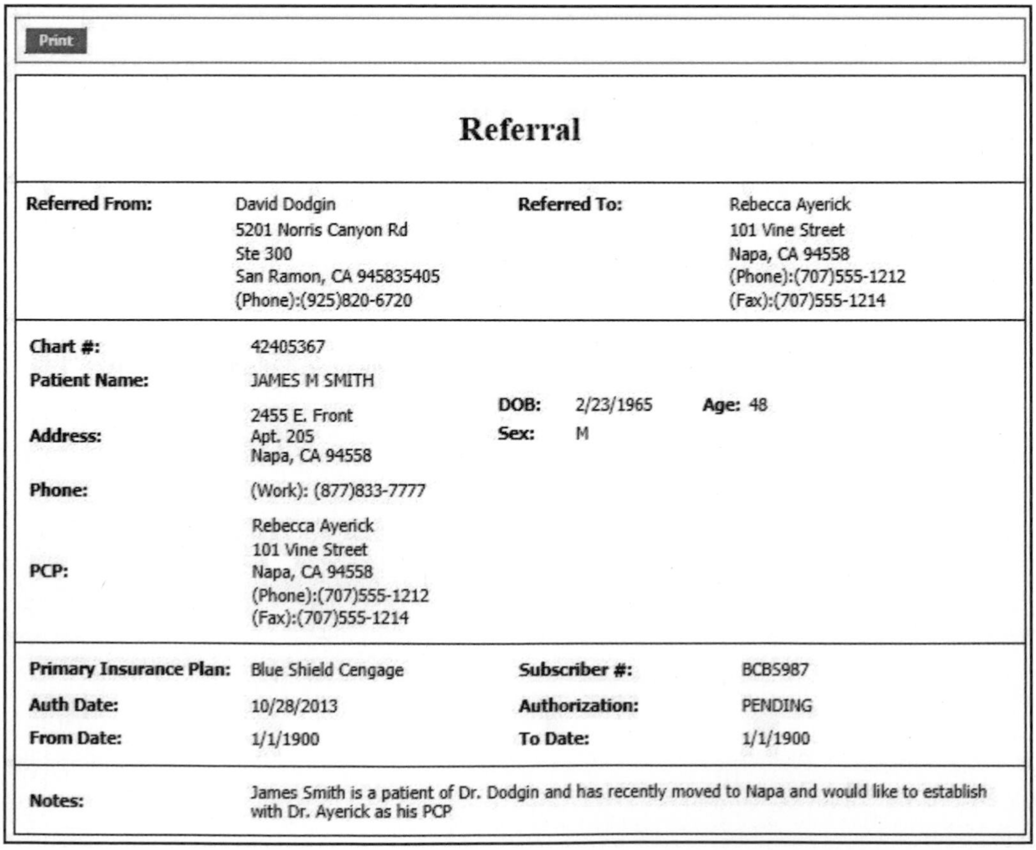

Figure 7-53   Incoming Referral Print Box

FYI

Alternatively, you can send the referral created in a *ToDo* by clicking the *Message Center* icon in the *Clinical Toolbar* and selecting *New ToDo* from the drop-down menu. Harris CareTracker EMR displays the *New ToDo* dialog box, enabling you to enter the required information and click *OK*. By default, the *Type* list displays "EHR." Change the selection in the *Reason* list to "Referral-Follow Up" in the *ToDo* dialog box. Print the *ToDo* by clicking *Print*.

Print the Incoming Referral by clicking the Print button in the Referral Print dialog box, or by right-clicking your mouse and selecting Print from the menu. Label it "Activity 7-18" and place it in your assignment folder.

You can generate a report in Harris CareTracker PM and EMR to help manage patient referrals and authorizations. For more information on generating referral authorization reports, see *Reports* module > *Patient Reports* > *Referral Authorizations Report* in the *Help* system.

Now that you have completed the tasks assigned, review Jane Morgan's *Progress Note* for the encounter you created in Chapter 6. Scroll down to the bottom and confirm that all orders, immunizations, referrals, and educational materials ordered in the A&P have been completed (Figure 7-54). You note that the patient is to return in 10 days for a follow-up UA and blood pressure check.

ASSESSMENT AND PLAN
HYPERTENSION
URINARY TRACT INFECTION
Stat lab test - "Urinalysis dipstick panel by Automated test strip"
Send Urine out for lab test "Urinalysis microscopic panel [#volume] in urine by automated count"
Give patient educational handouts for UTI and Hypertension
Bactrim DS Oral Tabs (800-160 mg), Sig 1 tab bid for 5 days, No refills
Patient to return in 10 days for a Follow/Up UA and BP check
Set patient up for a referral with a urologist
PREVENTION GOALS:
Patient to have her first Hepatitis B shot today
Set patient up for a mammogram
Dysuria (788.1, R30.0)

Orders Written Today:
Patient information entered into a reminder system with a target due date for the next mammogram (RAD)
Urinalysis dipstick panel in Urine by Automated test strip
Urinalysis microscopic panel [#/volume] in Urine by Automated count

Prescriptions Written Today:
Bactrim DS Oral Tablet 800-160 MG
Take 1 tablet twice a day for 5 day(s)
Refills: No Refills
Rx quantity: 10

Immunizations Given Today:
Hep B, adult

Patient Education Given Today:
Patient Education Provided: (Controlling High Blood Pressure),02/13/14 5:05 PM EST,
Patient Education Provided: (Urinary Tract Infections in Women),02/13/14 5:05 PM EST

Courtesy of Harris CareTracker PM and EMR

Figure 7-54 Completed A&P for Jane Morgan

Schedule Follow-Up Appointment for Jane Morgan

Make a follow-up appointment for Jane Morgan with Dr. Raman for 10 days from her original encounter (Figure 7-55). (Refer to Chapter 4, Activity 4-1, if you need to review the instructions for making an appointment.)

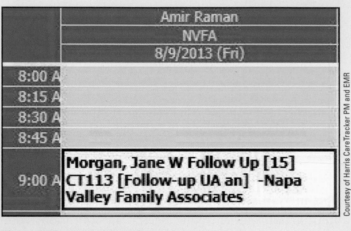

Figure 7-55   Jane Morgan Follow-Up Appointment

COMPLETING A VISIT FOR BILLING PURPOSES

Learning Objective 7: View and resolve open encounters and unsigned notes by completing the visit and signing the Progress Note.

In Chapter 6 you completed much of the patient work-up to the point of completing and printing the progress note. In order for a patient visit to be billable, any open encounters must be resolved and the visit must be completed and the note signed. The provider is the person who is responsible for signing the progress note; however, to enhance your understanding of workflows in the EMR, you will be completing the visit, resolving open encounters, and electronically signing the note.

Completing a Visit

To generate claims, charges must be captured for the patient's appointment. The *Visit* application allows you to capture charges and enter procedure, NDC, and diagnosis codes for a patient's appointment.

Visits can be entered into Harris CareTracker PM and EMR via several applications. Access the *Visits* application by one of the following methods:

- Left-click on a patient's appointment in the *Book* application and select *Visit* from the pop-up mini-menu.
- Pull a patient into context, click the *Appts* button in the *Name Bar,* pull the appointment into context, and select *Visit* from the *Actions* menu.
- Click the *Appointments* link under the *Appointments* section of the *Dashboard* tab in the *Home* module, pull the patient appointment into context, and then select *Visit* from the *Actions* menu.

Tip Box

If a patient is flagged as VIP in the *Demographic* application of the *Patient* module, the patient name displays as **VIP** in the appointment list unless you have the VIP overrides assigned to your profile. The overrides include *VIP Patient Access Break Glass* or *VIP Patient Access*. The VIP status is set in the *Demographic* application of the *Patient* module and overrides in the *Operators & Roles* application of the *Administration* module.

- Click the *Visits* link from the *Actions* drop-down list for a patient listed in the *Appointments* application of the *Clinical Today* module.
- Click the *Visit* icon on the *Clinical Toolbar* within the *Medical Record* module.

The *Visit* window contains a number of applications, but to save a visit you only need to enter the procedure and diagnosis code(s). Please note that a visit can only be edited prior to becoming a charge. For our first *Visit* activity, refer to patient Christina Stoned's appointment on May 14, 2013, with Dr. Brockton. Access the *Assessment* and *Plan* tabs in the *Progress Note* (Figure 7-56), and capture the *Visit*.

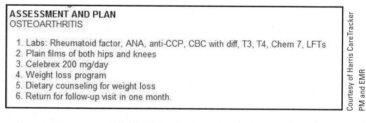

ASSESSMENT AND PLAN
OSTEOARTHRITIS

1. Labs: Rheumatoid factor, ANA, anti-CCP, CBC with diff, T3, T4, Chem 7, LFTs
2. Plain films of both hips and knees
3. Celebrex 200 mg/day
4. Weight loss program
5. Dietary counseling for weight loss
6. Return for follow-up visit in one month.

Courtesy of Harris CareTracker PM and EMR

Figure 7-56 Christina Stoned A&P

ACTIVITY 7-19: Capture a Visit

1. Click the *Scheduling* module. Harris CareTracker PM and EMR opens the *Book* application by default.

2. Move the schedule to display the date of service for which you want to confirm an appointment. This can be done by manually entering in the date in the *Date* box, by clicking the *Calendar* 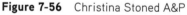 icon, or by selecting a time period from the *Move* list. (Enter "May 14, 2013" in the *Date* box.) You will need to set the *Resource* drop-down to "All Resources" for the full schedule and all providers to display. Click *Go*.

3. Left-click the appointment for which you want to enter visit information and select *Visit* from the mini-menu. (Select Christina Stoned's appointment.) The application displays the *Visit* window (Figure 7-57). When you first bring up the *Visit* window it automatically displays the procedures section (*Procedures* tab located at the top of the window)

4. The *Procedures* screen contains a list of procedure codes that mirror the CPT® codes on the encounter form. Verify that the checkboxes next to each code associated with the patient's appointment are selected: codes 99213, 73565, 73520, and 36415. (**Note:** If no *Visit* had yet been entered for the patient,

the encounter form would display with no checkboxes next to procedures or diagnoses. If you see the code you want to select for the *Visit*, you can select the checkbox next to the code. Alternatively, you could enter either a code or key term in the *Procedure Search* box to locate the desired code.)

Source: Current Procedural Terminology © 2013 American Medical Association.

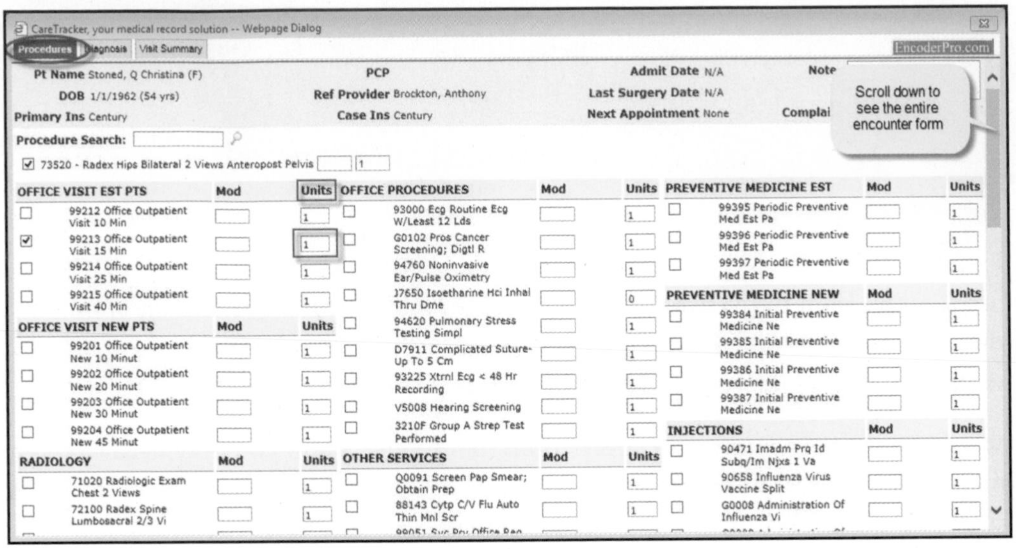

Courtesy of Harris CareTracker PM and EMR

Figure 7-57 Christina Stoned Visit Window

FYI

If you need to search for a CPT® code:

- Enter a partial code, complete code, or a keyword in the *Procedure Search* field, and then click the *Search* icon. The application opens the *Procedure Search* window.
- *(Optional)* To search for an NDC Code, select *NDC Code* from the *Search Type* list and then click *Search*.
- Click on the desired procedure to select it. The codes selected from the search are added to the patient's *Visit* window and there is no limit to the number of codes you can select.

5. Enter any modifiers in the *Mod* field next to each selected procedure code, if applicable. (No modifier is required.)
6. If needed, enter the number of units in the *Units* field for each selected procedure code. (Number of units is "1" per CPT® code for this activity [as noted in Figure 7-57].)
7. Click the *Diagnosis* tab in the *Visit* window. The application displays the *Diagnosis* application.
8. The *Diagnosis* screen displays a list of codes that mirror the ICD codes on the encounter form. Because this visit took place prior to the implementation date of October 1, 2015 for ICD-10 codes, you will only be able to select ICD-9 codes. ICD-10 codes displaying on the *Diagnosis* tab will be grayed out. Select the checkbox next to each code associated with the patient's appointment. (Select ICD-9 code 715.09 as in Figure 7-58.)

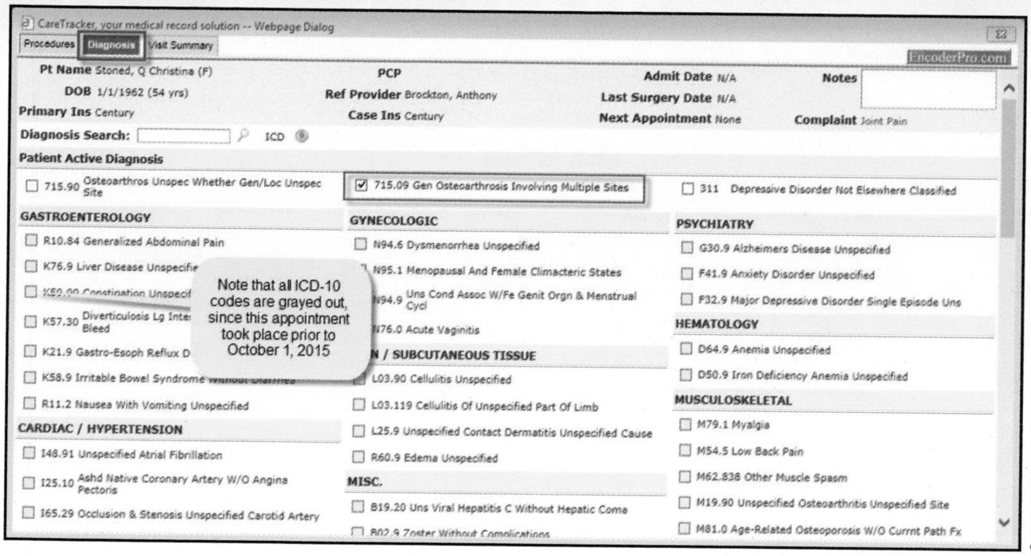

Courtesy of Harris CareTracker PM and EMR

Figure 7-58 Christina Stoned Diagnosis Codes

FYI

If you need to search for a diagnosis code:

- Enter a partial code, a complete code, or a keyword in the *Diagnosis Search* field, and then click the *Search* icon. The application opens the *Diagnosis Search* window.
- Click on the desired ICD-9/ICD-10 code to select it. The codes selected from the search are added to the patient's *Visit* window.

9. Click the *Visit Summary* tab in the top left corner of the *Visit* window. Harris CareTracker PM displays a summary of the visit information.
10. To check out the patient directly from the *Visit* application, select the *Check out Patient?* checkbox (Figure 7-59) at the bottom of the screen.
11. Review the screen (Figure 7-59) and verify the accuracy of the information including the *Location, Place of Service (POS), Referring Provider, Insurance, Billing,* and *Servicing Provider*.
12. (If applicable) To link the visit to a case you would select a case from the *Case* list. (There is no *Case* number associated with this visit.)
13. Select an authorization number from the *Authorization* list, if applicable (not applicable in this activity).
14. From the *Billing Type* list, select the billing type "Professional" at the bottom of the *Visit* screen (Figure 7-60).
15. *(Optional)* Click *EncoderPro.com* to obtain coding information from *EncoderPro*. This information can be used as a guide to correct the visit information.

Courtesy of Harris CareTracker PM and EMR

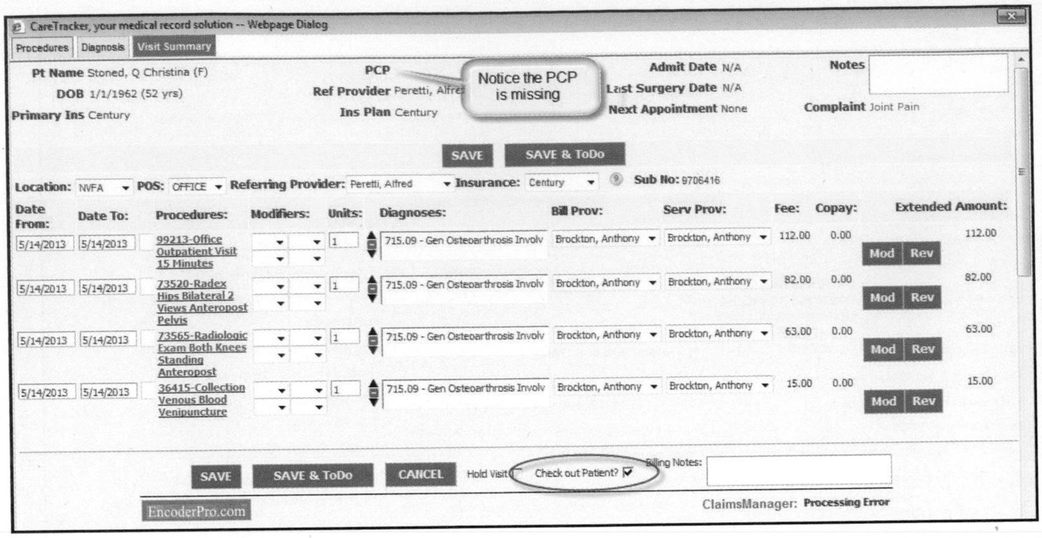

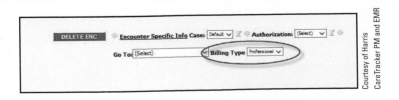

Figure 7-59 Christina Stoned Visit – Summary Window

Tip Box

The referring provider is pulled from the *Authorization*. If there is no authorization, the referring provider is pulled from the patient's demographic record and the "referred by" field. If there is no referring provider selected in the demographic, the referring provider is pulled from the batch (if the *Default Referral Provider* is set to "Yes" in the batch).

Tip Box

You can also create a new case by clicking the *Add* icon next to the *Case* list. If the visit is linked to a case and you need to enter additional billing information for the case, such as disability dates, authorizations, admission dates, and so on, click the *Edit* icon next to the *Case* list.

Courtesy of Harris CareTracker PM and EMR

Figure 7-60 Billing Type - Professional

> ## 📦 Tip Box
>
> If "Institutional" is selected as the *Billing Type*, the application will automatically prompt you to select a *Revenue Code*.

16. *(FYI Only)* If **Real Time Adjudication (RTA)** is available for the payer, click *RTA* to receive preliminary payment information. RTA refers to the immediate and complete adjudication of a health care claim upon receipt by the payer from a provider. **Adjudication** is the final determination of the issues involving settlement of an insurance claim, also known as a claim settlement.

> ## ADMINISTRATIVE SP⦿TLIGHT
>
> After Christina Stoned has been examined by her PCP for back and hip pain, she proceeds to check out. The medical assistant realizes that Ms. Stoned is a member of a health insurance plan operated by a payer that supports RTA. She logs into the payer's website and enters the information on the visit. The payer's system calculates the payment to the provider and the amount owed by Ms. Stoned, and then displays on the screen. The medical assistant (MA) then requests payment from Ms. Stoned for her share of the visit cost and records in the office practice management system the amount paid by the patient and the anticipated amount from the insurer. All of this occurs prior to Ms. Stoned leaving the office. The only remaining item is the payment from the insurer, which occurs the next day in an electronic funds transfer (EFT) payment deposited to the provider's bank account.

> ## 📦 Tip Box
>
> You must log a *ToDo* to Harris CareTracker PM and EMR *Support* to turn on RTA for your practice.

Print the Saved Visit screen. Label it "Activity 7-19" and place it in your assignment folder.

17. Click *Save* at the top or bottom of the screen. When the visit is saved, the coding information is sent to *ClaimsManager* for screening. In addition, Harris CareTracker PM and EMR automatically checks out the patient on the schedule and a check mark appears next to the patient's name confirming that the visit has been captured. Your *ClaimsManager* feature is not active in your student version of Harris CareTracker. Once you hit *Save*, you will receive a pop-up message (Figure 7-61) stating "An error occurred connecting to Claims manager. Transaction saved." Click *OK* on the pop-up.

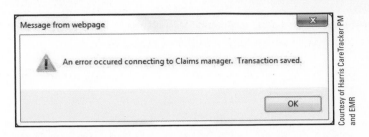

Figure 7-61 ClaimsManager Error Message

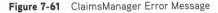

Tip Box

If the *ClaimsManager* screening triggers an edit, Harris CareTracker PM and EMR opens the *ClaimsManager Edit* window. By default, when a *ClaimsManager* edit is triggered, the visit is automatically held and moves to the *Visits On Hold* application. If an action option is not clicked, the *Hold Visit* checkbox is automatically selected and the visit information is held until further action is taken. If waiting for reports or additional information, you can select the *Hold Visit* checkbox to hold the visit and avoid further processing. The held visit is saved under the *Visits On Hold* application.

Visits to Charge. In Harris CareTracker PM and EMR, you have the option to save a visit directly as a charge. This eliminates the additional steps of either navigating to the *Charge* screen to save the charge from the previously created visit or from having to save *Bulk Charges* via the *Missing Encounters* link on the *Dashboard*.

Tip Box

You must log a *ToDo* to *Support* to have the *Visits to Charge* feature activated for your group. Additionally, the *Visit to Charge* button will only be available if the *Visit to Charge Privilege* is included in your operator role.

Open Encounters

An encounter is an interaction with a patient on a specific date and time. Encounter types include visits, phone calls, referrals, results of a test, and more. The *Open Encounters* application displays a list of appointment-based "visit"' type of encounters that do not have a corresponding clinical note and also identifies patients who have a clinical note for a specific date of service but no encounter billed for that same date. Additionally, the *Open Encounters* application displays customized encounters that require billing or a signed note. The *Open Encounters* application is accessible from the following locations:

- *Home* module > *Dashboard* tab > *Open Encounters* link (*Clinical* section) (Figure 7-62)

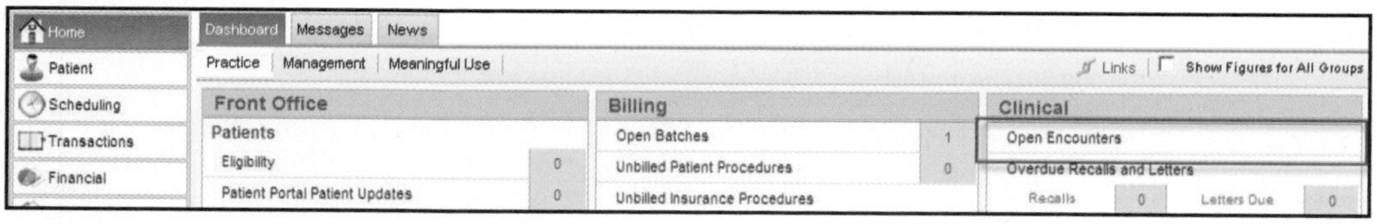

Figure 7-62 Open Encounters Link on Dashboard tab
Courtesy of Harris CareTracker PM and EMR

- *Clinical Today* module > *Tasks* tab > *Open Encounters* (from the *Tasks* menu on the right side of the window) (Figure 7-63)

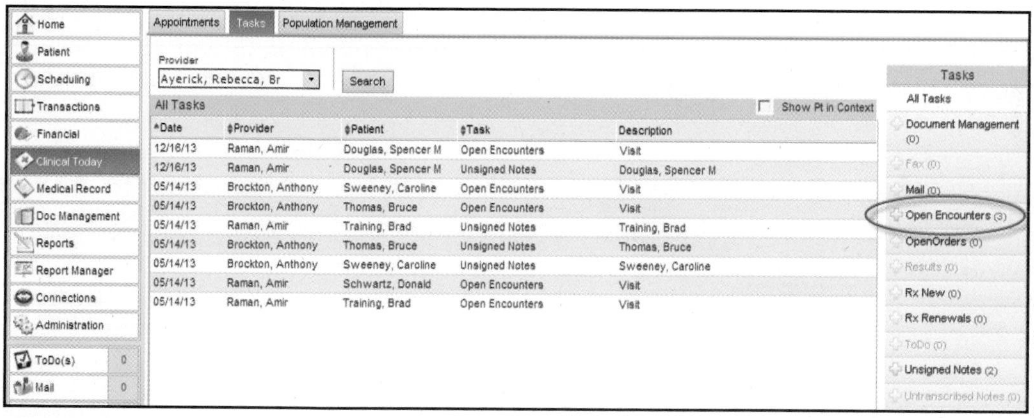

Courtesy of Harris CareTracker PM and EMR

Figure 7-63 Open Encounters from the Clinical Today module

Tip Box

An alternative method is to click the *Clinical Today* module and *Tasks* tab and view open encounter tasks in the *All Tasks* window. You can sort on the *Tasks* column to easily identify open encounter tasks.

Note: If a patient record is marked as VIP, the patient name displays as **VIP** in the open encounter list unless you have the VIP overrides (VIP Patient Access Break Glass or VIP Patient Access) assigned to your profile.

Table 7-12 describes the information displaying in the columns of the *Open Encounters* window. Refer to Figure 7-64 while reviewing Table 7-12.

Viewing a List of Open Encounters. Access the list of *Open Encounters* by going to your *Home* module > *Dashboard* tab > *Open Encounters* link (*Clinical* section). You may need to change the *Provider* to "All" using the drop-down arrow; otherwise the encounters might not display (Figure 7-65).

There are advanced features available in the *Open Encounters* application, such as the ability to filter the list of open encounters by clicking on the column header (e.g., Provider, Appointment Type/Complaint", etc.).

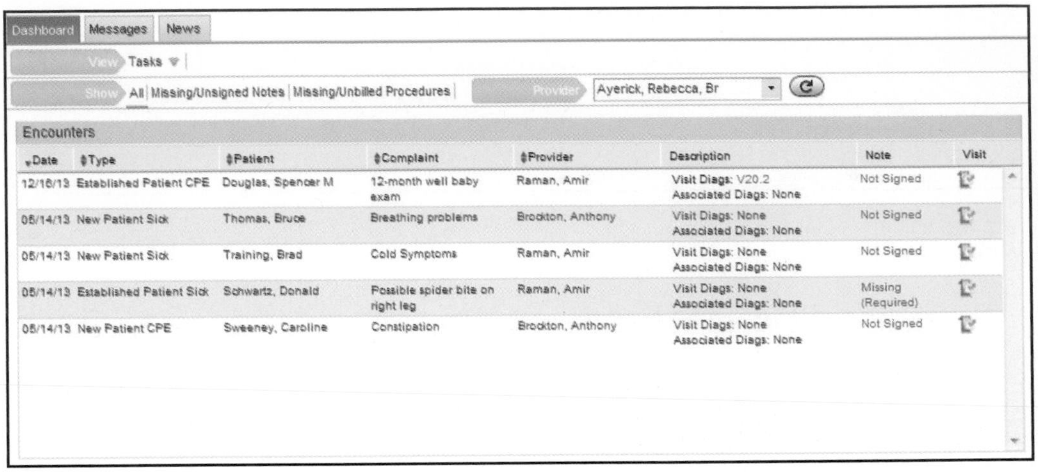

Figure 7-64 Open Encounters Window

TABLE 7-12	Open Encounters Columns
Column	**Description**
Date	The date of the encounter.
Type	The type of encounter.
Patient	The name of the patient with an open encounter.
Complaint	The complaint recorded on the appointment associated with the encounter.
Provider	The name of the billing provider associated with the encounter.
Description	The diagnoses associated with the encounter. You can point to the diagnoses codes to view the associated descriptions. • Visit Diags: Displays diagnosis codes selected in the *Visit* application in the order of priority. • Associated Diags: Displays diagnosis codes selected from the progress note template.
Note	A note can have four different statuses that include *Not Signed, Missing (Required), Missing (Not Required),* or *Complete*. It is important to focus on notes that are in the *Not Signed* or *Missing (Required)* statuses and complete the note (by clicking the *Progress Notes* icon on the *Clinical Toolbar* of the *Medical Record* module). Additionally, if a note consists of an untranscribed file, you must first transcribe the note prior to signing. When the note is signed the *Note* column displays the *Show Note* icon.
Visit	This column displays a *Visit* icon if visit information is required. When the appropriate CPT and ICD codes are saved and the visit is complete, the *Visit* icon displays a check mark on the visit. If an encounter does not require visit information, the *Visit* icon appears dimmed.

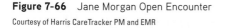

Figure 7-65   Open Encounters - Select All Providers

Courtesy of Harris CareTracker PM and EMR

Resolve Open Encounters.   The *Open Encounters* application helps resolve appointment-based "visit" type of encounters by entering the visit information, reviewing, transcribing (if the note contains an untranscribed file), signing the note, and then billing. All tasks related to the note can be completed via the *Progress Note* application in the *Medical Record* module. *Visit* information is captured by entering the appropriate CPT® and ICD codes using the *Visit* application. For this activity, you will want to view the *Progress Note* and confirm (resolve) that all items in the A&P for the encounter have been completed. If there are any outstanding items, complete them before you sign the note.

ACTIVITY 7-20:   Resolve an Open Encounter

1. Access the *Open Encounters* application from the *Home* module > *Dashboard* tab > *Open Encounters* link (*Clinical* section). If the encounter you are looking for does not display, use the drop-down feature next to *Provider*, select *All*, and then click the *Change Resource* icon.

2. Find the encounter you want to resolve (Figure 7-66). (Locate the encounter you created for Jane Morgan.)

| 04/06/16 | Established Patient Sick | Morgan, Jane W | Urinary symptoms | Raman, Amir | Visit Diags: None
Associated Diags: None | Not Signed | |

Figure 7-66   Jane Morgan Open Encounter

Courtesy of Harris CareTracker PM and EMR

ADMINISTRATIVE SP⬤TLIGHT

An open encounter with an unsigned note, untranscribed file, is billable if visit information is captured; however, it is recommended to enter, transcribe, and sign the note, and then complete the billing.

3. Under the *Note* column, click the *Not Signed* link. The *Progress Note* application displays, enabling you to complete and sign the note.

4. Confirm (resolve) that all items in the *A&P* for the encounter have been completed. Do not sign the note.

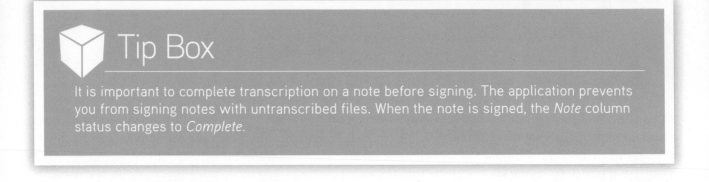

Tip Box

It is important to complete transcription on a note before signing. The application prevents you from signing notes with untranscribed files. When the note is signed, the *Note* column status changes to *Complete.*

5. Click on the *Visit* icon in the *Clinical Toolbar*. The *Visit* application will display. Enter the appropriate CPT® (99213 and 90746) and ICD-10 codes (N39.0, R30.0, and I10 (be sure a check mark is placed next to each ICD-10 code you selected)), then click the *Visit Summary* tab. On the *Visit Summary* screen (Figure 7-67), click *Save.* When the visit information is saved, the icon in the *Visit* column changes to "Complete". (**Note:** Refresh the *Open Encounters* screen to see the updated *Visit* column entry.)

Source: Current Procedural Terminology © 2013 American Medical Association.

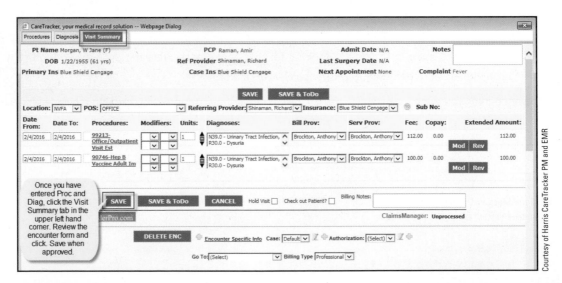

Figure 7-67   Morgan Visit Summary Screen

Print a screenshot of the updated Open Encounters window, label it "Activity 7-20," and place it in your assignment folder.

6. You will sign the note in Activity 7-21. After both the note and billing process is complete, the encounter is deleted from the *Open Encounters* application and is saved under the *Encounter* section of the patient's medical record for reference. Harris CareTracker PM and EMR updates the status of the *Note* and *Visit* columns to "Complete," and "Visit Complete."

> ## 📦 Tip Box
>
> Copies of billable open encounters are saved with other unbillable encounters in the *Encounters* section of the *Medical Record* module. Therefore, you can also resolve an open encounter for a patient using the *Encounter* application in the *Medical Record* module.

Unsigned Notes

The *Unsigned Notes* application displays a list of progress notes that are not signed or require a co-signature by the provider set in the batch. A co-signature is required when a progress note is documented by a non-physician provider such as a physician assistant (PA) or a nurse practitioner (NP). Co-signing for activities performed by others helps determine who is responsible for the supervision and quality of care.

> ## 🧠 Critical Thinking
>
> To determine the scope of practice and legal requirements regarding nurse practitioners that would apply to the NVFHA practice, log on to the website of the State of California Department of Consumer Affairs and select the "General Information: Nurse Practitioner Practice" document at http://www.rn.ca.gov/pdfs/regulations/npr-b-23.pdf. Determine if Gabriella Torres, the NP at NVFHA, requires supervision and a co-signature on the *Progress Note*. What actions would you need to take in Harris CareTracker PM and EMR? Write a summary of the actions required in Harris CareTracker and a one-page paper on NP status in the state of California. Submit to your instructor for class discussion.

Additionally, the *Unsigned Notes* application works the same as the *Progress Note* application and allows you to edit, preview, sign, attach the note to a *ToDo*, print, and view the activity log. The *Unsigned Notes* application (Figure 7-68) is accessible from the following locations:

- *Clinical Today* module > *Tasks* tab > *Unsigned Notes* (from the *Tasks* menu on the right side of the window) or click an unsigned notes task in the *All Tasks* window. You can sort on the *Tasks* column to easily identify unsigned note tasks. (Note: If the Unsigned Note is not displaying, change the provider to "All" and click the refresh icon.)
- An alternative method is to click the *Clinical Today* module, and then click *Un-Signed Notes* from the *Quick Tasks* menu (on the right side of the window).

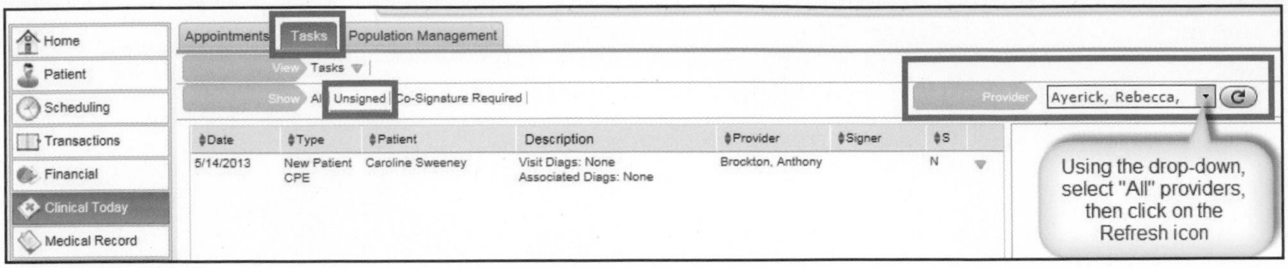

Figure 7-68   Unsigned Notes Application

Table 7-13 describes the columns of the *Unsigned Notes* window. Refer to Figure 7-68 as you review Table 7-13.

TABLE 7-13   Unsigned Notes Columns

Column	Description
Date	The date of the encounter associated with the note.
Type	The type of encounter or the short name for the appointment type. If the encounter type is linked to an appointment, the column displays the appointment short name only. If the encounter type is not linked to an appointment, the column displays the encounter type.
Patient	The patient name associated with the note.
Description	The diagnoses associated with the encounter. You can point to the diagnoses codes to view the associated descriptions. • Visit Diags: Displays diagnosis codes selected in the *Visit* application in the order of priority. • Associated Diags: Displays diagnosis codes selected from the progress note template.
Provider	The author of the note.
Signer	Both the provider signature and the co-signature. The co-signature is indicated with "(CS)" next to the name.
Signed	Indicates that the document requires a signature. The *Signed* column displays one of two statuses that include "N" or "CS." "N" indicates that the note is not signed and "CS" indicates that the note requires a co-signature.
Action	The *Action* menu allows you to do the following: • *Edit Note*: Allows you to edit the note. • *ToDo*: Allows you to attach the note to a *ToDo*. • *Print*: Allows you to print the note. • *Log*: Allows you to view activity related to the note.

View and Filter the List of Unsigned Notes.   The *Unsigned Notes* application enables you to filter the list of progress notes by provider and the signed status. You can sort on the *Tasks* column to easily identify unsigned notes tasks and filter the list of unsigned notes based on your requirements.

Tip Box

The notes that display under each tab are based on the provider selected in your list and the setup for your company.

Sign Notes.   The *Unsigned Notes* application lists notes that the treating and supervising provider must review and sign. You can sign the note directly from the following locations:

- *Unsigned Notes* application
- *Progress Note* application

It is important to know that once a *Progress Note* is signed, you can no longer make changes to it, and any open items/orders that were not completed prior to signing the note will not display within the A&P. When a note is signed, the provider's name displays at the bottom of the progress note as the treating provider with a signature and date stamp. If the note requires a co-signature, the *Signed* column displays "CS" until signed off by the supervising provider. In addition, the provider can make changes to the signed note until it is signed by the supervising provider.

Tip Box

The *Co-signature* maintenance application allows practices to set up providers requiring a co-signature on progress notes. You can assign one or more supervising providers who are authorized to provide a co-signature.

When the supervising provider signs the note, the signature is appended to the end of the note. In addition, the *Signed* column changes to "Y" and the supervising provider name displays under the *Signer* column with "CS" in parentheses. This locks the note by making *Edit* unavailable to prevent from making changes. However, either provider can add an addendum to the locked note if necessary. Table 7-14 indicates the information that must display in the *Signed* and *Signer* columns during the signing process.

TABLE 7-14 Progress Note Signing Workflow

Sign Requirement	Signed Column	Signer Column
(For Single Provider Signing) Note Created and Saved	N (Not Signed)	—
(For Single Provider Signing) Note Signed	Y (Signed)	Treating provider name
(For Notes Requiring Co-Signature) Note Created and Saved	N (Not Signed)	—
Treating Provider Signs the Note	CS (Indicates that a co-signature is required	Treating provider name
Supervising Provider Signs the Note	Y (signed and co-signed)	Treating provider name; Supervising provider name (CS)

Courtesy of Harris CareTracker PM and EMR

ACTIVITY 7-21: Sign a Note

Having confirmed that all tasks outlined in the *A&P* are completed:

1. Access the *Unsigned Notes* application by clicking on the *Clinical Today* module > *Tasks* tab > *Unsigned Notes* (from the *Tasks* menu on the right side of the window) or clicking an unsigned note task in the *All Tasks* window. You can sort on the *Tasks* column to easily identify unsigned note tasks.

2. Click the note to sign. The note launches on the right side of the pane. (Click the note for Jane Morgan's encounter.)

3. Review the note on the right pane and click the *Sign* ✎ icon. A message prompts to confirm the action (Figure 7-69). Click *OK*. (**Note:** Alternatively, you could point to the *Arrow* icon in the *Action* menu and click *Edit Note* to open the note in a new window, review, make changes, and sign or co-sign the note.) Once the *Progress Note* is signed, it will disappear from the *Unsigned Notes* application.

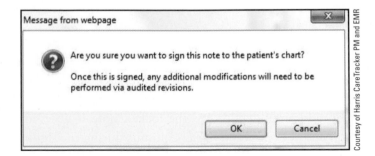

Figure 7-69 Sign Note Pop-Up Window

4. With patient Jane Morgan in context, click on the *Medical Record* module.

5. Click on *Progress Notes* from the *Patient Health History* pane, and select the progress note you created for Jane Morgan. The note launches on the right side of the pane.

6. Click the *Print* 🖫 icon on the *Progress Note* (Figure 7-70). A dialog box will display where you can select *Print* or *PDF*. Select *PDF*, then *Open* or *Save* the PDF as indicated in the *View Downloads* screen. Close the dialog box when you have finished printing.

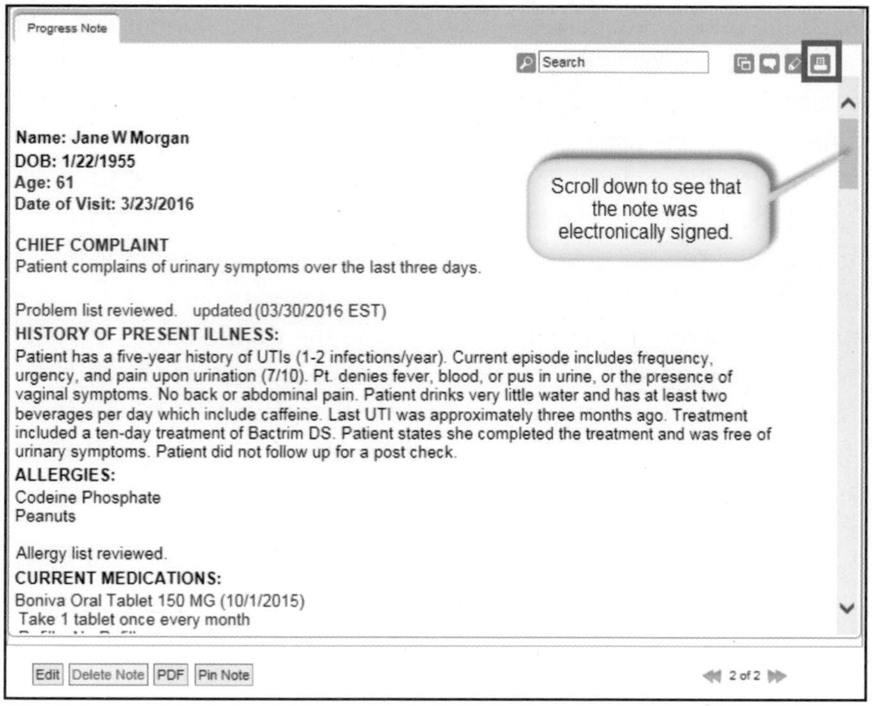

Figure 7-70   Progress Note with Print Icon

Print the signed Progress Note. Label it "Activity 7-21" and place it in your assignment folder.

7. Now access the *Open Encounters* application again from the *Home* module › *Dashboard* tab › *Open Encounters* link (*Clinical* section). Using the drop-down feature next to *Provider*, select *All*, and then click the *Change Resource* icon to refresh the screen. You will note that Jane Morgan's encounter is no longer listed in the *Open Encounters* link.

SUMMARY

Congratulations on completing the patient work-up: placing *Orders*, *Prescriptions*, *Immunizations*, and *Referrals* and completing the *Visit* and signing the *Progress Note*. This simulates the actual EMR workflows in a medical practice combined with practice management features, enhancing the coordination and quality of patient care. This chapter provides in-depth knowledge, practice, and application of the EMR functions in Harris CareTracker PM and EMR.

In summary, the *Orders* application is where you manage and track orders such as laboratory, radiology, pathology, and physical therapy directly from the patient's medical record. This ensures that all orders placed are followed up by the office for patient compliancy. The *Medications* application consists of the past and current medications the patient is taking. The list also includes medications prescribed, medications administered, and samples given to the patient. In addition you used the *Rx* feature to manage favorites, search for pharmacies, create, and print prescriptions. The list of newly administered immunizations, immunizations administered in the past, and immunizations the patient refused to have administered, are found in the *Immunizations* application.

You learned to search for patient educational materials through the *Patient Education* application using keywords, ICD or CPT® codes, or by searching for material by navigating the tree structure. The *Letters* application was used to search for and create letters for patients.

The *Referrals and Authorizations* application enables providers to create inbound and outbound referrals and associated authorizations directly via the patient's medical record. Use of electronic referrals provides the data about the patient's condition and needs, referring and referred-to provider details, treatment authorization data, and referral dates and ranges. Using the *Referrals* application enables you to track patient compliance with the referral instructions and eliminates paperwork.

To wrap up the patient encounter, you learned to complete the visit, resolve open encounters, and electronically sign the note. Having signed the *Progress Note*, you will no longer be able to make changes or add orders. Chapter 8 will instruct you on how to unsign and to make addendums to the *Progress Note* when needed. In addition you will be introduced to other advanced features such as recording results for open *Orders*, recording telephone calls, creating and updating patient *Recall Letters,* and using the *Clinical Export* feature to run an immunization report.

Check Your Knowledge

Select the best response.

_____ 1. Which is a method to access the *Medical Record* module?

    a. Pull the patient into context and click the *Appointments* module

    b. Click the patient's name in the *Appointments* application and select *Open*

    c. Pull the patient into context, and then click the *Medical Record* module

    d. Click the patient's name in the *Administration* tab, *Open Encounters*

_____ 2. Which icon indicates that an order includes multiple tests?

    a. Orders icon   c. Results icon

    b. Expand icon   d. Notes icon

_____ 3. Open orders in the *Open Activities* section displays a test that is overdue in:

    a. Italics   c. Highlights

    b. Gray   d. Red

_____ 4. If no interactions were returned in the *Medication* column *Actions,* the *Interactions* icon appears:

    a. Green   c. Dimmed

    b. Gray   d. Italicized

_____ 5. What is the only method to process a controlled (scheduled) drug prescription?

    a. Print   c. Fax

    b. Via electronic transmission   d. *ToDo*

_____ 6. Generic versions of drugs are displayed in _____ for easy identification.

    a. italics   c. gray

    b. green   d. red

_____ 7. Which application provides access to the Centers for Disease Control and Prevention (CDC) website?

    a. *Open Orders*   c. *Immunizations*

    b. *Medications*   d. *Clinical Today*

_____ 8. A *Visit* can only be edited:

    a. Prior to becoming a charge

    b. Before procedure and diagnosis codes are entered

    c. Before payment is received

    d. None of the above

_____ 9. In *Open Encounters*, a *Note* can have four different statuses. Which of the following is not one of the four statuses?

   a. Not signed   c. Counter signature (required)
   b. Missing (required)   d. Complete

_____ 10. You can sign the note directly from which of the following locations?

   a. *Unsigned Notes* application and *Progress Notes* application
   b. *Encounter* and *Medical Records* pane
   c. *Dashboard, Unsigned Notes* application
   d. None of the above

mini-case studies

Note: Case studies must be completed in every chapter since future chapter activities build upon them.

If the demographic pop-up alerts you to missing information when you pull the patient into context, it is best practice to update as necessary. Update patient's PCP, subscriber numbers, and confirm (Y) to Consent, HIE, and NPP as needed.

Case Study 7-1

Update the missing demographic information for patient Christina Stoned, as indicated by the pop-up alert.

Print a copy of the updated demographic screen for Christina Stoned, label it "Case Study 7-1," and place it in your assignment folder.

Case Study 7-2

Referring to Activity 7-2, and using the information that follows, complete an *Order* for a mammogram referral for patient Jane Morgan.

- *Order Type:* Diag. Imaging
- *Ordering Physician*: Dr. Raman
- *Due Date*: The date of the encounter
- *Diagnosis*: Encounter for screening mammogram for malignant neoplasm of breast (Z12.31) (**Note:** Search under "Mammogram.")
- *Test*: Patient information entered into a reminder system with a target due date for the next mammogram (RAD) (**Note:** Search for and select this test from the database. Do not add your own entry.)

Print the mammogram order for Ms. Morgan. Label it "Case Study 7-2" and place it in your assignment folder.

Case Study 7-3

a. Using steps you learned throughout this chapter, complete the outstanding orders for patient Adam Thompson. To accurately complete the order, refer to the information contained in the A&P of the *Progress Note* you created for Mr. Thompson's encounter in Chapter 6.

- *ABN given to Pt:* Yes
- *Due Date:* The date of the encounter
- *Tests:* 1) CBC W Auto Differential panel in Blood; 2) Electrolytes 1998 panel in Serum or Plasma

b. Referring to Activity 7-19, and using the information that follows, capture the visit for Adam Thompson.

- *CPT® Codes:* 99213; 71020; 94760; 93000
- *ICD-10 Codes:* J18.9; K21.9; I10; M19.90

Source: Current Procedural Terminology © 2013 American Medical Association.

c. Once the visit has been captured, sign the *Progress Note* for Adam Thompson.

🖊 **Print a copy of the order and label it "Case Study 7-3A." Print a screenshot of the completed visit and label it "Case Study 7-3B." Print the signed *Progress Note* and label it "Case Study 7-3C." Place all three documents in your assignment folder.**

Case Study 7-4

a. Using steps you learned throughout this chapter, complete the outstanding orders for patient Ellen Ristino. To accurately complete the order, refer to the information contained in the A&P of the *Progress Note* you created for Ms. Ristino's encounter in Chapter 6.

   - *Due Date:* The date of the encounter
   - *Tests:* 1) CBC W Auto Differential panel in Blood; 2) Heterophile Ab [Titer] in Serum by Agglutination

b. Referring to Activity 7-19, and using the information below, capture the visit for Ellen Ristino.

   - *CPT® Codes:* 99213; 3210F; 36415; 94760; 86308
   - *ICD-10 Codes:* J06.9; J02.9
   Source: Current Procedural Terminology © 2013 American Medical Association.

c. Once the visit has been captured, sign the *Progress Note* for Ellen Ristino.

🖊 **Print a copy of the order and label it "Case Study 7-4A." Print a screenshot of the completed visit and label it "Case Study 7-4B." Print the signed *Progress Note* and label it "Case Study 7-4C." Place all three documents in your assignment folder.**

Case Study 7-5

a. Referring to Activity 7-19, and using the information that follows, capture the visit for patient Craig X. Smith. Refer to the encounter you created for Mr. Smith in Chapter 6.

   - *CPT® Codes:* 99213; J7650; 71020
   - *ICD-10 Code:* R06.2
   Source: Current Procedural Terminology © 2013 American Medical Association.

b. Once the visit has been captured, sign the *Progress Note* for Craig X. Smith.

🖊 **Print a screenshot of the completed visit and label it "Case Study 7-5A." Print the signed *Progress Note* and label it "Case Study 7-5B." Place both documents in your assignment folder.**

Case Study 7-6

a. Referring to Activity 7-19, and using the information that follows, capture the visit for patient Barbara Watson. Refer to the encounter you created for Ms. Watson in Chapter 6.

   - *CPT® Codes:* 99213; 94760
   - *ICD-10 Code:* R50.9
   Source: Current Procedural Terminology © 2013 American Medical Association.

b. Once the visit has been captured, sign the *Progress Note* for Barbara Watson.

🖊 **Print a screenshot of the completed visit and label it "Case Study 7-6A." Print the signed *Progress Note* and label it "Case Study 7-6B." Place both documents in your assignment folder.**

Case Study 7-7

a. Referring to Activity 7-19, and using the information that follows, capture the visit for patient Jordyn Lyndsey. Refer to the encounter you created for Ms. Lyndsey in Chapter 6.

   - *CPT® Code:* 99203
   - *ICD-10 Codes:* M54.5; M99.03; M99.05; I10; E11.9
   Source: Current Procedural Terminology © 2013 American Medical Association.

b. Once the visit has been captured, sign the *Progress Note* for Jordyn Lyndsey.

(Continued)

Print a screenshot of the completed visit and label it "Case Study 7-7A." Print the signed *Progress Note* and label it "Case Study 7-7B." Place both documents in your assignment folder.

Case Study 7-8

  a. Referring to Activity 7-19, and using the information that follows, capture the visit for patient Spencer Douglas's June 14, 2013, encounter. (Because these visits were in the year 2013, you will be selecting ICD-9 codes.)

  - *CPT® Code:* 99391
  - *ICD-9 Code:* V20.2

  Source: Current Procedural Terminology © 2013 American Medical Association.

  b. Once the visit has been captured, sign the *Progress Note* for Spencer Douglas's June 14, 2013, encounter.
  c. Now capture the visit for Spencer Douglas for his encounter dated September 16, 2013. (**Note:** Do not sign the Progress Note for this encounter at this time.)

  - *CPT® Code:* 99391
  - *ICD-9 Code:* V20.2

  Source: Current Procedural Terminology © 2013 American Medical Association.

  d. Now capture the visit for Spencer Douglas for his encounter dated December 16, 2013. (**Note:** Do not sign the *Progress Note* for this encounter at this time.)

  - *CPT® Code:* 99391
  - *ICD-9 Code:* V20.2

  Source: Current Procedural Terminology © 2013 American Medical Association.

Print screenshots of the completed visits and label them "Case Study 7-8A," "Case Study 7-8C," and "Case Study 7-8D." Print the signed *Progress Note* and label it "Case Study 7-8B." Place all the documents in your assignment folder.

Resources

The Harris CareTracker PM and EMR Help home page represents a wealth of information for the electronic health record (https://training.caretracker.com/help/CareTracker_Help.htm).

Centers for Medicare and Medicaid Services (CMS). Glossary. Accessed from the CMS website at http://www.medicare.gov/glossary/f.html

General information: Nurse practitioner practice. (2011, April 13). Retrieved from http://www.rn.ca.gov/pdfs/regulations/npr-b-23.pdf

Health Information and Management Systems Society. (2008, August). *Real time adjudication of healthcare claims* (HIMSS Financial Systems Financial Transactions Toolkit Task Force White Paper). Retrieved from http://himss.files.cms-plus.com/HIMSSorg/content/files/Line%2027%20-%20Real%20Time%20Adjudication%20of%20Healthcare%20Claims.pdf

Chapter 8
Other Clinical Documentation

Key Terms

addendum
progress note
titer

Learning Objectives

1. Access, view, edit, add an addendum, sign, and print a Progress Note.
2. Manually enter Results into the patient's medical record to view, customize, graph, and print those results.
3. Record messages in Harris CareTracker PM and EMR.
4. Create and update patient Recall Letters.
5. Run an immunization report using the Clinical Export feature.

Certification Connection

1. Utilize EMR and practice management (PM) systems.
2. Perform routine PM and clinical EHR tasks within a health care environment according to appropriate protocols.
3. Coordinate patient flow within the back office clinical setting (e.g., check-in, transfer to a room, record vital signs and patient history, create outgoing referrals, and check out patients).
4. Access, edit, and store patient information in the EHR database.
5. Enter live data into an EHR and assist clinicians with charting.
6. Acquire external patient data (labs, radiology reports, patient visit summaries, and more); edit the patient medical record in the EHR within your scope of practice.
7. Access the Internet to obtain patient- and practice-related information and transmit patient data for external use (e.g., insurance, pharmacies, other providers), complying with HIPAA and office protocol regarding security.
8. Locate requested information in the chart and complete tasks (orders) called out in the progress note.
9. Adhere to federal, state, and local laws relating to exchange and transmission of patient information for external use.
10. Describe how to use and find the most current ICD, CPT®, and HCPCS codes in an EMR.
11. Identify the impact of HIPAA for the medical assistant; adhere to rules pertaining to the confidentiality and release of PHI.
12. Demonstrate time management principles to maintain effective office workflows and patient care follow-up.
13. Purge, archive, and secure electronic charts; create an action plan for data recovery in case of downtime or a catastrophic event.

Adapted from national standards of the National Healthcareer Association (NHA), Commission on Accreditation and Allied Health Education Program (CAAHEP), and Accrediting Bureau of Health Education Schools (ABHES)

INTRODUCTION

This chapter expands on other clinical documentation in the EMR. Moving forward, you will perform advanced features in an EMR that streamline workflows and promote continuity of patient care. You will complete activities that simulate real-world office workflows of a medical assistant, which include navigating the *Progress Notes*, *Results*, and *Messages* applications and creating *Recall Letters* and using the *Export* tool.

Your activities will include viewing and entering patient's lab results via the *Results* application. In addition, you will customize, graph, and print patient results. You will expand on the *ToDos* activities that were reviewed in earlier chapters, now focusing on the clinical side of Harris CareTracker PM and EMR. In the *Messages* application you will record messages; create new mail messages; access and view mail messages; reply to, move, and manage your inbox.

The final features introduced are the *Recalls* application and the *Clinical Export* feature. *Recalls* are reminders to patients that an appointment needs to be booked. Harris CareTracker PM and EMR tracks all recalls, enabling you to generate recall letters at the appropriate time intervals.

The *Clinical Export* feature provides you the ability to export a batch of patient clinical data in PDF. You can select the time period to cover and the level of patient information to include. You will use the *Immunization Export* application to generate a record of all vaccinations given during a specified time period, monitor inventory, and provide a database of information should there be a recall of a medication.

Upon completion of this chapter's activities, you will have gained useful knowledge and application skills using Harris CareTracker EMR—a transferable skill to a wide variety of EMR products available in the market.

THE PROGRESS NOTES APPLICATION

Learning Objective 1: Access, view, edit, add an addendum, sign, and print a Progress Note.

The *Progress Notes* application allows you to navigate the list of notes saved for the patient and click a note to view and manage from the right pane. A **progress note** is a document, written by the clinician or provider, that describes the details of a patient's encounter and is sometimes referred to as a chart note. To navigate and view the progress notes listed in a patient's medical record:

• Click *Next* and *Previous* buttons on the bottom of the *Progress Note* window to navigate through the list of notes (Figure 8-1).

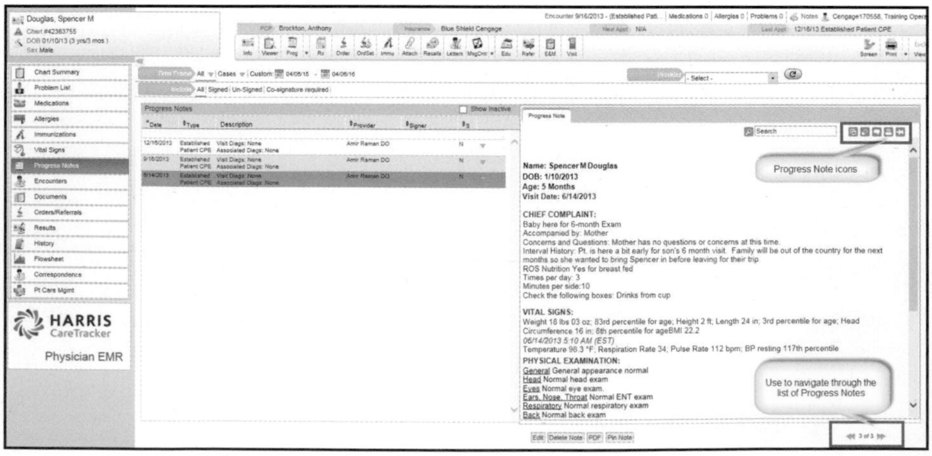

Figure 8-1 Progress Notes – Next and Previous Buttons

- Click the *Expand/Collapse* 🔲 icon in the upper-right-hand corner of your screen to maximize the view for readability.

 Various ways to manage the progress note include:

- *Edit* and *Overwrite* edits of a progress note
- Sign or unsign a note
- Add an addendum to a note
- ⬤ Create a PDF of the note
- Sign or print a note
- Pin/Unpin a note (Pinning a note will lock in a narrative to a progress note template, displaying the same narrative each time you access the template.)

> ## Tip Box
>
> **Important!!** It is important to complete and sign all progress notes before any billing information is submitted to the payers.

Access and View Progress Notes

The *Progress Notes* application displays a list of notes recorded during each patient appointment and progress note–type documents that are uploaded. Progress notes include information such as the patient's history, medications, allergies, as well as a complete record of all that happened during the visit. This information is required for medical, legal, and billing purposes.

 You can use the application to browse through all the patient notes, including uploaded notes, on the right pane of the window. When viewing uploaded notes, the right pane displays the document in the *Document Viewer* and fits the width of the pane. However, you can click the *Expand/Collapse* 🔲 icon to control the view.

ACTIVITY 8-1:   Access the Progress Notes Application

1. There are several ways to access the *Medical Record* module. Use one of the following methods:

   a. Pull the patient, Spencer Douglas, into context, and click the *Medical Record* module.

   b. If the patient has an appointment, click the patient's name in the *Appointments* application of the *Clinical Today* module. (Patient has appointments scheduled on 06/14/2013, 09/16/2013, and 12/13/2013.)

2. In the *Patient Health History* pane, click *Progress Notes*.

3. The *Progress Notes* window displays with a list of signed and unsigned notes for the patient (Figure 8-2).

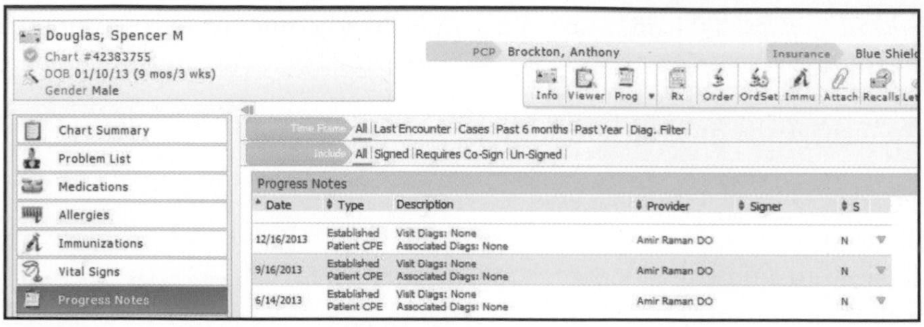

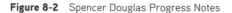

Figure 8-2 Spencer Douglas Progress Notes

Written Activity

On a blank sheet of paper write down the list of the signed and unsigned progress notes for the patient. Label the page "Activity 8-1" and place it in your assignment folder.

Table 8-1 describes the columns in the *Progress Notes* window. The documents that are attached or scanned to the application only display the information in the specific columns that are marked with an asterisk ("*") in the table. Refer to Figure 8-2 while reviewing Table 8-1.

In addition to the *Progress Notes* application, Harris CareTracker EMR provides quick access to progress notes via two other locations:

- *Progress Note* icon on the *Clinical Toolbar*
- *Select Encounter* dialog box

TABLE 8-1 Progress Notes Columns

Column	Description
*Date	The date of the encounter associated with the note or the document date selected when uploading the note via the *Document Management Upload* application.
*Type	The type of encounter or appointment. If the encounter type is linked to an appointment, the column displays the appointment type only. If the encounter type is not linked to an appointment, the column displays the encounter type. If the note is uploaded, the column displays the subtype selected when uploading the document.
*Description	The diagnosis associated with the encounter. You can point to the diagnoses codes to view the associated descriptions. This provides the flexibility of reviewing previous notes for a recurring problem or similar symptoms and helps reduce time to issue orders. • Visit Diags: Displays diagnosis codes selected in the *Visit* application • Associated Diagnosis: Displays diagnosis codes selected from the progress note template If the note is uploaded, the column displays the *Document* icon and the document name.
*Provider	The author of the note or the provider selected when uploading the document.
Signer	Both the provider signature and the co-signature. The co-signature is indicated with (CS) next to the name.

TABLE 8-1   *(Continued)*

*S	Indicates that the document requires a signature. The *Signed* column displays the following: • N: Indicates that the note is not signed and requires a signature • CS: Indicates that the note requires a co-signature by the supervising provider • Y: Indicates that the note is signed
*Action	The *Action* drop-down menu allows you to do the following: • *Edit Note*: Allows you to edit the note • *ToDo*: Allows you to attach the note to a *ToDo* • *Print*: Allows you to print the note • *Log*: Allows you to view activity related to the note The *Action* drop-down menu for uploaded documents displays the following options. • *View Document*: Allows you to view the document attached • *ToDo*: Allows you to attach the document to a *ToDo* • *Print*: Allows you to print the document • *Delete*: Allows you to delete the document

Tip Box

You can also access the *Progress Note* application by clicking the *Encounters & Progress Notes* section (Figure 8-3) title in the *Chart Summary*.

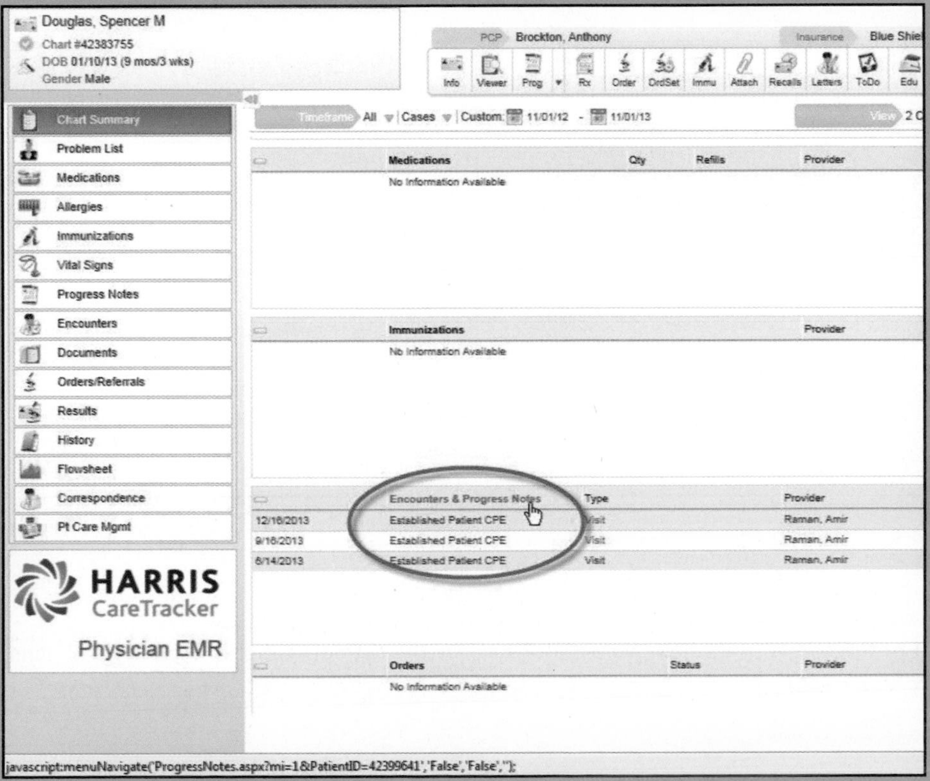

Figure 8-3   Douglas Encounters & Progress Notes Section

ACTIVITY 8-2: Access Progress Notes from the Clinical Toolbar

1. Pull patient Spencer Douglas into context and click the *Medical Record* module.
2. In the *Clinical Toolbar*, click the *Arrow* icon next to the *Progress Notes* icon. Harris CareTracker EMR displays the *Note* icon next to the encounters that have a progress note.

Tip Box

Important!! You must actually click on the *Note* icon, not just on the encounter date (Figure 8-4). If you click on the encounter date you will receive an error message.

3. Click the *Note* icon next to the encounter dated June 14, 2013. Harris CareTracker EMR displays the *Viewing Clinical Note* dialog box with the selected progress note to the right of the date (see Figure 8-4).

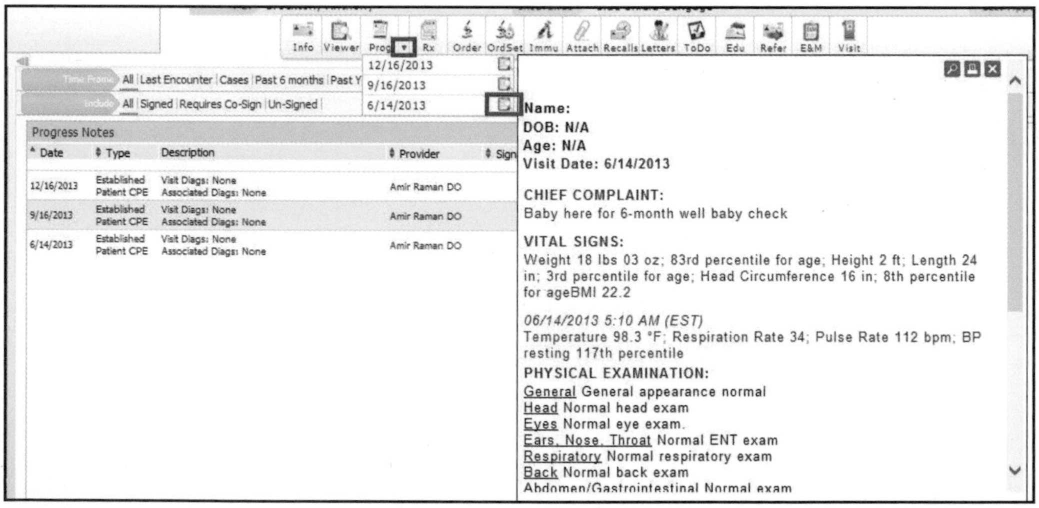

Courtesy of Harris CareTracker PM and EMR

Figure 8-4 Spencer Douglas Progress Note

Print a screenshot of the *Viewing Clinical Note* dialog box for the patient. Label it "Activity 8-2" and place it in your assignment folder.

4. Click "X" to close out of the *Viewing Clinical Note* dialog box.

Activity 8-3 instructs you to use the alternative method of accessing the *Progress Note* from the *Encounter* dialog box.

ACTIVITY 8-3: Access the Progress Note from the Encounter Dialog Box

1. Pull patient Jane Morgan into context and click the *Medical Record* module.
2. In the *Patient Detail* bar, click the *Encounter* link (Figure 8-5). Harris CareTracker EMR displays the *Select Encounter* dialog box (Figure 8-6). Encounters with progress notes display the *Note* icon next to the encounter.

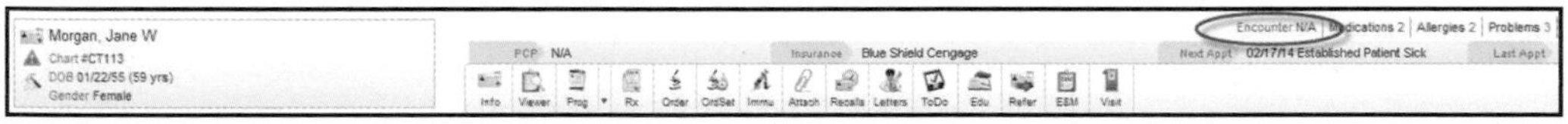

Figure 8-5 Encounter Link
Courtesy of Harris CareTracker PM and EMR

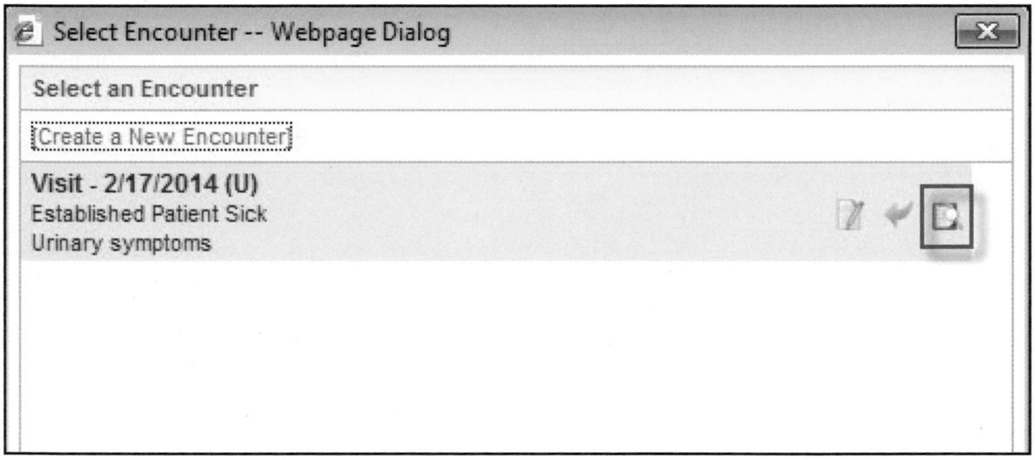

Courtesy of Harris CareTracker PM and EMR

Figure 8-6 Select Encounter Dialog Box

3. Click the *Note* icon next to the encounter you created for the patient in Chapter 6. Harris CareTracker EMR displays the *View Clinical Note* dialog box with the selected progress note (Figure 8-7).

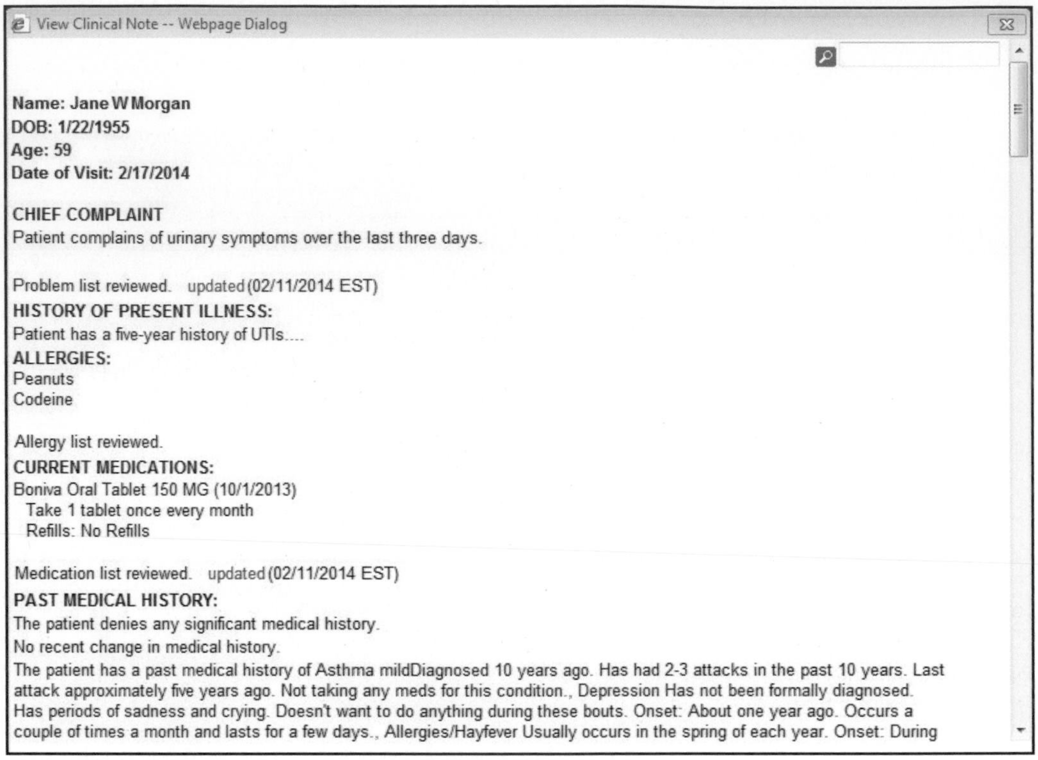
View Clinical Note -- Webpage Dialog

Name: Jane W Morgan
DOB: 1/22/1955
Age: 59
Date of Visit: 2/17/2014

CHIEF COMPLAINT
Patient complains of urinary symptoms over the last three days.

Problem list reviewed. updated (02/11/2014 EST)
HISTORY OF PRESENT ILLNESS:
Patient has a five-year history of UTIs....
ALLERGIES:
Peanuts
Codeine

Allergy list reviewed.
CURRENT MEDICATIONS:
Boniva Oral Tablet 150 MG (10/1/2013)
Take 1 tablet once every month
Refills: No Refills

Medication list reviewed. updated (02/11/2014 EST)
PAST MEDICAL HISTORY:
The patient denies any significant medical history.
No recent change in medical history.
The patient has a past medical history of Asthma mildDiagnosed 10 years ago. Has had 2-3 attacks in the past 10 years. Last attack approximately five years ago. Not taking any meds for this condition., Depression Has not been formally diagnosed. Has periods of sadness and crying. Doesn't want to do anything during these bouts. Onset: About one year ago. Occurs a couple of times a month and lasts for a few days., Allergies/Hayfever Usually occurs in the spring of each year. Onset: During

Courtesy of Harris CareTracker PM and EMR

Figure 8-7 View Clinical Note Dialog Box

Print a screenshot of the *View Clinical Note* dialog box for the patient. Label it "Activity 8-3" and place it in your assignment folder.

4. Click on "X" to close the *View Clinical Note* dialog box.

Filter Progress Note Templates

The *Progress Notes* application helps filter a list of notes documented during a patient encounter. You can filter the list of notes based on the approval status, document date, or the diagnoses associated with the note.

ACTIVITY 8-4: Filter the List of Notes

1. Pull patient Spencer Douglas into context and click the *Medical Record* module.
2. In the *Patient Health History* pane, click *Progress Notes*. The *Progress Notes* window displays with a list of signed and unsigned notes for the patient.
3. Practice filtering by doing each of the following (Figure 8-8), and then take a screenshot of each for your Activities folder:
   a. To filter the list of notes by approval status, click the *Signed, Un-Signed,* or *Co-signature required* tab.
   b. To filter the list of notes by documented date, select *Last Encounter, Past 6 months,* or *Past Year* from the *All* drop-down menu directly to the right of the *Time Frame* tab.

c. *(FYI Only)* To filter the list of notes by case:

   i. Click the second drop-down menu to the right of the *Time Frame* tab.

   ii. Select *Cases, All Cases* or *Default.*

Courtesy of Harris CareTracker PM and EMR

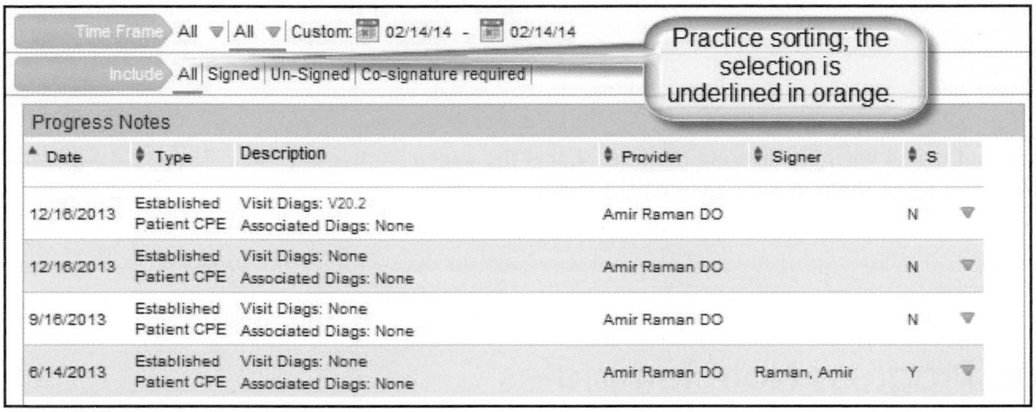

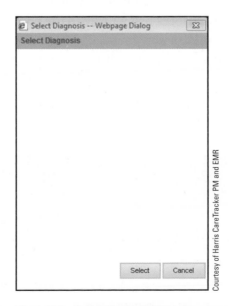

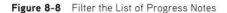

Figure 8-8 Filter the List of Progress Notes

d. To filter the list of notes by diagnoses selected in the *A&P* (Assessment) tab of a progress note:

   i. Select *Diag. Filter* from the *All* drop-down menu to the right of the *Time Frame* tab. Harris CareTracker EMR displays the *Select Diagnosis* dialog box (Figure 8-9). (**Note:** If no diagnoses have been entered in the *A&P* (*Assessment* tab) of the *Progress Note*, the dialog box will be blank. If a diagnosis appears, you would select the checkbox pertaining to the diagnosis you want.)

   ii. Click *Select.* Harris CareTracker EMR displays the notes associated with the selected diagnoses.

Courtesy of Harris CareTracker PM and EMR

Figure 8-9 Select Diagnosis Dialog Box

CLINICAL SP○TLIGHT

The *Diag. Filter* tab displays all diagnoses selected in the *A&P* (*Assessment*) tab of a progress note when documenting a patient encounter. It does not display the primary diagnosis selected via the *Visit* application.

Print a screenshot of the various Filtering methods. Label the pages "Activity 8-4a," "Activity 8-4b," and "Activity 8-4d" and place them in your assignment folder.

Manage Progress Note Templates

You will now perform various activities related to managing progress notes such as:

- *Edit* and *Overwrite* edits of a progress note
- Unsign a signed note
- Add an addendum to a note
- Send a *ToDo*
- Create a PDF of the note
- Sign or print a note

Edit a Progress Note.   Edits can be made to a progress note until it is signed by the provider. If the note requires a co-signature, it can be edited until the supervising provider signs the note. If a note is signed, the template is unavailable to prevent any changes being made to the note. However, the signing provider (you, in this case of student training) can unsign a note to make changes if necessary.

Harris CareTracker EMR provides a notification if the content of the note changes before the operator has a chance to save his or her edits. You can overwrite the edits by reviewing the options in the *Override Edits* box, selecting the edit you want, and clicking *Apply* (Figure 8-10).

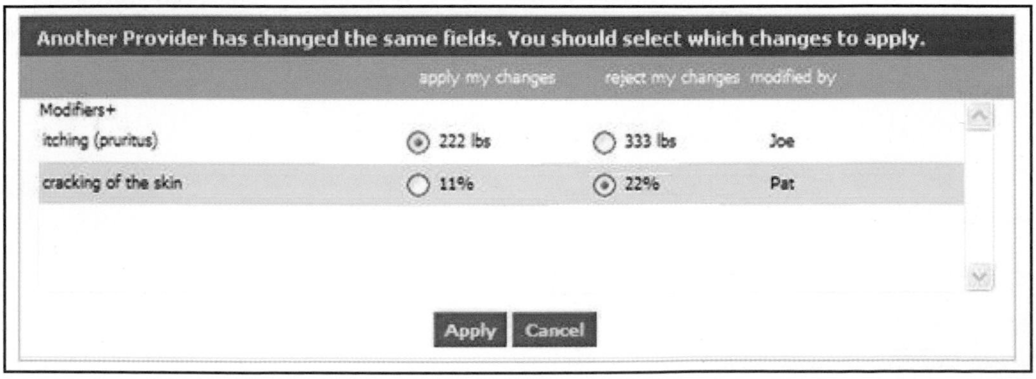

Courtesy of Harris CareTracker PM and EMR

Figure 8-10   Override Edits Box

ACTIVITY 8-5: Edit a Progress Note

1. In the *Clinical Today* module, set the calendar to September 16, 2013, and click on Spencer Douglas's name in the *Appointments* window. This will launch his medical record.

2. In the *Patient Health History* pane, click *Progress Notes*. Harris CareTracker EMR displays the *Progress Notes* window.

> ## Tip Box
>
> If you had previously signed the progress note, unsign it so that you can make edits (see Activity 8-9).

3. To edit from the *Actions* menu:

   a. Click the *Arrow* icon ▼ next to the note dated September 16, 2013, and then click *Edit Note*. In the *Copy prior note* dialog box, click *Cancel*. Harris CareTracker EMR displays the *Progress Note Template* window (Figure 8-11). In the *Template* field, select "9 Month Well Child Visit" if not already displaying.

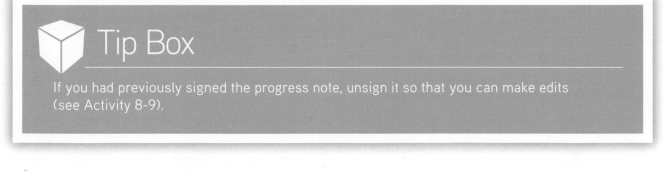

Figure 8-11 Progress Note Template Window

   b. Notice that there is no information in the *Progress Note*. Refer back to Chapter 6 and, using the steps outlined in Activity 6-15, edit the note using the information packet for Spencer Douglas on page 648 of Appendix A.

   c. Click *Save*.

   d. Sign the note (refer to Activity 7-20 if you need to review the steps).

4. To edit from the preview in the *Progress Notes* screen, repeat Steps 1 and 2 of this activity, but set the calendar to December 16, 2013:

   a. Click the progress note (not the *Actions Arrow* icon) you want to edit. Select the progress note dated December 16, 2013. The progress note displays on the right pane of the window.

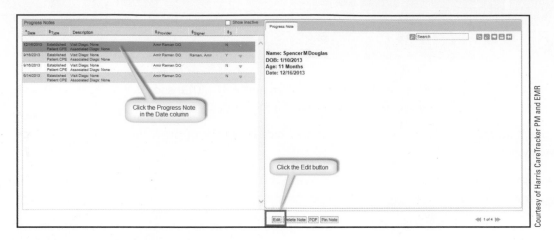

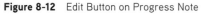

Figure 8-12 Edit Button on Progress Note

b. Click *Edit* at the bottom of the screen (Figure 8-12).

c. In the *Copy prior note* dialog box, click *Cancel*. The *Progress Note* window launches, enabling you to edit the unsigned note.

d. Notice that there is no information in the progress note. Using the steps outlined in Activity 6-15, edit the note using the information packet for Spencer Douglas on page 649 of Appendix A.

e. Click *Save*.

f. Now sign the note.

Print the edited progress notes. Label the September 16, 2013, progress note "Activity 8-5a" and the December 16, 2013, progress note "Activity 8-5b," and then place them in your assignment folder.

Delete a Progress Note. You can only delete unsigned notes. When a note is signed, *Delete Notes* appears dimmed.

ACTIVITY 8-6: Delete a Progress Note

1. Pull patient Donald Schwartz into context and click the *Medical Record* module.

2. In the *Patient Health History* pane, click *Progress Notes*. Harris CareTracker EMR displays the *Progress Notes* window.

3. Click the progress note you want to delete. Select the note dated May 14, 2013. The progress note displays on the right pane of the window.

4. Click *Delete Note* (Figure 8-13). Harris CareTracker EMR displays the *Void* dialog box.

5. Select *Delete Reason*: "Other" (Figure 8-13).

6. You will be prompted to enter a reason. Enter "Test Activity Chapter 8."

7. Click *Save*. (**Note:** It may take a few moments for the note to be deleted.)

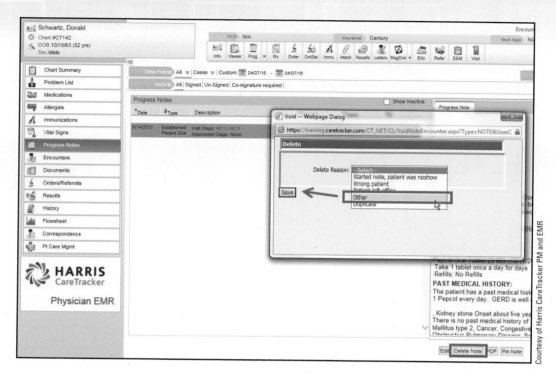

Figure 8-13   Void Dialog Box

Tip Box

A record of the deleted note is maintained in the *Clinical Log*. To access the *Clinical Log*, click the arrow next to the *View* ᏏᏏ icon at the top right of the *Chart Summary* screen, and then select *View Clinical Log*. The *View Log* dialog box will display (Figure 8-14).

View Clinical Logs

From Date	To Date	Type		Operator		
04/07/2016 ×	04/07/2016	-Select-	⌄	-Select-	⌄	Show Log

Date ⇕	User ⇕	Data ⇕	Event ⇕	Host IP ⇕
4/7/2016 12:22:40 AM (EST)	Cengage170558, Training Operator	Progress Notes List	Accessed	
4/7/2016 12:22:21 AM (EST)	Cengage170558, Training Operator	Clinical Note	Removed/Inactivated	
4/7/2016 12:18:35 AM (EST)	Cengage170558, Training Operator	Progress Notes List	Accessed	
4/7/2016 12:18:32 AM (EST)	Cengage170558, Training Operator	Patient Chart	Accessed	

Showing 1 - 4 of 4   1

Figure 8-14   View Log Dialog Box

Print a screenshot of the *Clinical Log*, which shows the deleted progress note (see Tip Box above). Label it "Activity 8-6" and place it in your assignment folder.

Add an Addendum to a Progress Note.   You can add an addendum to both a signed and an unsigned note to accommodate any clinical workflow your practice follows. An **addendum** is text that is added to a progress note after it is signed. The addendum displays at the end of the original progress note and helps track updates made to the note. Additionally, the "Addended By" label displays with the operator's name and the date and time of the addendum. This tracks changes made to the note and the person responsible for the change.

ACTIVITY 8-7:   Add an Addendum to a Progress Note

1. Pull patient Cristina Stoned into context and click the *Medical Record* module.

2. In the *Patient Health History* pane, click *Progress Notes*. Harris CareTracker EMR displays the *Progress Notes* window.

3. Click the progress note you want to addend. Select the note dated May 14, 2013. The progress note displays on the right pane of the window.

4. Click the *Add Addendum* 🗨 icon. Harris CareTracker EMR displays the *Add Clinical Note Addendum* dialog box. (**Note:** If you receive an error message, close the dialog box and click on the *Add Addendum* icon again until the prompt displays.)

5. Enter additional note: "Pt requests referral to Dr. Robert Rovner for Orthopaedic evaluation" (Figure 8-15). Click *Save*.

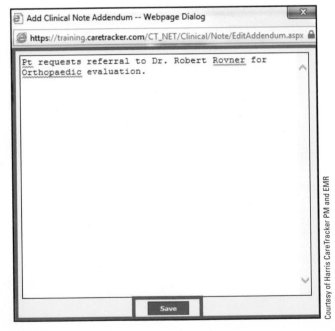

Figure 8-15   Add Clinical Note Addendum Dialog Box

CLINICAL SP🔘TLIGHT

You can also choose to dictate the addendum or use the quick text feature to enter additional notes.

6. In the right pane, scroll to the bottom of the progress note where the *Addendum* has been added (Figure 8-16).

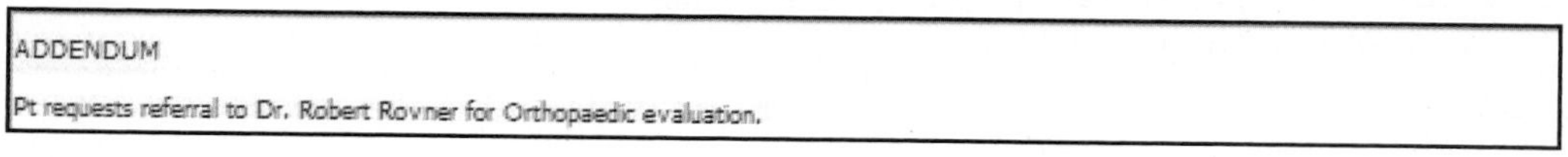

ADDENDUM

Pt requests referral to Dr. Robert Rovner for Orthopaedic evaluation.

Figure 8-16   Christina Stoned Addendum Added
Courtesy of Harris CareTracker PM and EMR

Print a screenshot of the progress note Addendum. Label it "Activity 8-7" and place it in your assignment folder.

Sign the Progress Note.   Having previously learned to sign the progress note in Chapter 7 (Activity 7-20 and related Mini-Case Studies), you will now sign the progress note(s) you have worked on in this chapter. (**Note:** Before you sign a progress note, be sure the visit has been captured with CPT® and ICD codes entered. Refer to Activity 7-19 and related Mini-Case Studies if you need to review these steps.)

ACTIVITY 8-8:   Sign a Progress Note

Tip Box

Before signing the progress note, with the encounter in context, first confirm that there is a captured *Visit* with the CPT® and ICD codes already entered (following instructions from Activity 7-19).

1. Pull patient Christina Stoned into context and click the *Medical Record* module.

2. In the *Patient Health History* pane, click *Progress Notes*. Harris CareTracker EMR displays the *Progress Notes* window.

3. Click the progress note you want to sign. Select the note dated May 14, 2013.

4. (Optional) Click on the *Expand* icon to maximize the readability of the progress note you are viewing. You can click the icon again to collapse the narrative.

5. After confirming all the orders outlined in the A&P have been completed, and the addendum to the note has been added, click the *Sign* icon on the right pane of the window to sign the note.

6. Harris CareTracker EMR will display a pop-up window asking "Are you sure you want to sign this note to the patient's chart?" Click *OK*.

7. Harris CareTracker EMR will update the status of the note. When complete, you will note the electronic signature stamp at the bottom of the progress note (Figure 8-17).

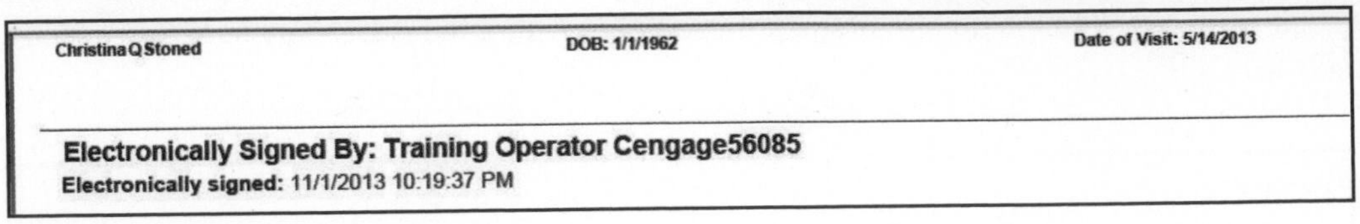

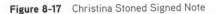

| Christina Q Stoned | DOB: 1/1/1962 | Date of Visit: 5/14/2013 |

Electronically Signed By: Training Operator Cengage56085
Electronically signed: 11/1/2013 10:19:37 PM

Figure 8-17 Christina Stoned Signed Note

Print a screenshot of the signed progress note. Label it "Activity 8-8" and place it in your assignment folder.

Unsign the Progress Note. You can unsign a signed note, if necessary. However, only the operator who signed the note is allowed to unsign a note, based on the operator's role. Enter a reason for unsigning the note if required to complete the action. For audit purposes, a copy of the original note is maintained in the patient's clinical log.

ACTIVITY 8-9: Unsign a Progress Note

1. After signing Ms. Stoned's progress note in the previous activity, you realize that Dr. Brockton is the provider who needs to sign the note, not you.

2. To unsign the note, pull patient Christina Stoned into context, and click the *Medical Record* module.

3. In the *Patient Health History* pane, click *Progress Notes*. Harris CareTracker EMR displays the *Progress Notes* window.

4. Click the progress note you want to unsign. Select the note dated May 14, 2013. The progress note displays on the right pane of the window.

5. Click the *Unsign* icon. Harris CareTracker EMR displays a confirmation message.

6. Click *OK* to unsign the note.

7. In the *Progress Notes* window, the note will now be listed as unsigned (Figure 8-18).

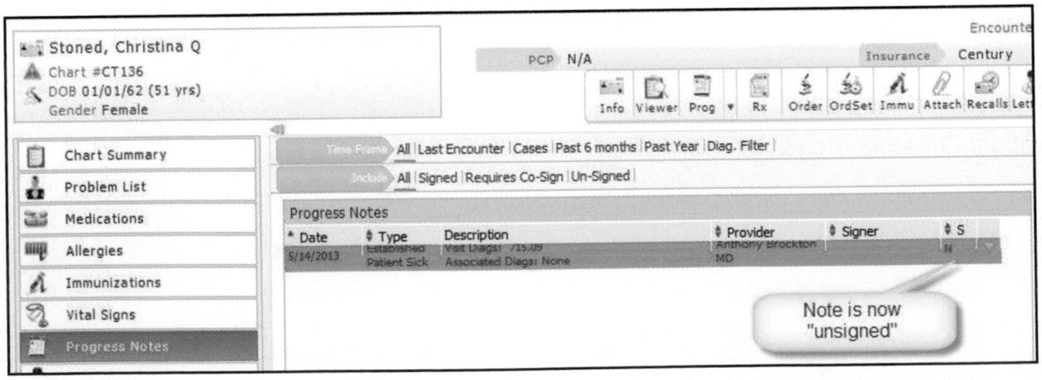

Figure 8-18 Progress Note Window – Unsigned Note

Print a screenshot of the unsigned progress note. Label it "Activity 8-9" and place it in your assignment folder.

8. Now sign the progress note once again and save it so you can use this encounter in later activities.

Print the Progress Note. To print the progress note, follow the instructions in Activity 8-10.

ACTIVITY 8-10: Print the Progress Note

1. With patient Christina Stoned in context click the *Medical Record* module.
2. In the *Patient Health History* pane, click *Progress Notes*. Harris CareTracker EMR displays the *Progress Notes* window.
3. With the May 14, 2013, progress note in context, use each of the following three print functions:
   a. Print from the *Actions* menu:
      i. Click the *Arrow* icon and click *Print*. Harris CareTracker EMR displays the *Clinical Note* dialog box.
      ii. Click *Print*. A copy of the notes prints to the printer attached to your computer.
   b. Print from the preview in the right pane:
      i. Click the progress note you want to print. The progress note displays on the right pane of the window.
      ii. Click the *Print* icon. Harris CareTracker EMR displays the *Clinical Note* dialog box.
      iii. Click *Print*. A copy of the note prints to the printer attached to your computer.
   c. Create a PDF of the progress note:
      i. Click the progress note you want to convert to PDF. The progress note displays on the right pane of the window.
      ii. Click *PDF* at the bottom of the screen. Harris CareTracker EMR creates a PDF version of the documented progress note. You can print or save a copy.

Tip Box

An alternative method is to click the *Print* icon, and then click *PDF* in the *Clinical Note* dialog box (Figure 8-19).

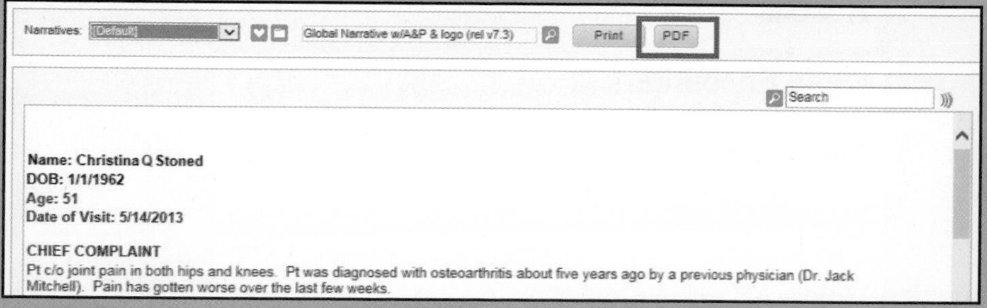

Courtesy of Harris CareTracker PM and EMR

Figure 8-19 PDF Button in Clinical Note Dialog Box

Print the progress note using each of the methods in the activity. Label the pages "Activity 8-10a," "Activity 8-10b," and "Activity 8-10c" and place them in your assignment folder.

ACCESS AND RECORD RESULTS

Learning Objective 2: Manually enter Results into the patient's medical record to view, customize, graph, and print those results.

The *Results* application is where lab and radiology results are displayed. The medical assistant should monitor results on a continuous basis, ascertaining that results are received, reviewed, and handled in an efficient manner. Results received electronically are saved in the following locations:

- *Home* module > *Dashboard* tab > *Clinical* section > *Results* link
- *Clinical Today* module > *Tasks* tab > *Results* (from the *Tasks* menu on the right side of the window)
- *Open Activities* section of the *Chart Summary*
- *Results* section of the *Chart Summary*.

Tip Box

An alternative method to view the results display is to click the *Clinical Today* module, and then click *Results* from the *Quick Task* pane on the right side of the window (Figure 8-20). Recall that *Quick Tasks* will only display for the provider in your *Batch*.

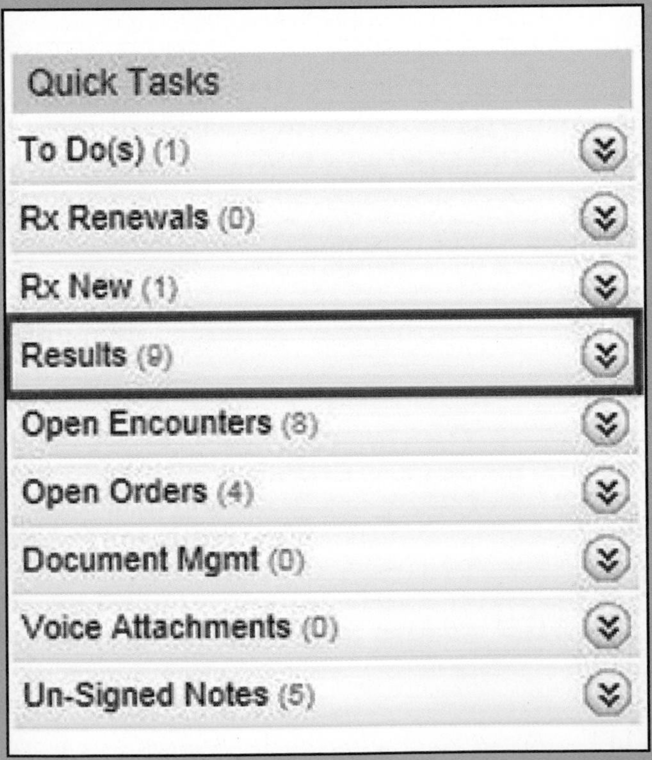

Figure 8-20   Results from Quick Tasks Pane

The results displaying in the *Medical Record* module are color coded based on the status of the results, as shown in Table 8-2.

TABLE 8-2 Results Statuses

Result Color	Status
Black	Final result
Gray	Preliminary result
Bright Red	Abnormal result **Note:** If any component within a result is returned with an abnormal value, the entire result is considered as an abnormal result.
Light Red	Preliminary Abnormal result

Courtesy of Harris CareTracker PM and EMR

Results received into Harris CareTracker EMR are automatically linked to the corresponding patient based on the demographic information and the order. If a result has an "Unmatched" status, the result is saved only in the *Results* application of the following locations:

- *Home* module
- *Clinical Today* module

Your student version of Harris CareTracker will not receive results electronically. However, you are able to manually enter lab results into the patient's medical record.

Manual results can be entered, scanned, or attached to the patient's medical record. If a result has an *Unmatched Patient* icon, it indicates that the computer was unable to find any patients with the same exact demographics, thus the result is saved only in the *Results* application.

FYI

Electronic results received into Harris CareTracker EMR automatically link to the corresponding patient based on the demographic information.

The result is not saved in the *Results* application in the *Medical Record* module unless it is manually matched. If a matching patient is not found, Harris CareTracker EMR displays the *Match* icon, enabling you to manually link the results to the corresponding patient. Additionally, any test result that falls outside of normal parameters displays the observation in red to alert you and get your immediate attention (Figure 8-21).

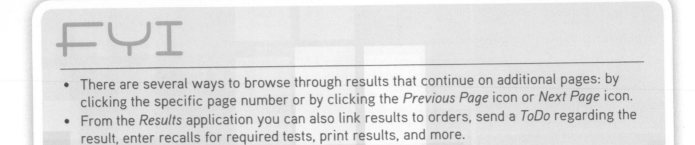

Figure 8-21   Abnormal Result Displayed in Red

FYI

- There are several ways to browse through results that continue on additional pages: by clicking the specific page number or by clicking the *Previous Page* icon or *Next Page* icon.
- From the *Results* application you can also link results to orders, send a *ToDo* regarding the result, enter recalls for required tests, print results, and more.

Entering Results Manually

The *Open Orders* application enables you to manually enter the results of lab tests into the system or automatically download them from the facility. If the delivery method of results includes fax, phone, paper, or download, you must manually enter the results for the specific order. This automatically updates the order status and the results in the patient's medical record. When the result is entered, both the order and the result are removed from the *Open Orders* application under *Quick Tasks* and the *Open Activities* section of the *Chart Summary* in the *Medical Record* module.

In Activity 8-11 you will manually record *Results* for patient Jane Morgan's urinalysis lab order you created in Chapter 7. Enter the results found in Source Document 8-1 in Appendix A.

ACTIVITY 8-11:   Enter Results Manually

1. With patient Jane Morgan in context, click on the *Medical Record* module.

2. In the *Patient Health History* pane, click on *Orders/Referrals*. This will launch the *Orders* window.

3. In the *Actions* menu, click the *Arrow* ▼ icon next to the order for which you want to enter results (urinalysis) and select "Enter Results" (Figure 8-22). Harris CareTracker EMR displays the *Manual Lab Results* dialog box.

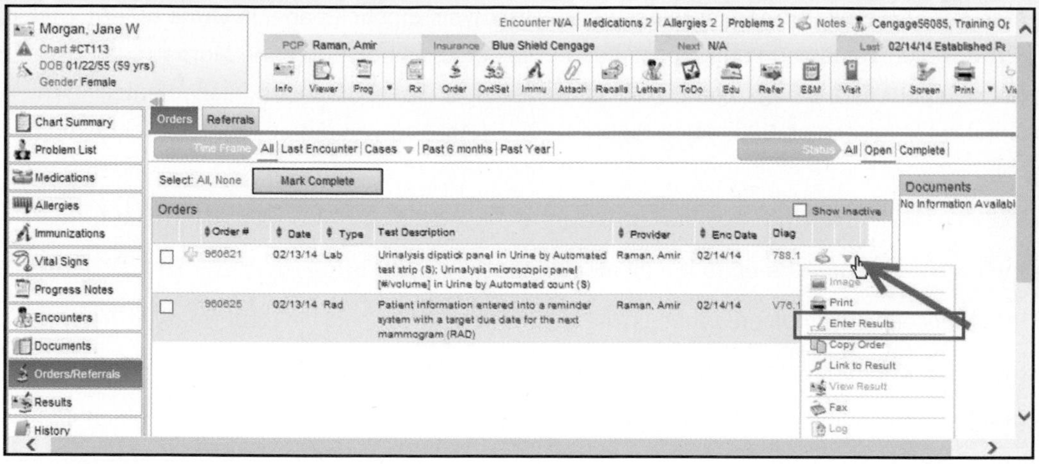

Courtesy of Harris CareTracker PM and EMR

Figure 8-22 Enter Results Link

4. Review the order information. The information is based on the entries made at the time of creating the order.

FYI

You also have the option of entering *Result Notes* and to add or delete result codes based on requirements or to use the existing codes to enter results (refer to Figure 8-24).

To remove result codes:

- Select the checkbox next to the result code you want to remove and click *Del*. The result code is removed from the list.

To add result codes:

- Click the *Add Item* icon.
- In the *Search Result Codes* box, enter a keyword and click *Search*. Harris CareTracker EMR displays a list of result codes matching the search criteria.
- Select the checkbox for the result code you want to add. The result code is added to the list, enabling you to enter results.

5. In the top part of the *Manual Lab Results* box, enter the selections at the time of the order (as listed in Source Document 8-1 in Appendix A):

a. *Laboratory:* Napa Valley Family Health Associates Laboratory (**Note:** Click on the *Show Favorite Labs* icon to access a drop-down menu of your favorite labs.)

b. *Ordering Provider:* Amir Raman

c. *Result Type:* Lab

d. *Filler Order #:* Leave blank

e. *Fasting or Non-Fasting:* Non-Fasting

f. *Collected Date:* Enter the date of the appointment you created for Jane Morgan in Activity 4-1

g. *Collected Time*: Enter a time that is 15 minutes after the start of Jane Morgan's appointment.

6. In the *Manual Lab Results* screen, scroll down to "Urinalysis dipstick panel in Urine by Automated test strip." Enter result values and units for the codes selected, as noted in Jane Morgan's lab result form (Source Document 8-1), using Figure 8-23 as a reference. When you have finished entering the results for this test, your screen should match Figure 8-24. (**Note:** You will notice that both tests and results are on one lab order.)

a. In the *Value* box, enter the "Results" or "Abnormal Results" entry from the lab result form.

b. In the *Units* box, enter the units if indicated on the lab result form.

c. In the *Abnormal* box, indicate whether the results were "Normal" or "Abnormal."

d. In the *Reference Range* box, enter the normal range for the test.

e. In the *Status* list, click the status of the result code. For example, if the result received states "incomplete," click *Incomplete* in the *Status* list; otherwise select *Final.* For Jane Morgan's results, select *Final.*

	Patient Name	DOB	Age	Gender			
	Morgan, Jane W	1/22/1955	58	F	Report Status:	**Final**	
	Ordering Provider				Reported:	**11/11/2013 10:07:05 PM**	
	Amir Raman DO				Accession:		
					Collected:	**7/30/2013**	

A	Test	Results	Abnormal Results	Units	Reference Range
	Urinalysis dipstick panel in Urine by Automated test strip				
A	**Clarity of Urine**		Cloudy		Clear
N	Ketones [Mass/volume] in Urine by Automated test strip	Negative			Negative
A	**Nitrite [Presence] in Urine by Automated test strip**		Positive		**Negative**
A	**Hemoglobin [Mass/volume] in Urine by Automated test strip**		Trace		**None**
N	pH of Urine by Automated test strip	7.5			5.0-9.0

Figure 8-23   Morgan Lab Results Form

Tip Box

You can enter partial results on panels by entering a value for the result under the *Value* column and selecting the correct option under the *Abnormal* column. **Example**: If the order is for a CBC (panel) and there are multiple individual tests that are part of that panel, you do not have to enter values for all tests to save the result.

7. Now scroll up and enter the results for the remaining test: "Urinalysis microscopic panel [#/volume] in Urine by Automated count." Refer to the lab results form (Source Document 8-1).

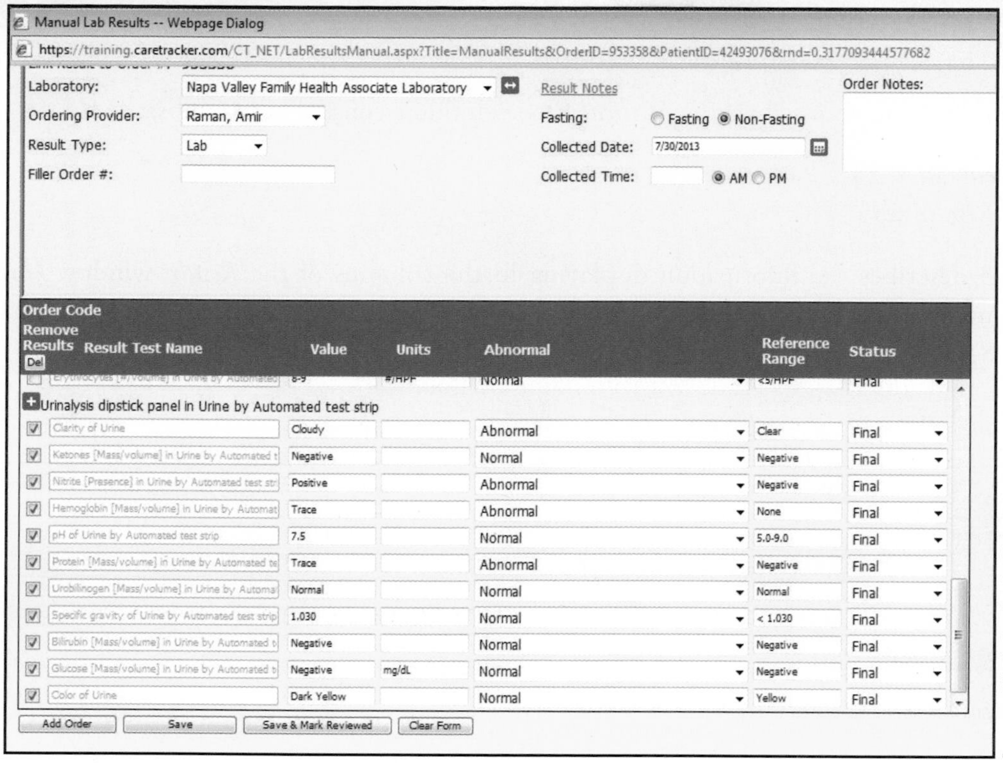

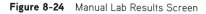

Figure 8-24   Manual Lab Results Screen

Print the Manual Lab Results screen for the Urinalysis Lab Order. Label it "Activity 8-11" and place it in your assignment folder.

8. Based on your requirements, click one of the following action buttons: *Add Order, Save, Save & Mark Reviewed,* or *Clear Form* (Figure 8-25). Select *Save*.

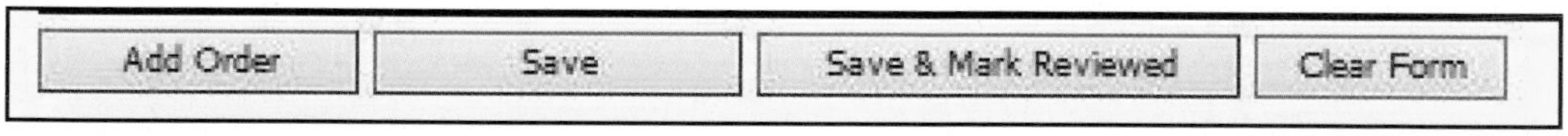

Add Order	Save	Save & Mark Reviewed	Clear Form

Figure 8-25   Results Action Buttons
Courtesy of Harris CareTracker PM and EMR

9. Once you click *Save*, you will receive a pop-up asking if you want to mark the order as complete (Figure 8-26). Select *No*. You will receive another pop-up stating "Update Successful." Click *OK*.

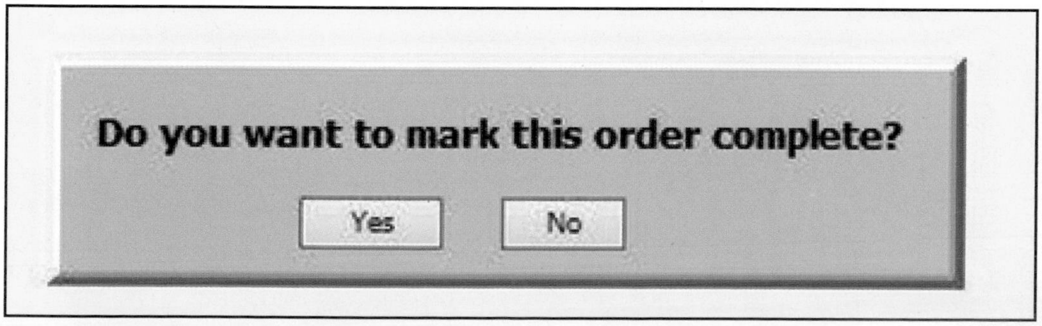

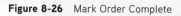

Do you want to mark this order complete?

Yes   No

Figure 8-26   Mark Order Complete

Viewing Results

The *Results* application accessed via the *Medical Records* module consists of two tabs:

- *List View* tab
- *Chart Results* tab

Table 8-3 describes the information displaying in the columns of the *Results* window (*List View* tab). However, manual results (attached or scanned) only display information in specific columns marked with an "*" in Table 8-3. Refer to Figure 8-27 while reviewing this table.

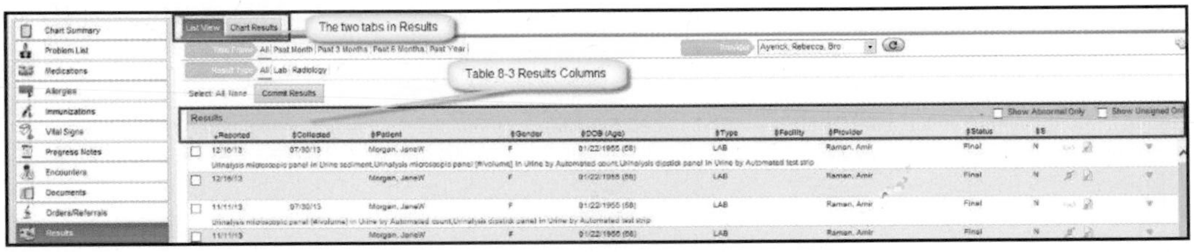

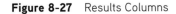

Figure 8-27   Results Columns

Courtesy of Harris CareTracker PM and EMR

TABLE 8-3	Results Columns
Column	**Description**
*Reported	The date and time the results were transmitted into Harris CareTracker EMR or selected when uploading the result via the *Document Management Upload* application.
	Additionally, the column displays the name of the result below the reported date. Manual results displays the *Document* icon to the left of the document name, the subtype in parentheses, and notes entered when uploading the document.
Collected	The date and time the specimen is collected.
Patient	The name of the patient.
Sex	The sex (gender) of the patient.
DOB (Age)	The patient's date of birth in mm/dd/yyyy format and the age of the patient.
Type	The type of the result.
Facility	The name of the facility.
*Provider	The name of the ordering provider or the provider selected when uploading the result document. Additionally, if a provider was copied on the result, the name displays below the ordering provider's name and is indicated with "CC."
	Note: The provider who was copied on the result can see the result only if the *Include Copy To* checkbox is selected.
*Status	The status of the result.

TABLE 8-3	*(Continued)*
*S	"S" represents whether or not the result has been reviewed and signed and can have one of two values. Results reviewed and committed to the patient's medical record are indicated with a "Y." Results that are not reviewed by the ordering provider are indicated with an "N."
*Linked to Order	Allows you to link the result to an order. When a result is linked to a document, the *Link to Order* icon is replaced by the *View* icon. You can click the *View Linked Order* icon to view the order linked to the result.
Link to Document	Allows you to link the result to a document associated with the patient. When a result is linked to the document, the *View Linked Order* icon displays, allowing you to view the document linked to the result. **Note:** The *Link to Document* icon appears dimmed if the result is an attached or scanned document.
Action	The *Action* menu allows you to do the following: • *Print:* Allows you to print the result. • *ToDo:* Allows you to attach the result to a *ToDo*. • *Log:* Allows you to view the *Result Activity Log*.
Observation (below the result row)	Comments about the result. *Abnormal* results display the specific test values in red in the observation row.
Notes (below the observation row)	Displays any comments you entered when signing the result.

Courtesy of Harris CareTracker PM and EMR

Customize Patient Results View.   The *Results* application enables you to create an operator-specific default view for both the *List View* and *Chart Results* tabs. You can select the time frame, result type, and the providers for the list view. You can select the default chart type and the reported date for the chart view.

ACTIVITY 8-12:   Create Customized Result Views

1. With patient Jane Morgan in context, click the *Medical Record* module.

2. In the *Patient Health History* pane, click *Results*. Harris CareTracker EMR displays the *Results* window with a list of patient results.

3. Click the *Settings* icon in the top right corner of the screen, which will open the *Set Results Default* window.

4. Select the options you want to set as the default in both the *List View Operator Defaults* and *Chart View Operator Defaults* sections (Figure 8-28).

   a. Set *Time Frame*, *Result Type*, and *Providers* to "All."

   b. Set *View* to "Graph" and *Reported Date* to "All."

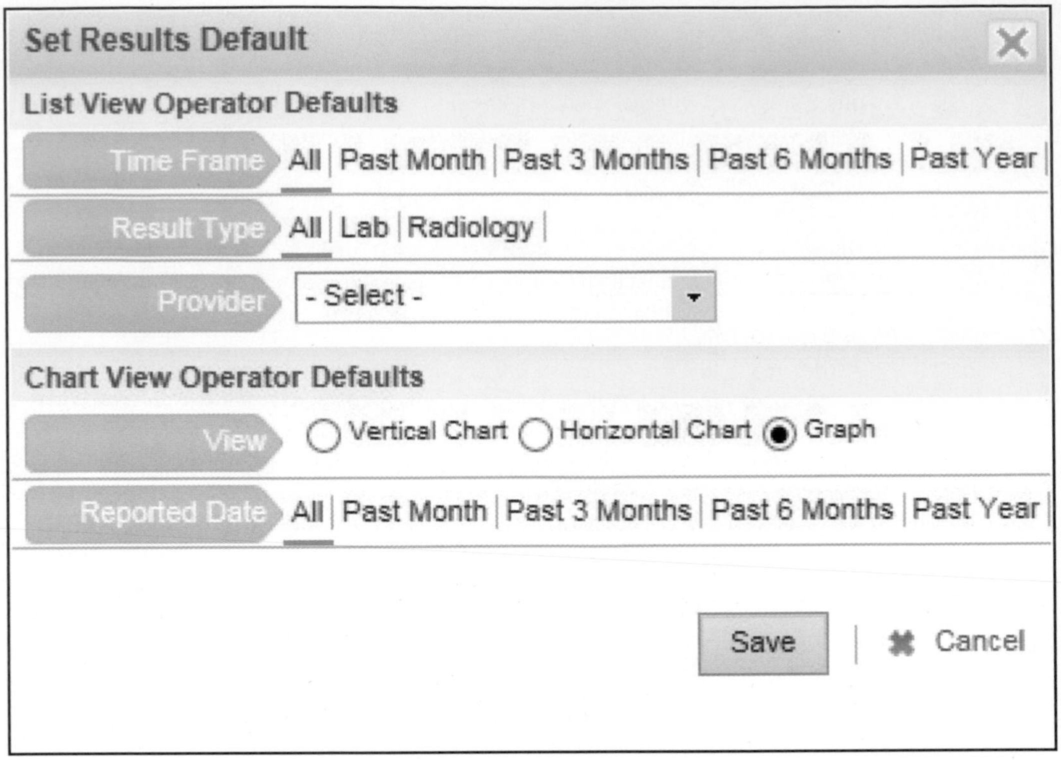

Courtesy of Harris CareTracker PM and EMR

Figure 8-28 Set Results Default Dialog Box

Print a screenshot of the Set Results Default box. Label it "Activity 8-12" and place it in your assignment folder.

5. Click *Save*. A "Success" message displays to confirm the action.
6. Click *Close*.

Filter Patient Results. The list of results pertaining to the patient can be filtered on the result type, date, or provider.

ACTIVITY 8-13: Filter the Patient's Result List

1. With patient Jane Morgan in context, click the *Medical Record* module.
2. In the *Patient Health History* pane, click *Results*. Harris CareTracker EMR displays the *Results* window with a list of patient results.
3. Complete each the following:
   a. You have the option to change the display of results based on the *Time Frame* of the result by selecting the *All, Past Month, Past 3 Months, Past 6 Months,* or *Past Year* tabs. Select *All* (Figure 8-29).

b. You can filter the results based on the *Result Type* by selecting the *All, Lab,* or *Radiology* tab. Select *All.*

c. You can view results pertaining to one or more providers by selecting the checkboxes in the *Provider* list. Click *All* so that you will view results pertaining to all providers.

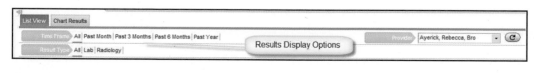

Figure 8-29   Results Display Options
Courtesy of Harris CareTracker PM and EMR

d. View abnormal results by selecting the *Show Abnormal Only* checkbox. An abnormal result displays the specific test values in red in the observation row. Now uncheck the box.

e. View the unsigned results by selecting the *Show Unsigned Only* checkbox. You can also sort signed and unsigned results by clicking on the *Signed* column. Now uncheck the box.

CLINICAL SPOTLIGHT

It is important that all results are signed and committed to the patient's chart in a timely manner.

Print a screenshot of each window that illustrates you have filtered the patient results as directed. Label them "Activity 8-13a," "Activity 8-13b," "Activity 8-13c," "Activity 8-13d," and "Activity 8-13e" and place them in your assignment folder.

Critical Thinking

A patient calls to inquire about some tests she had performed three days ago. She states that she checked the patient portal but no results are showing up. She is quite nervous about the testing. You check the patient's EMR but the results have not been uploaded. Where else in the EMR might you look for these results? What can be done if you are unable to locate the results?

Graph Patient Results.   The *Chart Results* tab in the *Results* application allows you to plot all or specific lab test values that pertain to a specific time period in three different views. The views include *Vertical Chart, Horizontal Chart,* and *Graph.* Results in chart or graph views are color coded based on the status of the result and display the measurements associated with each result as shown in Table 8-2. You can only graph results that were entered, not results that were scanned into the chart.

ACTIVITY 8-14: Graph Patient Results

1. With patient Jane Morgan in context, click the *Medical Record* module.

2. In the *Patient Health History* pane, click *Results*. The *List View* tab opens by default. Click on the *Chart Results* tab.

3. In the *Lab Test Values* list, you have the option of selecting *All* or selecting the checkbox of the results you want to include in the chart. Select *All*.

4. In the *Reported Date* list, click the time period you want. Select *Past Year*.

5. In *View*, you have the option to select *Vertical Chart*, *Horizontal Chart*, or *Graph* (Figure 8-30). Select *Vertical Chart*.

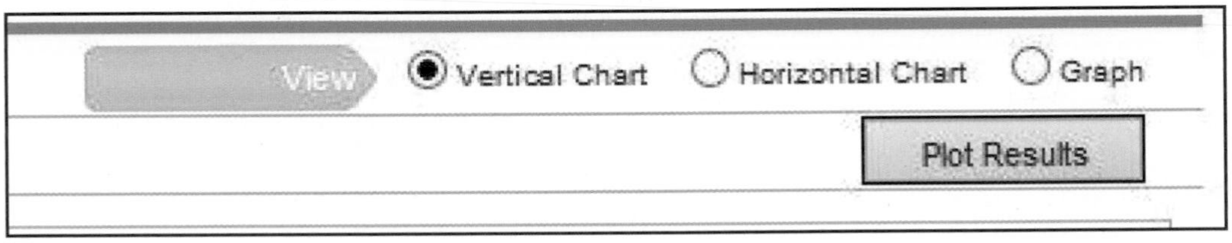

Figure 8-30   Results View Options

6. Click *Plot Results*. Your screen will look like Figure 8-31.

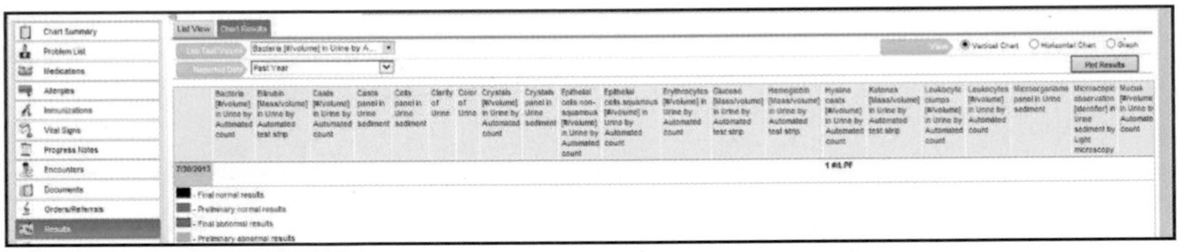

Figure 8-31   Results of Vertical Chart View

7. Repeat step 6 and plot the results in *Horizontal Chart* and *Graph* view as well.

Print a screenshot of each of the charts (Horizontal and Vertical) as well as the Graph view screen. Label them "Activity 8-14a," "Activity 8-14b," and "Activity 8-14c" and place them in your assignment folder.

Print Patient Results.   The *Results* application helps print test result records to give to the patient and other entities such as specialists and hospitals that are treating the patient. Fewer laboratory tests will be ordered because health practitioners across the provider network will have the results of earlier tests, eliminating the need to reorder tests that were previously completed. The *Results* application provides two methods to print a specific result: you can use the *Action* menu in the *Result* application or open the result to print.

ACTIVITY 8-15: Print a Single Result

1. With patient Jane Morgan in context, click the *Medical Record* module.

2. In the *Patient Health History* pane, click *Results.* Harris CareTracker EMR displays the *Results* window with a list of patient results.

> ### Tip Box
>
> For each printing option, clicking *Print* will open a new screen with the printable results. Click *Print* on the shortcut menu to print the result.

3. Do each of the following:

   a. Click the result (urinalysis lab order) to open it and then click *Print* in the *Lab Results Report* dialog box (Figure 8-32A).

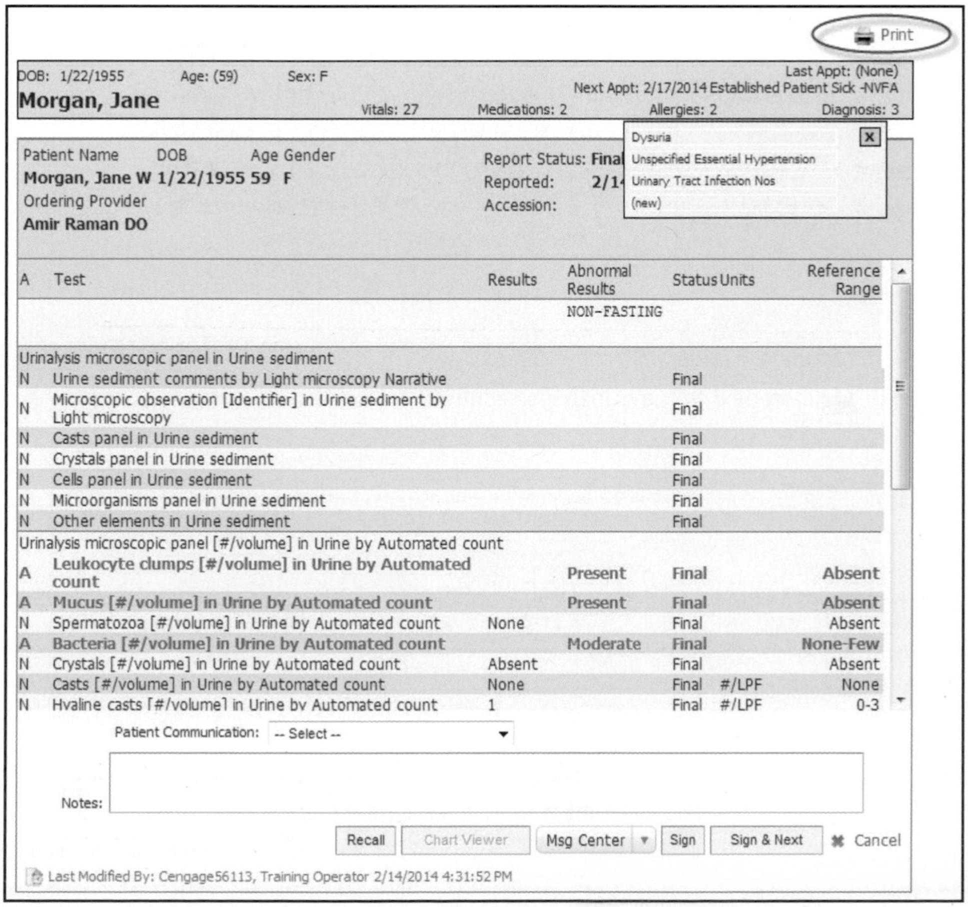

DOB: 1/22/1955	Age: (59)	Sex: F		Last Appt: (None) Next Appt: 2/17/2014 Established Patient Sick -NVFA	
Morgan, Jane		Vitals: 27	Medications: 2	Allergies: 2	Diagnosis: 3

Patient Name DOB Age Gender		Report Status: Final
Morgan, Jane W 1/22/1955 59 F		Reported: 2/14
Ordering Provider		Accession:
Amir Raman DO		

Dysuria
Unspecified Essential Hypertension
Urinary Tract Infection Nos
(new)

A	Test	Results	Abnormal Results	Status Units	Reference Range
			NON-FASTING		
	Urinalysis microscopic panel in Urine sediment				
N	Urine sediment comments by Light microscopy Narrative			Final	
N	Microscopic observation [Identifier] in Urine sediment by Light microscopy			Final	
N	Casts panel in Urine sediment			Final	
N	Crystals panel in Urine sediment			Final	
N	Cells panel in Urine sediment			Final	
N	Microorganisms panel in Urine sediment			Final	
N	Other elements in Urine sediment			Final	
	Urinalysis microscopic panel [#/volume] in Urine by Automated count				
A	Leukocyte clumps [#/volume] in Urine by Automated count		Present	Final	Absent
A	Mucus [#/volume] in Urine by Automated count		Present	Final	Absent
N	Spermatozoa [#/volume] in Urine by Automated count	None		Final	Absent
A	Bacteria [#/volume] in Urine by Automated count		Moderate	Final	None-Few
N	Crystals [#/volume] in Urine by Automated count	Absent		Final	Absent
N	Casts [#/volume] in Urine by Automated count	None		Final #/LPF	None
N	Hyaline casts [#/volume] in Urine by Automated count	1		Final #/LPF	0-3

Patient Communication: -- Select --

Notes:

Recall   Chart Viewer   Msg Center ▾   Sign   Sign & Next   ✳ Cancel

Last Modified By: Cengage56113, Training Operator 2/14/2014 4:31:52 PM

Figure 8-32A   Print from the Lab Results Report Dialog Box

   b. In the *Results* window, click the *Arrow* ▼ icon (Figure 8-32B) beside the urinalysis order and click *Print*.

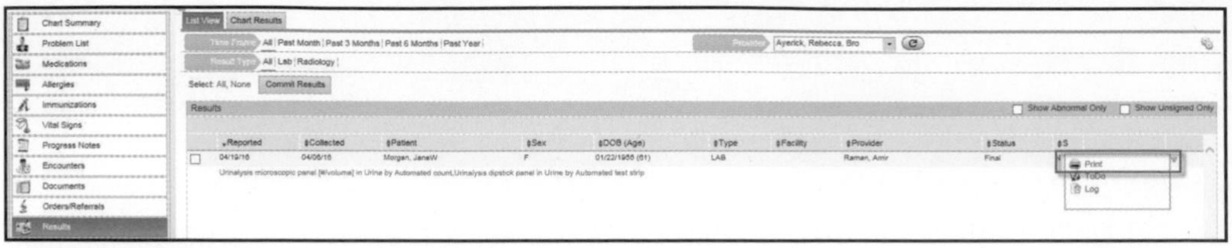

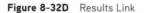

Figure 8-32B Print from the Actions menu

c. Go to the *Clinical Today* module > *Quick Tasks* pane. Click the arrow next to the *Results* link (Figure 8-32C). (**Note:** If there are no *Results* showing, check your *Batch* and make sure the ordering provider is displaying.) Click on the result, which opens a new screen, and click the *Print* icon at the top right of the screen.

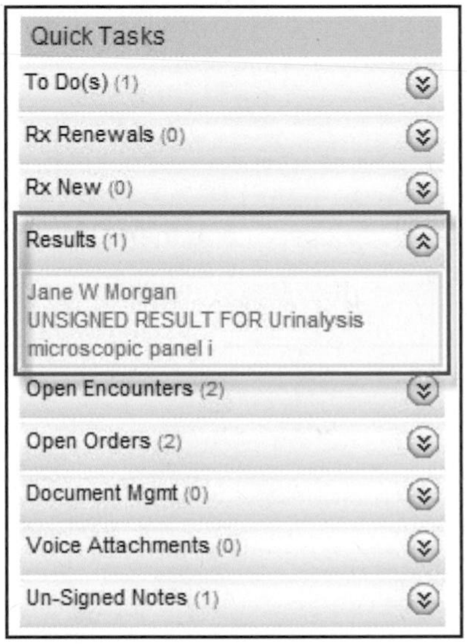

Figure 8-32C Print from Quick Tasks Tab

d. Go to the *Home* module > *Dashboard* tab > *Clinical* section > *Results* link (Figure 8-32D), and then click the *Print* icon next to the urinalysis results.

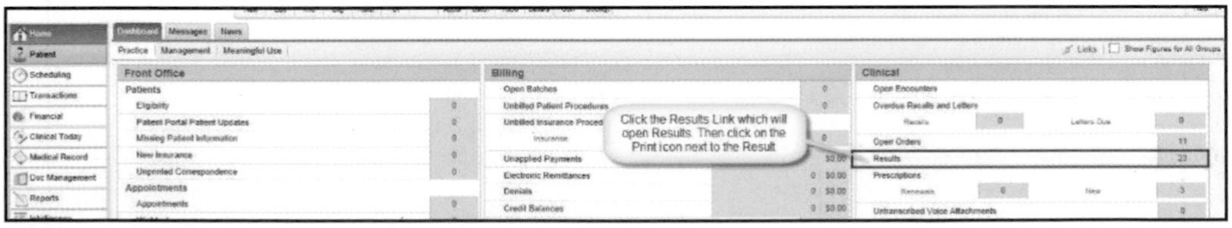

Figure 8-32D Results Link

Print the patient's result using each method in Activity 8-15. Label them "Activity 8-15a," "Activity 8-15b," "Activity 8-15c," and "Activity 8-15d" and place them in your assignment folder.

RECORDING MESSAGES

Learning Objective 3: Record messages in Harris CareTracker PM and EMR.

In Chapter 2 you were introduced to the *Message Center* where you created *ToDos* and *Mail* messages and viewed *Queues* and *Fax* options. In this chapter, we expand on your previous activities, simulate the office environment and workflows, and record patient messages in Harris CareTracker PM and EMR.

Message Center Templates

The *Messages* application is a communication tool accessed via the patient's medical record that allows you to manage customer, staff, and patient communications. The application supports the clinical workflow by providing the ability to create a *ToDo* by attaching PDF documents or image files (jpg, gif, tif, etc.) and links with patient information. This helps the provider coordinate patient care activities during a patient visit and electronically communicate that information in real-time to front office and clinical staff in your practice. This also helps the clinical staff monitor and complete tasks efficiently as a patient goes through the visit and ensures that no important tasks are left undone.

When a patient checks out from an appointment, the patient is automatically pulled into context, and all *ToDos* for orders, prescriptions, referrals, educational handouts, and the chart summary display as patient *ToDos*, enabling the person responsible to manage and complete the tasks efficiently. Patient-related *ToDos* also display in the *Correspondence* and *Open Activities* sections of the patient's medical record. The *Messages* application is a combination of *ToDos, Mail, Queues,* and *Fax.*

Use the steps outlined in Activity 8-16 to access the *Messages* application each time you are instructed to create a *ToDo* or *Mail* message.

ACTIVITY 8-16:   Access the Messages Application

1. Pull patient Jane Morgan into context and click the *Medical Record* module.

2. In the *Clinical Toolbar,* click the drop-down arrow next to *Msg Cntr* ☑ and select *New ToDo.* Harris CareTracker EMR displays the *New ToDo* dialog box. Click "X" in the top right corner of the window to close it.

Tip Box

The *ToDo* application is also accessible by clicking the *ToDo* ☑ icon or the *ToDo* button in other applications accessed via the patient's medical record.

You can use templates to create preformatted content for *ToDos*, faxes, and mail messages. For example, you can create a standard mail message used for outgoing referrals. Anytime that template is selected the mail message is automatically populated with the text in the template. (Templates are discussed in detail in Chapter 2.)

ToDos

ToDos are Harris CareTracker PM and EMR's internal messaging system that serves two primary functions: assigning a co-worker a task and communicating with the Harris CareTracker PM and EMR support team. You can also view *ToDos* for a patient if the *Messages* application is accessed when a patient is in context.

Create a ToDo. In Chapter 2 you created a "test" *ToDo* (see Activity 2-18). Now you will create a clinical *ToDo* related to EMR.

ACTIVITY 8-17: Create a ToDo

1. Pull patient Christina Stoned into context and click the *Medical Record* module.
2. Click on the *Msg Center* icon in the *Clinical Toolbar*. This will launch the *New ToDo* window.
3. By default, the *From* list displays your operator name.
4. Table 8-4 describes the options available in the *To* list. Select "Operator."

TABLE 8-4 The "To" List

Field	Description
Operator	Enables you to select an Harris CareTracker user from your company.
Queue	Enables you to select a work queue set up for the practice to redirect the *ToDo* to a queue. For example, you can send a *ToDo* to the Practice queue (e.g., Front Desk, Nursing, etc.) and an operator in the queue will respond to the *ToDo*.
Participant	Enables you to select a participant in the *ToDo*. This can be a person or a queue that participated in the *ToDo*.

Courtesy of Harris CareTracker PM and EMR

5. If a patient is in context when sending a *ToDo*, the patient's name displays in the *Patient* box. If no patient is in context, click the *Search* icon next to the *Patient* list. The *Patient Search* dialog box displays, enabling you to enter the required parameters to search for the patient.

CLINICAL SPOTLIGHT

You can click on the *At A Glance* icon to view more information about the patient. However, the patient information does not include advance directive information. To delete a patient from context in the message, click the *Remove* icon.

6. By default, the *Subject* box displays information based on the selection in the *Type* and *Reason* lists. However, you can change the subject if necessary. Leave as is.

7. In the *Due Date* and *Due Time* boxes, enter the date and time by which the *ToDo* must be completed. This is important to track overdue items. Change to the date Ms. Stoned called the office requesting the referral (June 5, 2013). Leave *Due Time* box blank.

8. (Optional) From the *Template* list, select the template you want to use. (You must select a macro before selecting a template.) Leave blank.

9. From the *Category* list, select the appropriate *ToDo* category. (For example, if the *ToDo* created is for the Harris CareTracker PM and EMR *Support* entity, select "Support Center" from the *Category* list.) Select "Interoffice."

10. By default, the *Type* list displays "EHR". Leave as is.

11. By default, the *Reason* list displays "Other." However, you can click a different reason for creating the *ToDo*. Select "Phone Call (Patient)."

12. In the *Severity* list, click the priority of the *ToDo*. Select "Medium."

Tip Box

Click the *Info* icon to view a description of each severity level.

13. By default the *Status* list is set to "Open." Leave as is.

14. Leave the *Duration* box blank.

FYI

Additional/Optional *ToDo* Features:
- (Optional) You can click *Chart Viewer* to access clinical information for the patient in context. The *Chart Viewer* button displays only if you have the EHR-Mid and EHR-Provider roles or have the *ToDo – Chart Viewer* override included in your operator profile. The *Chart Viewer* button is active only if a patient is attached to the *ToDo*.
- (Optional) Click the *Add Attachments* link to attach a document to the *ToDo*. The *Document Management Upload* dialog box displays, enabling you to attach or scan a document or link a voice attachment to the *ToDo*. (This feature is not available in your student environment.)
- (Optional) You can click the attachment name to view the document in the document viewer. All markups made to a document attached to a *ToDo* can be saved by clicking *Save*. However, if you edit the document information, you must click *Upload* to save the changes made.
- If a patient is in context, Harris CareTracker PM and EMR displays the *Link Patient Data* link. You can click the link to attach other documents for the patient using the *ToDo Attachments/Links* dialog box.

15. In the *Notes* box, enter additional notes pertaining to the *ToDo*. You can format the note and spell-check the note entered. This is similar to the formatting toolbar in MS Word®. Enter the text from Figure 8-33, regarding referral to Dr. Rovner.

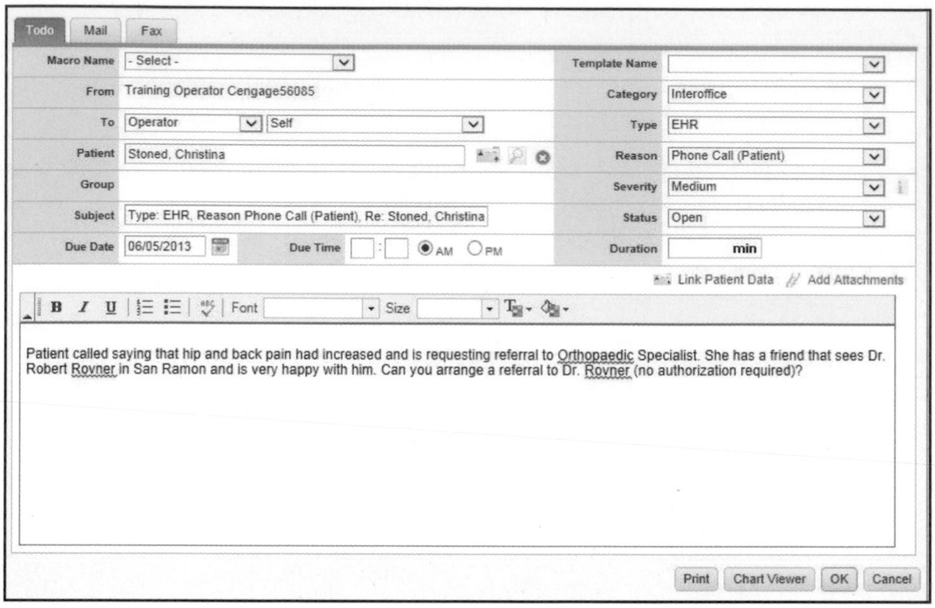

Figure 8-33 Christina Stoned ToDo Requesting Referral

16. Click *OK*.

CLINICAL SP⬤TLIGHT

If the *ToDo* is for a patient, it is saved under the *Correspondence* application of the Financial module when the patient is in context, and the *Correspondence* and *Open Activities* section of the patient's medical record. In addition, all *ToDos* are also saved in the *ToDo* list of the people involved in the *ToDo*, the owner of the *ToDo*, and the person who was assigned the *ToDo*.

17. Refresh your *Home* module screen. The *ToDo* will be listed in the bottom left corner of the screen. Click on the *ToDo* link to view the *ToDo List* window (Figure 8-34).

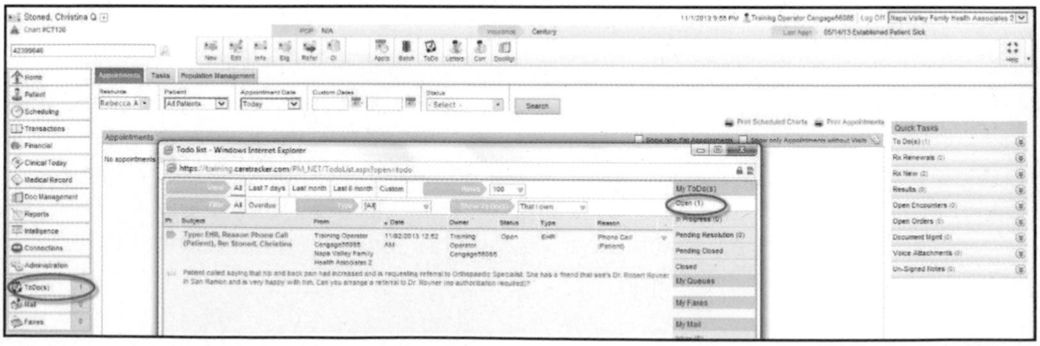

Figure 8-34 ToDo List Window

18. Now repeat the activity and create *ToDos* as listed in Table 8-5. For each *ToDo* in Table 8-5 use the *Category* "Interoffice," *Type* "EHR," and *Reason* "Phone Call (Patient)."

TABLE 8-5	New ToDo Messages				
From	**To**	**Subject**	**Severity**	**Notes (message)**	**Patient**
You	You (Provider: Raman)	Fall/Refer to X-ray	High	Patient fell at home and hand is in extreme pain. He wants to know if he can get an X-ray in the office today, or if he should go to Urgent Care. Please call on cell phone ASAP. OK to leave message.	Domenic Scott
You	You (Provider: Raman)	Medication Question	Medium	Patient wants to know if he can take a multivitamin while he is taking Coumadin. Please advise, and I can return call to patient. Thank you.	Bradley Torez
You	You	Referral/ Authorization Status	Medium	Patient called and wants to know if her request for referral and authorization for MRI has been ordered. Please call patient at home phone between 3:00 and 5:00 PM. OK to leave message on voicemail.	Kimberly Johnson

Print a screenshot of the contents of the *ToDo*s you created. Label them "Activity 8-17a," "Activity 8-17b," "Activity 8-17c," and "Activity 8-17d" and place them in your assignment folder.

Critical Thinking

What would happen if you closed a *ToDo* that had not been resolved? For example, MA Sally closed a *ToDo* sent to her by Dr. Raman regarding patient Mr. Scott before she called him back with instructions to go immediately to the hospital (call 911) and to follow up regarding his status, and make follow-up office visit. Where does the original message go? Who would know it was not completed or that MA Sally had not followed Dr. Raman's instructions? What are the ramifications of closing *ToDo* messages? Write a one-page paper answering these questions, and then prepare another document creating what you consider to be "Best Practice" instructions for closing *ToDos*. Submit to your instructor for discussion.

Mail

The *Mail* application is similar to any standard e-mail application and allows you to send, receive, organize, and reply to mail messages. In Chapter 2, Activity 2-19, you created a "Test Mail Message." This chapter expands by creating new *Mail* messages that mimic clinical workflows.

Create a New Mail Message.   The *Mail* application allows you to communicate electronically with staff members, providers in your *Provider Portal,* and patients activated in the *Patient Portal.* The mail feature works similarly to other e-mail applications, enabling you to open, view, create, send and receive, and delete messages. In Harris CareTracker PM and EMR, the mail application is a secure messaging system that users can participate in by invitation only and allows a user to send secure messages outside of the Harris CareTracker system to patients through the patient portal or to referring doctors who are part of the referral network. This is different from e-mail because it is on a secure server, but the use and functions within the mail system are similar to standard e-mail. In addition, you can link attachments such as patient encounter notes, documents, results, referrals, and authorization forms and set priorities and more. As a general rule, the *Mail* feature should only be used when sending a message to someone outside the practice, for example, to refer to providers (outside the practice), or to patients active in the *Patient Portal.* Figure 8-35 lists the tabs available to use when selecting a mail recipient (*My Company, Provider Portal,* or *Patients*). (**Note:** For your training environment, you will use only the *My Company* tab.)

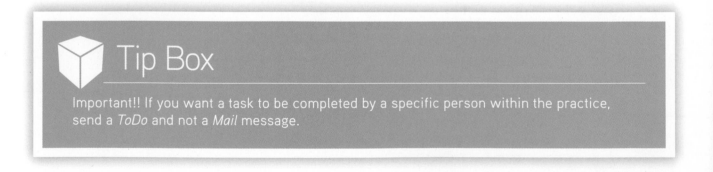

Figure 8-35   Select Mail Recipient

Tip Box

Important!! If you want a task to be completed by a specific person within the practice, send a *ToDo* and not a *Mail* message.

Tip Box

You can use the *Mail Message Templates* to create preformatted content for mail messages. For example, you can create a standard mail message used for outgoing referrals. Anytime that template is selected, the mail message is automatically populated with the text in the template. *Templates* are created in the *Event Manager* application of the *Administration* module.

ACTIVITY 8-18: Create Mail Message

FYI

This will be a simulated activity because your student version of Harris CareTracker does not include an active *Patient Portal* or *Provider Portal*. For this activity you will remain in the *My Company* tab.

1. With no patient in context, click the *Home* module and then click the *Messages* tab. The *Messages Center* opens and displays all of your open *ToDos*.
2. Click *Send Mail* in the bottom right corner of the screen (Figure 8-36), which opens the *New Mail* dialog box.

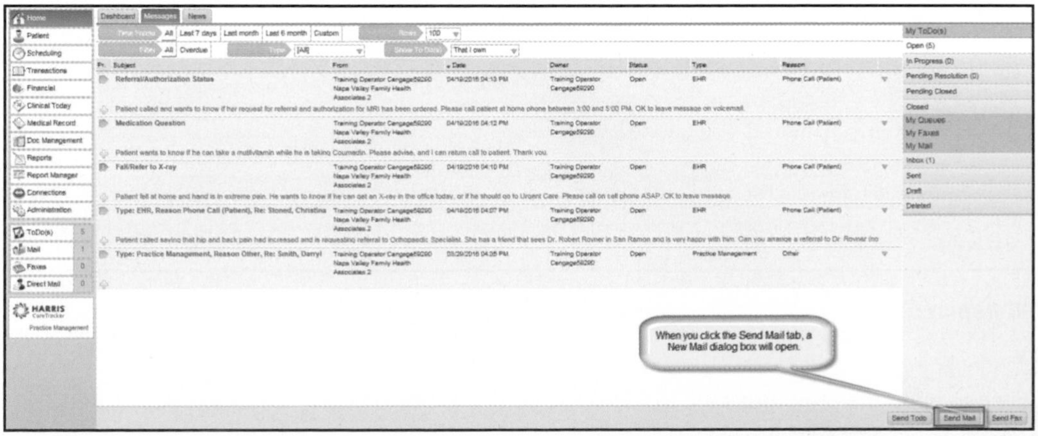

Courtesy of Harris CareTracker PM and EMR

Figure 8-36 Send Mail Button

3. (FYI) The *From* list defaults to the operator creating the mail message (you) and cannot be edited.

4. In the *To* field, click the *Search* 🔍 icon. Harris CareTracker PM and EMR opens the *Select Operators* dialog box. You will be the only operator available to select (along with any operators you have created). In a live environment you would select the most appropriate person (this could also be a provider or a patient). Check the box next to your operator name and click *Select* at the bottom of the screen.

LEGAL SP⬤TLIGHT

If sending *Mail* messages to a patient, be sure to follow HIPAA policy and protocol.

5. If a patient is in context, the patient's name displays in the *Patient* box. However, you can also send a mail message about a different patient by clicking on the *Search* 🔍 icon. You can delete a patient from the list by clicking the *Remove Patient* ⊗ icon. There should be no patient in context, so leave the *Patient* field blank.

6. In the *Subject* box, enter "Cardiology Group Presentation." If the subject is patient related, be sure the correct patient's name displays in the *Subject* box. If the message does not relate to a patient, be sure to remove the patient's name. Remove any patient from the *Subject* box.

7. By default, the *Severity* list displays "Medium." However, you can change the priority of the mail message if necessary. Leave as is.

8. In the *Notes* box, enter the message and format the information as directed in Figure 8-37. (Sign the note with your operator number.)

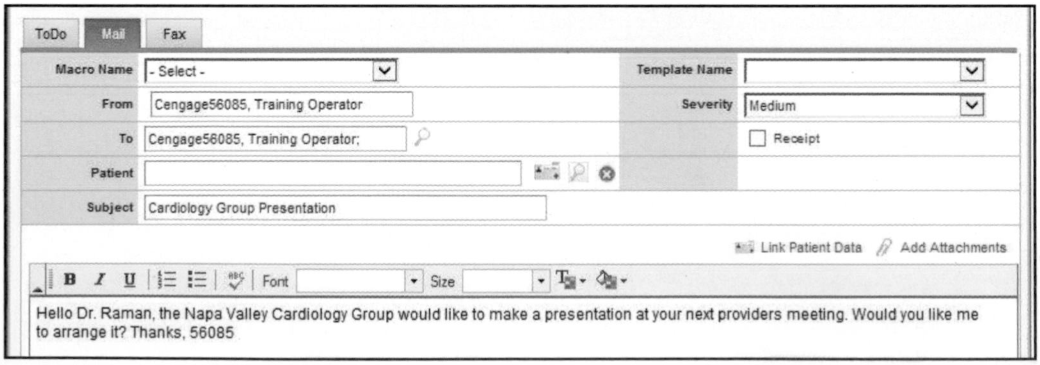

Figure 8-37   Mail Message – Cardiology Group

9. Click *Send* to send the mail message to the selected operators. The message(s) you created will now appear in your *Inbox* (see Figure 8-40).

10. Repeat these steps to create the *Patient Portal* and Office Holiday Party messages in Figures 8-38 and 8-39. Figure 8-40 shows your *Inbox* with all these messages.

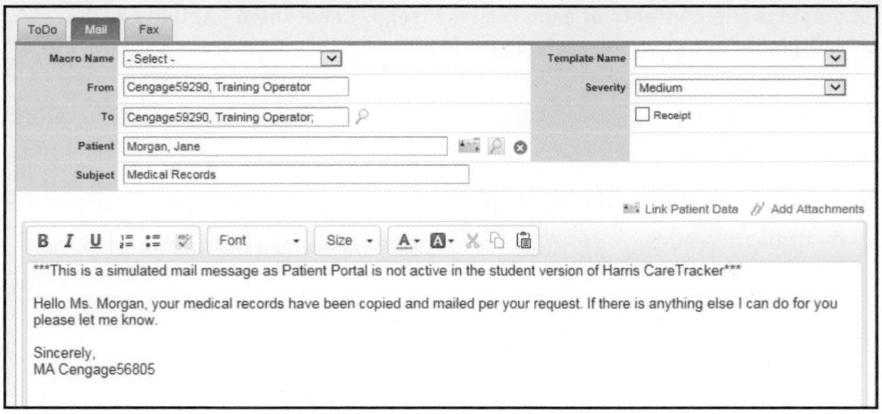

Courtesy of Harris CareTracker PM and EMR

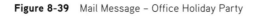

Figure 8-38 Mail Message – Patient Portal

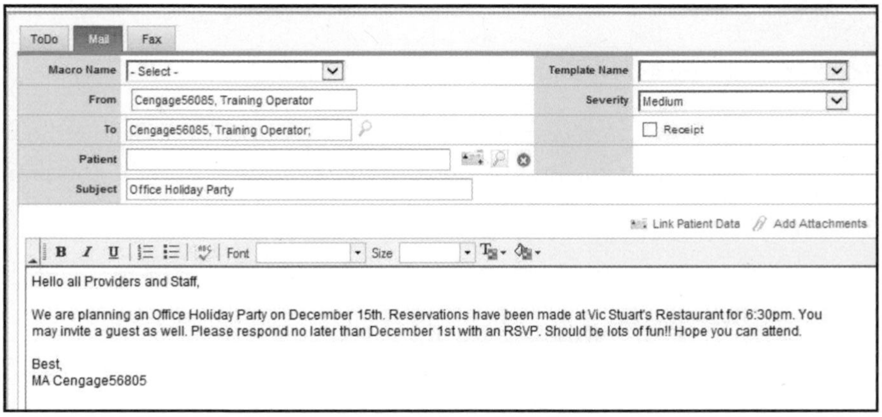

Courtesy of Harris CareTracker PM and EMR

Figure 8-39 Mail Message – Office Holiday Party

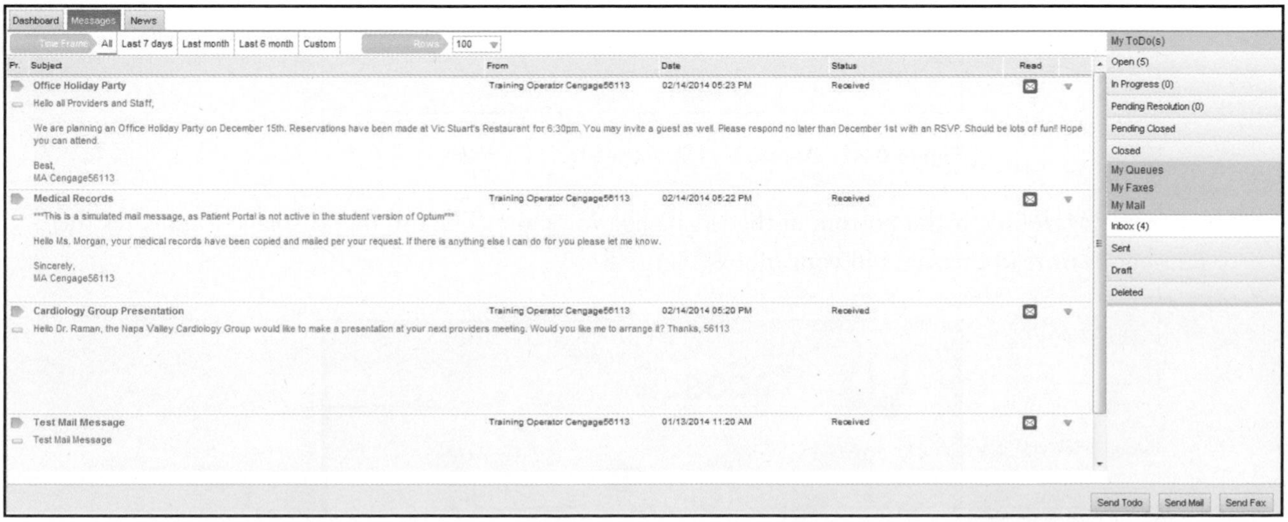

Courtesy of Harris CareTracker PM and EMR

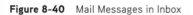

Figure 8-40 Mail Messages in Inbox

Print the screen that displays the contents of each mail message. Label them "Activity 8-18a," "Activity 8-18b," and "Activity 8-18c" and place them in your assignment folder.

Manage Mail. Similar to any standard e-mail application, the *Mail* application allows you to send, receive, organize, and reply to mail messages. *Managing Mail* consists of:

- Accessing *Mail* Messages
- Viewing *Mail* Messages
- Moving *Mail* Messages
- Replying to a *Mail* Message
- Forwarding a *Mail* Message
- Deleting a *Mail* Message
- Working with Attachments

Accessing Mail Messages. There are two ways to access your mail:

- In the *Home* module, click the *Messages* tab and then click the *Inbox* link below the *My Mail* section on the right side of the window. The number next to the *Inbox* indicates the total number of unread mail messages (Figure 8-41).

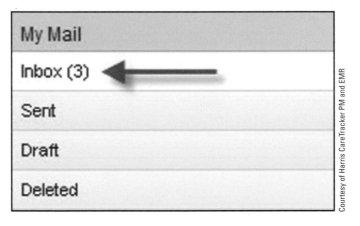

Figure 8-41 Access Mail Messages from the Inbox Link

- Click the *Mail* link at the bottom of the left navigation pane. The number displayed indicates the number of unread messages in your inbox (Figure 8-42).

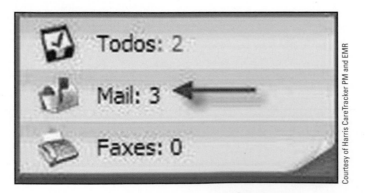

Figure 8-42 Access Mail Messages from the Mail Link

View Mail Messages. The *Mail* application displays all mail messages sent to you. A mail message is used as a method of sharing information and may or may not require a return action. The functionality is similar to any other e-mail application such as *Outlook*®, *Outlook Express*®, *Yahoo!*, and *Gmail*. The inbox is easy to customize (Figure 8-43):

- Click any of the column headings to sort the messages in the inbox by *Priority, Subject, Date*, and so on.
- Click the filters at the top of the page to view mail messages based on the time period (*Last 7 days, Last month*, etc.), or click the *Custom* tab to enter a specific date range.
- Click the *Rows* list to select the number of messages to display.

Filters
Click headings to sort
View
All
Last 7 days
Last month
Last 6 month
Custom
Rows: 100
Pr.
Subject
From
Date
Status
Read
Actions
Fw: Johnson, Geoffery
Re: Johnson, Geoffery
The patient needs to reschedule his appointment for 6/1/10 at 12:30.
Re: Johnson, Geoffery
I rescheduled the appointment and I will call the patient ot confirm.

Courtesy of Harris CareTracker PM and EMR

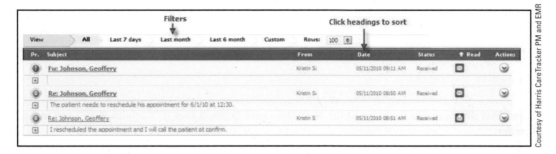

Figure 8-43 Customize Inbox

ACTIVITY 8-19: View Mail Messages

1. Access your mail messages from the *Home* module.
2. Click the *Messages* tab and then click the *Inbox* link below the *My Mail* section on the right side of the window. (**Note**: You may have to refresh your screen for the recent activity to display.)
3. Click on the plus sign [+] next to the messages to quickly review the message thread without opening the message. Now click the minus sign [-] to close the thread (Figure 8-44).

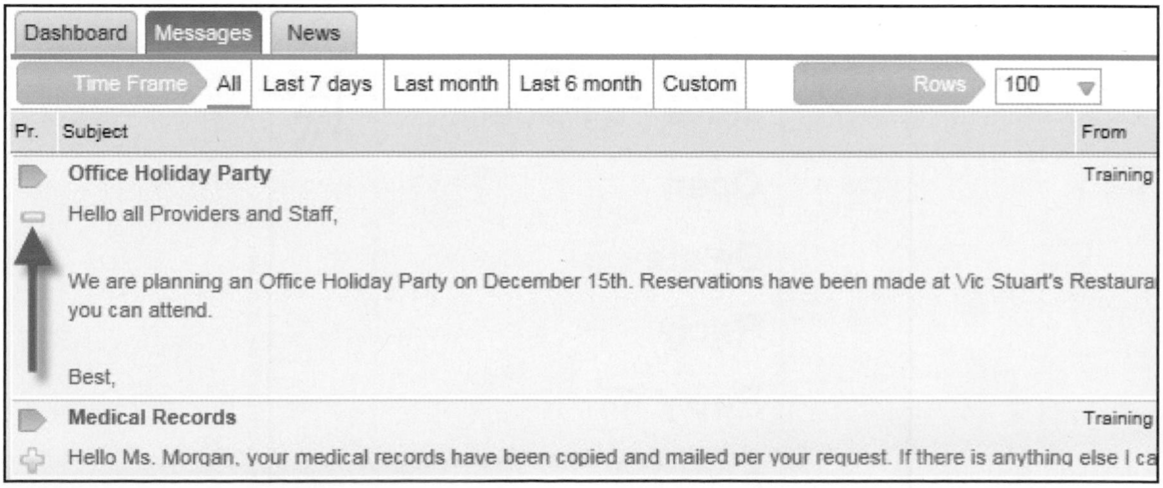

Dashboard
Messages
News
Time Frame
All
Last 7 days
Last month
Last 6 month
Custom
Rows
100
Pr.
Subject
From
Office Holiday Party
Training
Hello all Providers and Staff,
We are planning an Office Holiday Party on December 15th. Reservations have been made at Vic Stuart's Restaura
you can attend.
Best,
Medical Records
Training
Hello Ms. Morgan, your medical records have been copied and mailed per your request. If there is anything else I ca

Courtesy of Harris CareTracker PM and EMR

Figure 8-44 Review Mail Message Thread

4. To open the mail message, either click on the *Subject* line or point to the *Arrow* ▼ icon at the far right end of the row, and then select "Open." Harris CareTracker PM and EMR opens the message.

5. From the *Actions* column you can choose to reply to, forward, or delete the mail message (Figure 8-45). (You will move, reply, forward, and delete messages in later activities.)

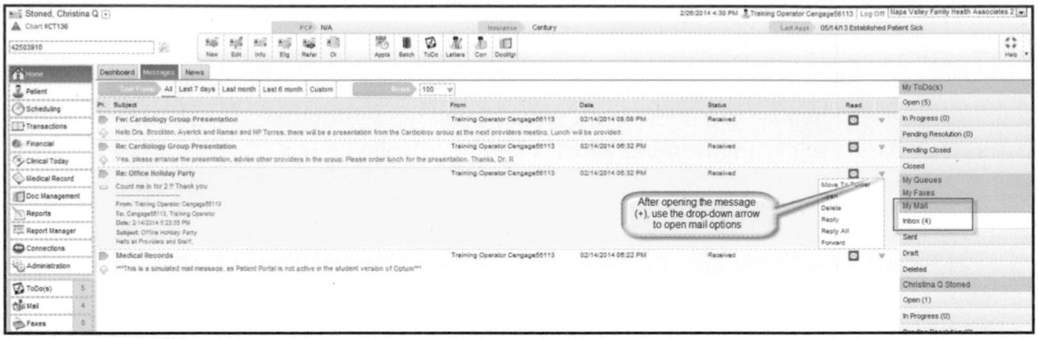

Figure 8-45   Mail Options

🌿 **Print the screen that displays the contents of the Mail Messages Inbox. Label it "Activity 8-19" and place it in your assignment folder.**

Moving Mail Messages.   You have the option to move mail messages to the *Inbox, Sent, Draft*, and *Deleted* folders.

ACTIVITY 8-20:   Move a Mail Message

1. Access your mail messages. You will be moving the message "Test Mail Message."

2. In the "Test Mail Message" row, point to the *Arrow* ▼ icon and then select "Move To Folder" (Figure 8-46). Harris CareTracker PM and EMR displays the *Select Folder* dialog box (Figure 8-47).

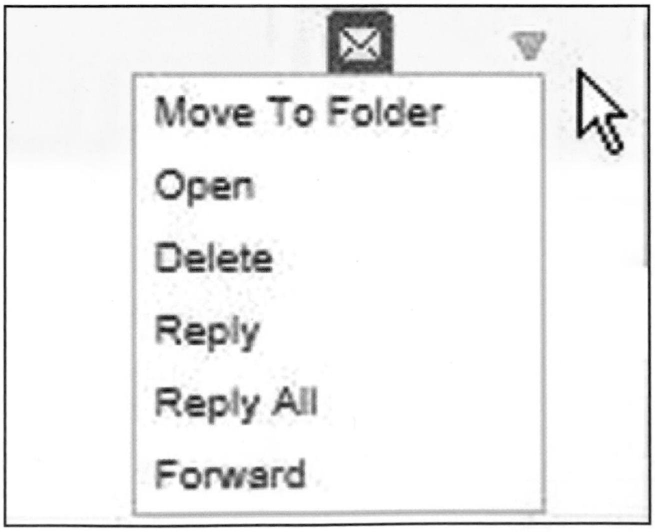

Figure 8-46   Action Column Options

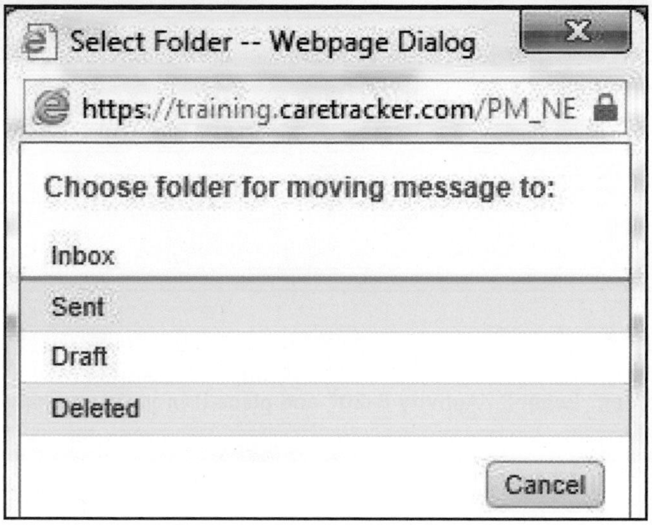

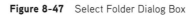

Figure 8-47   Select Folder Dialog Box

3. Click on the folder you want to move the mail message to. Move to "Deleted." The mail is moved to the selected folder.

4. Under *My Mail,* click the *Deleted* link (Figure 8-48). The message you deleted will display (Figure 8-49).

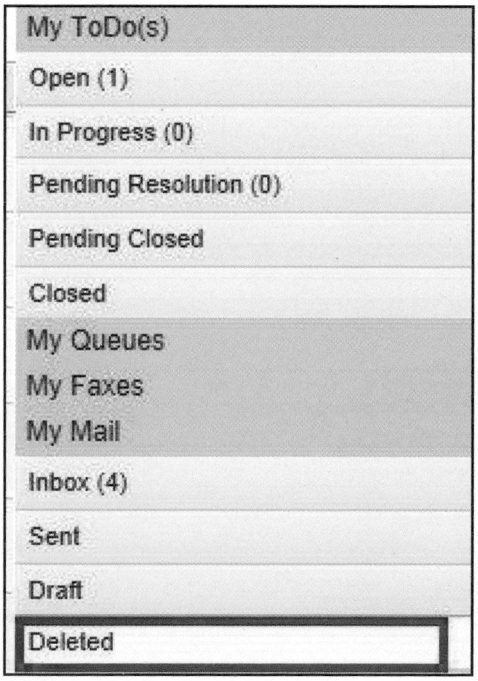

Figure 8-48   My Mail Deleted Link

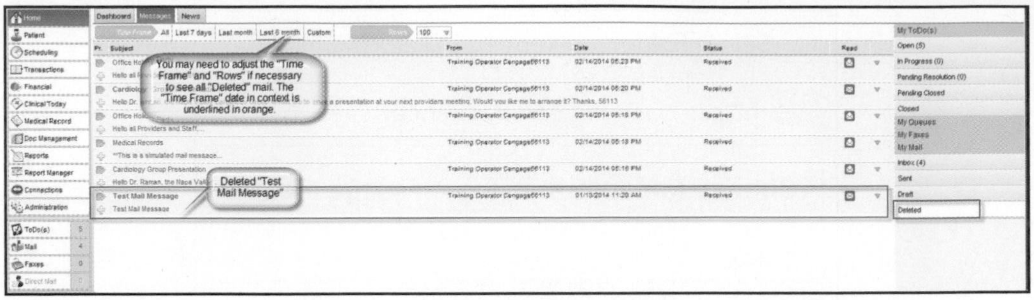

Figure 8-49 Deleted Mail Messages

Print the Deleted message screen. Label it "Activity 8-20" and place it in your assignment folder.

Replying to a Mail Message. To reply to a mail message, follow the instructions in Activity 8-21.

ACTIVITY 8-21: Reply to a Mail Message

1. Access the mail messages in your *Inbox.* You will reply to the mail message "Office Holiday Party."

2. To reply to only the sender, point to the *Arrow* ▼ icon in the *Actions* column and then click "Reply."

Tip Box

If there are multiple recipients on a mail message, you can reply to all of the recipients by pointing the *Arrow* ▼ icon in the *Actions* column and clicking *Reply All.*

3. Type the reply message as noted in Figure 8-50.

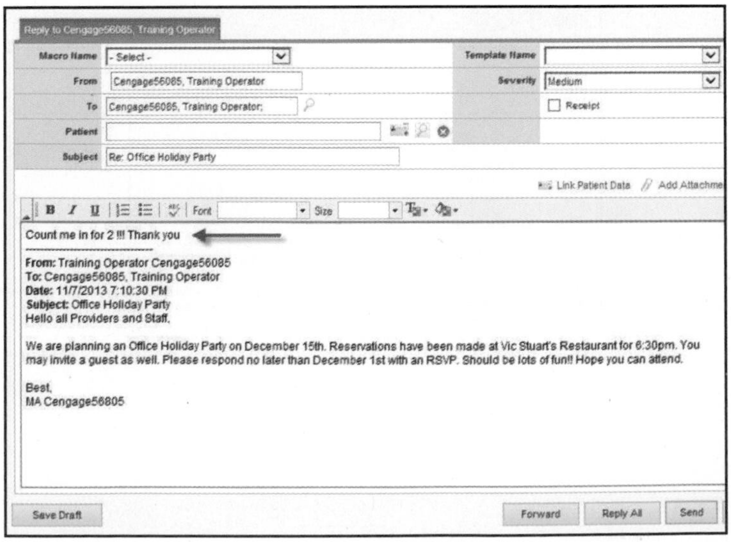

Figure 8-50 Office Holiday Party Reply Message

4. Click *Send*. You may need to refresh your screen before the message appears in your *Inbox*.

5. Repeat the activity and reply to the "Cardiology Group Presentation." Type the reply message as noted in Figure 8-51 and click *Send*.

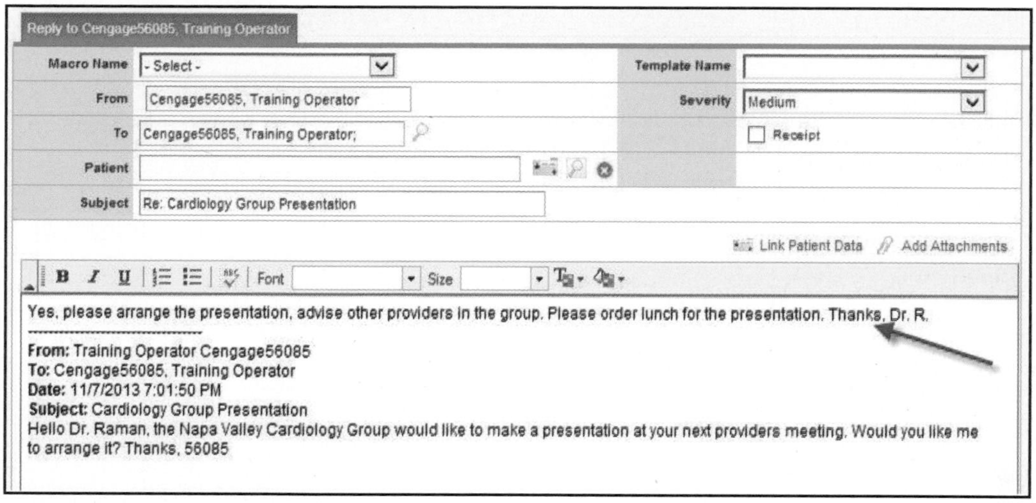

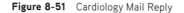

Reply to Cengage56085, Training Operator				
Macro Name	- Select - ▾	Template Name		▾
From	Cengage56085, Training Operator	Severity	Medium	▾
To	Cengage56085, Training Operator; 🔍	☐ Receipt		
Patient	🔍 ⊗			
Subject	Re: Cardiology Group Presentation			

🔲 Link Patient Data   🖉 Add Attachments

B *I* U ≣ ≣ ᴬᴮᶜ Font [   ] ▾ Size [   ] ▾ T̲ ▾ ◊ ▾

Yes, please arrange the presentation, advise other providers in the group. Please order lunch for the presentation. Thanks, Dr. R.

From: Training Operator Cengage56085
To: Cengage56085, Training Operator
Date: 11/7/2013 7:01:50 PM
Subject: Cardiology Group Presentation
Hello Dr. Raman, the Napa Valley Cardiology Group would like to make a presentation at your next providers meeting. Would you like me to arrange it? Thanks, 56085

Courtesy of Harris CareTracker PM and EMR

Figure 8-51   Cardiology Mail Reply

Print each screen that displays the mail message reply. Label them "Activity 8-21a" and "Activity 8-21b" and place them in your assignment folder.

Forwarding a Mail Message.   Forwarding allows you to send the original mail message to a new recipient.

ACTIVITY 8-22:   Forward a Mail Message

1. Access your *Inbox*. You will forward the mail message "Cardiology Group Presentation."

2. In the *Actions* column, point to the *Arrow* ▼ icon and then select "Forward." Harris CareTracker PM and EMR displays the *Forward Message* window.

3. In the *To* field, click the *Search* 🔍 icon. The *Select Operators* dialog box displays. In this training environment, you will be the only operator listed (along with any operators you have created).

4. Select the checkbox next to the person (you) to whom you want to forward the message.

5. Click *Select*. Harris CareTracker PM and EMR closes the *Select Operators* dialog box. Free text the message to forward (see Figure 8-52 for text entry).

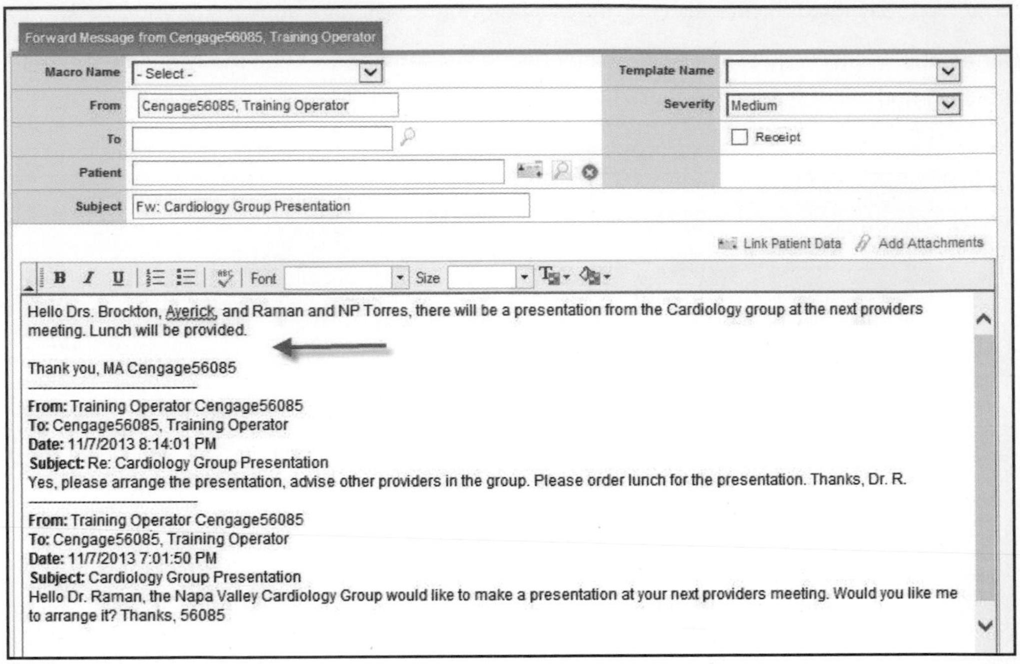

Forward Message from Cengage56085, Training Operator

Macro Name	- Select - ⌄			Template Name	⌄
From	Cengage56085, Training Operator			Severity	Medium ⌄
To	⌕				☐ Receipt
Patient		🔲 🔍 ⊗			
Subject	Fw: Cardiology Group Presentation				

🔲 Link Patient Data   🖉 Add Attachments

B *I* U | 1≡ ≡ | ᵃᵇᶜ | Font [⌄] Size [⌄] Tₐ ▾ ◒ ▾

Hello Drs. Brockton, Averick, and Raman and NP Torres, there will be a presentation from the Cardiology group at the next providers meeting. Lunch will be provided.

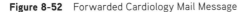

Thank you, MA Cengage56085

From: Training Operator Cengage56085
To: Cengage56085, Training Operator
Date: 11/7/2013 8:14:01 PM
Subject: Re: Cardiology Group Presentation
Yes, please arrange the presentation, advise other providers in the group. Please order lunch for the presentation. Thanks, Dr. R.

From: Training Operator Cengage56085
To: Cengage56085, Training Operator
Date: 11/7/2013 7:01:50 PM
Subject: Cardiology Group Presentation
Hello Dr. Raman, the Napa Valley Cardiology Group would like to make a presentation at your next providers meeting. Would you like me to arrange it? Thanks, 56085

Courtesy of Harris CareTracker PM and EMR

Figure 8-52   Forwarded Cardiology Mail Message

6. Click *Send*. The message is forwarded to the selected recipients.

⬤ **Print the screen that displays the forwarded mail message. Label it "Activity 8-22" and place it in your assignment folder.**

Deleting a Mail Message.   Once you finish with a mail message it is best practice to clean up your mail box. This means you should delete messages that no longer require attention or a response.

ACTIVITY 8-23:   Delete a Mail Message

1. Access your *Inbox*. You will delete the original "Office Holiday Party" and "Cardiology Group Presentation" messages.

2. In the *Actions* column for each message, point to the *Arrow* ▼ icon and then select "Delete." Harris CareTracker PM and EMR deletes the message from the list.

3. Click the *Deleted* link under *My Mail* to view your deleted message. Figure 8-49 represents the *Deleted Mail Messages* in your *My Mail* tab.

⬤ **Print the screen that displays the deleted mail messages. Label it "Activity 8-23" and place it in your assignment folder.**

Working with Attachments.   If a *ToDo, Mail* message, or *Fax* contains an attachment, you can save the attached file in the *Document Management* application (Figure 8-53). The *Document Management* feature is not available in your student version of Harris CareTracker PM and EMR.

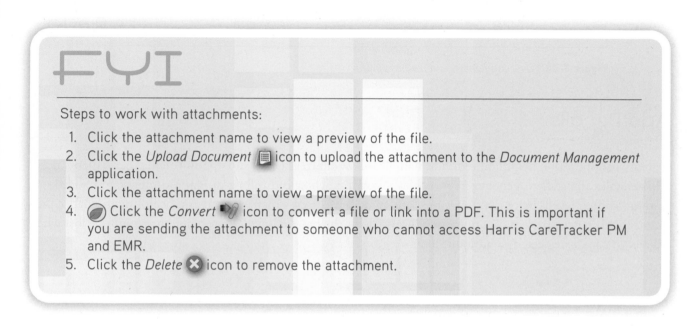

Figure 8-53   Working with Attachments

FYI

Steps to work with attachments:

1. Click the attachment name to view a preview of the file.
2. Click the *Upload Document* 📄 icon to upload the attachment to the *Document Management* application.
3. Click the attachment name to view a preview of the file.
4. ⬤ Click the *Convert* 📎 icon to convert a file or link into a PDF. This is important if you are sending the attachment to someone who cannot access Harris CareTracker PM and EMR.
5. Click the *Delete* ✖ icon to remove the attachment.

RECALL LETTERS

Learning Objective 4: Create and update patient Recall Letters.

Recalls are reminders to patients that an appointment needs to be booked. Rather than scheduling a future appointment, a recall date is set for the appointment in the *Scheduling* module. Harris CareTracker PM and EMR tracks all recalls, enabling you to generate recall letters at the appropriate time intervals. The *Recalls/ Letters Due* application allows you to generate and print letters and labels for the following:

- Appointment Recalls
- Appointment Reminders
- Missed/Cancelled Appointments

Recalls are categorized by recall type and age. A recall is considered overdue if the recall has not been linked to a patient appointment prior to the date of the recall. When a patient calls to schedule an appointment, his or her recall will be linked to the appointment and will be removed from the *Recall* application.

Harris CareTracker PM and EMR automatically generates an appointment reminder for any patient entered into the *Recall* application and generates letters and envelope labels for printing. This application helps the office to keep track of patient visits and provide proper medical care.

For example, when a patient schedules an appointment, you can manually link the recall to the appointment if necessary. If the appointment type scheduled is the same as the existing recall, Harris CareTracker PM and EMR links the appointment to the recall, making it inactive. If the patient cancels an appointment linked to a recall, the recall changes to an active recall and displays on the *Overdue Recalls and Letters* link on the *Dashboard* (Figure 8-54). The *Recall* application helps review, add, and update recalls saved for the patient.

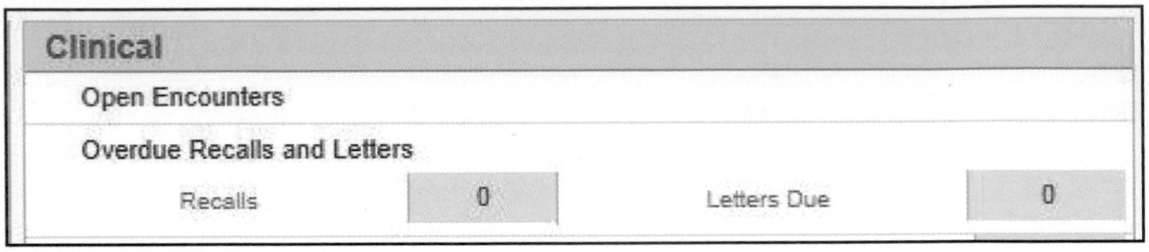

Figure 8-54   Overdue Recalls and Letters Link

Add Recalls

The *Recall* application helps add reminders about follow-up treatments and appointments that patients need. This enables the staff to generate reports about patients who need follow-up appointments and additional testing. Adding recalls helps develop robust and responsive disease management and health maintenance programs for enhanced patient care outcomes. It also helps the practice generate revenue that might be lost when follow-up care is neglected or appointments are missed.

ACTIVITY 8-24:   Add Recalls

1. Pull patient Caroline Sweeney into context. If the pop-up alert advises missing information, update her demographics screen.

2. Click the *Medical Record* module. You see that Ms. Sweeney's last appointment displayed was May 14, 2013, New Patient CPE (Figure 8-55).

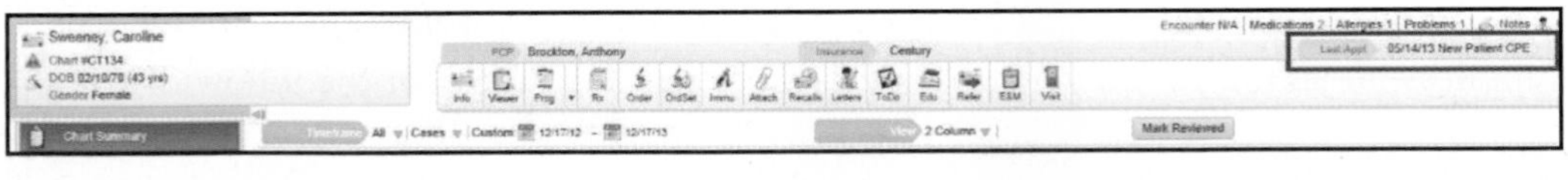

Figure 8-55   Last Appointment Displayed for Caroline Sweeney
Courtesy of Harris CareTracker PM and EMR

3. In the *Clinical Toolbar*, click the *Recalls* icon.

4. If an encounter is in context, Harris CareTracker EMR displays the *Recalls* dialog box. If an encounter is not in context, Harris CareTracker EMR displays the *Select Encounter* dialog box. Select the encounter dated May 14, 2013.

5. Click *+ New Recall* (Figure 8-56). Harris CareTracker EMR displays the *Add Patient Recall* dialog box.

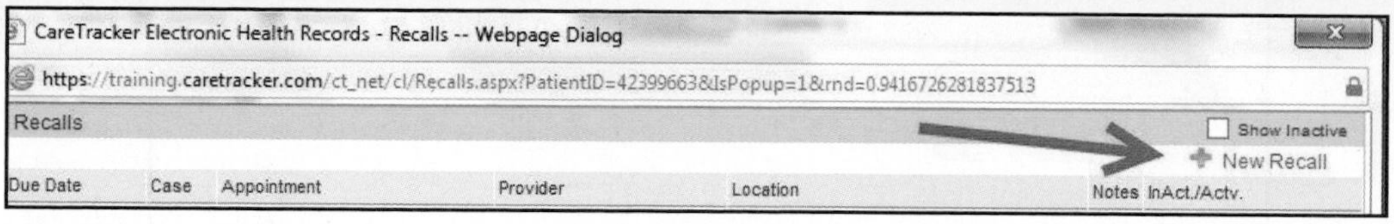

Figure 8-56   Add New Recall

6. In the *Time Frame* list, click the time interval when the patient is expected to return to the office. Select "2 Years".

7. In the *Appointment Type* list, click the reason for the patient recall. Select "Established Patient CPE."

8. In the *Resource* list, click the provider assigned to the recall (Dr. Brockton). This is the preferred provider the patient wants to see during the appointment. (**Note:** If there is no preference, select "Any Provider" from the list.)

9. In the *Location* list, click the preferred location for the appointment. If there is no preference, click "Any Location" from the list. Select "Napa Valley Family Associates."

10. (*FYI*) In the *Case* list, click the case associated with the recall. If no case is associated with a recall, click "Default." A case list would apply in the case of workers' compensation. No case list applies.

Tip Box

If a recall is associated with a case, it is linked to the appointment when scheduled. For example, you can link workers' compensation and auto accident cases to an appointment.

11. By default, the *EMR Alert Status* is set to "No Alert." If required, add an alert to the recall by clicking either "Soft Alert" or "Pop-Up Alert." Select "Soft Alert."

Tip Box

The *pop-up alert* ! displays when the patient's medical record is launched. The alert displays each time the patient's medical record is accessed and stops displaying when the alert is closed. You can also click the *Alert* icon next to the patient's chart number on the *Patient Detail* bar to view both soft and pop-up alerts.

12. In the *Recall Notes* box, enter additional comments for the recall. Enter "Schedule CPE and send Lab Order 30 days prior to appointment for complete panel." (Figure 8-57).

13. In the *Active* field, select "Yes".

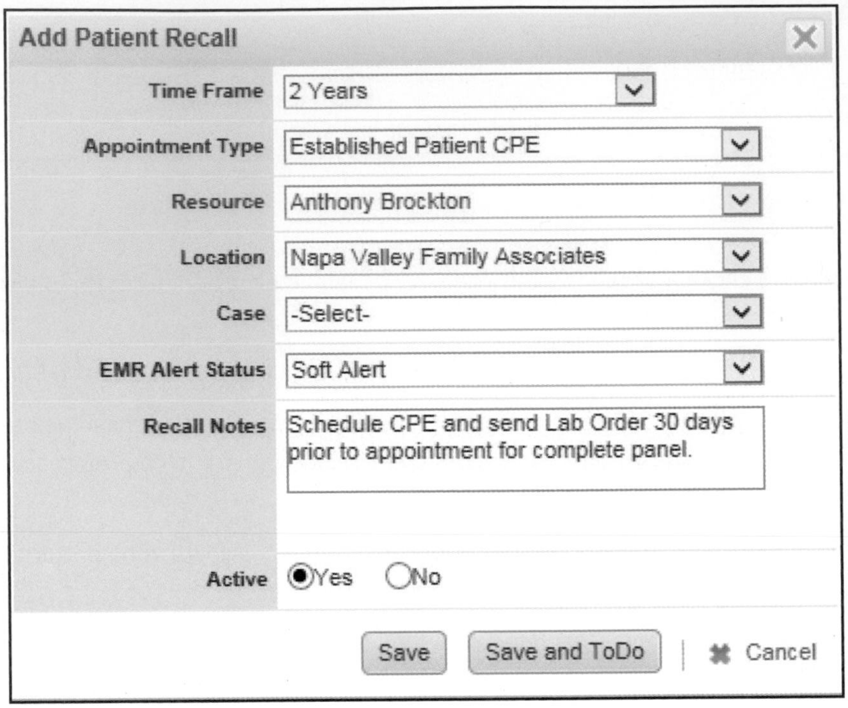

Courtesy of Harris CareTracker PM and EMR

Figure 8-57 Add Recall for Caroline Sweeney

14. Click *Save* to save the recall to the patient's record. (You could also click *Save and ToDo* to send a *ToDo* for the recall saved.) The *Recalls* dialog box displays with the recall just created (Figure 8-58).

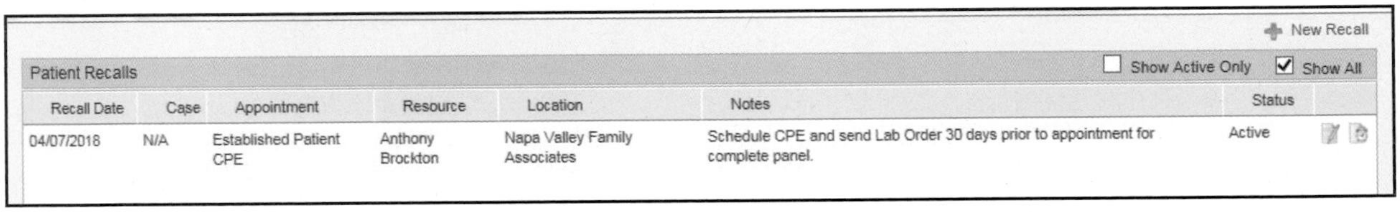

Courtesy of Harris CareTracker PM and EMR

Figure 8-58 Recalls Dialog Box

Tip Box

When creating an interoffice *ToDo* for a recall, the *Type* list displays "EHR" and the *Reason* list displays "Recall Follow-up." Additionally, Harris CareTracker PM and EMR helps generate and print recall letters by accessing the *Home* module and then clicking the *Overdue Recalls and Letters* link under the *Clinical* section. An alternative method is to click the *Administration* module, *Practice* tab, and then click the *Print Batch Letters* link under the *Daily Administration* section.

15. Now repeat the activity for the following patients, using each patient's PCP as provider:

   a. Bruce Thomas (recall for CPE due May 14 of next year). Include a note to send a lab order (complete panel) one month prior to CPE.

   b. Christina Stoned (recall for CPE due June 1 of next year). Include a note to send lab (complete panel) and mammogram orders one month prior to CPE.

Print a copy of each patient's recall. Label the recall summaries "Activity 8-24a," "Activity 8-24b," and "Activity 8-24c" and place them in your assignment folder.

Update Recall Details

The *Recall* application helps update recall details recorded for the patient.

ACTIVITY 8-25:   Update Recall Details

1. Pull patient Caroline Sweeney into context and click the *Medical Record* module.

2. In the *Clinical Toolbar,* click the *Recalls* icon.

3. If an encounter is in context, Harris CareTracker PM and EMR displays the *Recalls* dialog box. If an encounter is not in context, Harris CareTracker PM and EMR displays the *Select Encounter* dialog box. Select the encounter dated May 14, 2013.

4. Find the recall you want to update ("Established Patient CPE" you created in Activity 8-24).

5. Click on the *Edit* icon next to the recall and make the necessary changes to the available information. Dr. Brockton is having his non-Medicare patients see NP Torres for CPEs. Change the provider to NP Torres.

6. Click *Save*. The existing recall for the patient is updated.

> ## Tip Box
>
> To deactivate an open recall, click the *Edit* icon and change the *Active* field to "No." To activate a recall, click the *Edit* icon and change the *Active* field to "Yes."

Print a copy of the updated recall, label it "Activity 8-25," and place it in your assignment folder.

RUNNING AN IMMUNIZATION LOT NUMBER REPORT

Learning Objective 5: Run an immunization report using the Clinical Export feature.

There are many reasons to run immunization lot number reports. For example, occasionally you will receive a notice that certain lot numbers of a product have been recalled by the Food and Drug Administration (FDA). Lot numbers provide a source of comfort during a recall because each immunization is recorded in the EMR and various reports can be run to track which patients received the immunization. In addition, a practice can monitor inventory and expiration of immunizations on hand and also use the report for internal audit purposes.

Immunization Export

The *Immunization Export* application allows a practice to generate a record of all vaccinations given during a specified time period. This application pulls the Harris CareTracker PM and EMR data into a state-specific format that can be downloaded and then sent to the state's department of health.

In Activity 8-26 you will take the appropriate steps after your practice has received a letter from a drug company recalling a specific lot number. The *Immunization* records will be generated on the report so that you can contact any patient who received the immunization. You would then relay to the patient that the drug may not be effective and that it is recommended that the patient come in to have a **titer** (labs drawn). A titer determines how much antibody is present in the patient's blood to fight a specific antigen (disease-causing agent). If the levels are at an acceptable level to protect the patient, the test results will indicate that the patient has reached full immunity against the disease. In this case, it would mean that the immunization given reached its desired effect. However, if the test results indicate that the patient is not immune, the patient will need to return for another immunization to reach full immunity.

FYI

Export Immunization Data
Your student version of Harris CareTracker PM and EMR is not associated with an immunization registry; therefore, you cannot export data. However, in a live practice, the steps to *Export Immunization Data* are as follows:

1. Click the *Administration* module and then click the *Clinical* tab.
2. Click the *Immunization Export* link. Harris CareTracker PM and EMR launches the application.
3. In the *Start Date* and *End Date* fields, click the calendar icon and select the date range for which you want to export immunization records. Select start date January 1, 2013, and end date "today." Click the *Clock* icon to populate the box with today's date.
4. In the *State Formats* section, select the checkbox next to each state for which you want to export immunization records. Select "Arizona."
5. (*Optional*) The *Exclude previously downloaded patients* checkbox is selected by default. Deselect the checkbox to include patients who were previously downloaded.

6. Click *Build My File*(s). Harris CareTracker PM and EMR generates the immunization form(s) and displays download links at the bottom of the window (Figure 8-59).

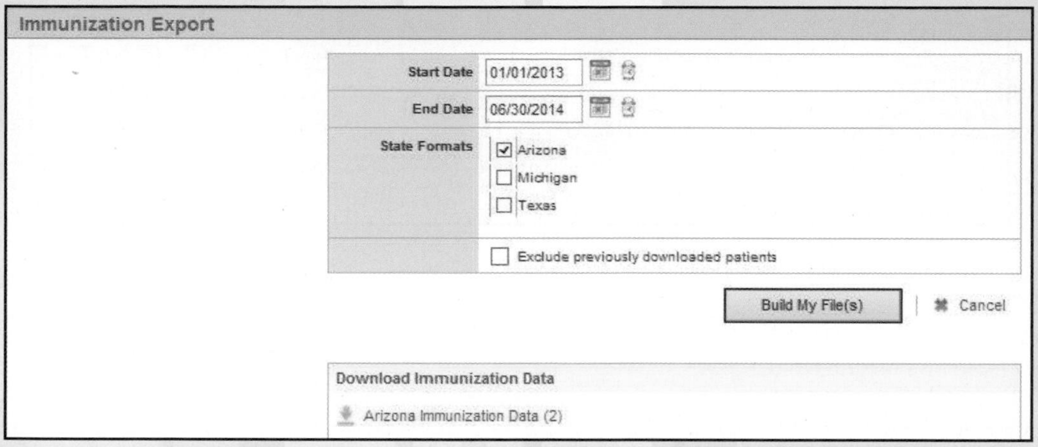

Immunization Export

Start Date	01/01/2013
End Date	06/30/2014
State Formats	☑ Arizona
	☐ Michigan
	☐ Texas
	☐ Exclude previously downloaded patients

Build My File(s)   ✖ Cancel

Download Immunization Data

⬇ Arizona Immunization Data (2)

Courtesy of Harris CareTracker PM and EMR

Figure 8-59   Immunization Export Results

Tip Box

When downloading records for Michigan, Harris CareTracker PM and EMR will prompt you to enter the Michigan Care Improvement Registry (MCIR) Site ID number.

7. In the *Download Immunization Data* section, click the state links to save the file(s) locally. This may take a moment depending on the size of the downloaded file. If you attempt to run this report, you will receive an error message.

Immunization Lot Number Report

Now that you have learned the steps to run the *Immunization Export* report, you will run an *Immunization Lot Number* report.

ACTIVITY 8-26:   Run an Immunization Lot Number Report

1. With no patient in context, click on the *Reports* module and then click the *Reports* tab.

2. Under *Medical Reports*, click on the *Other Reports* link.

3. Click the *Report* drop-down menu and select "Global – Immunization by Lot Number" (Figure 8-60).

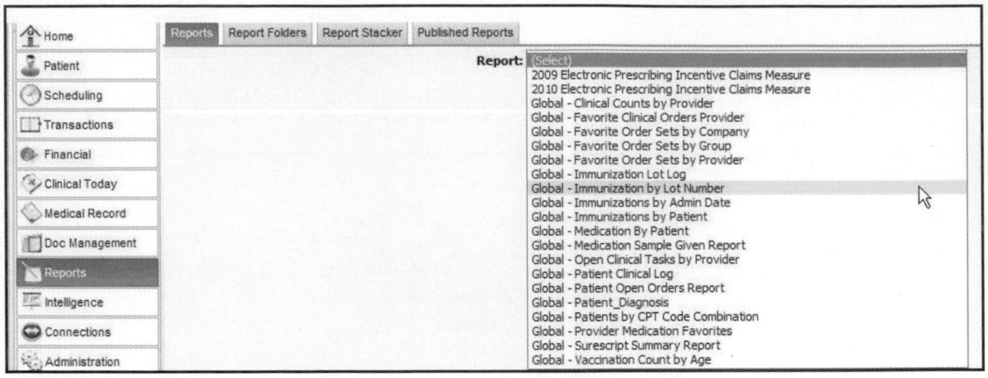

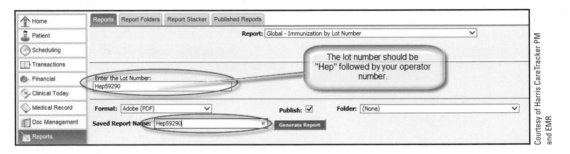

Figure 8-60 Select Global – Immunization by Lot Number

4. Enter the lot number you created in Activity 7-7 in the *Enter the Lot Number* box and also in the *Saved Report Name* box (Figure 8-61).

5. Click *Generate Report*.

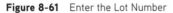

Figure 8-61 Enter the Lot Number

6. In the lower-left-hand corner of your screen "The report has been sent to the Queue" will display (Figure 8-62).

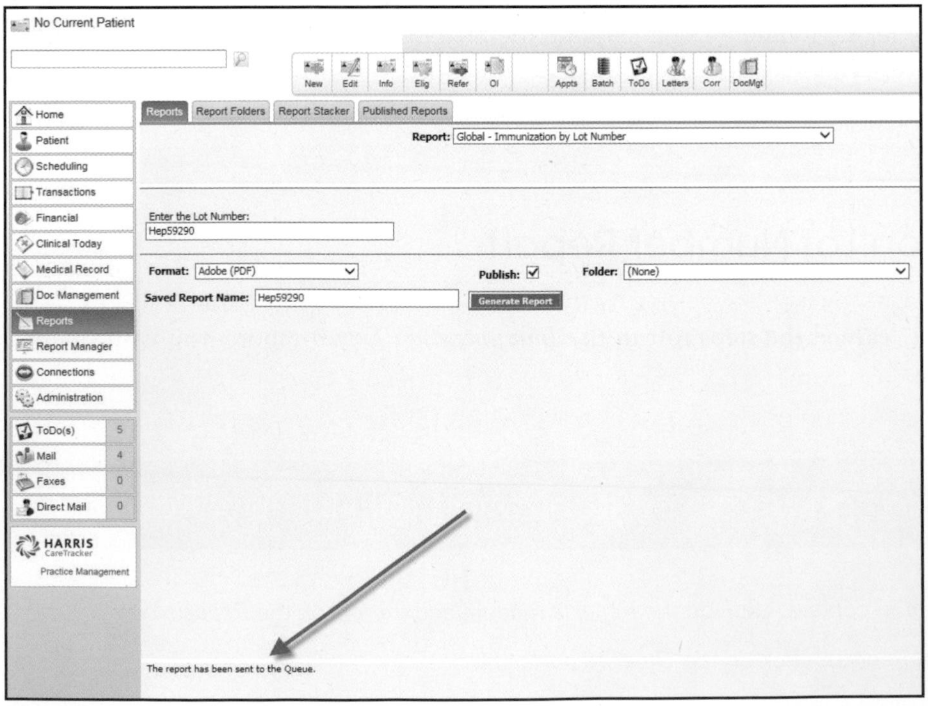

Figure 8-62 Report Sent to Queue

7. Click on the *Published Reports* tab of the *Reports* module, and click on the PDF format for the first report listed (noted in Figure 8-63). (**Note**: You may need to refresh your screen for the report to display.)

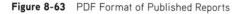

Home	Reports	Report Folders	Report Stacker	Published Reports

Patient
Scheduling
Transactions   All Groups   Show Archived Reports   Select All for Printing   Deselect All for Printing   Print Selected Files   Delete Marked Reports   Unmark All Reports
Financial
Clinical Today

If you would like to keep a file indefinitely, click on the 'Archive' button to the right of the file.
To move a report to another group or make it available to all groups, click on the 'Move' button to the right of the file.

Medical Record
Doc Management   **Napa Valley Family Health Associates 2**

Name	Date/Time	Type	Size	Print			
Hep59290_20160419172220_31165_5	4/19/2016 5:22:23 PM	Adobe Acrobat Document	34KB	☐	Archive	Move	Delete ☐
Global - Company Details_20130305122404_5809_3	3/9/2013 8:56:03 PM	Adobe Acrobat Document	58KB	☐	Archive	Move	Delete ☐

Reports
Report Manager

Figure 8-63   PDF Format of Published Reports

8. A pop-up window will display asking if you want to *Open* or *Save* the PDF report. Select *Open* and the report will display.

9. Click on the *Print* icon in the PDF to print the report.

10. Now repeat the activity, this time selecting the "Global – Immunizations by Admin Date" report using the begin date of 01/01/2013 and today's date as the end date. Generate and print the report.

Print a copy of the Immunization by Lot Number report and label it "Activity 8-26a." Print a copy of the Immunizations by Admin Date report and label it "Activity 8-26b." Place both copies in your assignment folder.

SUMMARY

This chapter has focused on other clinical documentation and advanced features in Harris CareTracker EMR. You learned to navigate the *Progress Notes* application, which allows you to view and manage the list of notes saved for the patient, and complete advanced activities.

The *Results* application was also introduced. Although results are not received electronically in your student version of Harris CareTracker EMR, you learned to manually enter lab results and to customize, graph, and print patient results.

We expanded on the knowledge you learned from earlier chapters and completed activities related to the *ToDo* application, focusing now on the clinical side of Harris CareTracker. Activities performed that mimic a medical assistant's clinical responsibilities included creating new *ToDos* and *Mail* messages, accessing and viewing mail messages, as well as replying to, moving, and managing your inbox. We also reviewed advanced features of Harris CareTracker EMR such as generating *Recall Letters* and running *Immunization Lot* reports.

Congratulations on completing Practice Management and EMR components, functions, and activities in your student version of Harris CareTracker PM and EMR! You will now advance to the *Billing* and *Collections* features in Chapters 9 and 10.

Check Your Knowledge

Select the best response.

_____ 1. The *Progress Notes* application displays a list of notes recorded during each patient appointment. *Progress Notes* include information such as:

   a. Patient's history
   b. Medications
   c. Allergies
   d. All of the above

_____ 2. In addition to the *Progress Notes* application, you have quick access to progress notes via other locations. Which is not one of the alternate ways to access progress notes?

   a. *Quick Picks*
   b. *Select Encounter* dialog box
   c. *Progress Notes* icon in the *Clinical Toolbar*
   d. *Progress Notes* application

_____ 3. When can you make edits to a progress note after it has been signed by the provider and supervising provider?

   a. Never
   b. At any time
   c. If the signing provider unsigns the note first
   d. When there is no addendum on the progress note

_____ 4. Which statement is true regarding deleted progress notes?

   a. Progress notes can never be deleted.
   b. You can only delete an unsigned note.
   c. You can only delete a signed note.
   d. None of the above.

_____ 5. Who can "unsign" a progress note?

   a. An operator with "Break the Glass" privileges
   b. The operator who signed the note
   c. The supervising physician
   d. Any operator with access to the progress note

_____ 6. If a progress note requires a co-signature, the *Signed* column displays:

   a. "Y"
   b. "CS"
   c. *Edit* icon
   d. *Pencil* icon

_____ 7. If a *Result* has an "unmatched status," the result is saved only in the *Results* application of which of the following locations?

   a. Patient alerts
   b. *Home* module
   c. *Clinical Today* module
   d. Both b. and c.

_____ 8. The *Action* menu in the *Results* column allows you to do the following:

    a. Print the result
    b. Attach the result to a *ToDo*
    c. Delete the result
    d. All of the above

_____ 9. When a patient checks out from an appointment, the patient is automatically pulled into context. What displays upon checkout?

    a. All *ToDos* for orders, prescriptions, referrals, educational handouts, and the chart summary
    b. Patient alerts
    c. *Scheduling* module
    d. Patient insurance balance due

_____10. Which of the following is not a type of *Recall Letter* available when using the *Recalls/Letters Due* application?

    a. Appointment recalls
    b. Outstanding orders
    c. Appointment reminders
    d. Missed/cancelled appointments

_____11. Which of the following is a reason to run an *Immunization Lot* report?

    a. Product recall
    b. Monitory inventory
    c. Monitor expiration dates
    d. All of the above

mini-case studies

Note: Case studies must be completed in every chapter since future chapter activities build upon them.

Case Study 8-1
Patient: Adam Thompson

  a. For Adam Thompson's encounter created in Chapter 6, repeat Activity 8-11 and enter results for the *Open Lab Orders* found in Source Document 8-2 in Appendix A.
  b. Following the instructions in Activity 8-7, add an *Addendum* to the patient's progress note as follows: "Patient went to ED and was admitted to NVGH for treatment."

 Print screenshots of the screens that illustrate you entered the results and addendum. Label them "Case Study 8-1a" and "Case Study 8-1b" and place them in your assignment folder.

Case Study 8-2
Patient: Spencer Douglas

  a. Repeat Activity 8-7 and create an addendum for the patient's encounter dated September 16, 2013, as follows: "Mother called to inquire if any vaccinations are required for overseas travel. Sent CDC recommendations for traveling to South America."

 Print a screenshot that illustrates you entered the addendum. Label it "Case Study 8-2a" and place it in your assignment folder.

  b. Repeat Activity 8-7 and create an addendum for the patient's encounter dated December 16, 2013, as follows: "Mother called to say Spencer is refusing to eat solid foods; asked her to bring him into office for immediate follow-up. She will go to Urgent Care for after-hours visit."

Print a screenshot that illustrates you entered the addendum. Label it "Case Study 8-2b" and place it in your assignment folder.

(Continued)

Case Study 8-3

Patient: Ellen Ristino

 a. For Ellen Ristino's encounter created in Chapter 6, repeat Activity 8-11 and enter results for the *Open Orders* found in Source Document 8-3 in Appendix A.
 b. Unsign the *Progress Note.* Enter "Negative" into the *Rapid Strep* field at the top of the *Tests* tab of the *Progress Note.*
 c. Sign the progress note created for the patient's encounter.

 Print screenshots of the screens that illustrate you completed the orders, entered the result in the progress note and signed the progress note. Label them "Case Study 8-3a," "Case Study 8-3b," and "Case Study 8-3c" and place them in your assignment folder.

Case Study 8-4

Repeat Activity 8-26 and run the *Immunization by Lot Number* report for the immunization lot you created in Activity 5-12. (**Note:** The immunization lot name should be "MMR" followed by your operator number.)

 Print the *Immunization by Lot Number* report. Label it "Case Study 8-4" and place it in your assignment folder.

Case Study 8-5

Before ending this chapter, be sure to sign the *Progress Notes* for patients with encounters that have visits captured. Follow the instructions in Activities 7-18, 7-19, 7-20 and 7-21 to complete this case study.

 1. Click on the *Home* module > *Dashboard* tab > *Practice* tab > *Clinical* heading > *Open Encounters* link. Select *All* providers and click on the refresh icon.
 2. The screen will display any unsigned notes and whether or not the visit has been captured. Sign all of the progress notes for the patients with captured visits. This will allow you to complete the *Billing* and *Collection* activities in Chapters 9 and 10.

Print a screenshot of the *Open Encounters* screen before signing any unsigned notes, and another screenshot that illustrates you signed any unsigned notes. Label them "Case Study 8-5a" and "Case Study 8-5b and place them in your assignment folder.

Resource

The Harris CareTracker PM and EMR Help homepage represents a wealth of information for the electronic health record (https://training.caretracker.com/help/CareTracker_Help.htm).

Chapter 9

Billing

Key Terms

batch
clearinghouse
crosswalk
explanation of benefits (EOB)
explosion codes
Healthcare Common Procedure Coding System (HCPCS)
mnemonics
modifier
scrub
variance

Learning Objectives

1. Create a batch for financial transactions.
2. Manually enter a charge.
3. Edit an unposted charge.
4. Generate electronic and paper claims.
5. Demonstrate knowledge of and perform activities related to electronic remittance including: posting payments and adjustments; reconciling insurance payments; matching unmatched transactions; and printing EOBs, paper claims, billing statements, and batch deposits.

Certification Connection

1. Utilize a computerized office billing system (e.g., Harris CareTracker PM).
2. Identify types of insurance plans and enter coding and billing information in the EHR.
3. Demonstrate understanding of under-coding and up-coding and why to avoid these practices.
4. Describe how to use and find the most current ICD, CPT®, and HCPCS codes in an EMR.
5. Abstract and enter diagnoses and procedural descriptions from the patient's paper chart into the electronic medical record.
6. Generate insurance verification reports, patient statements, patient receipts, and encounter forms.
7. Describe common periodic financial reports.

Adapted from national standards of the National Healthcareer Association (NHA), Commission on Accreditation and Allied Health Education Program (CAAHEP), and Accrediting Bureau of Health Education Schools (ABHES)

INTRODUCTION

Harris CareTracker PM and EMR provides a secure environment to ensure that the billing process goes smoothly and the quality of the information sent to insurance carriers is clean. The *Billing* feature crosses many modules, applications, and functions. The normal flow for a claim in Harris CareTracker PM and EMR starts with a patient appointment, followed by checking in the patient where patient information is confirmed and updated. At the end of the patient visit, the services are recorded and reviewed before the claims are sent out.

Harris CareTracker PM and EMR will **scrub** the claim before it is sent to payers. Claim scrubbing ensures that claims are correctly coded before being sent to the insurance company, which reduces denials and increase payments to the practice. *ClaimsManager,* the claim scrubber in Harris CareTracker PM, provides a comprehensive set of coding and technical edits. Each individual edit may be enabled or disabled completely for a specific claim type or for an individual payer. Most claims are sent electronically in Harris CareTracker PM and any claims that have been identified as having a problem that would prevent them from being paid will show up on a *Worklist* list to be resolved.

This chapter introduces you to billing activities in Harris CareTracker PM and EMR. Having learned the concept and created a batch in Chapter 4, you will build upon activities previously completed. The **batch** is the essential component required before entering and posting any financial transaction such as charges, payments, adjustments, and refunds. In this chapter you will perform billing functions, enter and edit charges, run a journal to verify your batch and entry information, view all open batches, and then post your batch into the system.

Once charges are entered, you will learn how to generate an insurance claim by using (or by simulating) the electronic remittance features of Harris CareTracker PM. Activities include posting payments and adjustments, reconciliation, matching unmatched transactions, and working denials and credit balances. An **explanation of benefits (EOB)** (Figure 9-1) is the insurance company's written explanation to a claim, showing the amount paid by the insurance company, any contractual write-off amounts, and any balance that the patient must pay.

UnitedHealthcare

A UnitedHealth Group Company

United HealthCare of New England, Inc.

P.O. BOX 31361
SALT LAKE CTY UT 84131
Phone: 8778423210

Date: 03/06/2009
Payment Number: 12808957
Payment Amount: $545.36

KYLE DUNN MD
PO BOX 6300
PROVIDENCE   RI 02904

PROVIDER
EXPLANATION OF
BENEFITS

Account Number	Patient Name				Subscriber ID		Claim Number			
DATES OF SERVICE	DESCRIPTION OF SERVICE	AMOUNT CHARGED	NOT COVERED	PROV ADJ DISCOUNT	AMOUNT ALLOWED	DEDUCT/ COINS/ COPAY	PAID TO PROVIDER	ADJ REASON CODE	RMK CODE	PATIENT RESP
1732059X17980724	Pitt, Brad				51001976579529		PVS0626477000			
02/11/2009-02/11/2009	HC:99213	$110.00	$0.00	-$64.04	$45.96	$15.00	$30.96	45		$15.00
Subtotal		$110.00	$0.00	-$64.04	$45.96	$15.00	$30.96			$15.00

45 - Charges exceed your contracted/ legislated fee arrangement.

Total Paid to Provider : $30.96

Courtesy of Harris CareTracker PM and EMR

Figure 9-1 Example of an EOB

CREATE A BATCH

Learning Objective 1: Create a batch for financial transactions.

As discussed in Chapter 4, you must create a batch to enter any financial information into Harris CareTracker PM and EMR, for example, charges, payments, and adjustments. For this learning objective, you will create a new batch for billing activities.

Setting Operator Preferences

In order to perform any financial transactions, you must create a batch or have a batch open. Harris CareTracker PM will prompt you to create a batch unless you have already created a batch that has not yet been posted. You can view open batch(es) by clicking on the *Home* module > *Dashboard* tab > *Billing* header > *Open Batches* link (Figure 9-2). Activities related to searching for a patient or scheduling a patient do not require that a batch be created. You begin by setting the operator preferences that you completed in Chapter 4, Activity 4-15. Following the instructions in Activity 9-1, create a *Batch* as instructed to begin your activities in this chapter.

Figure 9-2   Open Batches Link

ACTIVITY 9-1:   Create a Batch for Billing and Charges

1. Prior to creating a batch, you will need to open the fiscal period for which you will be entering activities. Go to the *Administration* module > *Practice* tab > *System Administration, Financial* headers > *Open/Close Period* link (Figure 9-3).

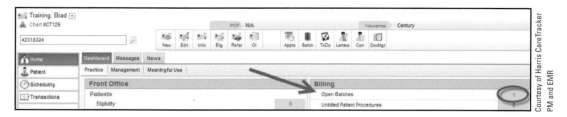

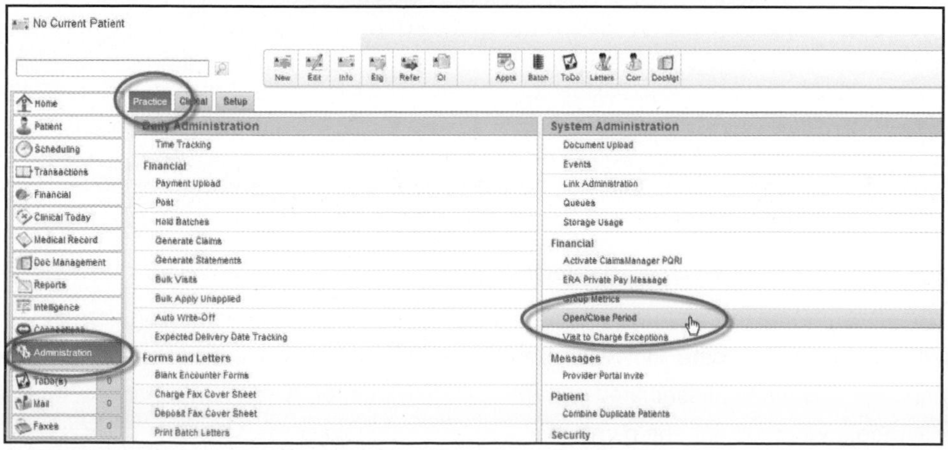

Figure 9-3   Open/Close Period Link

2. Open the period for the activities you are posting (June 2013), and then click *Save* (Figure 9-4).

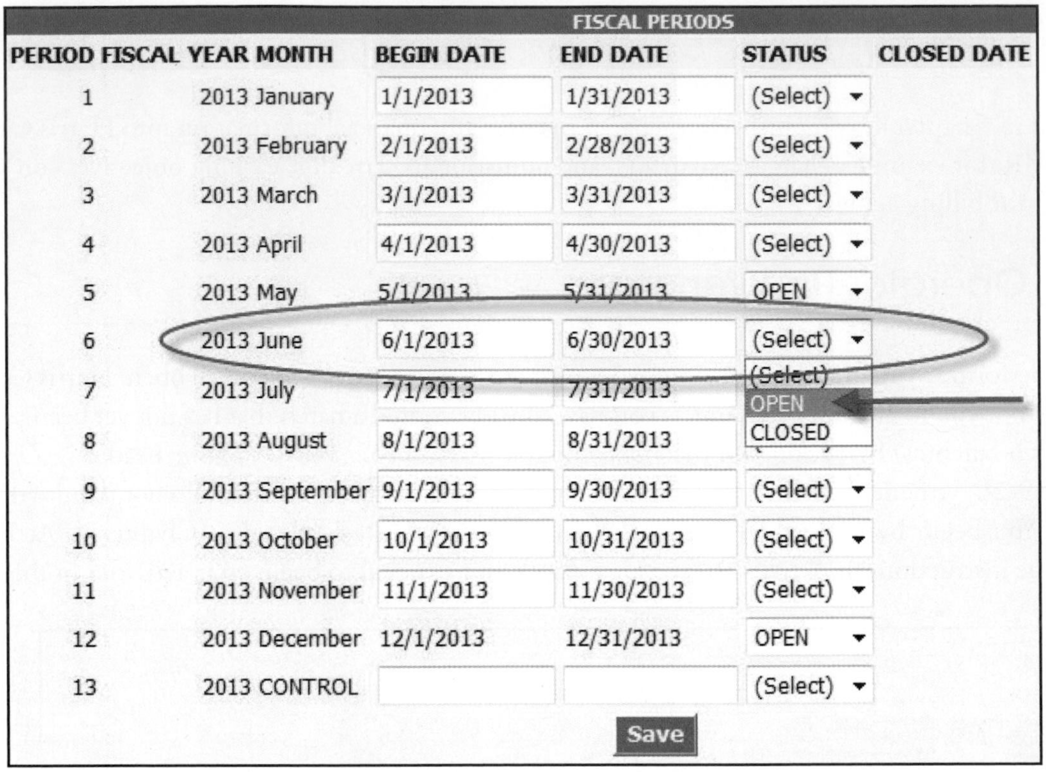

FISCAL PERIODS					
PERIOD	**FISCAL YEAR MONTH**	**BEGIN DATE**	**END DATE**	**STATUS**	**CLOSED DATE**
1	2013 January	1/1/2013	1/31/2013	(Select) ▾	
2	2013 February	2/1/2013	2/28/2013	(Select) ▾	
3	2013 March	3/1/2013	3/31/2013	(Select) ▾	
4	2013 April	4/1/2013	4/30/2013	(Select) ▾	
5	2013 May	5/1/2013	5/31/2013	OPEN ▾	
6	2013 June	6/1/2013	6/30/2013	(Select) ▾	
7	2013 July	7/1/2013	7/31/2013	(Select) OPEN CLOSED	
8	2013 August	8/1/2013	8/31/2013		
9	2013 September	9/1/2013	9/30/2013	(Select) ▾	
10	2013 October	10/1/2013	10/31/2013	(Select) ▾	
11	2013 November	11/1/2013	11/30/2013	(Select) ▾	
12	2013 December	12/1/2013	12/31/2013	OPEN ▾	
13	2013 CONTROL			(Select) ▾	

Save

Courtesy of Harris CareTracker PM and EMR

Figure 9-4   Open Fiscal Period for June 2013

Tip Box

Because you will have been working in various activities in more than one period, always work in the "current" period (e.g., if you begin an activity in September, complete all the related activities in that period. If you start a new activity unrelated to a previous period [e.g., in December], you would then use the new period [December]). Although you will be instructed to complete activities and post batches, *never* close a period. In Chapter 11, Applied Learning Case Studies, you will conclude with closing period(s) once all activities have been completed.

3. Click the *Batch* ▌ icon on the *Name Bar* and the *Operator Encounter Batch Control* dialog box will display (Figure 9-5).

4. Click *Edit* and then click *Create Batch*. The *Batch Master* dialog box displays (Figure 9-6).

5. By default, the *Batch Name* box displays a batch identification name. The name consists of your user name followed by the current date. However, you can edit the batch name if necessary to identify the types of financial transactions associated with the batch. Name the batch "Ch9Charges" (Figure 9-7). Do not use symbols when editing the name.

6. By default, the *Group Id* displays the name of your group.

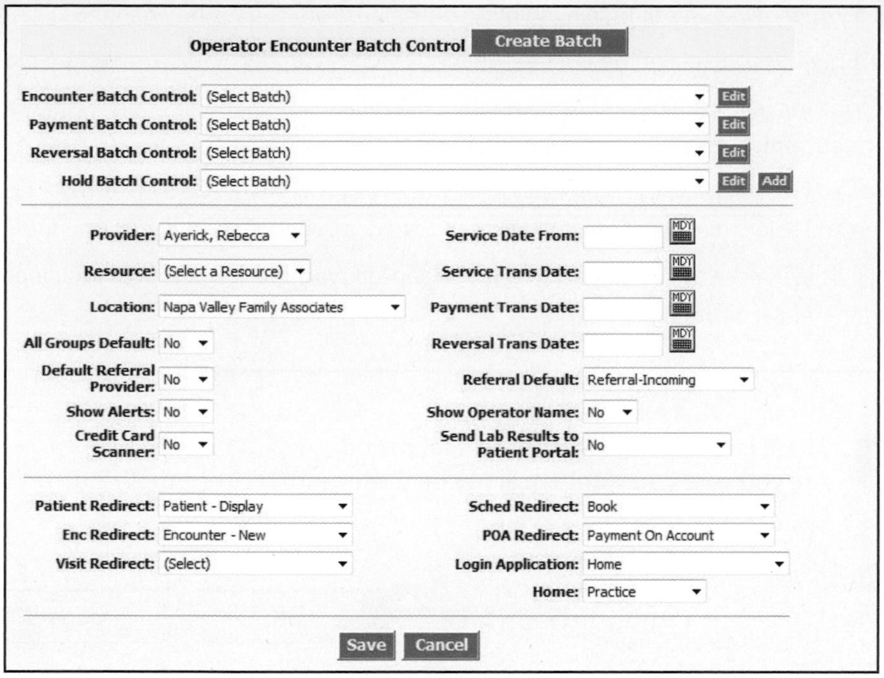

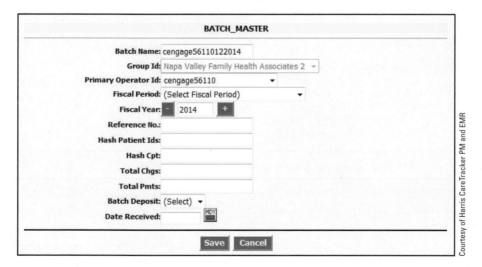

Figure 9-5   Operator Encounter Batch Control Dialog Box

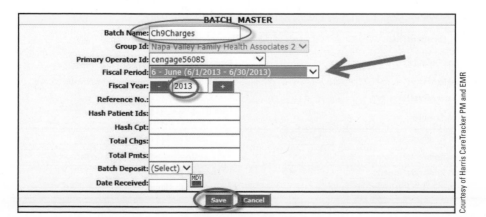

Figure 9-6   Batch Master Dialog Box

Figure 9-7   Change Batch Name

7. By default, the *Primary Operator Id* displays your user name. This cannot be changed.
8. By default, the *Fiscal Year* displays the current financial year set up for your company. Select "2013."
9. In the *Fiscal Period* list, click the period to post financial transactions. The list only displays fiscal periods that are currently open. Select "June 2013" as the *Fiscal Period*.
10. In the *Date Received* box, enter the date the encounter was created in MM/DD/YYYY format or click the *calendar* icon and select the date. Select the date of Spencer Douglas's first appointment (June14, 2013).
11. Click *Save*. If you have more than one period open, a pop-up warning (Figure 9-8) will appear asking you to confirm the fiscal period. Click *OK*.

Courtesy of Harris CareTracker PM and EMR

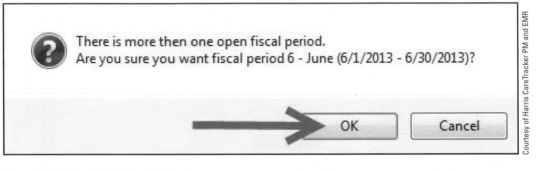

Figure 9-8 Fiscal Period Pop-Up Warning

12. Harris CareTracker PM and EMR displays the *Operator Encounter Batch Control* dialog box with the new batch information (Figure 9-9).
13. You can further *Edit* your batch by using the drop-down arrow next to each field and updating the provider, resource, location, and so on, if needed. Confirm that the *Provider* and *Resource* noted in the batch match with patient Spencer Douglas. Select "Anthony Brockton."
14. Click *Save*.

Courtesy of Harris CareTracker PM and EMR

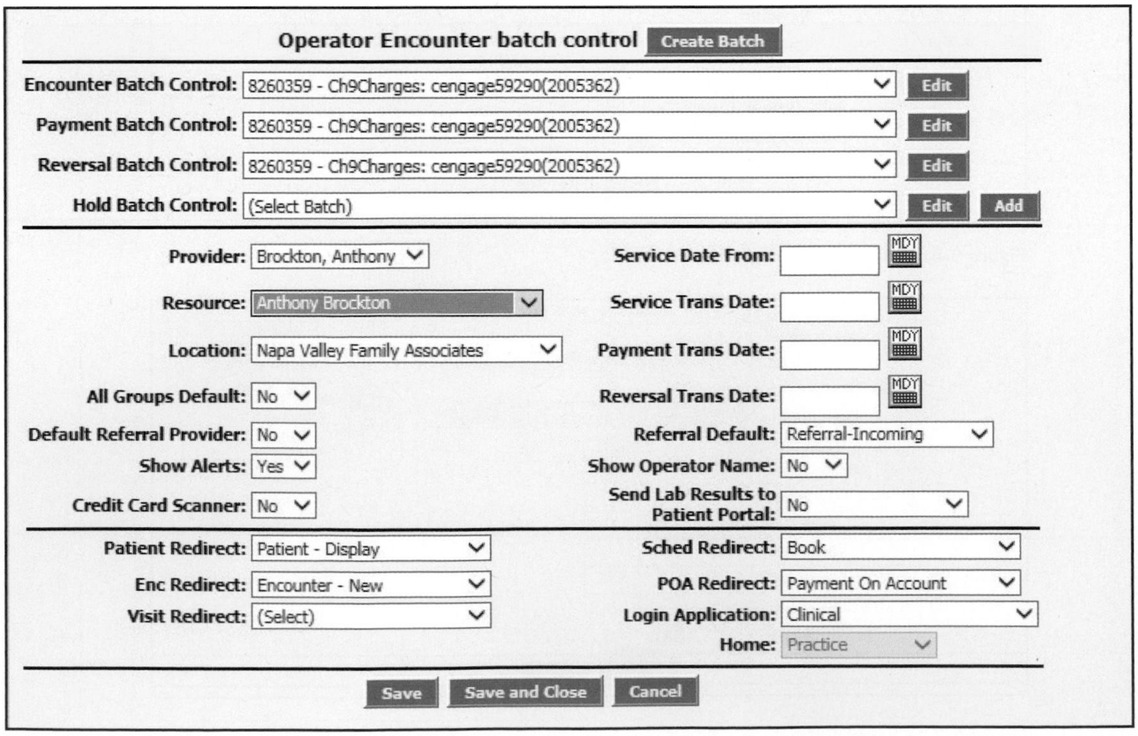

Figure 9-9 Ch9Charges Batch Information

15. Write down your "Encounter Batch Control No." for future reference (should include "Ch9Charges").
_____

Print the Operator Encounter Batch Control screen, label it "Activity 9-1," and place it in your assignment folder.

16. Click the "X" in the upper-right corner to close the dialog box.

MANUALLY ENTER A CHARGE

Learning Objective 2: Manually enter a charge.

Charges are financial transactions that require a batch to be created before entering and saving a charge. Having created your batch in Activity 9-1, complete Activity 9-2 to post a patient payment.

ACTIVITY 9-2:   Posting a Patient Payment

1. If not already done, open the fiscal year/period in which you are entering a charge (see Figure 9-4) from the _Administration_ module > _Practice_ tab > _Open/Close Period_ link.

2. Pull patient Spencer Douglas into context.

3. Open the _Transactions_ module. The _Charge_ application displays by default.

4. Click on the _Pmt on Acct_ tab.

5. In Chapter 4 you learned how to enter and print copay receipts for patients. Following the instructions in Activity 4-17, enter the copay amount for patient Spencer Douglas (refer to the patient demographics or click on the _At A Glance_ 🔲 icon to determine the amount of copay required [$30]). Enter check number "4434", and the appointment date to be applied to Spencer's payment (June 14, 2013). Your screen should look like Figure 9-10. (**Note:** Be sure to check the "Copay?" box.)

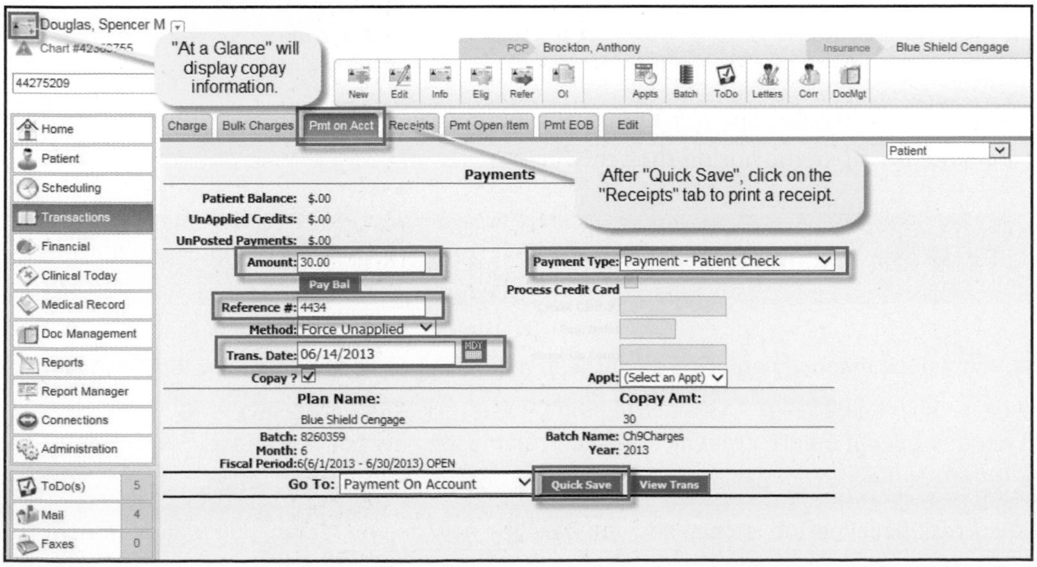

Figure 9-10   Spencer Douglas Payment on Account

6. Click *Quick Save.*

7. Click on the *Receipts* tab and print a receipt for Spencer Douglas.

Print the receipt, label it "Activity 9-2," and place it in your assignment folder.

You will not post the batch at this time because you will complete additional activities before running a journal and posting a batch.

> ## Tip Box
>
> If you were through with billing activities and wanted to post the batch, you would click on the *Home* module > *Practice* tab > *Billing* section > *Open Batches* link (Figure 9-11). You would then click the checkbox next to the batch you want to post (Figure 9-12) and select *Post Batches.*

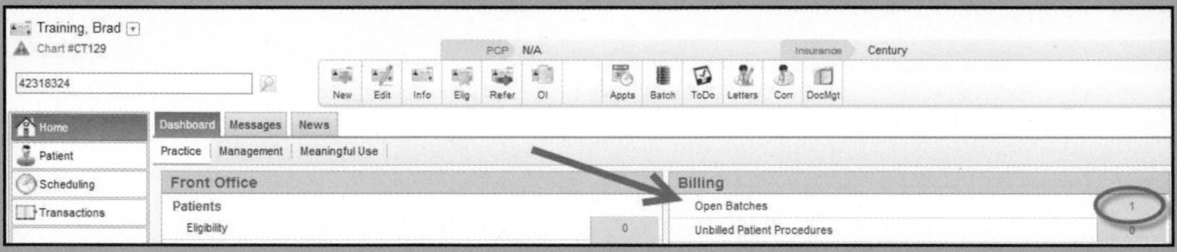

Figure 9-11   Open Batches Link

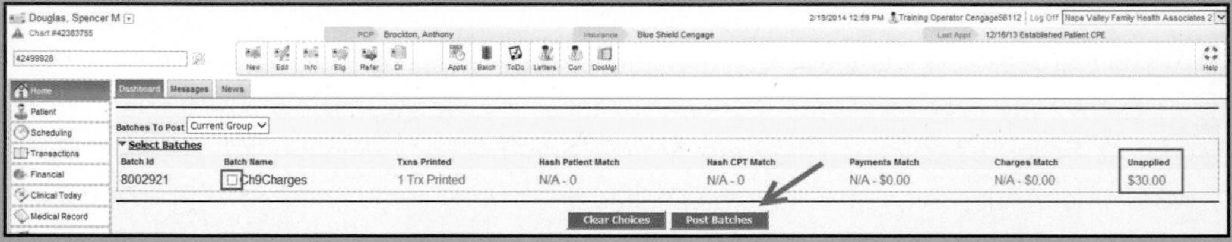

Figure 9-12   Post Copay Batch

Having entered the co-pay for Spencer Douglas in Activity 9-2, continue your billing activities by manually entering a charge for a patient not on the schedule.

ACTIVITY 9-3:   Manually Enter a Charge for a Patient

1. Because you will be manually entering a charge in a different period, follow the steps in Activity 9-1 to create a new batch using today's current month and year. (**Note:** If the fiscal period is not already open, you will need to open it before creating the batch.) Name the new batch "LyndseySNF". Set the batch defaults to reflect the current period, PCP for patient Jordyn Lyndsey, and so on.

2. After the current fiscal period is open and you have the new batch created, pull patient Jordyn Lyndsey into context.

3. Open the *Transactions* module. The *Charge* application displays by default, displaying the charge screen.
4. Manually enter a "Skilled Nursing Facility" charge using the following charge-related information:
    a. Using the *Location* drop-down, select "NVSNF."
    b. Using the [Tab] key will automatically populate the *POS* with "SKILLED NURSING FACILITY".
    c. Enter *Ref Provider* "Dr. Raman".
    d. If a service date was not selected when you created your batch, it must be entered in the *Date* and *Date To* fields. The date must be within the open period in your current batch. A date can either be entered manually in MM/DD/YYYY format or can be selected from the *Calendar* function. In the *Date* and *Date To* fields, enter today's date (Figure 9-13).

Courtesy of Harris CareTracker PM and EMR

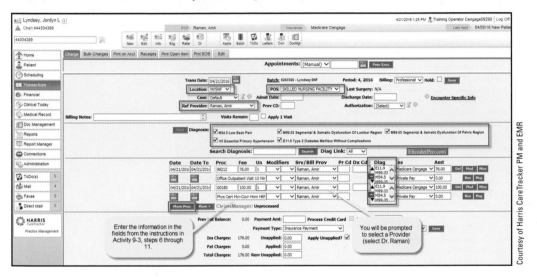

Figure 9-13 SNF Charge

5. *Visit Diagnosis* (Figure 9-14) will be grayed out in the student environment in the center of the screen.

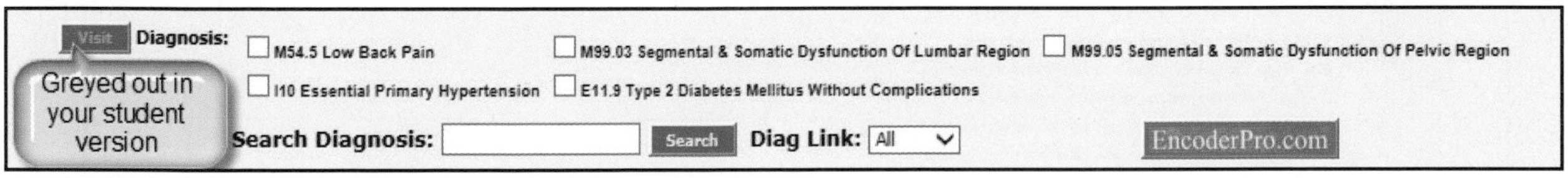

Figure 9-14 Visit Diagnosis
Courtesy of Harris CareTracker PM and EMR

6. If there have been previous ICD codes entered for this patient, you can place a check mark by the desired code to select it. If the code is not listed, type the code (enter "E11.9") in the *Search Diagnosis* field, and then click *Search* (it may take a few moments to populate). Harris CareTracker PM will pull in the diagnosis code of E11.9 (Type 2 diabetes mellitus without complications) to the *Diag* field (Figure 9-15).

Courtesy of Harris CareTracker PM and EMR

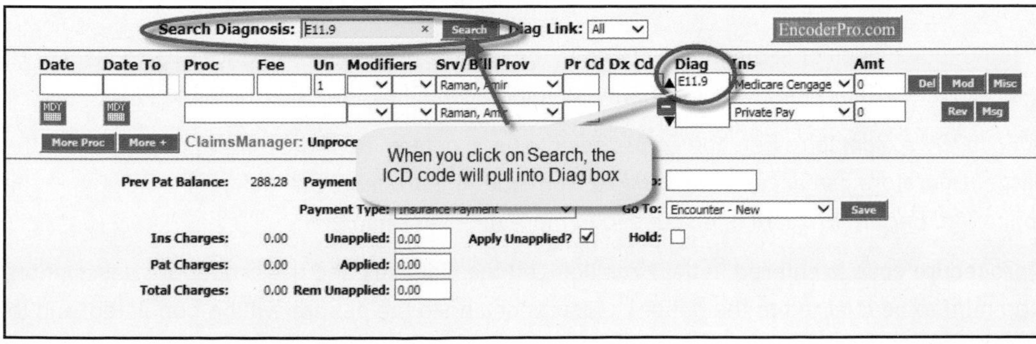

Figure 9-15 Search Diagnosis

FYI

If you need to search for a diagnosis code, enter a partial code or a keyword (enter "Diabetes") in the *Search Diagnosis* box, and then click *Search*. The application opens the *Code Search* window (Figure 9-16). Click on the desired ICD-9 or ICD-10 code to select it. The application pulls the selected code into the *Diag* box.

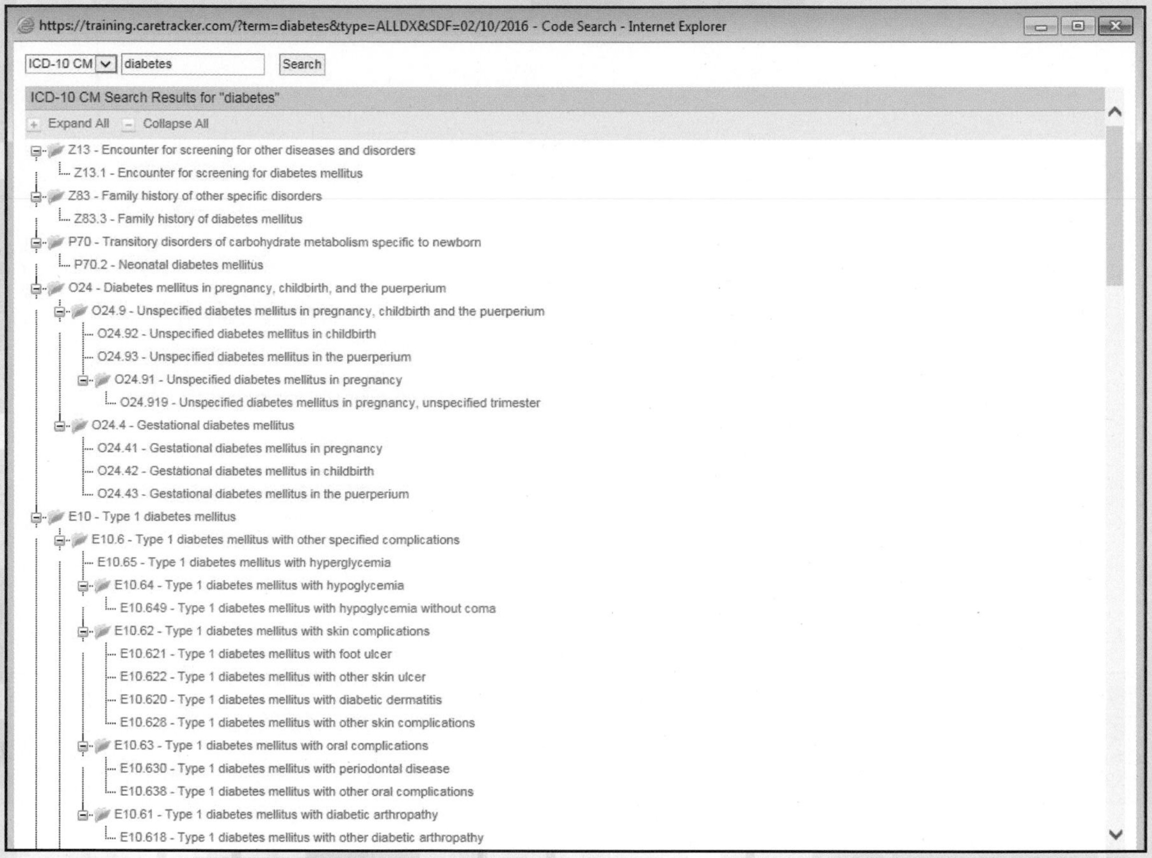

Courtesy of Harris CareTracker PM and EMR

Figure 9-16 Diagnosis Search Window

7. Repeat step 6 to add additional diagnosis codes to the *Diag* box if needed. Add ICD-10 codes: M99.03, M99.05, M54.5, and I10 by searching for them using the *Search* box (see Figure 9-14).
8. Click on *EncoderPro.com* to review the codes selected and determine if they are appropriate for the visit/charge. Operators can access *EncoderPro* from both the procedure and diagnosis pages in the *Visit* application. *EncoderPro.com* is discussed in more detail in Chapter 1.
9. When a procedure code is entered in the *Proc* field, hit the [Tab] key and the procedure description, fee, and the amount to be charged to the patient's insurance and to the patient will be populated, and the

Tip Box

ICD-9 codes are internationally recognizable 3- to 5-digit code sets, representing medical conditions or signs and symptoms. ICD-9 was replaced by the ICD-10 code set on October 1, 2015. To accommodate the change to ICD-10, Harris CareTracker has a *View Mappings* link (Figure 9-17) that will enable you to find the ICD-10 code as needed. The *Visit Diagnosis*, *Visit Summary*, and *Claim Edit* screens for visits after October 1, 2015 now display a code set ⑩ icon next to the insurance field that indicates if the insurance company or plan is configured to receive ICD-9 or ICD-10 diagnosis codes (Figure 9-18). A diagnosis code in the *Diag* box can be removed by double-clicking on the code. The order of multiple codes can also be changed in the *Diag* box by highlighting the code to move up or down and then clicking on the corresponding up or down black arrow next to the *Diag* box.

Code	Description
✔ 692	Contact dermatitis and other eczema
692.0	Due to detergents
692.1	Due to oils and greases
692.2	Due to solvents
692.3	Due to drugs and medicines in contact with skin
692.4	Due to other chemical products
692.5	Due to food in contact with skin

ICD-9 V1   poison   Search   ⑩ View Mappings   Select

ICD-9 V1 Code Section (692-692.9)

Courtesy of Harris CareTracker PM and EMR

Figure 9-17 View Mappings

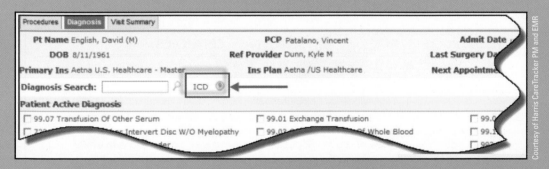

Procedures | Diagnosis | Visit Summary

Pt Name English, David (M)   **PCP** Patalano, Vincent   **Admit Date**
DOB 8/11/1961   **Ref Provider** Dunn, Kyle M   **Last Surgery Da**
Primary Ins Aetna U.S. Healthcare - Master   **Ins Plan** Aetna /US Healthcare   **Next Appointme**
Diagnosis Search: [   ] ICD ⑨
Patient Active Diagnosis
☐ 99.07 Transfusion Of Other Serum   ☐ 99.01 Exchange Transfusion   ☐ 99.0
☐ ... Intervert Disc W/O Myelopathy   ☐ 99.0... Of Whole Blood   ☐ 99.1
☐ ...   ☐ 99.

Courtesy of Harris CareTracker PM and EMR

Figure 9-18 Diagnosis Code Set

Mapping Screen

The ICD mapping screen is accessed by clicking the *View Mappings* link at the top of the search results. This screen acts as a basic mapping tool, allowing the operator to see which ICD-10 codes map to the current ICD-9 codes (Figure 9-19) and vice versa. Basic mapping is available for:

- ICD-9-CM Vol. 1 to ICD-10-CM
- ICD-10-CM to ICD-9-CM Vol. 1

(Continues)

(Continued)

The mapping screen contains several columns with information about the relationship between the ICD-9 and ICD-10 codes.

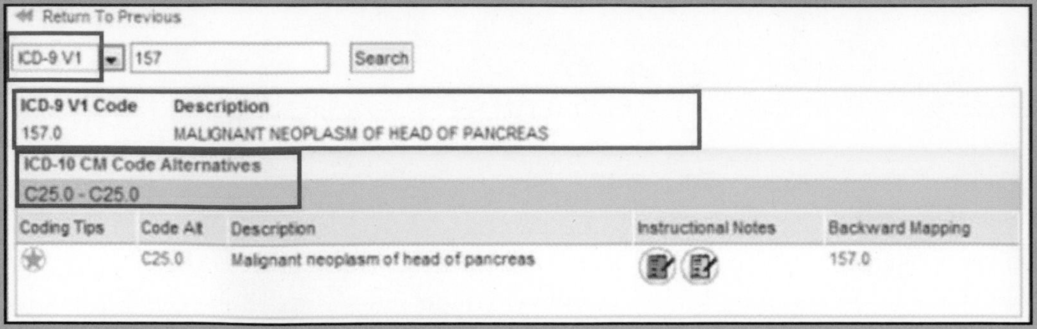

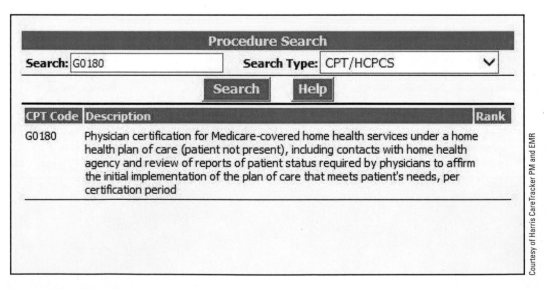

Figure 9-19 ICD-9 to ICD-10 Mapping

Modifiers field will become the active field. Enter the code "99212" in the *Proc* field, hit the [Tab] key, and a $76 *Fee* will automatically populate from the fee schedule.

10. Click on the *More Proc* button, which brings up another billing line. Enter CPT® code "G0180" in the *Proc* field. Hit the [Tab] key and the *Procedure Search* pop-up box will appear (Figure 9-20). Click on the code or description and the procedure will be pulled in to the charge box.

<table>
<tr><th colspan="3">Procedure Search</th></tr>
<tr><td>**Search:** G0180</td><td>**Search Type:**</td><td>CPT/HCPCS ∨</td></tr>
<tr><td colspan="3" align="center">Search   Help</td></tr>
<tr><th>CPT Code</th><th>Description</th><th>Rank</th></tr>
<tr><td>G0180</td><td>Physician certification for Medicare-covered home health services under a home health plan of care (patient not present), including contacts with home health agency and review of reports of patient status required by physicians to affirm the initial implementation of the plan of care that meets patient's needs, per certification period</td><td></td></tr>
</table>

Figure 9-20 G0180 Procedure Search Window

11. Enter $100 in the *Fee* field because this CPT® code is not on the NVFHA fee schedule.

12. Enter the provider's name (Dr. Raman) in the *Srv/Bill Prov* field from the drop-down list, if not already selected (Figure 9-21).

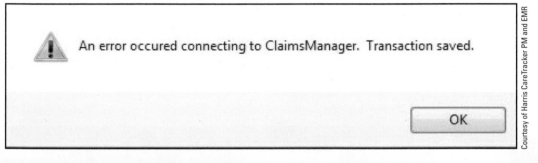

Date	Date To	Proc	Fee	Un	Modifiers	Srv/Bill Prov	Pr Cd Dx Cd	Diag	Ins	Amt			
04/21/2016	04/21/2016	99212	76.00	1	▼ ▼	Raman, Amir ▼		▲ E11.9 M99.03	Medicare Cengage ▼	76.00	Del	Mod	Misc
MDY 📅	MDY 📅	Office Outpatient Visit 10 Min			▼ ▼	Raman, Amir ▼		⊟ M54.5 ▼ M99.05	Private Pay ▼	0.00		Rev	Msg
04/21/2016	04/21/2016	G0180	100.00	1	▼ ▼	Raman, Amir ▼		▲ E11.9 M99.03	Medicare Cengage ▼	100.00	Del	Mod	Misc
MDY 📅	MDY 📅	Phys Cert Mcr-Covr Hom Hlth			▼ ▼	Raman, Amir ▼		⊟ M54.5 ▼ M99.05	Private Pay ▼	0.00		Rev	Msg
More Proc	More +	ClaimsManager: **Unprocessed**											

Figure 9-21 SNF Charge

Print the Charge Screen, label it "Activity 9-3," and place it in your assignment folder.

13. Click *Save*. You will receive an error message (Figure 9-22) because your student version is not connected to *Claims Manager*. However, the transaction will be saved, and the patient is taken out of context. (**Note:** It may take a few moments for this task to save. Wait until you receive the "error" message "Transaction Saved" before moving on.)

14. Click *OK* and the patient is removed from context and "Encounter Added" displays on your screen.

15. Your manually entered charge is now saved.

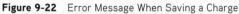

> ⚠ An error occured connecting to ClaimsManager. Transaction saved.
>
> OK

Figure 9-22 Error Message When Saving a Charge

Tip Box

A **modifier** is a two-character code added to a CPT® or **Healthcare Common Procedure Coding System (HCPCS)** (pronounced "hick picks") code that is used to help in the reimbursement process. For example, a modifier is used to explain that a procedure is not normally covered when billed on the same day as another, but is actually a separate and significant process, or that it is a rural health procedure that gets higher reimbursement. Up to four modifiers can be attached to each CPT® code, although in most cases only one or two are used. HCPCS (level II) is managed by the Center for Medicare and Medicaid Services (CMS) and classifies durable medical equipment (DME), injectable drugs, transportation services, and other services not classified in CPT®.

A common modifier in an outpatient setting is Modifier 25, which is defined as a significant, separately identifiable evaluation and management service by the same physician on the same day of the procedure or other service (e.g., an office visit for a facial lesion and a separate charge for destroying the lesion, vaccination(s) given at time of office visit, etc.). Refer to Figure 9-23 for modifier selections in Harris CareTracker PM and EMR.

(Continues)

(*Continued*)

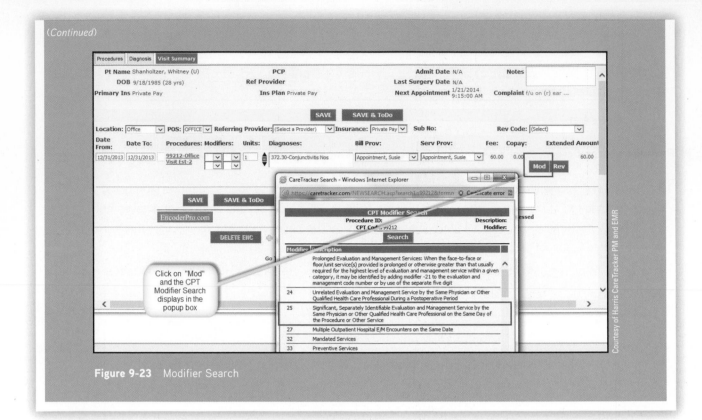

Figure 9-23 Modifier Search

PM SP●TLIGHT

In Harris CareTracker PM and EMR, explosion codes can be built to include multiple CPT codes, which eliminates the need to enter each procedure individually. For example, in cardiology practices, the same three CPT® codes are used to bill every echocardiogram (93307, 93320 and 93325). Creating one explosion code for this procedure reduces the amount of time it takes to enter the charge into the system. Valid modifiers for each procedure code can also be linked to them. Explosion codes are practice-specific and you can determine the descriptive name of the code set along with the CPT® codes it will include. There is no limit to the number of different explosion code sets you can build for your practice.

Tip Box

When a patient has both Medicare and a commercial insurance, always use the HCPCS code when billing injectables, DME, and others. If the HCPCS code is linked via a **crosswalk** code set to the CPT® code, the application will automatically pull the corresponding CPT® code onto the claim when the claim goes to the commercial insurance. Crosswalk (sometimes referred to as a "link") refers to a relationship between a medical procedure (CPT®/HCPCS code) and a diagnosis (ICD code). Not all HCPCS codes are linked via a crosswalk code set to CPT® codes.

FYI

Alternate Workflow for Checking Procedure and Diagnosis Codes

- When all procedure and diagnosis codes have been entered, click on the *EncoderPro.com* button at the top of the screen to verify that all the codes you have entered will be paid. Clicking the *EncoderPro.com* button displays basic information on all procedure codes that pertain to the charge. *EncoderPro* is Harris CareTracker's partner for online code verification, which can be run to verify all the procedures, diagnoses, and modifiers entered for a patient. Running *EncoderPro* helps to ensure that correct coding information is entered and that claims are processed and paid quickly.

- When *EncoderPro* has finished code verification, click *Save* at the bottom of the *Charge* screen. When the *Save* button is clicked, the associated procedures, diagnoses, and modifiers are sent to *ClaimsManager* instantly for screening. (If you click *Save* in your student environment you will receive an error message because the *ClaimsManager* feature is not active in your student version.) The screening can result in one of three statuses that include "Passed," "Failed," or "Warning" (Figure 9-24). If the screening results in the "Passed" status, the patient's charge is saved in Harris CareTracker PM and EMR.

CLAIMSMANAGER SCREENING STATUS		
Color	**Status**	**Description**
☐	**Not Processed**	Not processed status indicates that the item has not been screened by the ClaimsManager.
▪	**Passed**	Passed status indicates that the item has passed the ClaimsManager screening.
▫	**Warning**	Warning status indicates that the item may fail or the ClaimsManager has suggested edits.
▪	**Failed**	Failed status indicates that the item does not meet the rules set by ClaimsManager and further edits are required.
▨	**CMS Edits**	This status indicates that the claim was flagged for CMS edits. **Note:** The CMS Edits status is deactivated by default. You must send a ToDo to CareTracker Support to request this feature.

Courtesy of Harris CareTracker PM and EMR

Figure 9-24   Claims Manager Screening Status

Tip Box

When the *Save* button is clicked, an *alert* will display if a charge for the same procedure codes on the same date of service for the same provider has already been entered into Harris CareTracker PM and EMR, preventing the creation of duplicate charges.

- If the *ClaimsManager* screening triggers an edit, Harris CareTracker PM and EMR opens the *ClaimsManager Edit* window. (See "*ClaimsManager Edits for Charges*" for a detailed description of each status and edit option in the *Help* section.) All edits are categorized into **mnemonics** for easy identification and each edit is color coded to indicate its severity (Figure 9-25). Mnemonics, defined as assisting memory, are added in the *Administration* module > *Setup* tab > *Financial* section > *Provider Mnemonics* link.

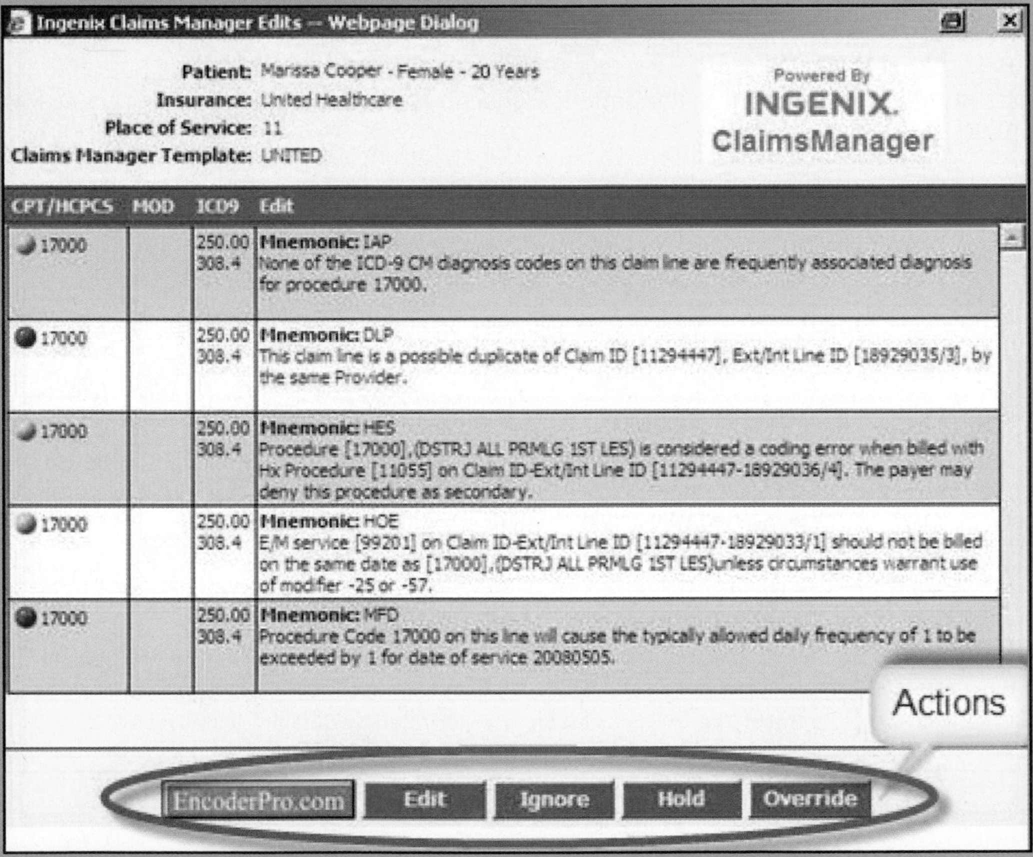

Figure 9-25 Claims Manager Edits

- If an action option is not clicked when a *ClaimsManager Edit* is triggered, the *Hold* checkbox is automatically selected and the charge is held until further action is taken. If waiting for reports or additional information, you can select the *Hold* checkbox manually to hold the charge and avoid further processing.

Critical Thinking

Coding is quite detailed, and improper coding can be considered "fraudulent billing," subjecting you, the practice, and providers to monetary and criminal penalties. In addition, "under-coding," which is often the result of coders using a "cheat-sheet" of common codes, leaves substantial reimbursement to the provider/practice on the table.

Examine and interpret the chart notes and/or ICD and CPT® codes selected for patient Bruce Thomas, encounter date 5/14/2013. Identify and justify the proper code, analyze, and question the code(s) entered on the encounter form to ensure that the most appropriate and accurate code(s) have been selected. Provide your rationale for selecting the code: How did you reach your conclusion, and did you consider other code(s) that would also be appropriate?

EDIT AN UNPOSTED CHARGE

Learning Objective 3: Edit an unposted charge.

Although it is not required to edit charges, there will be times when you will find it necessary to edit an unposted charge (e.g., a biller is reviewing a charge and sees that the incorrect CPT® code was assigned to the claim). Using the charge entered in Activity 9-3, edit the unposted charge.

ACTIVITY 9-4: Reversing a Charge

1. Pull patient Jordyn Lyndsey into context. (Review the batch screen to confirm you are still working in the "LyndseySNF" batch.)
2. Click the *Transactions* module. Harris CareTracker PM and EMR opens the *Charge* application.
3. Click on the *Edit* tab. When *Edit* is clicked all of the procedures entered in the patient's account along with each financial transaction linked to it will display (Figure 9-26) beginning with the most recent

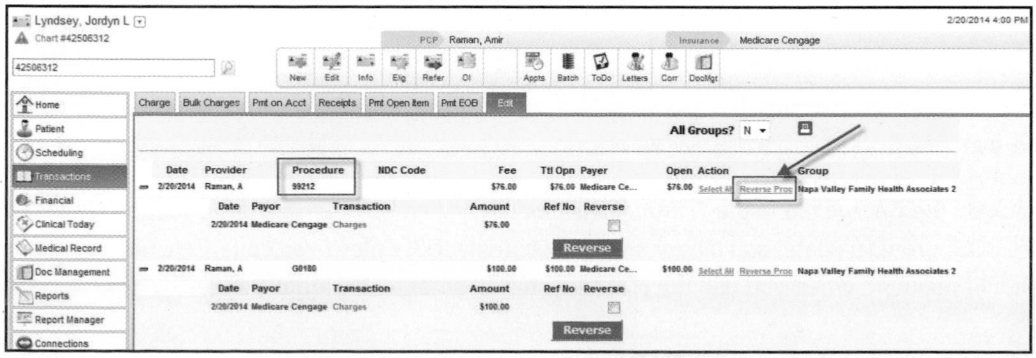

Figure 9-26 Edit Unposted Charge for Jordyn Lyndsey

Courtesy of Harris CareTracker PM and EMR

date of service. Locate the procedure that needs to be entirely reversed on the patient's account. (**Note:** You may need to scroll down the screen to locate the charge in question.) As biller, you have noticed that CPT® code 99212 is incorrect, and want to change it to CPT® code 99214.

Tip Box

You can edit any active field, including *Location, Pos, Case, Referring Provider, Date, Modifiers, Servicing Provider, Billing Provider,* and *Diag.*

---

4. On the procedure line that needs to be entirely reversed, you can click on either the *Select All* link or the *Reverse Proc* link. Select the *Reverse Proc* link on the 99212 charge (see Figure 9-26).

FYI

If you click on the *Reverse* button, all of the selected transactions are reversed.

---

5. You will receive a pop-up warning message (Figure 9-27) asking "Are you sure you want to reverse the selected Financial Transactions?" Click *OK.* The transaction will be reversed (see Figure 9-28). (**Note:** If you receive the error message "The Reversal Date must be within Period Start and End Dates: xx/xx/20xx and: xx/xx/20xx" it may be due to a "compatibility" issue with your browser. Click on the compatibility icon in your web browser so that functionality is restored.)

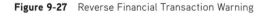 **Print the Edit Unposted Charge screen, label it "Activity 9-4a," and place it in your assignment folder.**

> ? Are you sure you want to reverse the selected Financial Transactions?
>
> OK   Cancel

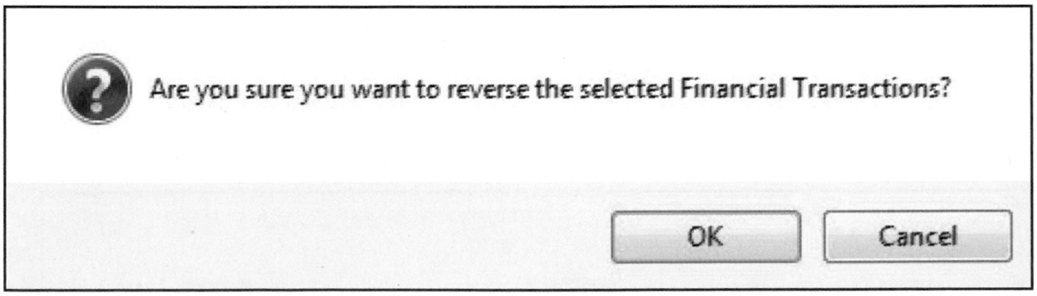

Courtesy of Harris CareTracker PM and EMR

Figure 9-27 Reverse Financial Transaction Warning

6. Click back on the *Charge* tab in the *Transactions* module and complete the charge screen for the same location, POS, provider, date, and diagnoses as in Activity 9-3. Enter *Proc* code "99214." The amount of $245 should populate when you use the [Tab] key. If not, enter "$245" into the *Fee* field.

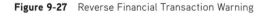 **Print the Charge screen, label it "Activity 9-4b" and place it in your assignment folder.**

7. Click on *Save* to save the charge.

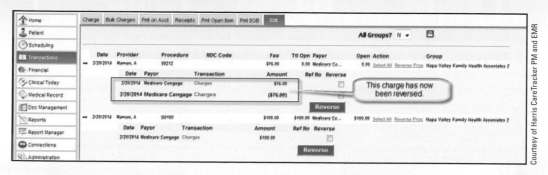

Figure 9-28 Reversed Charge

Tip Box

If a patient has a managed care insurance plan, the patient will be required to have a referral from his or her PCP. The referring provider is pulled from the *Authorization*. If there is no authorization, the referring provider is pulled from the patient's demographic record. If there is no referring provider selected in the demographic record, the referring provider is pulled from the batch (if the *Default Referral Provider* is set to "Yes" in the batch).

FYI

- For hospital visits, you would enter an admission and discharge date in the *Admit Date* and *Discharge Date* fields. Dates must be entered in MM/DD/YYYY format (Figure 9-29).

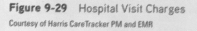

Figure 9-29 Hospital Visit Charges
Courtesy of Harris CareTracker PM and EMR

- For encounters with a set number of visits linked to an authorization (e.g., physical therapy), you would select *Apply 1 Visit* if the charge is for an authorized visit. Harris CareTracker PM and EMR will automatically deduct the visit from the total number of authorized visits.
- (Optional feature) Click the *Encounter Specific Info* link to enter additional claim information specific to the charge, such as injury date, LMP, attachment types, and so on. The information entered applies only to this encounter and is not carried forward in the default case information.

Many tasks in Harris CareTracker PM and EMR have more than one way to complete the function. One such alternate workflow scenario for editing charges would be to assume that the provider has entered the CPT® and ICD codes in the *Clinical* application. In this case, the biller would do the following:

- Go to the *Home* module > *Dashboard* tab > *Visit* header > *Missing Encounters* > *Charges* link (Figure 9-30).

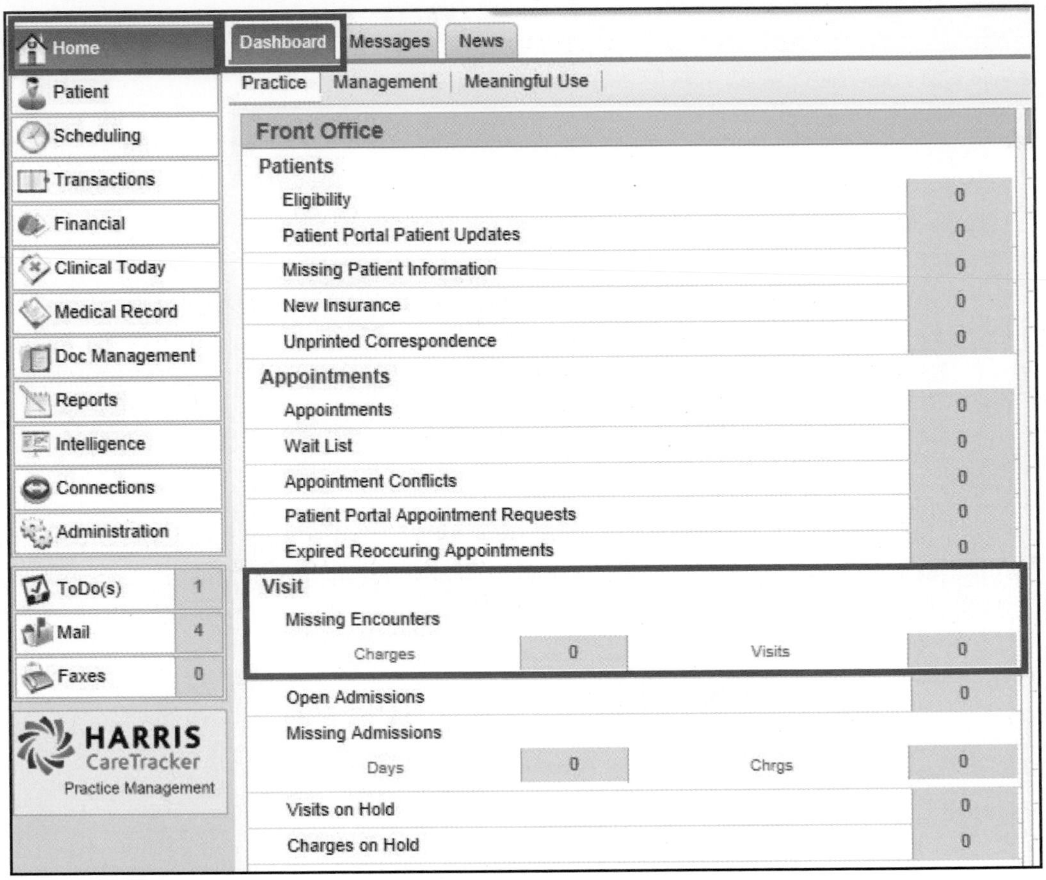

Courtesy of Harris CareTracker PM and EMR

Figure 9-30 Missing Encounters/Charges Link

- Change the beginning date to January 1, 2013, and then click *Go* (Figure 9-31).

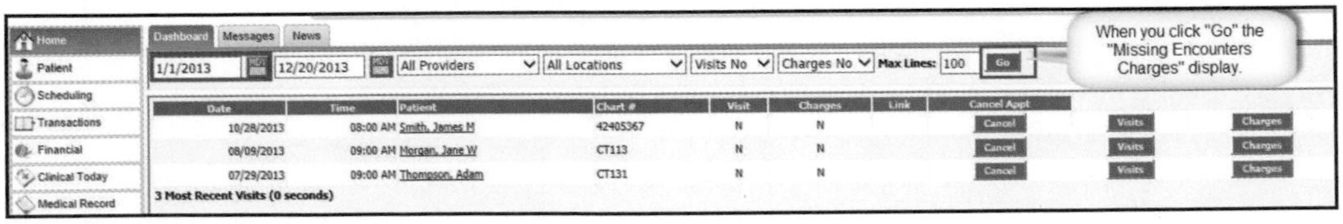

Courtesy of Harris CareTracker PM and EMR

Figure 9-31 Missing Encounters Display

- Review the charges by clicking on the *Charge* link, then *Go* on the left-hand side of the screen. The missing charge will display. (Be sure to scroll all the way down the screen to review all charges. We will assume here that the charges look OK.)
- Click *Save* on the left (Figure 9-32).

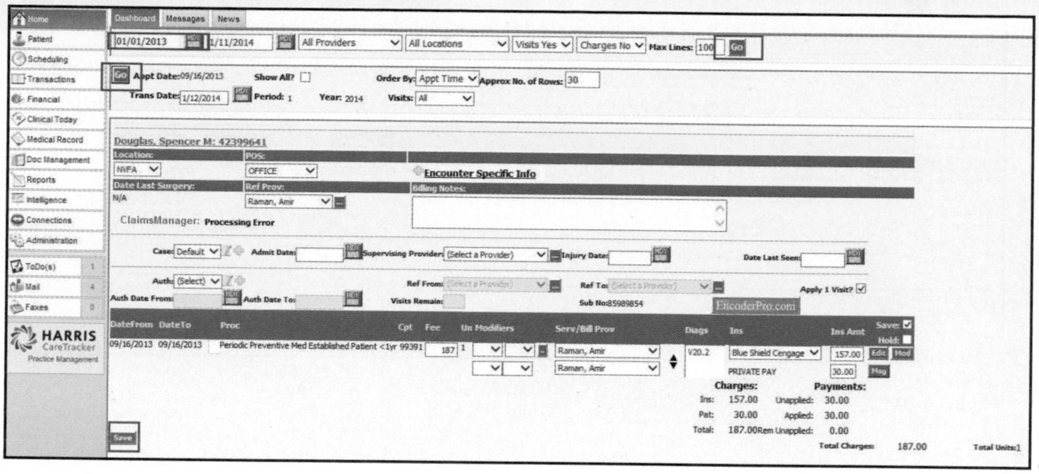

Figure 9-32 Missing Encounters Charges

Now that you have manually entered and edited unposted charges, complete the process by running a journal and posting your batch. Once you have verified your balance with your journal by completing Activity 9-5, you will post the batch(es) in Activity 9-6.

Journals

When you have finished entering data into your batch, you will run a journal to verify your batch and entry information. It is best practice to run a journal (as in Activity 4-19) prior to posting your batch to verify that you have entered all the financial transactions correctly in Harris CareTracker PM.

ACTIVITY 9-5: Run a Journal

1. Go to the *Reports* module > *Reports* tab > *Financial Reports* header > *Today's Journals* link (Figure 9-33).

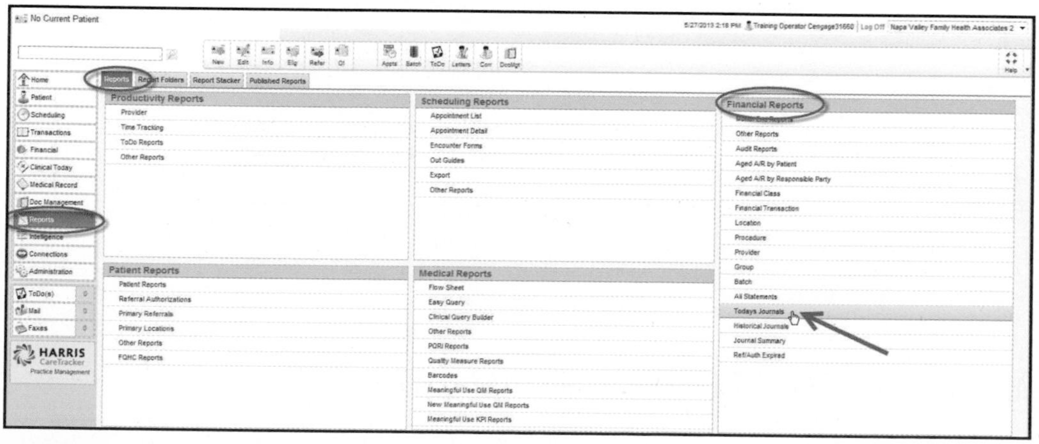

Figure 9-33 Today's Journals Link

2. Harris CareTracker PM displays the *Todays Journal Options* screen. All of your group's open batches are listed in the *Todays Batches* box. You may need to click on the [+] sign to expand the *Batches* field (see Figure 9-34).

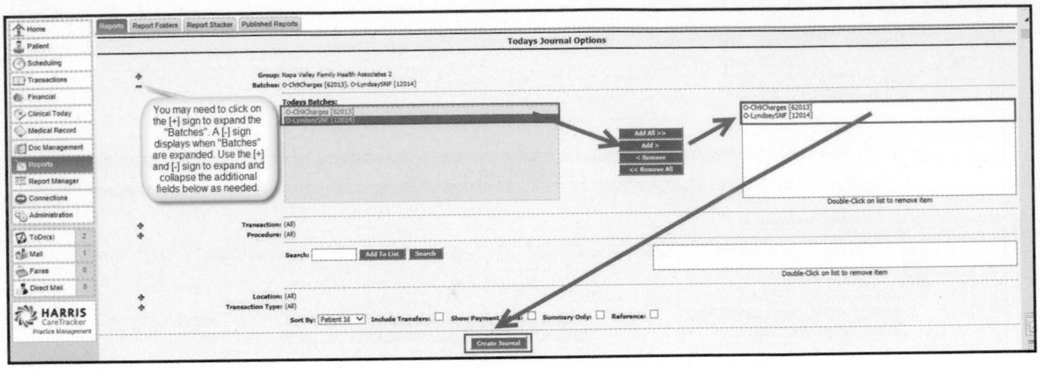

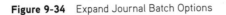

Figure 9-34 Expand Journal Batch Options

3. Select a batch to include in the journal either by double-clicking on the batch name or by clicking on the batch and then clicking *Add >*. Harris CareTracker PM adds the selected batches to the box on the right. Select batches "Ch9Charges" and "LyndseySNF".

4. Scroll down to the bottom of the screen. From the *Sort By* drop-down list, select "Entry Date" (Figure 9-35).

5. Select the *Show Payment Totals* checkbox.

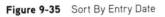

Figure 9-35 Sort By Entry Date

6. Click *Create Journal*. Harris CareTracker PM generates the journal (Figure 9-36).

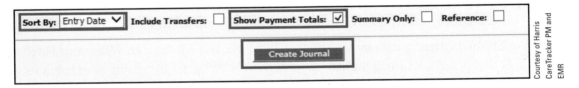

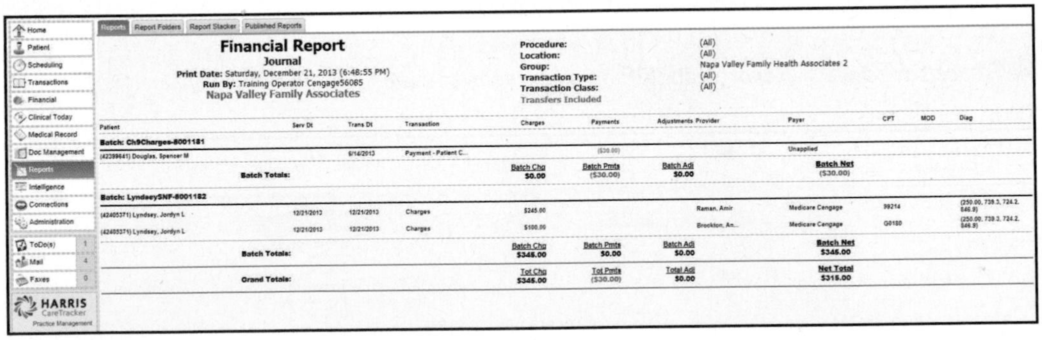

Figure 9-36 Financial Report

7. To print, right-click on the journal and select *Print* from the shortcut menu.

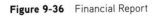 Print the journal, label it "Activity 9-5," and place it in your assignment folder.

Having generated a journal for the batch(es) you would like to post, review and identify any transactions errors that may have been made, and correct them prior to posting (using the steps in Activity 9-4, Edit an Unposted Charge). We will assume that there are no errors in the *Journal Report* created in Activity 9-5. Having balanced the money in your journal, post your open batch(es) in Activity 9-6.

ACTIVITY 9-6: Post a Batch

1. Go to the *Administration* module > *Practice* tab > *Daily Administration* section > *Financial* header > *Post* link (Figure 9-37). Harris CareTracker PM displays a list of all open batches for the group (Figure 9-38).

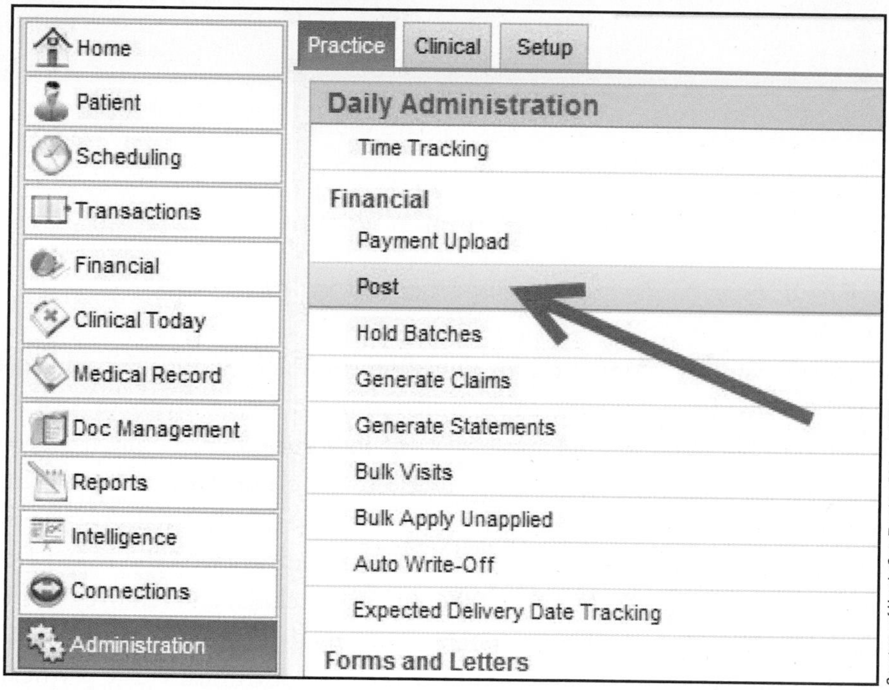

Courtesy of Harris CareTracker PM and EMR

Figure 9-37 Post Link from Practice Tab

ADMINISTRATIVE SPOTLIGHT

An alternate way to access and post batches is through the *Home* module > *Dashboard* tab > *Billing* header > *Open Batches* link (see Figure 9-2).

2. Check the box next to the batch(es) you want to post, and then click *Post Batches.* Select the batch "Ch9Charges" (Figure 9-38). The batch "LyndseySNF" should not be posted at this time.

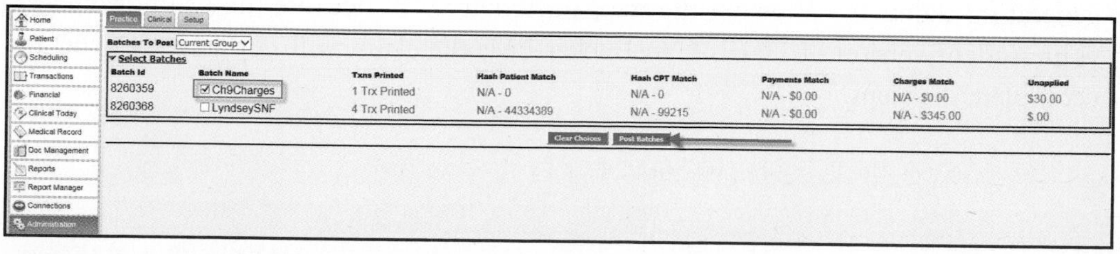

Courtesy of Harris CareTracker PM and EMR

Figure 9-38 Post Batches

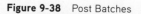

Print the Post Batches screen, label it "Activity 9-6," and place it in your assignment folder.

> ## Tip Box
>
> Although not required, it is recommended to only post a batch after a journal has been generated and balances verified. The total number of open batches for your group displays next to the *Open Batches* link.

GENERATE CLAIMS

Learning Objective 4: Generate electronic and paper claims.

Harris CareTracker PM transmits electronic claims directly to insurance companies and to **clearinghouses**. After an electronic claim batch has been received by either an insurance company or a clearinghouse, Harris CareTracker PM will receive an electronic acknowledgement indicating that the file has been accepted. After the insurance company or clearinghouse has reviewed the electronic claims batch, Harris CareTracker PM will then receive a report indicating whether the claims have been accepted or rejected. Any claims that have been rejected must be corrected and rebilled. After you have received and reviewed the report from the insurance company or clearinghouse, the electronic claim batch should then be closed and removed from your *Dashboard*. In the medical field, a clearinghouse is a private or public company that provides connectivity and often serves as a "middleman" between physicians and billing entities, payers, and other health care partners for transmission and translation of claims information (primarily electronic) into the specific format required by payers.

Claims can only be generated after your batch has been posted. Most claims in a medical practice are transmitted electronically to a clearinghouse or directly to an insurance company; however, some claims will need to be printed out and mailed. To manually print out paper claims in Harris CareTracker PM, you would go to the *Home* module > *Dashboard* tab > *Billing* header > *Unprinted Paper Claim Batches* link. Because *ClaimsManager* is not active in your student version, you will not be able to perform this function.

Electronic Submission of Claims

In a live environment, after completing the activities of posting payments, charges, running the journal, and posting the batch, Harris CareTracker PM will electronically submit the claims through *ClaimsManager*. You will simulate generating claims by following the steps in Activity 9-7. Because the *ClaimsManager* feature is not active in your student version of Harris CareTracker PM, the claim will not actually generate, but you will be able to complete the steps.

ACTIVITY 9-7: Workflow for Electronic Submission of Claims

1. Go to the *Administration* module > *Practice* tab > *Daily Administration* section > *Financial* header > *Generate Claims* link (Figure 9-39). Harris CareTracker PM launches the *Generate Claims* application.

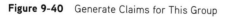

Figure 9-39 Generate Claims Link

2. Click *Generate Claims For This Group* (Figure 9-40). You will receive an error message (Figure 9-41) because the *ClaimsManager* feature of your student version is not active.

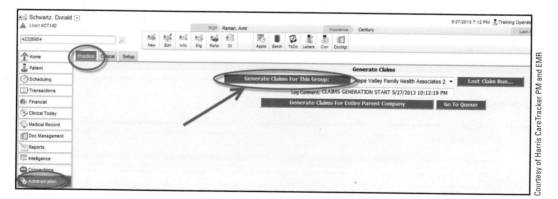

Figure 9-40 Generate Claims for This Group

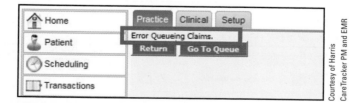

Figure 9-41 Error Queuing Claims

3. In a live environment, your screen would look like Figure 9-42, which states "Claims are Queued for all Groups under this Parent Company." Even though you have received an error message, click on *Go to Queue* and a report will generate. Figure 9-43 represents an example of the *Claims Queue* in a live environment which displays the *Claims Worklist* (see Figure 9-44). Since you are working in a student environment, all of your queues will be empty.

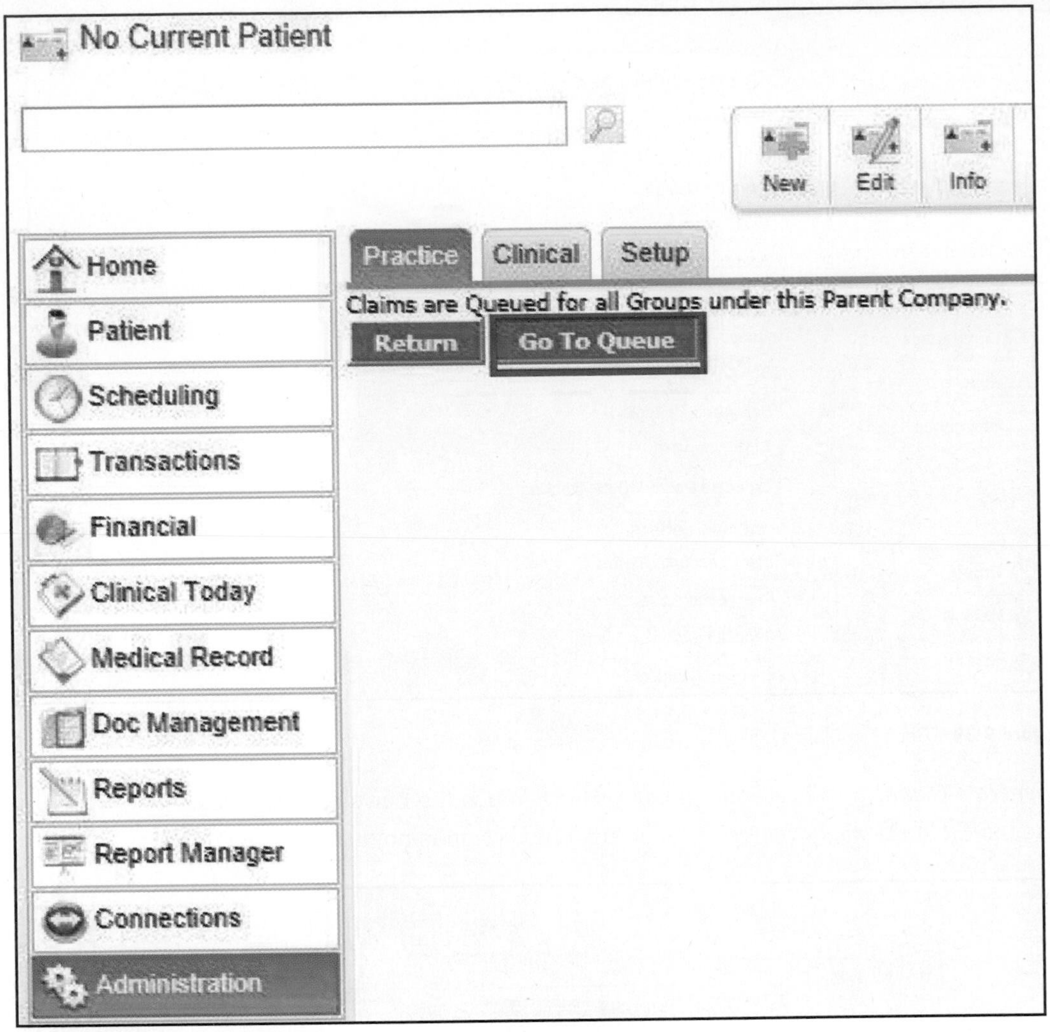

Courtesy of Harris CareTracker PM and EMR

Figure 9-42 Generated Claims

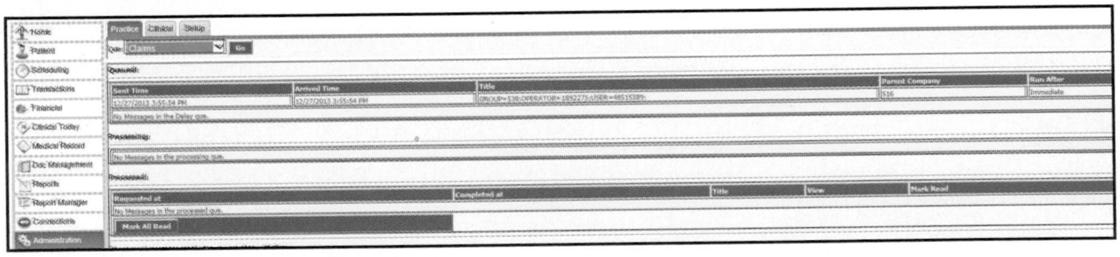

Courtesy of Harris CareTracker PM and EMR

Figure 9-43 Claims Queue

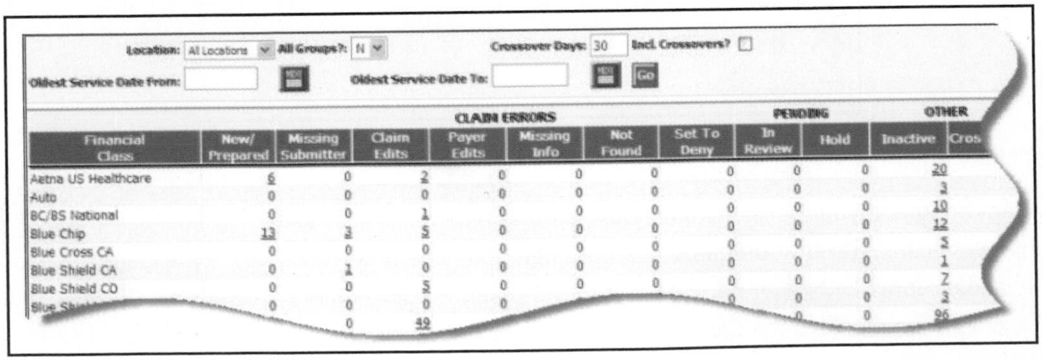

Courtesy of Harris CareTracker PM and EMR

Figure 9-44 Claims Worklist

4. Click back on the *Administration* module to exit the claims queue.

PM SP●TLIGHT

Claims wait in *Queue* to be processed at 5 P.M.

FYI

In a live environment, the claims would be electronically transmitted to their intended payer. A typical workflow would be:

- For claims transmitted electronically, you would receive a *Report* response back from the insurance company that needs to be reviewed. This can be done by clicking on the *Open Electronic Claim Batches* link on the *Dashboard* tab in the *Home* module.
- Your *Dashboard* should be reviewed daily; however your student version of Harris Care-Tracker PM will not show a *Report* back.
- On the day after you have generated your claims, you would check to see if any claims that were supposed to be transmitted or dropped to paper were unable to be billed out by Harris CareTracker PM. You would do this by clicking on the *Claims Worklist* link under the *Billing* section of the *Dashboard* tab in the *Home* module.
- The system would separate electronic vs. paper claims with *ClaimsManager*.
- As a biller, you would see what dropped to paper and then generate a paper claim.

Paper Claim Batches

Although paper claims are rare, there are occasions when you will need to send one. In Harris CareTracker PM, paper claims are generated by way of the method outlined in Activity 9-9. To print paper claims, you must first apply print settings, as in Activity 9-8.

ACTIVITY 9-8: Apply Settings to Print Paper Claims

There are two ways to apply print settings in Harris CareTracker. For this activity, use the Harris CareTracker *Dashboard*.

1. In Harris CareTracker PM and EMR, go to the *Home* module > *Dashboard* tab > *Billing* section > *Unprinted Paper Claim Batches* link. The application displays the *Print Options* window.

2. Click the *Print Options* button in the upper-right corner of the screen.

3. Locate the desired claim form ("1500 CMS Paper Form") in the list and then enter the margin size for the form in the corresponding *Offset Top* field (enter "10") and *Offset Left* field (enter "10") if not already populated (Figure 9-45).

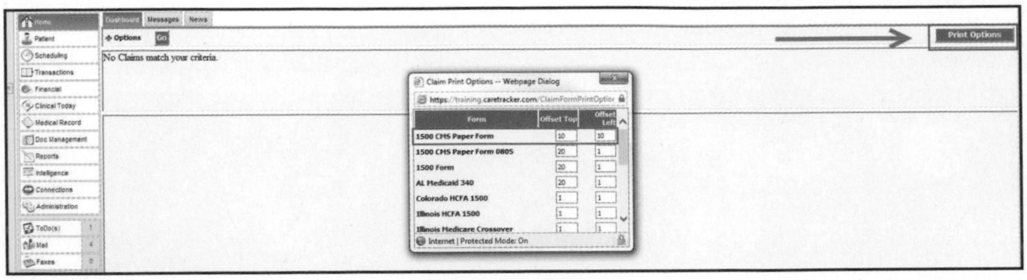

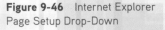

Figure 9-45 Apply Settings to Print Paper Claims

Print the Claim Print Options window, label it "Activity 9-8," and place it in your assignment folder.

4. Scroll to the bottom of the dialog box and click *Update.* You must log out and then log back in to Harris CareTracker PM and EMR before the setting takes effect.

FYI

The alternative method is to open an *Internet Explorer* browser window and launch the *Page Setup* from the menu bar; however this method may require more adjustments than using the Harris CareTracker *Dashboard.* To apply a setting through *Internet Explorer*, click the following links to view browser-specific instructions:

- For *Internet Explorer 8, 9,* and *10*: Select the *File* drop-down menu and then click *Page Setup* (Figure 9-46). **(Note:** Harris CareTracker no longer supports IE7.)
- In the *Page Setup* dialog box, remove any entries from the *Header* and *Footer* boxes. These boxes should be empty. For *Internet Explorer 8,* select *Empty* in each of the *Header* and *Footer* fields.
- In the *margins* section, set the Left, Right, Top, and Bottom margins to "0" (Figure 9-47). Click *OK.*

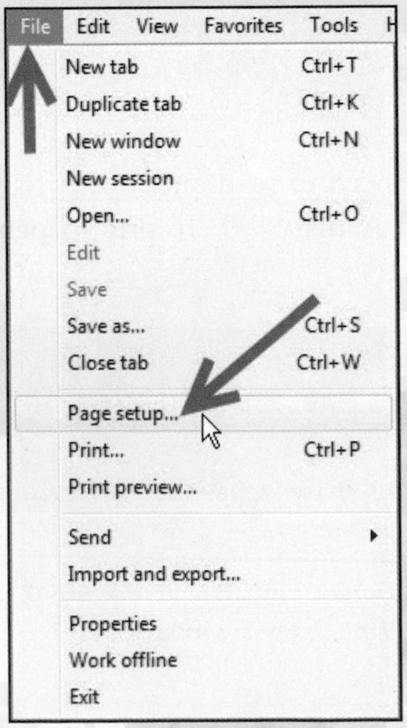

Figure 9-46 Internet Explorer Page Setup Drop-Down

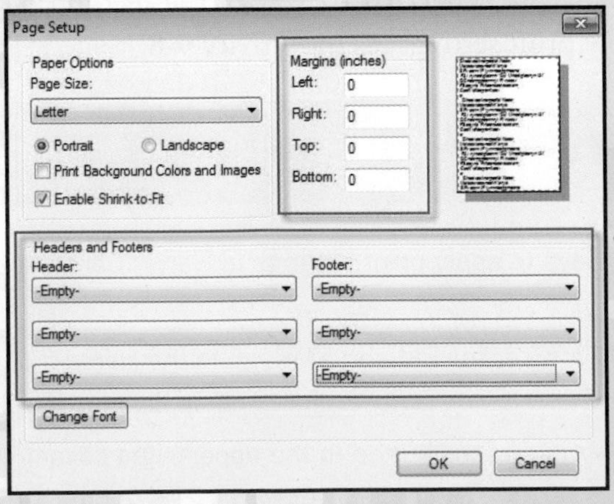

Figure 9-47 Internet Explorer Page Setup Screen

Tip Box

For the 1500 Form, Mass Health Form, or UB92 Form, you may have to adjust the *Offset Top* and *Offset Left* settings several times to get the form to line up properly.

Now that you have entered your print settings, you will be set to generate paper claims. Harris CareTracker PM sends all electronic claims to the appropriate insurance company clearinghouse and captures all paper claims that cannot be transmitted electronically in the *Unprinted Paper Claim Batches* application. The paper claim batches should be printed and marked as printed in a timely fashion, per practice protocol.

Practices have the option to automatically update the status of batch paper claims when the *Print Forms* button is used. This eliminates the need to manually mark each claim as printed. For this feature to be activated, the practice would send a *ToDo* to its support entity.

Tip Box

Harris CareTracker PM provides the ability to do real-time claim status checks from any application in Harris CareTracker PM and EMR where the Claim Summary screen displays. If your practice does not use the *Claims Status* application the billing staff should call the insurance companies two weeks after claims are mailed to verify that the claims have been received, are on file, and are set to pay.

ACTIVITY 9-9: Generate a Paper Claim

1. Pull patient Jordyn Lyndsey into context.
2. Click the *OI* tab in the *Name* bar.
3. Click on *Instant Claim* in the *First Clm* column (Figure 9-48) for each claim that you want to generate a paper claim for (select the charge you created in Activity 9-4 [99214]). Harris CareTracker PM displays the *Claims Summary* in the lower frame of the screen.

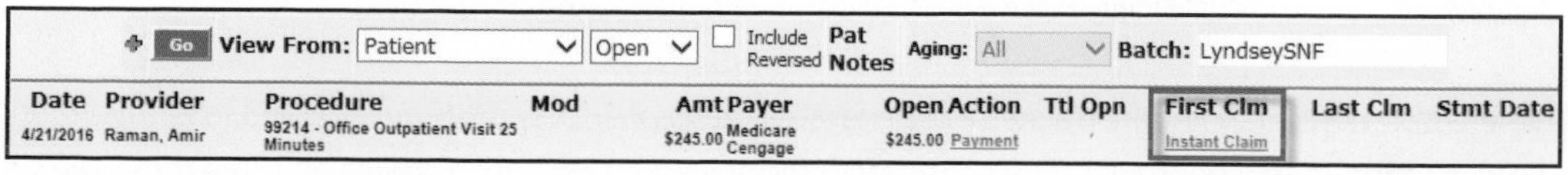

Figure 9-48 First Clm Column
Courtesy of Harris CareTracker PM and EMR

4. Place a check mark next to the claim you want to rebill to paper (select "99214" and "G0180"), and then click *Build Claim*. You will then note that the date you performed the activity is listed in the *First Clm* column.

5. Click on the date in the *First Clm* column (Figure 9-49) for which you want to generate a paper claim (select the charge you created in Activity 9-4 [99214]). Harris CareTracker PM displays the *Claims Summary* in the lower frame of the screen.

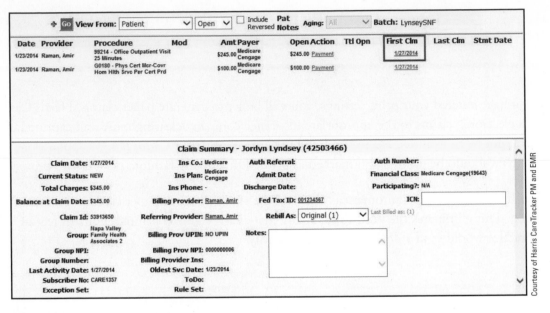

Figure 9-49 Select First Clm Date

6. Scroll down and click the *Rebill To= = >* drop-down list at the bottom of the screen and select "Paper 1500." Click *Rebuild Paper* (Figure 9-50).

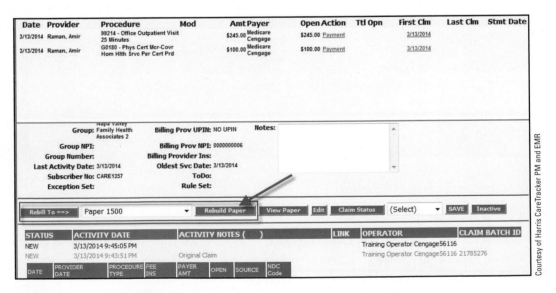

Figure 9-50 Select Rebuild Paper Claim

7. In a live environment, Harris CareTracker PM generates the *HCFA 1500 CMS Paper Form* in a new window. Your student version will not generate a paper 1500 form; instead, you will receive an error message on your screen (Figure 9-51). (**Note:** You can click "X" to close out of the error message and *Open Items* screens.)

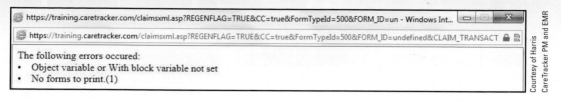

Figure 9-51   Paper Claim Error Message

8. In a live environment your screen would look like Figure 9-52. To print the form, you would right-click on the form and select *Print* from the shortcut menu. Figures 9-53 and 9-54 provide examples of the HCFA and Workers Comp HCFA forms.

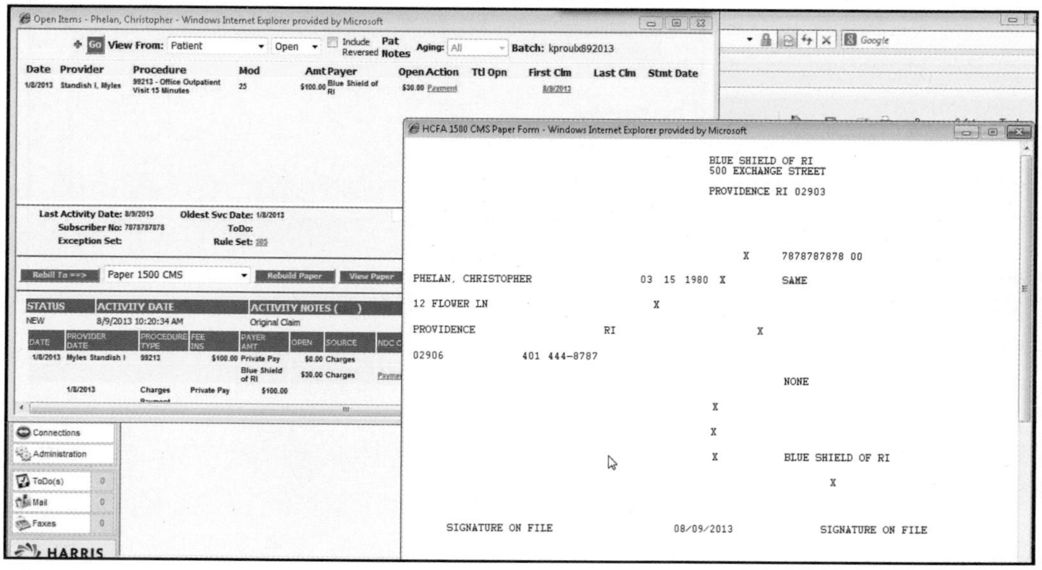

Figure 9-52   Paper Claim to 1500

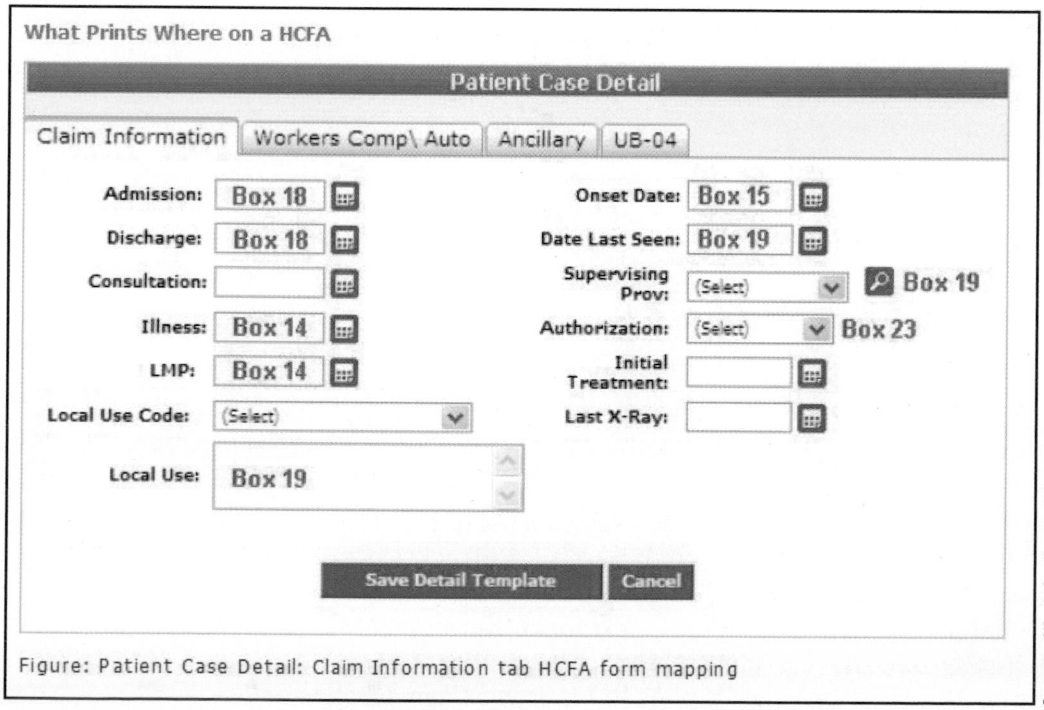

Figure 9-53   What Prints Where on an HCFA

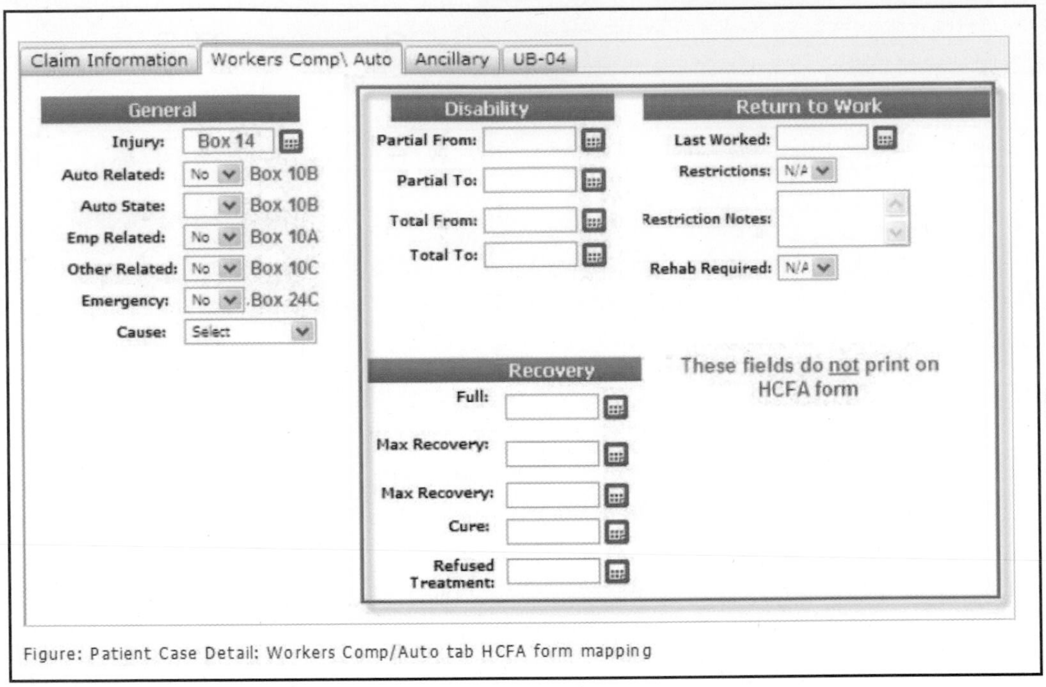

Figure: Patient Case Detail: Workers Comp/Auto tab HCFA form mapping

Figure 9-54 Workers Comp/Auto HCFA

Tip Box

HCFA is an acronym for the Health Care Financing Administration. HCFA references the insurance claim form that a health care provider submits to an insurance company, the CMS-1500 Form.

FYI

To print paper claim batches:

1. Go to the *Home* module > *Dashboard* tab > *Billing* section > *Unprinted Paper Claim Batches* link.
2. Click *Go*. Harris CareTracker PM displays a list of paper claim batches that need to be printed. In your student version of Harris CareTracker it will display "No Claims match your criteria".
3. (Optional) Click the plus sign [+] next to the word *Options* to display a set of filters (Figure 9-55). Use the filters to customize the list of paper claim batches displayed. (**Note:** The *Links Only* field applies to *Electronic Claim* batches only.)

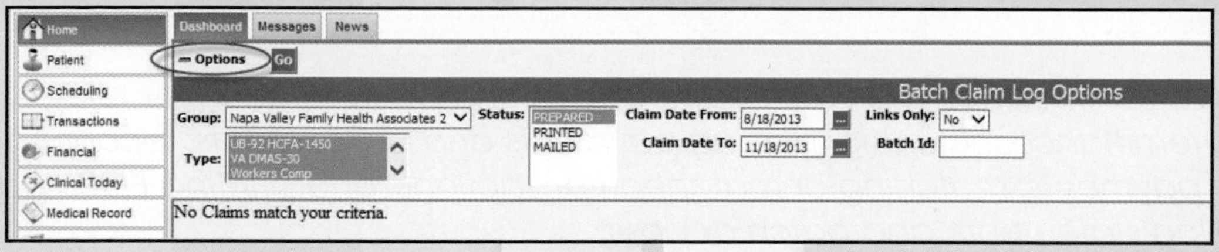

Courtesy of Harris CareTracker PM and EMR

Figure 9-55 Batch Claim Log Options

Tip Box

You can also submit a secondary paper claim form with an explanation of benefits (EOB) by collating secondary CMS-1500 paper forms in to a separate batch. This avoids having to browse through a list of CMS-1500 forms and reduces time and labor required to print secondary claim forms.

- Click on a paper claim batch line. The application displays the *Claim Activity Log* for the selected paper claim batch.
- (Optional) Click *View* to review claims before printing. Click *Back* to return to the previous view.
- Click *Print Forms.* The application displays the CMS-1500 form in the lower frame of the screen.
- Right-click on the CMS-1500 form and select *Print* from the pop-up menu. (At the practice, make sure laser CMS-1500 forms are loaded into the selected printer.)

Note: If you are having difficulty aligning the form properly, please see *Applying Print Settings* in the *Help* section.

- After printing the paper claims, click on the paper claim line under the *Paper Claim Batches* heading again and then click *Add*. The application displays additional fields in the lower frame of the screen.
- From the *Status* list, select *Printed.*

PM SPOTLIGHT

Practices have the option to automatically update the status of batch paper claims when the *Print Forms* button is used. This eliminates the need to manually mark each claim as printed. The practice would send a *ToDo* to its support entity to activate this feature.

4. If necessary, enter any notes regarding the printed paper claims in the *Notes* field.
5. Click *Save.*

ELECTRONIC REMITTANCE

Learning Objective 5: Demonstrate knowledge of and perform activities related to electronic remittance including: posting payments and adjustments; reconciling insurance payments; matching unmatched transactions; and printing EOBs, paper claims, billing statements, and batch deposits.

Remittances received electronically in Harris CareTracker PM are identified in the *Electronic Remittances* application in the *Billing* section of the *Dashboard* (Figure 9-56). Harris CareTracker PM matches the transactions on the electronic remittance to a specific patient, date of service, CPT® code, and charge amount.

Courtesy of Harris CareTracker PM and EMR

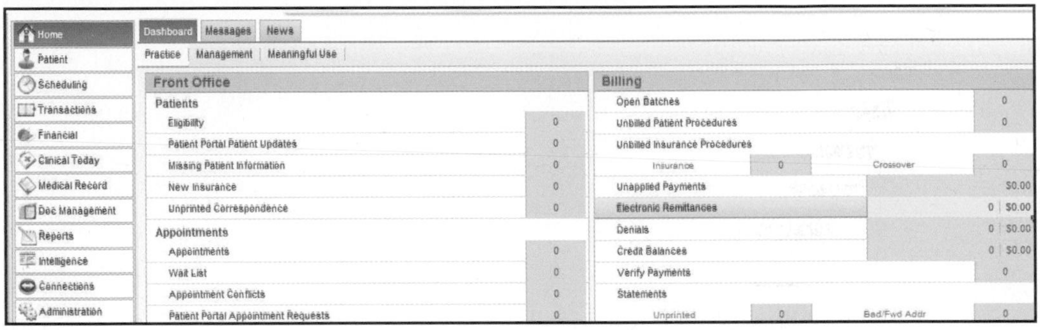

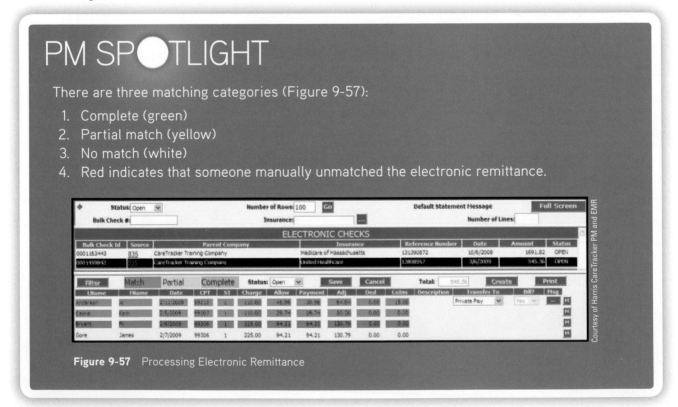

Figure 9-56 Electronic Remittances Link

PM SPOTLIGHT

There are three matching categories (Figure 9-57):

1. Complete (green)
2. Partial match (yellow)
3. No match (white)
4. Red indicates that someone manually unmatched the electronic remittance.

Courtesy of Harris CareTracker PM and EMR

Figure 9-57 Processing Electronic Remittance

Only complete matches will be processed electronically; partial and no matches must be manually matched before they can be processed. If they are not matched the payment will need to be manually posted into Harris CareTracker PM via the *Payments Open Items* application (Figures 9-58 and 9-59). In *Electronic Remittances*, statement messages can be added for individual patients that will print on their statements generated from Harris CareTracker PM.

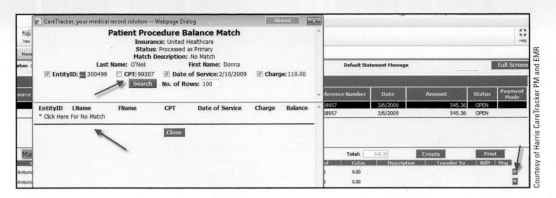

Figure 9-58 Patient Procedure Balance Match

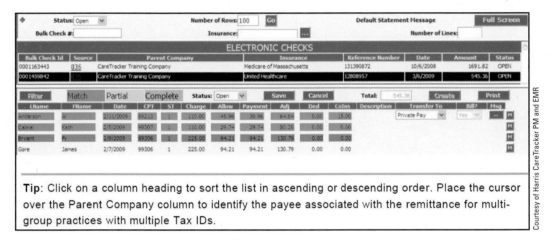

Figure 9-59 Filter Patient Procedure Balance Match

Post Payments and Adjustments

Harris CareTracker PM provides a rich environment to record payments and ensures that these claims are being paid appropriately. *Transactions, Reports, Admin, Financial, Messages,* and *Scheduling* are the modules used in Harris CareTracker PM when entering and processing payments. Several applications within each module are made use of as well.

There is a normal flow of payment activity in Harris CareTracker PM that begins when a patient pays his or her copayments. Copayments are entered in Harris CareTracker PM when the patient checks in or checks out (depending on the office workflow). Next, a claim is sent to the insurance company. In Harris CareTracker PM, most claims are transmitted electronically; however, paper forms are sometimes mailed. When bills are transmitted electronically, the payment is received electronically or on a paper EOB. Paper EOBs received in the mail from primary or secondary insurers are entered in the *Transactions* module. If payments are not received, Harris CareTracker PM provides a work list of unpaid claims that need to be reviewed and followed up. Once a payment has been accepted in full, Harris CareTracker PM verifies the payment and the adjustment entered is based on contractual tables that can be loaded into the system for specific payers.

Open Items. *Open Items* is an application in the *Financial* module. There is an identical application accessed via the *Pmt Open Item* tab in the *Transactions* module, and this application can also be accessed as a window by clicking the *OI* button on the *Name Bar*. The *Open Items* application is used to view all dates of service and the associated procedures, financial transactions, and claims activity (Figure 9-60). In this application you can enter many different types of financial transactions including patient payments, insurance payments, third-party payments, transfer balances, refunds, and apply unapplied money. You can also view the procedure details of each procedure, enter denial descriptions, attach statement messages to appear on patient statements, view a claim history, potentially rebill a claim, view electronic responses received from insurance companies, and view EOBs attached to payments.

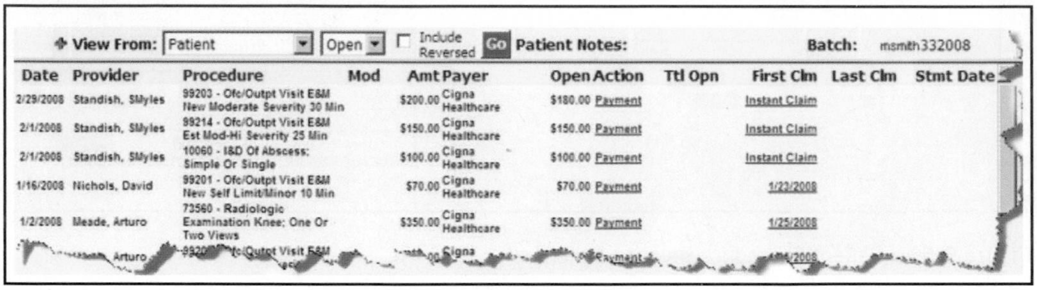

Courtesy of Harris CareTracker PM and EMR

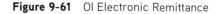

Figure 9-60 Open Items

Tip Box

You can access *Open Items* in the following ways:

- Left-click on an appointment in the *Book* application and select *Open Items*
- Click the *Appts* button in the *Name Bar*, and for any appointment listed select *Actions > Pmt Open Items.*
- Click the *OI* button on the *Name Bar*.
- Click the *Pmt Open Item* tab in the *Transactions* module.

Processing Electronic Remittances. The total number and sum of remittances received electronically into Harris CareTracker PM displays on the *Dashboard* and a list of the received remittances that need to be posted into the system is accessed by clicking on the *Electronic Remittances* link. Electronic remittances should only be posted after the check is received from the insurance company. Using electronic remittances will change the process for posting payments. After payments have been posted electronically, you must work credit balances and denials as a separate process. Typically, credit balances and denials are handled as an EOB is processed.

Before posting payments via *Electronic Remittances*, select one patient from the remittance, pull the patient into context, click the *OI* button on the *Name Bar*, and verify that the date of service is still open in Harris CareTracker PM (Figure 9-61).

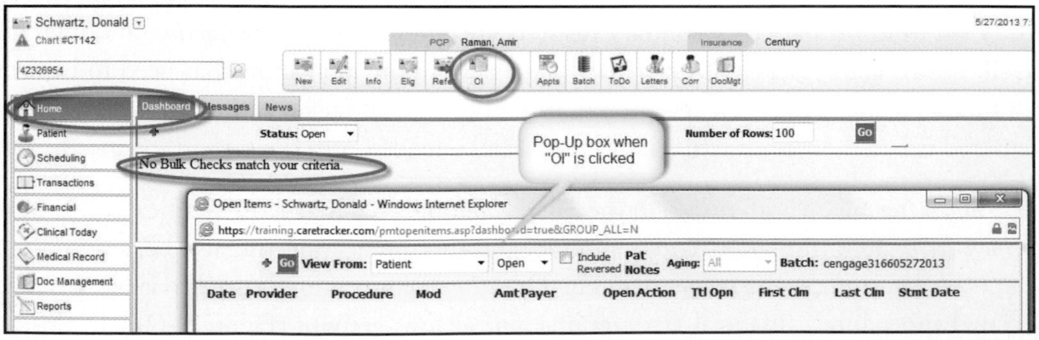

Courtesy of Harris CareTracker PM and EMR

Figure 9-61 OI Electronic Remittance

FYI

The *ClaimsManager* feature of Harris CareTracker PM is not active in your student version; however, the workflow to process electronic remittances in a live practice would be as follows:

1. Go to the *Home* module > *Dashboard* tab > *Billing* section > *Electronic Remittances* link. Harris CareTracker PM displays a list of electronic checks (Figure 9-62).

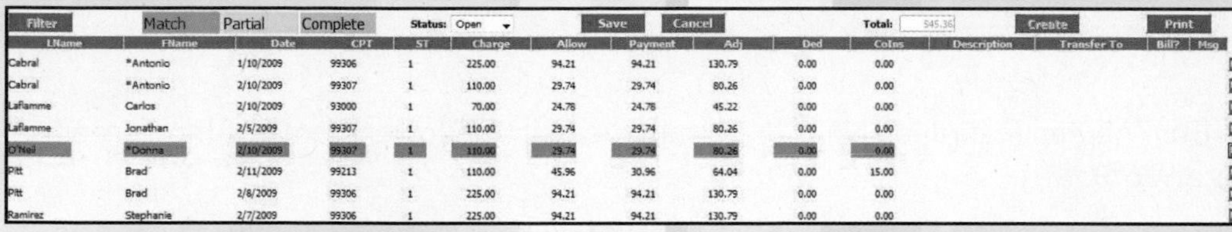

Courtesy of Harris CareTracker PM and EMR

Figure 9-62 Electronic Remittance Screen

2. Click the *plus sign* [+] to display the search fields (Figure 9-63). You would populate the desired search fields (Figure 9-64) as instructed in Table 9-1, Electronic Remittance Search.

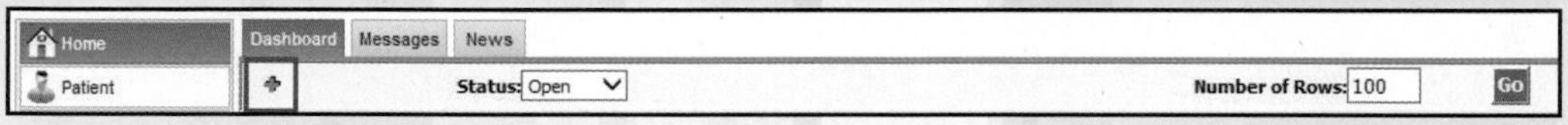

Figure 9-63 Electronic Remittance Plus Sign

Courtesy of Harris CareTracker PM and EMR

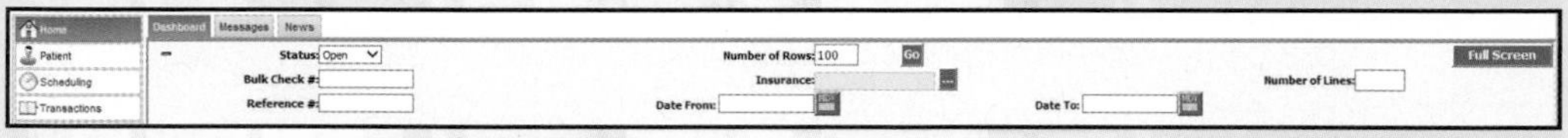

Figure 9-64 Electronic Remittance Search Fields

Courtesy of Harris CareTracker PM and EMR

TABLE 9-1 Electronic Remittance Search

Search Field	Description
Status	Select the status of remittances you want to access.
Number of Rows	Enter the number of remittances you want to return in the search. Limiting the number of rows increases system response times.
Default Statement Message	Place your cursor over this field to view the default statement messages. Messages can be added for individual patients that will print on their statements generated from Harris CareTracker PM. (**Note:** You will not see the "Default Message" tab if you had not yet set this up in the *Administration* module.)
Bulk Check #	Enter the check ID number.
Reference #	Enter the system generated reference number.
Number of Lines	Enter the number of check lines you want to work. Specifying a number of lines increases the response time by preventing the systems from loading all the lines from the electronic remittance. (**Note:** Limit the number of lines to 150 when processing large remittances.)
Date From/Date To	Enter the date range of the payments you want to access.

Courtesy of Harris CareTracker PM and EMR

(*Continues*)

(Continued)

PM SPOTLIGHT

You can update the default statement message in the *ERA Private Pay Message* application in the *Administration* module.

3. Click *Go*. The application displays the remittances in the lower frame of the screen (Figure 9-65).

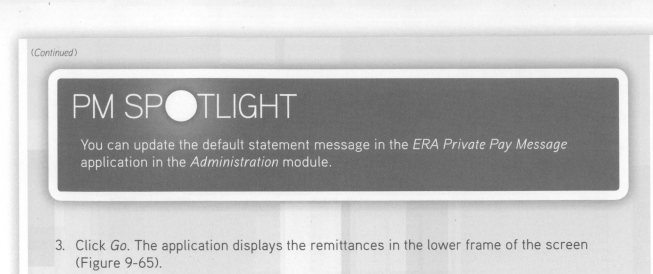

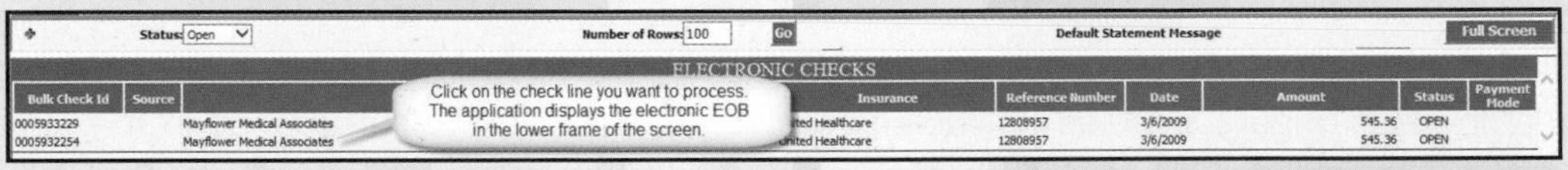

Figure 9-65 Electronic Checks

Courtesy of Harris CareTracker PM and EMR

4. Click the check line you want to process. The application displays the electronic EOB in the lower frame of the screen (Figure 9-66).

Courtesy of Harris CareTracker PM and EMR

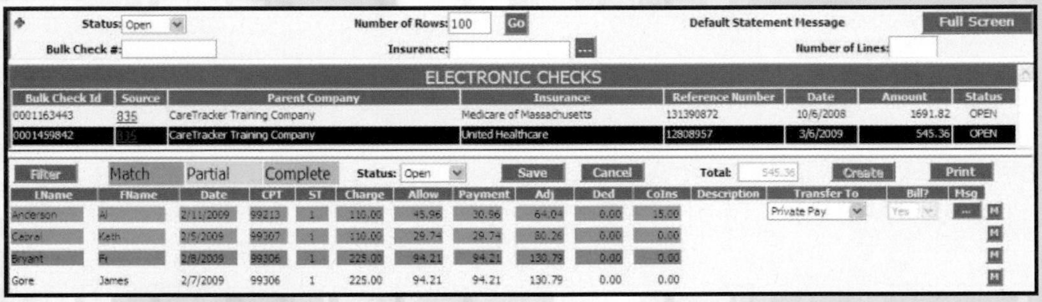

Figure 9-66 Payment Window

Tip Box

Click on a column heading to sort the list in ascending or descending order. Place the cursor over the *Parent Company* column to identify the payee associated with the remittance for multi-group practices with multiple tax IDs.

5. Click *Save*. Harris CareTracker PM will automatically match as many unmatched transactions as possible, which is especially useful if you have received checks from secondary payers.
6. Manually match any remaining partial or unmatched transactions and then click *Save*.
7. You can transfer any balances to either a secondary payer or to private pay by selecting payer from the list in the *Transfer To* column. For balances transferred to private pay, Harris CareTracker PM automatically includes the default message set up in the *ERA Private Pay Message* application in the *Administration* module, *Practice* tab. **Note:** You will not see the "Default Message" tab if you had not yet set this up.

PM SP⬤TLIGHT

If the practice has not set up a default message, and you would like to select a different message, or add a new message:

- Click the ellipses (...) button in the *MSG* column. The application displays the *Statement Message* dialog box.
- In the *Msg Code* box, enter the message code or select a message from the *Stmt Msg* list.
- (Optional) Click *Msg* to view the entire message.
- Click *Save* to save the message and close the dialog box. The ellipses (...) button changes to a *MSG* button indicating that a message has been added.

8. Click *Create*. The application displays your current open batch information in a dialog box. **WARNING:** Do not click the *Create* button more than once.
9. Verify that the batch information is correct and then click *Confirm*. The application creates the financial transactions and displays a confirmation message in the lower frame of the screen.
10. Click on the highlighted check line. All of the payments created are highlighted in gray.
11. Click *Print*. The application displays a print options dialog box that displays the payments listed, the total of the check, and the reference number entered on the batch.
12. In the window, click the *Print* button to print out the document, and attach it to the EOB. This document will replace your journal for payments processed via electronic remittances.

Tip Box

If there are yellow or white lines on the remittance that were not manually matched, these payments are not posted; therefore the payment amount on the EOB will not match the total payments on this document.

(Continues)

(Continued)

13. From the *Status* list, change the status to *Close* and click the *Save* button which indicates that the remittance has been processed and removes it from open items. The status of manually posted remittances should be changed to "Inactive."
14. Click on the *Filter* button and de-select all options except "No Match" and "Partial Match." Click the *Accept* button, click the *Print* button, and then a list of all payments that were not posted will print. These partial or unmatched payments will need to be posted manually from the *Open Items* application in the *Financial* module.
15. Post your batch in Harris CareTracker PM.
16. Then work credit balances and denials.

You will now process a simulated remittance in Activity 9-10.

ACTIVITY 9-10: Process a Remittance

1. Create a new batch and name it "PostEOBs". Update the provider to Jordyn Lyndsey's provider and PCP, and use the same service and payment dates as the appointment you scheduled for her in Activity 4-1.
2. Pull patient Jordyn Lyndsey into context.
3. Click on the *OI* button in the *Name Bar*.
4. All captured visits for the date entered will display. Find the date for which you want to process a remittance (select the appointment you created in Activity 4-1). Click on the *Payment* link in the *Action* column next to Procedure 99203. Harris CareTracker PM displays the payment window in the lower frame of the screen (Figure 9-67). (**Note:** If you do not see Procedure 99203 listed in the *Open Items* window, follow the steps in the *Tip Box* on pages 501–502. Then, before continuing on to Step 5, repeat Activity 9-9 and generate a paper claim for Procedure 99203.)

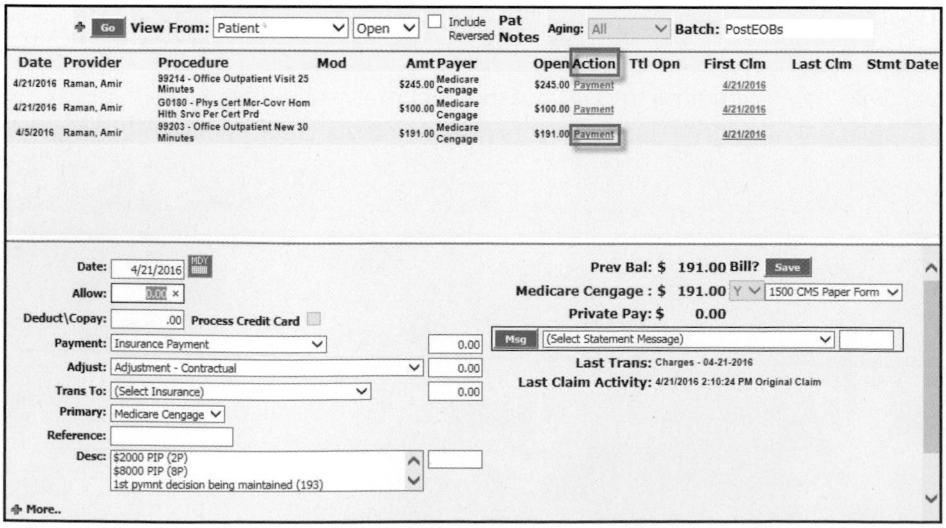

Courtesy of Harris CareTracker PM and EMR

Figure 9-67 OI for Jordyn Lyndsey

Tip Box

Important!! If you do not see the charge in *OI* for the visit you entered in Activity 4-1, you will need to follow these instructions. Go to *Home* module > *Dashboard* tab > *Visit* header > *Missing Encounters/Visits* link (Figure 9-68) and you will see that the *Visit* has not been saved (Figure 9-69).

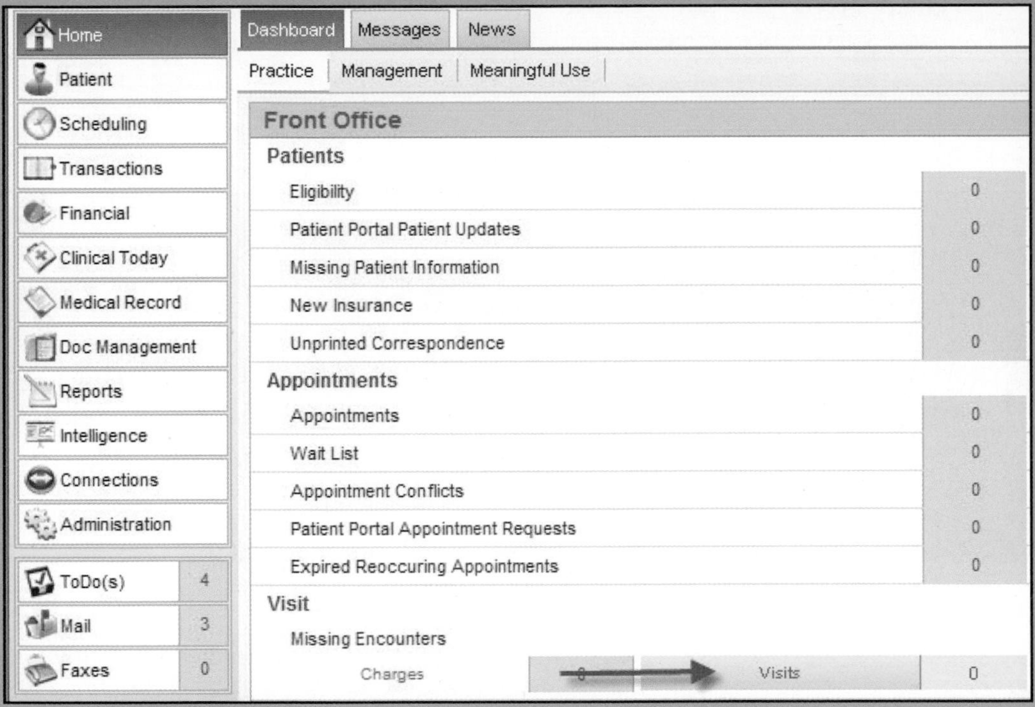

Courtesy of Harris CareTracker PM and EMR

Figure 9-68 Missing Encounters/Visits Link

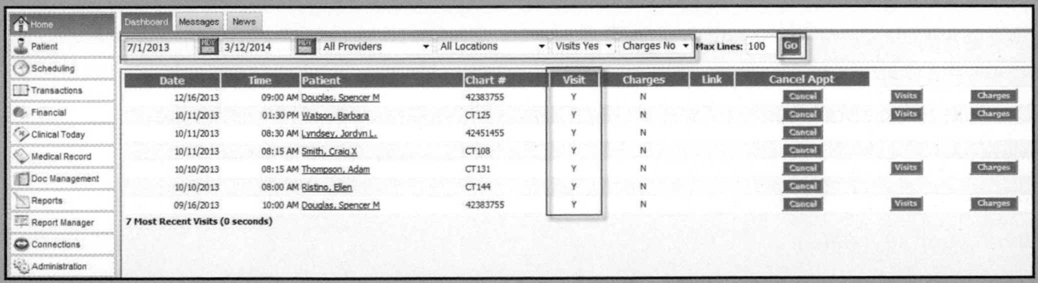

Courtesy of Harris CareTracker PM and EMR

Figure 9-69 Visits Not Saved

To save the *Charges*, set the fields as follows:

- Include the date of the patient encounter.
- Select *All providers*.
- Select *All locations*.
- Select *Visits Yes*.
- Select *Charges No*.
- Click *Go*.

(*Continues*)

(Continued)

Scroll up and locate the date of service (DOS) for the patient you are working on. You will see the *Visits* and *Charges* buttons (Figure 9-70). When you are working in *OI*, if more than one charge (e.g., multiple patient visits) appear on the same date, *Visits* will be saved for all patients.

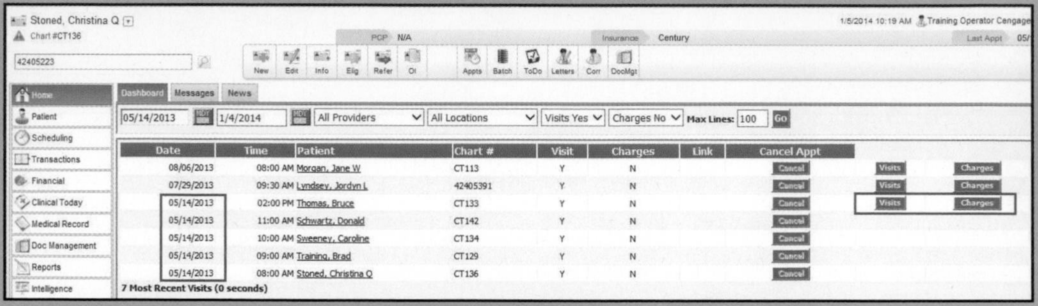

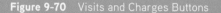

Figure 9-70   Visits and Charges Buttons

- Click on the *Charges* button on the right side of your screen for the DOS.
- Click *Go* on the left side of your screen. The charges for all patient encounters on the DOS display.
- Scroll down and click *Save* on the bottom left of your screen (**Note:** If more than one charge [e.g., multiple patient visits] appear on the date, the *Visits* will be saved for all patients).
- **Important!!** You must wait until the "Transaction Saved" message appears before the charges will appear in the *Open Items* window.

5. In the payment window, enter the information from Jordyn Lyndsey's EOB (Source Document 9-1 in Appendix A) for the *Visit* you created in Activity 4-1 and related charge you created in Case Study 7-7. You will note that the EOB also contains information for the charge you entered in Activity 9-3. **Important:** Only enter the EOB information for the visit created in Activity 4-1 (*Visit* captured in Case Study 7-7) at this time (Procedure 99203). You will enter the denial for the charge created in Activity 9-3 in a later activity. Enter the EOB information as listed below. Your completed screen should look like Figure 9-71.

   a. *Date:* This should match the date of the appointment you created in Activity 4-1 and Case Study 7-7 *Visit* capture.

   b. *Allow:* Enter the information from the *Amount Allowed* column on the EOB. Now hit the [Tab] button on your keyboard.

   c. *Deduct/Copay:* Enter the information from the *Deduct/Coins/Copay* column on the EOB. Now hit the [Tab] button and this will populate the amount in the *Adjust* and *Transfer* To fields based on the information entered in the *Demographics* screen.

   d. *Payment*: Confirm that "Insurance Payment" is selected

   e. *Adjust*: Confirm that "Adjustment – Contractual" is selected

   f. *Trans To:* Confirm that "Private Pay" is selected

   g. *Primary:* Confirm that "Medicare Cengage" is selected

   h. *Reference:* Leave blank

   i. *Desc:* Leave as is

   j. *Msg:* Enter "CO" in the blank box to the right of the drop-down menu and hit the [Tab] key.

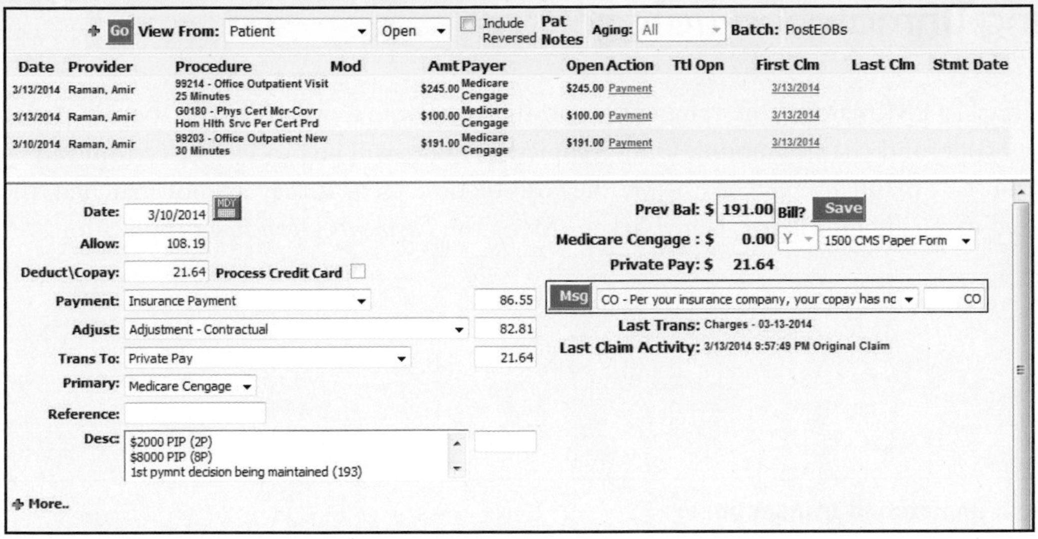

Courtesy of Harris CareTracker PM and EMR

Figure 9-71 OI for Jordyn Lyndsey

Print the Process Remittance (OI screen), label it "Activity 9-10," and place it in your assignment folder.

6. Once you have entered the EOB information, click *Save*. Your transaction will be saved and the claim disappears.
7. (FYI Only) If you were working multiple charges, you would repeat steps 5 and 6 for each of the charges listed on the EOB. **Note**: Do not enter the additional payments at this point.
8. Close out of the *Open Items* window by clicking the "X" in the upper-right corner of the window.

Late charges, interest payments, and "take backs" are not processed from *Electronic Remittance* and must be applied manually via the *Payment Open Items* application. Post all primary before secondary checks (e.g., Medicare checks before Blue Shield checks in the case of a Medicare primary patient).

Insurance Payment Reconciliation and Follow-Up

Credit balances are created when either a patient or an insurance company pays more money for a specific procedure for a specific date of service than what was billed. Credit balances can be identified by the *Credit Balances* link under the *Billing* section of the *Dashboard* on the *Home* page for a specific batch or group. A credit balance should either be refunded to the patient or an insurance company or it can be applied to another date of service.

Tip Box

After you post payments via electronic remittances, it is best practice to work credit balances for the batch you were working on before posting the batch.

Matching Unmatched Transactions

Harris CareTracker PM matches the transactions on the electronic remittance to a specific patient, date of service, CPT® code, and charge amount. Only complete matches will be processed electronically; partial and no matches must be manually matched before they can be processed. If they are not matched, the payment must be posted manually into Harris CareTracker PM via the *Payments Open Items* application.

FYI

To match unmatched transactions:

1. Double-click on a white or yellow line, or click on the *M* button at the end of one of these lines (Figure 9-72).

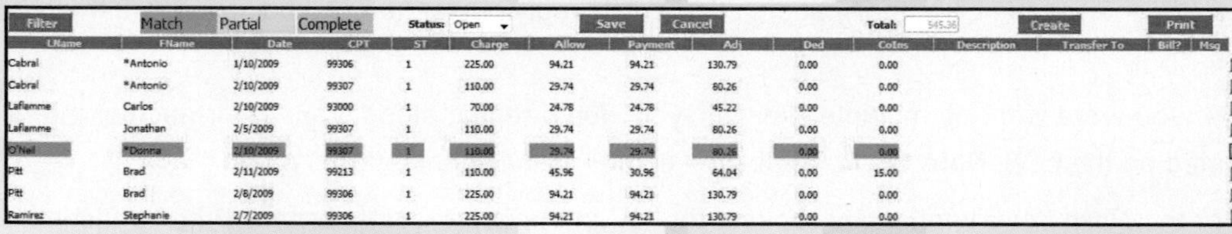

Figure 9-72 Electronic Remittance Screen

2. When a line is selected, the *Patient Procedure Balance Match* window displays, showing the insurance, status of claim, match description, and the patient's last name, and first name. Harris CareTracker PM's four matching options: patient ID number, CPT® code, date of service, and charge display as checked off in the pop-up, indicating that these options have been used as the matching criteria. Click on the *Search* button.

3. When you deselect one of the checkboxes and then click *Search*, all of the transactions entered in Harris CareTracker PM that match only the selected matching criteria display in the lower frame of the pop-up window.

Tip Box

If a matching transaction does not appear, try de-selecting a different match criteria and clicking on the *Search* button again.

4. Click on the transaction that matches the electronic remittance.

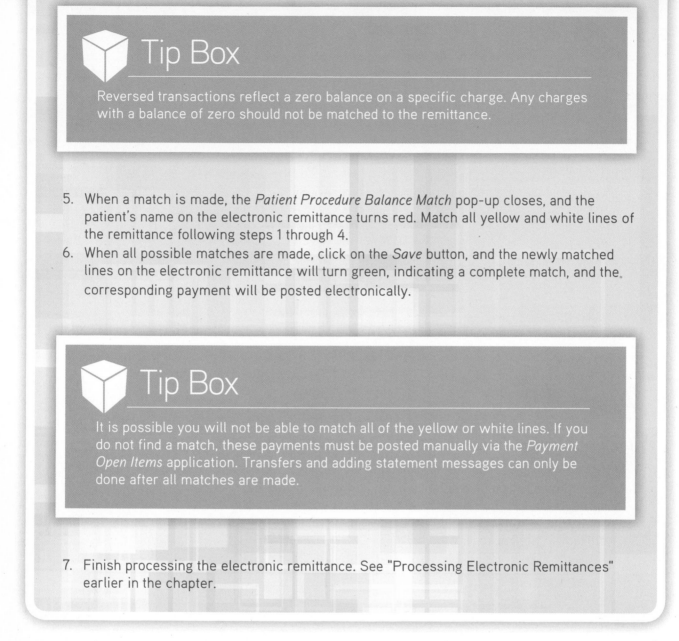

Tip Box

Reversed transactions reflect a zero balance on a specific charge. Any charges with a balance of zero should not be matched to the remittance.

5. When a match is made, the *Patient Procedure Balance Match* pop-up closes, and the patient's name on the electronic remittance turns red. Match all yellow and white lines of the remittance following steps 1 through 4.
6. When all possible matches are made, click on the *Save* button, and the newly matched lines on the electronic remittance will turn green, indicating a complete match, and the corresponding payment will be posted electronically.

Tip Box

It is possible you will not be able to match all of the yellow or white lines. If you do not find a match, these payments must be posted manually via the *Payment Open Items* application. Transfers and adding statement messages can only be done after all matches are made.

7. Finish processing the electronic remittance. See "Processing Electronic Remittances" earlier in the chapter.

Print Insurance EOBs

From *Electronic Remittances,* Harris CareTracker PM can also print paper EOBs. Harris CareTracker PM has payer-specific EOBs that mimic payers' customized EOBs. Although not an active feature in your student version, in a live environment payer-specific EOBs can be printed for the payers listed in Table 9-2.

A generic EOB can be printed for all other payers. A generic EOB does not mimic a payer's customized EOB, but does include standard information such as patient name, allowed amount, paid amount, deductible/copayment, and adjustment. Generic EOBs are printed the same way as payer-specific EOBs.

TABLE 9-2   Harris CareTracker Payer-Specific EOBs

Medicare	United Healthcare
Aetna	Medicaid of Rhode Island
Blue Cross Blue Shield of Massachusetts	Blue Cross Blue Shield of Rhode Island
Harvard Pilgrim	Medicaid of Massachusetts
Blue Shield of Texas	Tufts
Railroad Medicare	DME
Cigna, Unicare (GIC Indemnity)	Connecticare
Tricare (North Region)	GHI

FYI

The workflow to print insurance EOBs in a live environment:

1. Access the *Home* module > *Dashboard* tab > *Billing* section > *Electronic Remittances* link.
2. Select the electronic remittance that you want to print. The application displays the EOB in the lower frame of the screen. (**Note:** Your screen will display "No Bulk Checks match your criteria" (Figure 9-73) because *ClaimsManager* is not active in your student version of Harris CareTracker PM.)

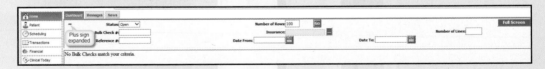

Figure 9-73   No Bulk Checks

3. Click *Print*. The application displays the *Print* window.
4. Click *Print EOB* to print the entire EOB. This will be a complete EOB without page breaks between patients. Figure 9-74 is representative of a generic EOB, not one that would be electronically generated in Harris CareTracker.
5. To print an EOB for a patient or multiple patients, click on the corresponding patient's name in the *Associated Patient* box and then click *Add*.

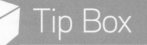 Tip Box

If a selection is made in error, click on the patient listed in the *Selected* box and then click the *Remove* button.

6. Click *Print EOB*. The application displays the *File Download* window.
7. Click *Open*. Adobe Acrobat opens the EOB in a window.
8. From the Adobe Acrobat menu, click *File > Print*.

Note: If printing multiple EOBs, each will print on a separate page by default.

Aetna

P.O. BOX 500
ALFRED NY 14802-0500
(800) 555-5000

CINDY MATTESON
5 GREENE ST
ALFRED NY 14802

DATE: 10/01/YYYY
ID #:   BLS123456789
ENROLLEE: CINDY MATTESON
HICN: 123XYZ
BENEFIT PLAN: COMMERCIAL

EXPLANATION OF BENEFITS

SERVICE DETAIL

PATIENT/RELAT CLAIM NUMBER	PROVIDER/ SERVICE	DATE OF SERVICE	AMOUNT CHARGED	NOT COVERED	AMOUNT ALLOWED	COPAY/ DEDUCTIBLE	%	PLAN BENEFITS	REMARK CODE
ENROLLEE 5629587	A SMITH OFFICE VISIT	09/01/YY	875.00		367.00	18.00	100	349.00	D1
						PLAN PAYS		349.00	

*THIS IS A COPY OF INFORMATION SENT TO THE PROVIDER. THANK YOU FOR USING THE PARTICIPATING PROVIDER PROGRAM.

REMARK CODE(S) LISTED BELOW ARE REFERENCED IN THE *SERVICE DETAIL* SECTION UNDER THE HEADING *REMARK CODE*
(D1)   THANK YOU FOR USING A NETWORK PROVIDER. WE HAVE APPLIED THE NETWORK CONTRACTED FEE. THE MEMBER IS NOT RESPONSIBLE FOR THE DIFFERENCE BETWEEN THE AMOUNT CHARGED AND THE AMOUNT ALLOWED BY THE CONTRACT.

BENEFIT PLAN PAYMENT SUMMARY INFORMATION
A SMITH $349.00

PATIENT NAME	MEDICAL/SURGICAL DEDUCTIBLE		MEDICAL/SURGICAL OUT OF POCKET		PHYSICAL MEDICINE DEDUCTIBLE	
	ANNUAL DEDUCT	YYYY YEAR TO-DATE	ANNUAL MAXIMUM	YYYY YEAR TO-DATE	ANNUAL DEDUCT	YYYY YEAR TO-DATE
ENROLLEE	$850.00	$875.00	$2500.00	$1699.50	$1250.00	$0.00

THIS CLAIM WAS PROCESSED IN ACCORDANCE WITH THE TERMS OF YOUR EMPLOYEE BENEFITS PLAN. IN THE EVENT THIS CLAIM HAS BEEN DENIED, IN WHOLE OR IN PART, A REQUEST FOR REVIEW MAY BE DIRECTED TO THE KEYSTONE PLAN AT THE ALFRED ADDRESS OR PHONE NUMBER SHOWN ABOVE. THE REQUEST FOR REVIEW MUST BE SUBMITTED WITHIN 60 DAYS AFTER THE CLAIM PAYMENT DATE, OR THE DATE OF THE NOTIFICATION OF DENIAL OF BENEFITS. WHEN REQUESTING A REVIEW, PLEASE STATE WHY YOU BELIEVE THE CLAIM DETERMINATION OR PRE-CERTIFICATION IMPROPERLY REDUCED OR DENIED YOUR BENEFITS. ALSO, SUBMIT ANY DATA OR COMMENTS TO SUPPORT THE APPEAL.

THIS IS NOT A BILL.

Figure 9-74 Generic EOB

Denials

Denials are claims that an insurance company has determined it will not pay, such as when a patient has not met his or her deductible. The *Denials* application identifies both the total number of denials and the total monetary value of the denials for a specific period, batch or group. The application is updated overnight. In this application you can work denials to adjust off balances. By working your denials separately from posting payments, you will improve the workflow and efficiency in your practice. Your student version of Harris CareTracker PM will not post *Denials* in your *Dashboard* because *ClaimsManager* is not active. If you were working in a live *Practice Management* system, best practice would be to work *Denials* after your batch has been posted. The *Dashboard* only shows *Denials* for the month. *Denials* are only tallied on the *Dashboard* if:

- The denial code or description was manually entered in the *Description* field in the *Open Items* application.
- Payments were posted electronically via *Electronic Remittances*. *Electronic Remittances* posted in Harris CareTracker PM will automatically post any denials. *Denials* remain in the *Denials* link on the *Dashboard* until they are paid or adjusted off.

Tip Box

Denials can be organized by assigning custom denial categories. Each category is linked to one or more denial transaction types. Company-specific *Denial Categories* are created and maintained in the *Denial Categories* maintenance application on the *Setup* tab in the *Administration* module. **Note:** You must have the *Denials* security privilege included in your operator profile to access the *Denials* application.

Denial Details. Clicking on a denial in the work list displays the *Denial Details* tab (Figure 9-75). From the *Details* screen you can:

- Click the denial to display the *Procedure Line Item Details* in a new window
- Adjust procedure denials individually or in bulk
- Transfer one or more denial balances to private pay
- Launch the *Open Items* application for a denial
- View the *Claim Summary* for the denial
- Click the *Microsoft Excel*® icon at the bottom of the work list to export the denial details to a *Microsoft Excel*® file.

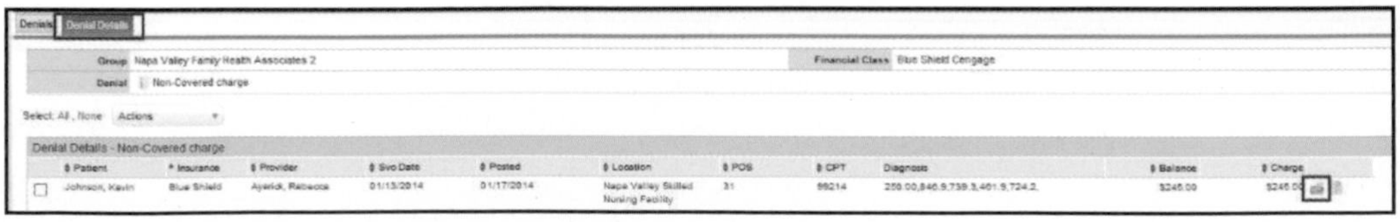

Figure 9-75 Denial Details Tab

Courtesy of Harris CareTracker PM and EMR

The *Denials* screen can be accessed by going to the *Home* module > *Dashboard* tab > *Billing* header > *Denials* link (Figure 9-76).

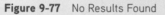

Figure 9-76 Denials Link

FYI

The workflow to view and export denials in a live environment:

1. Access the *Home* module > *Dashboard* tab > *Billing* header > *Denials* link.
2. The application displays the denials work list. **Note:** You may have to reset the criteria such as *Groups, Transaction Date Range, Fiscal Period,* and *Fiscal Year.* If no *Denials* fit the selected criteria, your screen will update and display "No results found" (Figure 9-77).

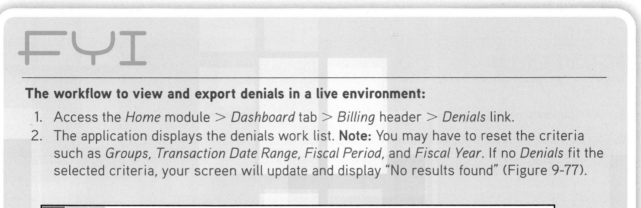

Figure 9-77 No Results Found

3. Select the desired search criteria and then click *Search.* The application returns the results (Figure 9-78). (See *Searching Denials* in *Help* for more information.)

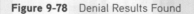

Figure 9-78 Denial Results Found

4. Click on a denial line to display the *Denial Details.*
5. Click on a denial detail line to view the procedure details.

(Continues)

(Continued)

6. To view the *Claim Summary*:
   a. Click the *Claim Summary* 📇 icon. The application displays the *Claim Details* in a new window. You can add a note to the claim, edit the claim, rebill the claim, flag the claim as missing information, or flag the claim as in review if needed.
7. To export denials:
   a. Click the *Microsoft Excel®* icon at the bottom of the denial details work list. The application displays a *File Download* dialog box.
   b. Click *Save*.
   c. Select a location to save the file and then click *Save*.

Using the same patient from Activity 9-10 (Jordyn Lyndsey), you will now post a denial and additional remittance to her account.

ACTIVITY 9-11: Enter a Denial and Remittance

1. With patient Jordyn Lyndsey in context, click on the *OI* 🗔 button on the *Name Bar*.
2. All captured visits for the date entered will display. Scroll down to display Jordyn Lyndsey's SNF edited charge you entered in Activity 9-4 (for Procedure 99214) and you will see the visit and charge captured.

📦 Tip Box

Important!! If you do not see the edited SNF charge you entered in Activity 9-4, go to the *Home* module > *Dashboard* tab > *Visit* header > *Missing Encounters/Visit* link (see Figures 9-69 and 9-70) and you will see that the *Visit* has not been saved.
To save the *Charges*, set the fields as follows:

- Include the date of the patient encounter.
- Select *All providers*.
- Select *All locations*.
- Select *Visits Yes*.
- Select *Charges No*.
- Click *Go*.

See Tip Box on pages 501-502 for complete instructions on saving the *Charges*.
Important!! You must wait until the "Transaction Saved" message appears before the charges will appear in the *Open Items* window.

3. In the *Open Items* dialog box, click the *Payment* link under the *Action* header for the 99214 charge and enter the *Denial* information from Jordyn Lyndsey's EOB (the amount that displays in the *Not Covered* column) (see Source Document 9-1 in Appendix A), as described next. (**Note:** If you are not currently working in a batch, you will be prompted to enter your batch information and redirects in the lower portion of the batch screen as displayed in Figure 9-79. You should still be working in the "PostEOBs" batch created in Activity 9-10.)

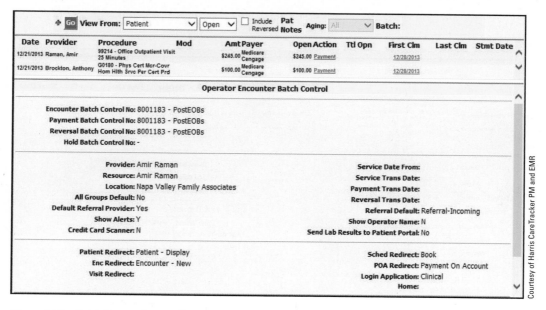

Figure 9-79   Batch Prompt Screen OI

a. *Date*: Leave the date as entered.

b. *Allow*: Leave blank.

c. *Deduct/Copay*: Leave blank.

d. *Payment*: Leave blank.

e. *Adjust*: Select "Adjustment – Contractual."

f. *Transfer To*: Use the drop-down and select "Private Pay." This will automatically populate the amount field to the right of *Trans To*, as well as the *Prev Bal* and *Private Pay* fields.

g. *Primary*: Leave blank (or it can remain "Medicare Cengage.")

h. *Reference*: Leave blank.

i. *Desc*: Type "96" in the blank box to the right of *Desc* and hit [Tab]. This will select "Non-Covered charge (96)."

j. In the *Msg* field, use the drop-down list and select "SEE BILLING NOTE."

Print the Denied Charge screen, label it "Activity 9-11," and place it in your assignment folder.

k. Click *Save*. Your transaction will be saved and the claim disappears.

June 5, 2017

4. In the *Open Items* window, click the *Payment* link under the *Action* header for the G0180 charge and enter the remittance information from Jordyn Lyndsey's EOB. (**Note:** Refer to Step 5 in Activity 9-10 to process this remittance.)

5. You have now saved all the *Denial* and *Remittance* information from the EOB related to the SNF charge you created in Activities 9-3 and 9-4 for Jordyn Lyndsey (as noted in Figure 9-80). Once your transaction is saved (Figure 9-81) the claim disappears. (You may have to close out of the *OI* screen and re-open it before the claim disappears.) **Note:** You must be sure to enter the charge in the period/year of the service as originally entered.

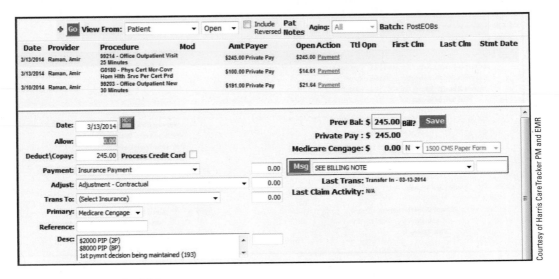

Figure 9-80 Lyndsey Denial Screen

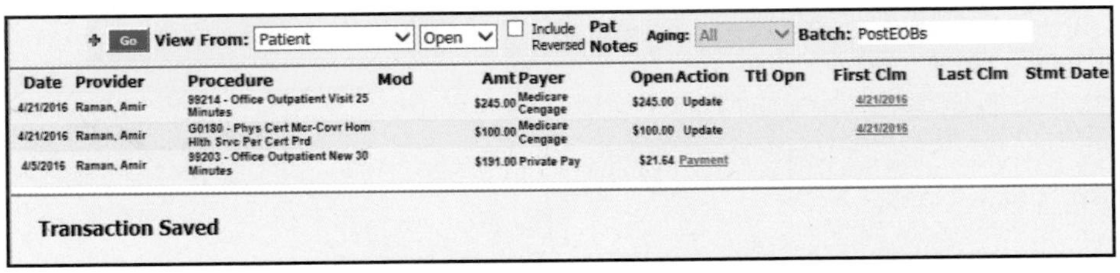

Figure 9-81 Lyndsey Transaction Saved

6. Do not post the "PostEOBs" batch at this time. You will be instructed to post it later.

Having entered the denial in Activity 9-11, the balance has now been transferred to private pay. **Note:** It is important to remember that it takes 24 hours for *Denials* to display in the *Dashboard* in a live environment. You can adjust your filters to set your display options. The *Dashboard* only shows *Denials* for the month. If you were to transfer a balance to Private Pay other than when posting a denial, you would follow the instruction in the FYI box.

FYI

The Workflow to Transfer a Denial Balance to Private Pay in a Live Environment:

1. You would create a new batch. Before saving your batch, review the location (place of service) and confirm that it is correct.
2. Access the *Home* module > *Dashboard* tab > *Billing* header > *Denials* link. The application displays the denials work list.
3. Click on the *Advanced Search* link and the *Advanced Search* dialog box will display. Change *Procedure Paid* and *Recent Activity* to "Yes," and then click on *Search* and the *Procedure Count by Reason* list will display the charge (Figure 9-82). (**Note:** If it does not display, click on the *Operator Maintenance* ⚙ icon and the *Default Operator Setting* dialog box displays. Change recent activity to "Yes"; leave procedure paid as "No." Click *Save* and the *Procedure Count by Reason* list will display the charge.)

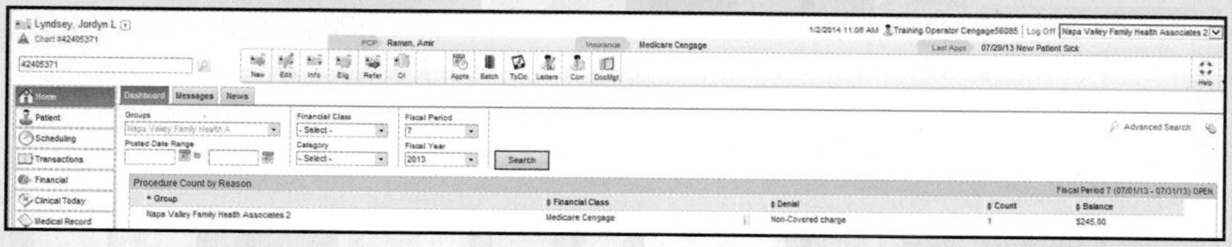

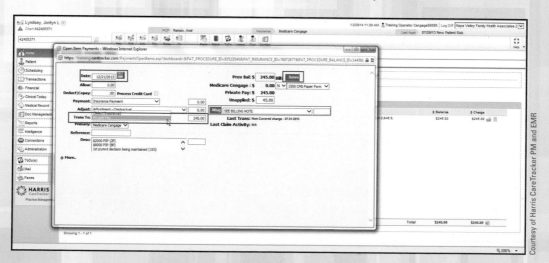

Figure 9-82   Denials Balance

4. Click on the denial line, and the *Denial Details* tab will display.
5. Click on the *Payment* 🗋 icon to the right of the *Charge* column and the *Open Item Payments* window displays.
6. Scroll down to the *Trans To* field and select "Private Pay" (Figure 9-83). You will note that the amount of the denial now displays in the *Private Pay* fields.

Figure 9-83   Transfer to Private Pay

7. Add the statement message "CO" in the blank box to the right of the *Msg* field.
8. Click *Save*.
9. Now post the batch.

Now that you have entered the EOB and transferred the remaining balance to Private Pay, a typical workflow would be to adjust the denial balance. For instance, if after you transferred the balance to Private Pay you determined that the CPT® code used should not have been billed, you would then adjust the denial balance to reflect the change.

FYI

The Workflow to Adjust a Denial Balance in a Live Environment:

The following steps represent an example of how to adjust a denial balance:

1. Create a batch and confirm that the appropriate *Date, Provider, Resource,* and *Location* are used.

2. With a patient in context, go to the *Home* module > *Dashboard* tab > *Billing* header > *Denials* link.

3. Select the desired search criteria and then click *Search.* The application will return the results of your search. If no results are returned, click on the *Advanced Search* button (Figure 9-84). In the *Advanced Search* pop-up dialog box, first confirm that *Procedure Paid* and *Recent Activity* radio dials are set to "Yes," and then click *Search.* If the *Procedure Count by Reason* does not display, click on the magnifying glass in the *Advanced Search* dialog box. In the *Search* box, you would enter at least two letters of the associated batch (for example enter "TR" and then click *Search.* (Be sure a check mark is placed next to *Include Closed Batches* and *All Groups.*)

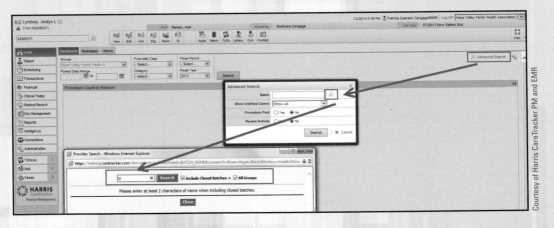

Courtesy of Harris CareTracker PM and EMR

Figure 9-84 Advanced Search

4. The pop-up will display the batch(es) (Figure 9-85). Click on the batch posted containing the denial, and it will be pulled into your pop-up *Advanced Search* box (Figure 9-86).

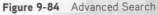

BATCH NAME	BATCH ID	ACTIVE	OPERATOR	PERIOD	FISCAL_YEAR	STATUS	GROUP
TrPrivatePay	8001237	N	cengage56085	December 2013		Closed	Napa Valley Family Health Associates 2

Courtesy of Harris CareTracker PM and EMR

Figure 9-85 Popup Provider Search - TrPrivatePay

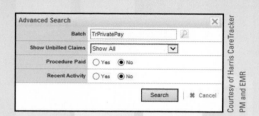

Figure 9-86   Advanced Search Batch Display

5. Click on the denial line to display the *Denial Details* item and select the CPT® code you want to adjust (for example, 99214).
6. Select the checkbox next to the denials you want to adjust, for example CPT® code 99214.
7. From the drop-down arrow in the *Actions* list, select "Adjust." The application displays the *Adjust Denial Detail* dialog box.
8. From the *Adjustment Code* list, select the adjustment type. Select the appropriate adjustment type to fit the reason for adjusting the denial.
9. In the *Amount* box enter the dollar amount you want to adjust. For example, enter "245.00."
10. The *Transaction Date* defaults to the current date. Click the *Calendar* icon to change the transaction date, if needed.
11. Click *Save* and your denial balance will be adjusted (Figure 9-87).

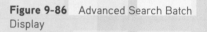

Figure 9-87   Denial Balance Adjustment

12. Post the batch.

Credit Balances

Working credit balances by batch should be done immediately after an electronic remittance has been posted in Harris CareTracker PM. Credit balances are created when either a patient or an insurance company pays more money for a specific procedure for a specific date of service than what was billed. Credit balances can be identified by the *Credit Balances* link under the *Billing* section of the *Dashboard* in the *Home* module for a specific batch or group (Figure 9-88). After you post payments via electronic remittances, it is best practice to work credit balances for the batch you were working in before posting the batch.

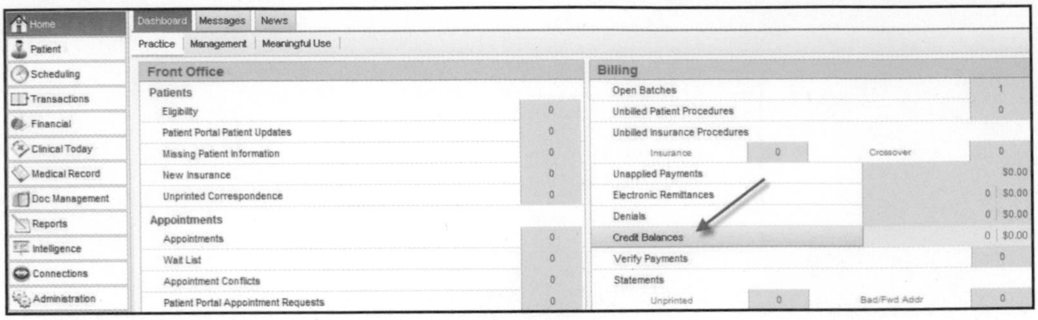

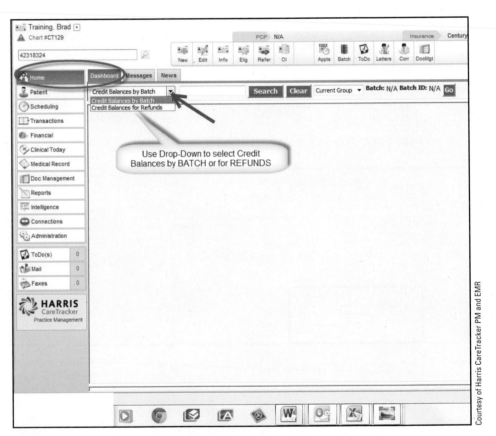

Figure 9-88 Credit Balances Link

There are two ways to work credit balances: *by Batch* or *for Refunds* (Figure 9-89). Once you post the batch, this will create a charge on the patient's account. You can then post a payment to create the credit balance.

Figure 9-89 Credit Balance by Batch or for Refund

Tip Box

There is a big difference between a "Credit" and an "Unapplied Credit." A credit is an overpayment on an account, and an unapplied credit is only a patient payment (not insurance) that has not been attached to a DOS.

ACTIVITY 9-12: Work Credit Balances

In order to work a Credit Balance, you must first have a credit in the patient's account.

1. Click on a patient's name to pull him or her into context on the *Name Bar* (select "Jordyn Lyndsey.")
2. Using patient Jordyn Lyndsey, create a new batch and name it "CreditBalance".
3. Click on the *OI* button on the *Name Bar*. Harris CareTracker PM displays the *Open Items* application.
4. If you do not see a credit balance, you will need to post a payment to the patient's account first, following these instructions. The payment must be greater than the balance in the patient's account in *OI* in the *Amt Payer* column:
   a. Click on the *Payment* line in the *Open Action* column of her G0180 *Procedure* (which should be listed as "Private Pay" in the *Payer* column). The *payment* screen will display in the lower portion of the window.
   b. Using the *Payment* drop-down, select "Payment – Patient Cash (PATCSH)."
   c. In the amount field next to the *Payment* drop-down, enter a payment in the amount of $50.00 more than the OI balance of her account. In this instance, her OI balance displays as $14.61, so you would add $50.00 to that amount for a total entry of $64.61. (**Note:** Do not enter the dollar sign.) You will see the *Private Pay* balance change to "$ -50.00."
   d. In the *Msg* drop-down select "Select Statement Message". Your screen should look like Figure 9-90.

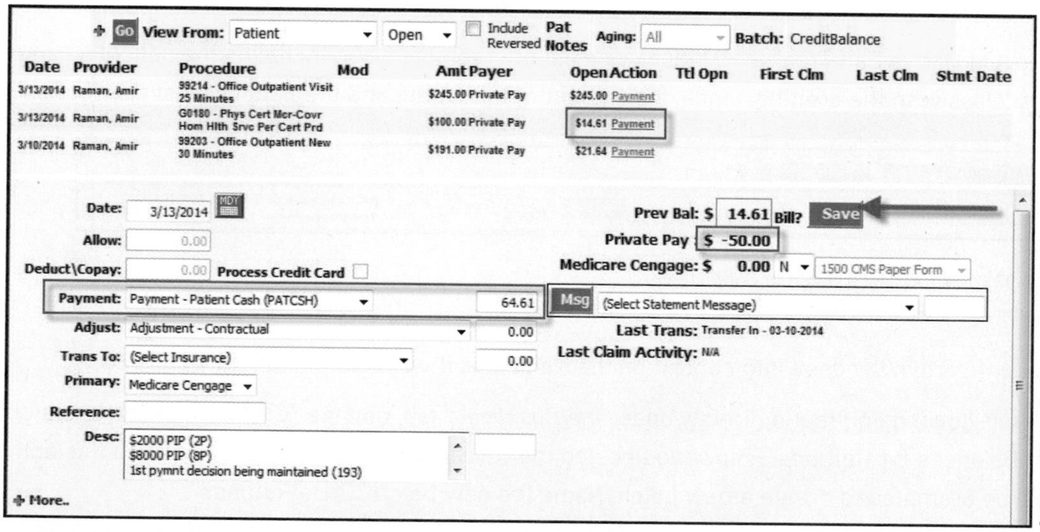

Courtesy of Harris CareTracker PM and EMR

Figure 9-90 OI Credit Balance Screen

   e. Click *Save*. To close the *Open Items* screen, click "X".
   f. Post the "CreditBalance" batch.
5. Go to the *Home* module > *Dashboard* tab > *Billing* header > *Credit Balances* link (see Figure 9-88).
6. Click on the *Search* button and Harris CareTracker PM displays a list of batches in the *Provider Search* dialog box (Figure 9-91).

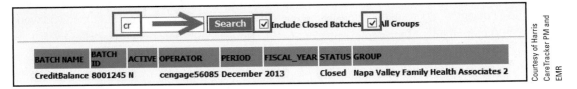

Figure 9-91   Provider Search

a. (FYI Only) If you had not posted your batch, in the *Provider Search* box you could click on the batch you want to view (select "CreditBalance"). Harris CareTracker PM populates the *Batch* and *Batch ID* fields with the selected batch.

b. Since you did post your batch, in the *Provider Search* dialog box you will need to select the check-boxes next to *Include Closed Batches* and *All Groups* and enter "Cr" or "Credit" in your batch name *Search* field (Figure 9-92) and then click *Search*.

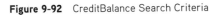

Figure 9-92   CreditBalance Search Criteria

6. Click on the "CreditBalance" batch and it is pulled into context (Figure 9-93).

7. Click *Go* and Harris CareTracker PM displays a list of credit balances including the patient's name, the financial class with the credit balance, the amount of the credit, and the patient's last transaction date.

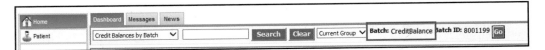

Figure 9-93   CreditBalance Batch in Context

Courtesy of Harris CareTracker PM and EMR

8. Pull patient Jordyn Lyndsey into context on the *Name Bar* if you have not already done so.

9. In the drop-down menu found directly under the *Dashboard* tab, change "Credit Balances by Batch" to "Credit Balances for Refunds". Since you posted the "CreditBalance" batch previously in this activity, you will be prompted to create a new batch. Name the new batch "CrBalRefunds".

PM SP⬤TLIGHT

If payments had been posted via electronic remittances, best practice would be to go into *Credit Balances* and search for the batch name associated with those payments, which will identify any credit balances created during the electronic payment process.

10. In the *Action* Column, use the drop-down and select "Refund-Patient (P)" (Figure 9-94). (**Note:** You may first need to adjust the *Date To* field to today's date and click *Go* for the screen to display.)

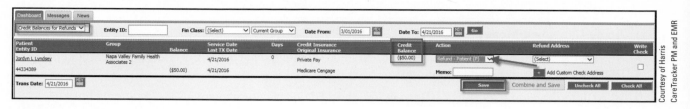

Figure 9-94 Credit Balance Refund

11. Click *Save*.

12. The *Credit Balance Transfer* dialog box will display. Click on *Write Transactions* (Figure 9-95).

13. The *Credit Balance Transfer* dialog box will confirm that the transaction has been saved (Figure 9-96).

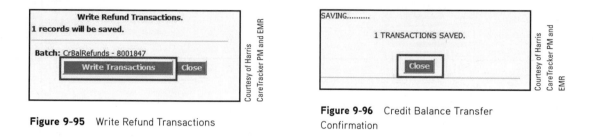

Figure 9-95 Write Refund Transactions

Figure 9-96 Credit Balance Transfer Confirmation

14. Click *Close*, and the credit balance is removed from your screen.

Print the Credit Balance for Refunds screen, label it "Activity 9-12," and place it in your assignment folder.

Unapplied Payments

When a patient makes a payment before services are rendered (such as a co-payment), or a payment is received that does not indicate a specific date of service, the payment is posted into Harris CareTracker PM as an *unapplied payment*. An unapplied payment is money that has been applied to a patient's account, but not to a specific date of service. The unapplied money can be applied automatically to the patient's charge through either the *Charges* or *Bulk Charges* application. If the unapplied money is not applied automatically you will be able to apply the unapplied amount manually. The *Unapplied* application on the *Dashboard* lists each patient with an unapplied balance, the amount of unapplied money and the patient's last transaction date. As best practice, this list should be reviewed and reconciled daily.

Applying Unapplied Money. A batch must be open to apply unapplied money and the patient must have a balance on his or her account.

FYI

Apply Unapplied Money

Not every Practice Management system has an *Apply/Unapplied* feature. Harris CareTracker PM does. To apply unapplied money you would follow these instructions:

1. Go to the *Home* module > *Dashboard* tab > *Billing* header > *Unapplied Payments* link.
2. In the drop-down menu, select "All Groups." Click *Go*. Harris CareTracker PM displays a list of all patients with *Unapplied* money (Figure 9-97).

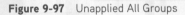

Patient	Unapplied	LastTXdate
Jordyn L Lyndsey (42 '05371)	$45.00	12/28/2013
Jane W Morgan (4239 '38)	$20.00	7/30/2013
Jeffrey Mills (42399643	$20.00	7/30/2013
Frank Powell (42399632	$35.00	7/30/2013
Barbara Watson (4239962	$20.00	7/29/2013
Ellen Ristino (42399655)	$20.00	7/29/2013
Spencer M Douglas (423996	$60.00	6/14/2013
Donald Schwartz (42399629)	$35.00	5/23/2013
Total:	$255.00	

> Use the drop-down to select "All Groups", then click "Go". The list displays. Select patient Frank Powell.

Courtesy of Harris CareTracker PM and EMR

Figure 9-97 Unapplied All Groups

3. Create a new batch. Update the batch to identify the selected patient's PCP as *Provider*, update the *Location* to the place of service, and use the same date as noted in the *LastTxDate* column.
4. Click on the patient's name in the *Patient* column. Harris CareTracker PM pulls the patient into context on the *Name Bar*.
5. Click the *OI* button on the *Name Bar*. Harris CareTracker PM launches the *Open Items* application.
6. Click *Go*. Harris CareTracker PM displays all of the patient's balances. **Note:** If there is no balance displayed for the patient it means there are no open charges on his or her account to apply the unapplied money.
7. Click the *Payment* link on a *Private Pay* procedure line with an open amount to which the unapplied money should be applied. Harris CareTracker PM displays the *Payment* fields at the bottom of the window.
8. The *Apply Unapplied* field displays the default financial transaction set up for your company. However, you can select a different financial transaction type if needed (Figure 9-98). (The *Apply Unapplied* field appears only if a balance is private pay.)
9. Click on the patient's name which brings the patient into context.
10. In the monetary box to the right of the *Apply Unapplied* field, use the drop-down and select *Payment – Patient Cash (PATCSH),* and then enter the amount of unapplied money you want to apply to this date of service. Enter the amount in the *Prev Bal* and *Private Pay* fields.
11. When you click or tab out of the monetary amount box, you will see the *Private Pay* amount is now $0.00 and the *Unapplied* amount is the remaining credit balance.

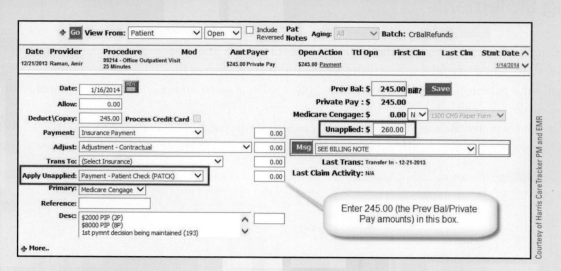

Figure 9-98   Apply Unapplied

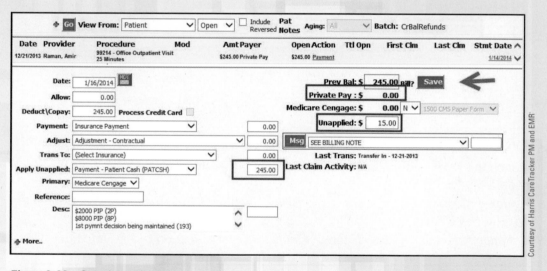

Figure 9-99   Open Items Apply Unapplied

Tip Box

The total amount of unapplied money saved on the patient's account is displayed in the *Unapplied* field. When a monetary amount is entered in the field next to *Apply Unapplied*, Harris CareTracker PM deducts that amount from the *Unapplied* box.

12. Click *Save* in the upper-right corner of the *Payment* screen and you will receive a "Transaction Saved" message. Close out the dialog box.

Billing Statements

Harris CareTracker PM generates and prints patient statements once a week; however, patients will only receive one statement every 30 days regardless of the number of services they have had. A statement will not be generated for a patient if the patient has an unapplied balance saved on his or her account equal to or greater than the current patient balance amount.

From the *Unprinted Statements* application you can identify the batch of patients who should receive a statement, print billing statements, and identify patient statements that were undeliverable or forwarded to a new address.

Tip Box

Undeliverable and forwarding addresses are gathered through Express Bill, the company Harris CareTracker PM uses to distribute patient statements.

FYI

The workflow to print unprinted statements would be:

1. Launch the batch statements application from either the *Reports* module or the *Home* module:
   a. *Home* module > *Dashboard* tab > *Billing* section > *Statements* > *Unprinted* link (Figure 9-100)
   b. *Reports* module > *Reports* tab > *Financial Reports* section > *All Statements* link

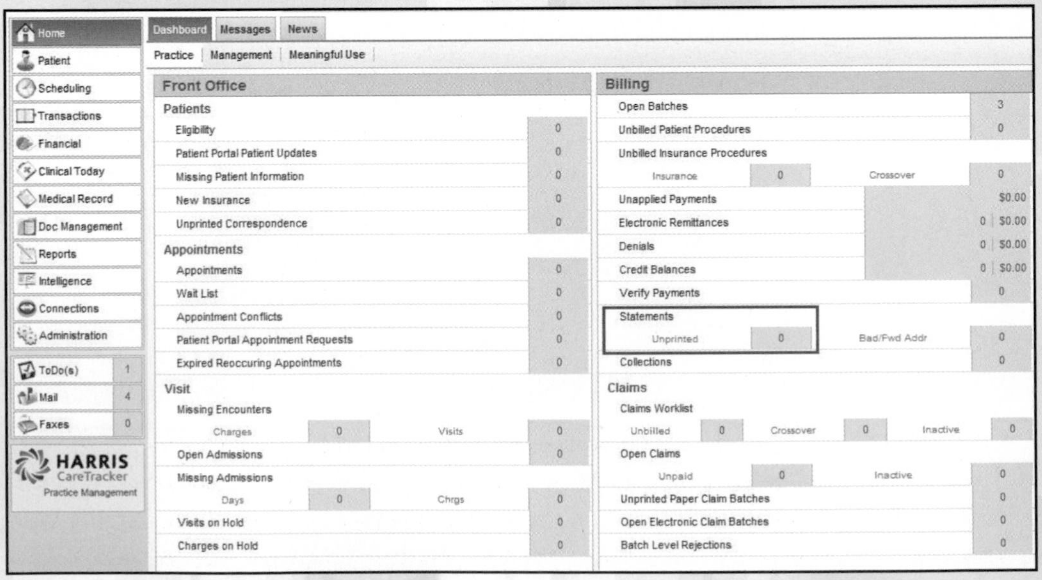

Courtesy of Harris CareTracker PM and EMR

Figure 9-100 Unprinted Statements Link

2. (Optional) Click the *plus sign* [+] next to the *Options* field to display *the Batch Statement Log Options*. Select the filters as needed. Select the most recent statement batch (if statements had already been generated). If no statements had been printed, there will be no results returned.

3. Click *Go*. The application displays a list of statement batches.

4. In the *Batch Statements* section of the page, select the checkbox in the *All* column next to each batch of statements that you want to print. If you want to select all of the batches listed, click *All*.

5. If statements had already been generated, scroll down to the bottom of the batch statement list and click *Print View*. (**Note:** It may take a few moments for the statements to populate.) The application displays all patient statements included in each selected statement batch (Figure 9-101). **Note:** If statements had not yet been generated, none will display.

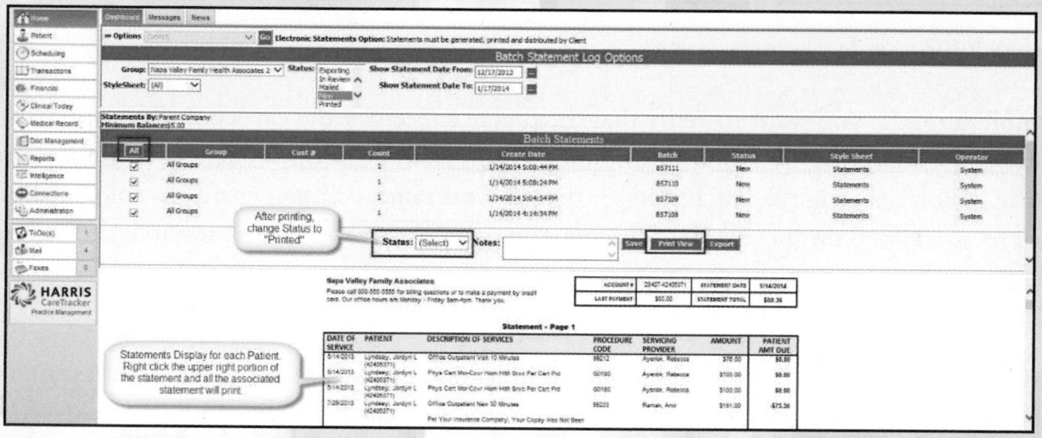

Figure 9-101   Patient Statements

6. Right-click on top of the first statement in the lower frame of the screen and select *Print* from the shortcut menu. The application displays a *Print* window.

7. Select the desired printer and then click *Print*. The application prints the statements.

8. When all the statements have printed, select *Printed* from the *Status* list. The application removes the printed statements from the batch statements list.

9. Click *Save* and the statements are removed from your screen.

Verify Payments

The *Verify Payments* application compares the actual amount paid by an insurance company for a claim to the expected allowed amount, as defined on the *Allowed Schedule* linked to the physician billing contract, and is payer specific. If the payment made by the insurance company is different than the allowed amount, then *Verify Payments* indicates the discrepancy. You can then view the details of the over- or underpayment and use the work area to override, adjust, rebill, or transfer payment amounts as necessary to resolve the variance (Figure 9-102).

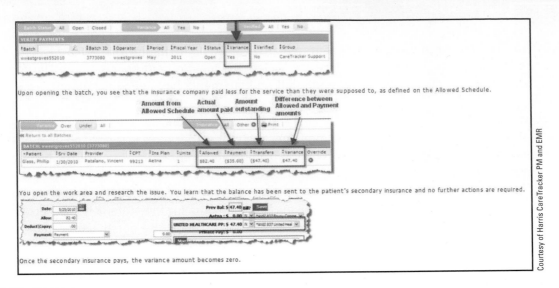

Figure 9-102 Verify Payments Example

For example, suppose you want to verify that the practice received the expected reimbursement for open payment batches. Using the *Verify Payments* application, you see that an open batch contains a payment item with a variance. Upon opening the batch, you see that the insurance company paid less for the service than it was supposed to, as defined on the *Allowed Schedule*. You open the work area and research the issue. You learn that the balance has been sent to the patient's secondary insurance and no further actions are required. Once the secondary insurance pays, the variance amount becomes zero.

Viewing Payment Variances. The *Verify Payments* application displays a list of open batches containing one or more payment items with a variance. You can filter, sort, and search batches with payment variances, and filter and sort payment variances within a particular batch.

FYI

To view batches with payment variances:

1. Go to the *Home* module > *Dashboard* tab > *Billing* section > *Verify Payments* link.
2. Change the *Batch Status*, *Variance*, and *Verified* tabs to "All". The *Verify Payments* application displays a list of all unverified batches containing one or more payments that differ from the allowed amount (Figure 9-103).

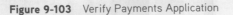

Figure 9-103 Verify Payments Application

3. Filter, sort, or search the list:
    a. To filter the list, click the filter options at the top of the page.
        -   *Batch Status.* By default, payment variances are displayed for both open and closed batches ("All"). Click "Open" or "Closed" to display variances for only opened or closed batches.
        -   *Variance.* By default, only batches with payment variances ("Yes") are displayed. Click "No" to display only batches that do not have variances or click "All" to display batches with and without payment variances, Figure 9-104 represents an example of payment variances in a live environment.

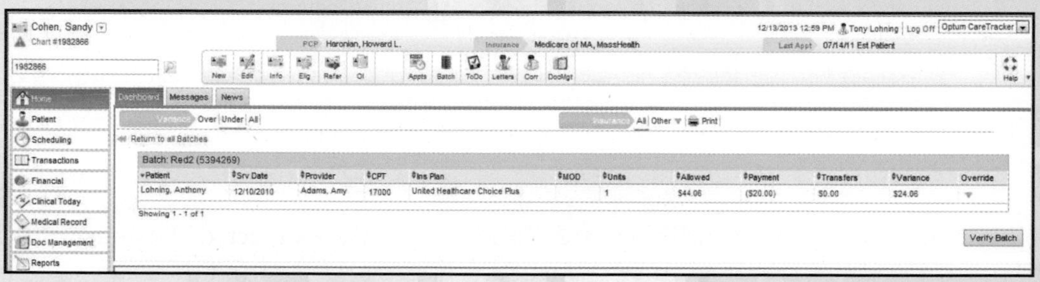

Figure 9-104   Payment Variance

        -   *Verified.* By default, only batches that are unverified ("No") are displayed. Click "Yes" to display only verified batches or click "All" to display both verified and unverified batches.
    b. To sort the list, click the name of the column by which to sort.
    c. To search for a specific batch within the list, enter the batch name or partial batch name in the *Batch* box and then click the *Search* 🔍 icon. Harris CareTracker PM displays the batches that match your search criteria.

Table 9-3 describes the variance details that are displayed for the Payment Item.

TABLE 9-3 Payment Item Variance Details	
Detail	**Description**
Patient	Name of the patient who received the service and incurred the charges.
Srv Date	Date on which the service was provided.
Provider	Physician responsible for providing the service.
CPT®	CPT® code identifying the service the patient received and for which the charge applies.
Ins Plan	Patient's primary insurance plan.
Units	Number of service units for which the charge applies.

(Continues)

TABLE 9-3 *(Continued)*

Detail	Description
Allowed	Negotiated amount of money the primary insurance is responsible for paying, as defined on the Allowed Schedule.
Payment	Amount of money received from the insurance company for the service to date.
Transfers	Amount of money outstanding. This is the total amount of money transferred to another party responsible for payment, such as a secondary insurance company, deductible or copay, and collections.
Variance	Difference between the Allowed and Payment amounts. This is the difference between the actual amount of money you received from the insurance company and the negotiated rate the insurance is responsible for paying. For example, Aetna's allowed amount for CPT® code 99213 is $82.40, but it paid only $35.00. Equation: Allowed − Payment = Variance Calculation: $82.30 − ($35.00) = $47.40 Therefore, the Variance is $47.40.
Override	If you want to allow the variance and verify the payment, then select a reason for overriding the variance. See the *Managing Payment Variances* section that follows for more information.

Courtesy of Harris CareTracker PM and EMR

You have the option to filter or sort the list. To filter the list, click the filter options at the top of the page.

- *Variance.* By default, only items that have been underpaid ("Under") are displayed. Click *Over* to display only items that have been over paid. Click *All* to display both under and over paid items and items with a variance that has been overridden.
- *Insurance.* By default, items for all insurance companies ("All") are displayed. To view only items for a particular company, click the company from the *Other* shortcut menu.

Managing Payment Variances. Managing payment variances involves first determining the cause and solution for the variance and then working the payment to resolve or override the variance. After resolving the variance, you can verify the payment batch.

Step 1 is to determine the cause and solution for a payment variance. Before you can work the payment to resolve the variance, you must first determine the cause of the variance and decide the appropriate way to resolve it. Determining the cause involves viewing the variance and looking at the item's payment history. When viewing the payment history for the item, you need to ask yourself questions about how to resolve the variance, such as:

- Does the payment need to be rebilled?
- Does the payment need to be adjusted?
- Will the payment be transferred to a secondary insurance?
- Is the patient responsible for the variance balance?

The way you will work the payment is determined by the answers to such questions, and is unique to the particular payment at hand.

Tables 9-4, 9-5, and 9-6 list scenarios, causes, and resolution details for payment variances. Each table contains variance details as they are displayed in the *Verify Payments* application. Underneath the variance details is a description of the variance scenario, how to determine the cause of the payment variance, and the steps you might take to resolve the variance.

TABLE 9-4   Scenario 1: Balance Transfer

Ins Plan	Allowed	Payment	Transfers	Variance
Medicare	$62.50	($50.00)	($12.50)	$12.50

Payment variance scenario:

A claim in the amount of $62.50 is submitted to the patient's primary insurance, Medicare. Medicare's allowed payment for the service is $62.50, but it paid only $50.00, leaving an under-variance of $12.50. The *Transfer* amount of $12.50 indicates that the balance may be transferred to a co-insurance, private pay, or other party.

Step 1: Determine the cause of the payment variance.

View the open item payment history and determine where the unpaid $12.50 was sent. If a co-insurance is responsible for the payment, then the variance will be adjusted once the payment is made. If the patient is responsible for the payment, then you need to work the payment and send a bill to the patient.

Step 2: Work the payment.

If the patient is responsible for the remaining $12.50, then you must *Transfer* the balance to the patient and generate a bill.

TABLE 9-5   Scenario 2: Insurance Denial

Ins Plan	Allowed	Payment	Transfers	Variance
Blue Cross	$50.00	($0.00)	($50.00)	$50.00

Payment variance scenario:

The lack of payment by the insurance company indicates that the insurance company may have denied payment, and the *Transfer* amount of $50.00 indicates that the amount may have been transferred to a co-insurance.

Step 1: Determine the cause of the payment variance.

View the open item payment history and determine why the insurance company did not pay its Allowed amount. You may need to take further steps to determine how to process the payment, such as contacting the insurance company to obtain more information about the payment status.

Step 2: Work the payment.

If the insurance company denied the claim, then you need to further process the payment. For example, you may need to bill the patient, override the variance, or resubmit the claim to the insurance company.

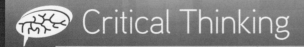

Critical Thinking

"Solve the problem." Referring to Scenario 2: Insurance Denial (see Table 9-5), brainstorm about reasons the insurance company denied the claim. Come up with ideas to solve the problem for this claim and prevent denials of future claims. Further analyze and debate findings and discuss how you reached your conclusions.

TABLE 9-6 Scenario 3: Copay Transfer

Ins Plan	Allowed	Payment	Transfers	Variance
Aetna	$50.00	($40.00)	($10.00)	$10.00

Payment variance scenario:

The under-variance of $10.00 implies that the primary insurance plus the patient copay equals 100% of the allowed amount.

Step 1: Determine the cause of the payment variance.

The $10.00 copay was transferred to private pay and therefore displays as a variance.

Step 2: Work the payment.

The remaining difference between the allowed amount and charge will be adjusted.

FYI

To view the payment history for an item with a payment variance:

1. Click the *OI* button on the *Name* bar. Harris CareTracker PM displays a list of the open items for the patient in a new window.
2. Click the payment item you are researching. Harris CareTracker PM displays the payment details for the item in the bottom pane of the window (Figure 9-105).

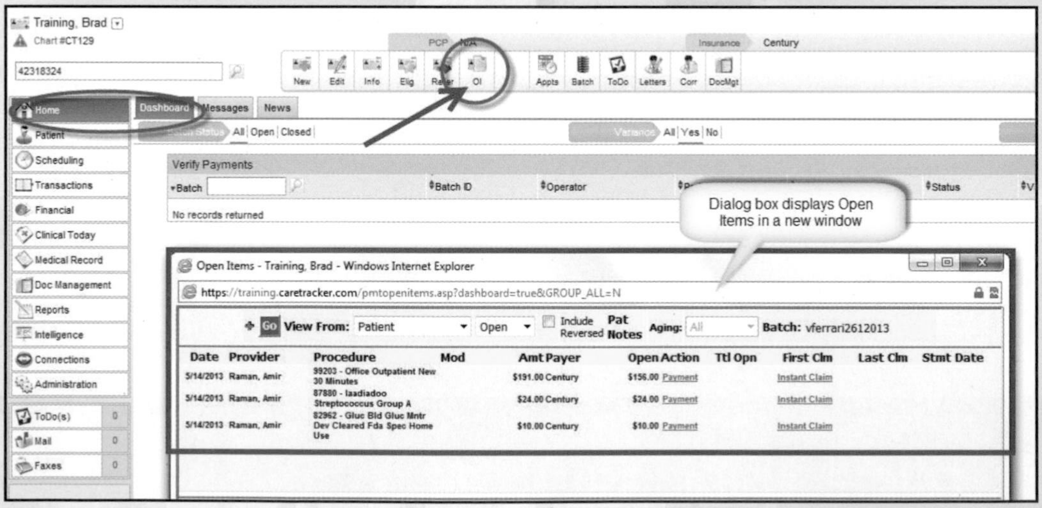

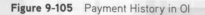

Figure 9-105 Payment History in OI

The next step of managing patient variances is to work the payment. After determining the cause of the variance and deciding the appropriate way to resolve it, you can work the payment to override or resolve the variance as necessary. To work the payment:

3. Display the payment variances for the batch you want to verify.
4. Override or resolve each variance, as necessary:
   - To allow the payment variance and mark it as verified, point to the *Arrow* ▼ icon in the *Override* column and then click the reason for overriding the variance. The payment item is removed from the list.
   - To resolve the variance, click the item in the list. Harris CareTracker PM displays the *Work Area* for the item.
     a. In the *Work Area*, change the necessary payment details to resolve the variance.
     b. Click *Save*. Harris CareTracker PM clears the details in the *Work Area* and displays a note stating that the transaction is saved.
5. Click *Verify Batch* to verify the batch.

View or Edit Batch Deposits

Although typically practices do not use the steps to view or edit batch deposits, it is helpful to know that this feature is available. The total amount of money your group has deposited for the current month displays to the *Batch Deposits* link on the *Management* dashboard and allows you to view details of each deposit, add deposits, and edit deposits (Figures 9-106 and 9-107).

Courtesy of Harris CareTracker PM and EMR

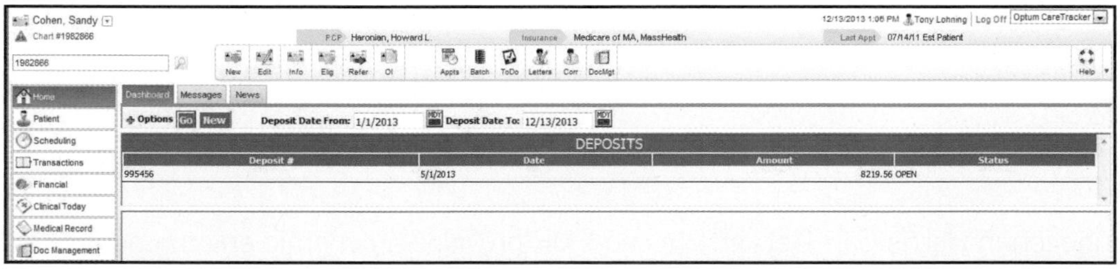

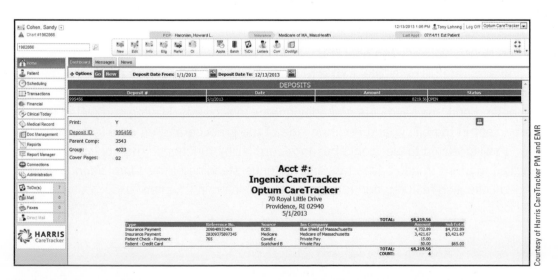

Figure 9-106 Deposits Application

Courtesy of Harris CareTracker PM and EMR

Figure 9-107 Deposit ID

FYI

View and Edit Batch Deposits

To view deposits entered into Harris CareTracker PM:

- Click the *Home* module.
- Click the *Dashboard* tab, and then click the *Management* tab. Harris CareTracker PM displays the *Management Dashboard*.
- Click the *Batch Deposits* link in the *Management* section of the *Dashboard*. Harris CareTracker PM displays the *Batch Deposits* application.
- If needed, click the [+] sign next to *Options* to expand the filters. Set the filters as needed to narrow the number of deposits that will display, and click *Go*. Harris CareTracker PM displays the batch deposit entered into Harris CareTracker PM including the batch deposit number, date of deposit, amount of money deposited, and status of the deposit.
- Click on a batch deposit line to view the details of a specific deposit. Harris CareTracker PM displays a deposit summary in the lower frame of the screen.

To edit a batch deposit:

- Click on a batch deposit line to view the details of a specific deposit. Harris CareTracker PM displays a deposit summary in the lower frame of the screen
- Click on the *Deposit ID*. Harris CareTracker PM displays the deposit details in edit mode.
- Edit the information as needed, and then click *Save*.

SUMMARY

The *Billing* function in Harris CareTracker PM and EMR provides a dynamic environment to ensure that the billing process goes smoothly and that the quality of the information sent to the insurance carriers is clean. The *Billing* function crosses many modules, applications, and functions.

The *batch* is the essential component required before entering and posting any financial transaction such as charges, payments, adjustments, and refunds. This helps identify transactions linked to the batch, the date of each transaction, and the operator who entered it into the system.

Prompt and accurate billing is vital to the revenue cycle and financial health of the medical practice. This chapter has provided instruction and activities that simulate workflows in a medical practice related to patient billing and entering payments and adjustments to accounts. Having completed this chapter, you should be proficient in the billing and revenue side of the practice and be able to demonstrate valuable knowledge and skills related to electronic health record billing functions. The application of skills related to the reconciliation of insurance payments, and the understanding of the *ClaimsManager* features leads to the advanced collection features and functions you will learn in Chapter 10.

Check Your Knowledge

Select the best response.

_____ 1. In *Batch Details*, the *Default Referral Provider* is set to "No." You should change the field to "Yes" if there is no referring provider in the patient's demographics or if there is no active referral/authorization for the patient. By changing the field to "Yes," who becomes the referring provider?

   a. None required
   b. Billing Provider
   c. Designated practice
   d. Resource

_____ 2. When manually entering a charge, how can you remove a diagnosis code in the *Diag* box?

   a. By left-clicking on the diagnosis code
   b. By clicking on the *EncoderPro* button
   c. By deleting the patient encounter
   d. By double-clicking on the diagnosis code

_____ 3. Once a batch has been posted, the transactions linked to it are locked in the system. How do you correct an error once the batch has been posted?

   a. Reverse the transaction in the *Edit* application of the *Transactions* module.
   b. Delete the line item in the *Transactions* module.
   c. Submit a *ToDo* to Harris CareTracker.
   d. Issue a refund to the patient or the insurance company.

_____ 4. All transactions must be posted before running any *Month End* report in Harris CareTracker PM. Periods cannot be closed:

   a. When open batches are linked to them
   b. When there are multiple periods open
   c. If you have not run a journal
   d. If there are multiple operators using the period

_____ 5. Remittances received electronically in Harris CareTracker PM are identified in the *Electronic Remittances* application on the *Dashboard*. Harris CareTracker PM matches the transactions on the electronic remittance to a specific patient, date of service, CPT® code, and charge amount. Which is not one of the three matching categories?

   a. Complete (green)
   b. Partial match (yellow)
   c. Error (red)
   d. No match (white)

_____ 6. A(n) _____ is created when either a patient or an insurance company pays more money for a specific procedure for a specific date of service than what was billed.

   a. error
   b. credit balance
   c. debit balance
   d. Both b and c

_____ 7. Claims that an insurance company has determined they will not pay are known as:

    a. Undercoded   c. Co-payments

    b. Overcoded   d. Denials

_____ 8. When a patient makes a payment before services are rendered (such as a co-payment), the payment is posted into Harris CareTracker as a(n):

    a. Unapplied payment   c. Bulk charge

    b. Credit balance   d. Credit balance transfer

_____ 9. When matching unmatched transactions, you double-click on a white or yellow line, or click on the *M* button at the end of one of these lines. When a line is selected, the *Patient Procedure Balance Match* window displays, showing:

    a. The insurance, status of claim, match description, the patient's last name, the patient's first name

    b. The patient ID number, CPT® code, date of service, and charge

    c. The pop-up check-off indicating the options to use as the matching criteria

    d. None of the above

_____ 10. Denials are only tallied on the *Dashboard* if:

    a. The denial code or description was manually entered in the *Description* field in the *Open Items* application

    b. Payments were posted electronically via *Electronic Remittances*

    c. Both a and b

    d. None of the above

_____ 11. When working a credit balance for a refund, if the *Memo* field is left blank, Harris CareTracker will:

    a. Reject the refund

    b. Apply to an outstanding service

    c. Print the patient's name and date of service on the refund check

    d. Refund the insurance company

_____ 12. To reverse an unapplied payment (such as $30), in the *Amount* box, how would you enter it in Harris CareTracker?

    a. 30   c. 60

    b. −30   d. −60

mini-case studies

Note: Case studies must be completed in every chapter since future chapter activities build upon them.

Case Study 9-1

1. Before beginning Case Study 9-1, create a new batch and name it "Ch9MCS-Remit".
2. Repeat Activity 9-9 and generate paper claims for all procedures listed for each patient. (**Note:** If a patient's charges are not showing on the *Open Items* window, follow the steps in the *Tip Box* on pages 501–502 to save all charges for the patient's date of service.)
3. For each patient, process the remittances and denials (Activities 9-10 and 9-11) for each encounter created in Chapter 6 and Case-Studies 7-3 through 7-6, Process the Remittances and Denials (EOBs) from Source Documents 9-2 through 9-6 in Appendix A.

   Patients:

   a. 9-1A: Jane Morgan
   b. 9-1C: Adam Thompson
   c. 9-1D: Ellen Ristino
   d. 9-1E: Craig X. Smith
   e. 9-1F: Barbara Watson

4. Upon completion run a journal and review. **Do not** post the "Ch9MCS-Remit" batch at this time.

Print the journal after completing all the 9-1 case studies, label it "Case Study 9-1," and place in your assignment folder.

Resources and Weblinks

The Harris CareTracker PM and EMR Help homepage represents a wealth of information for the Electronic Health Record (https://training.caretracker.com/help/CareTracker_Help.htm).

American Medical Association

National Healthcare Association. (n.d.). *Certified Electronic Health Records Specialist (CEHRS™).* Retrieved March 16, 2013, from http://www.nhanow.com/health-record.aspx

U.S. Department of Commerce, United States Census Bureau, American National Standards Institute (2013). Retrieved March 16, 2013, from http://www.census.gov/geo/www/ansi/ansi.html

Chapter 10

ClaimsManager and Collections

Key Terms

accounts receivable
adjudicate
aging
American National
  Standards Institute
  (ANSI)
crossover

EncoderPro
inactive claims
National Drug Code
  (NDC)
private pay
unpaid claims

Learning Objectives

1. Demonstrate understanding and use of the ClaimsManager feature.
2. Check status and work unpaid/inactive claims.
3. Generate patient statements.
4. Describe and identify components of the patient collection process.
5. Review collection status and transfer private pay balances.
6. Perform collection actions.
7. Create collection letters.
8. Generate collection letters.

Certification Connection

1. Utilize EMR and practice management (PM) systems.
2. Manage data and document accurately in the patient record using the electronic health record (EHR).
3. Compare and contrast manual and computerized billing systems used in ambulatory health care.
4. Describe period financial reports used in the EHR.
5. Utilize computerized billing software; prepare patient accounts for collections; explain both billing and payment options.
6. Discuss procedures for collecting outstanding accounts that have reached the established receivables aging.
7. Define the types of adjustments that may be made to a patient's account and the procedure to record payments and write-offs.
8. Apply unapplied balances to a patient's account; process refunds for overpayments.
9. Change the status of patient accounts to collections.
10. Discuss how guidelines are used in processing an insurance claim and remittance.
11. Compose professional and business (collections) letters.
12. Differentiate among private, federal, and state payers.
13. Execute administrative and clinical workflows within a health care facility.
14. Retrieve, store, and edit patient information from the EHR database.
15. Edit existing searchable databases (e.g., code changes, patient demographics, insurance carriers); transmit patient data for external use (e.g., insurance, pharmacies, other providers).
16. Generate patient statements.
17. Post payments to patient accounts.
18. Generate financial reports; aging reports by guarantor or carrier; financial analysis reports by provider, diagnosis, or procedure.
19. Adhere to federal, state, and local laws relating to exchange of information and describe elements of meaningful use and reports generated.

Adapted from national standards of the National Healthcareer Association (NHA), Commission on Accreditation and Allied Health Education Program (CAAHEP), and Accrediting Bureau of Health Education Schools (ABHES)

INTRODUCTION

This chapter continues many of the *Billing* and *ClaimsManager* features introduced in Chapter 9. The *ClaimsManager* and *Collections* applications in Harris CareTracker PM are where you begin the active process of reviewing and working claims, printing statements, and focusing collection efforts on patients with balances at least 30 days overdue.

Accounts receivable arises when a company provides goods or services on credit. For example, a medical practice may allow its patients to pay for services 30 days after they are provided and paid/adjusted by their insurance company. If patients do not pay as agreed, the practice could experience a cash flow problem. The term *aging* is often associated with a company's accounts receivable. **Aging** is the classification of accounts by the time elapsed after the date of billing or the due date. The aging of accounts receivable report will list each patient's outstanding balance and will then list the "age": current, 1–30 days past due, 31–60 days past due, 61–90 days past due, 91–120 days past due, and 120+ days past due. The aging of accounts receivable allows managers to quickly see which patients are behind in meeting the agreed-upon terms.

There are seven collection statuses in Harris CareTracker PM. Transferring private pay balances co-incides with changing a patient's collection status. Harris CareTracker PM automatically moves patients into *Collections* when their overdue balance reaches the aging level assigned in the group settings and automatically removes patients from collections when their overdue balance is paid.

Understanding the concepts and performing collection action tasks demonstrate how an EHR can streamline workflows. As a medical assistant you will perform routine EHR clinical and/or administrative duties relating to the collection process per facility protocol. Duties include the transfer of balances, moving accounts to/from collection, creating custom form letters, adding the letters to *Quick Picks*, and generating and printing collection letters.

Billing and collection functions are vital to the medical practice and its revenue cycle and help maintain the provider database for the continuity of care of patients. When a patient misses or late cancels an appointment, revenue and care can be compromised.

CLAIMSMANAGER

Learning Objective 1: Demonstrate understanding and use of the ClaimsManager feature.

The *ClaimsManager* application in Harris CareTracker PM electronically screens a claim and the associated CPT®, ICD, and HCPCS codes and modifiers at the time the claim is created. A claim cannot be generated and sent to payers until charges for patient visits are saved in Harris CareTracker. In Chapter 9 you learned to use the *Charge* application of the *Transactions* module. The *Charge* application is typically used to:

- Enter visit information and create charges for patient visits that are not booked in Harris CareTracker PM, such as hospital visits
- Create charges for a scheduled appointment
- *Edit* unposted charges

When entering a charge, the basic visit information needs to be entered, including location, place of service, referring provider, servicing provider, billing provider, and a case or authorization, if applicable.

Much of this information is pulled from the batch to which you are linking the charge and the patient's demographic.

The most important information that needs to be entered in the *Charge* application is the appropriate CPT® and ICD codes. Although there is no limit to the number of CPT® codes that can be entered for a charge, no more than four modifiers can be selected and no more than four ICD codes can be linked to each CPT® code.

Although *ClaimsManager* is not active in your student version, it is a very important tool for the medical practice. The instructions and screenshots included in this chapter provide useful information about the application. When the *Save* button is clicked during the claims process, the associated procedures (CPT®), diagnoses (ICD), and modifiers are sent to *ClaimsManager* instantly for screening. The screening can result in one of three statuses, including "Passed," "Failed," or "Warning" (Figure 10-1). If the screening results in a "Passed" status, the patient payment will be saved along with the charge and the two will be linked. If the *ClaimsManager* screening triggers an edit, the *ClaimsManager Edit* dialog box displays with detailed descriptions about the edits and provides action options to process the claim.

CLAIMSMANAGER SCREENING STATUS		
Color	**Status**	**Description**
	Not Processed	Not processed status indicates that the item has not been screened by the ClaimsManager.
	Passed	Passed status indicates that the item has passed the ClaimsManager screening.
	Warning	Warning status indicates that the item may fail or the ClaimsManager has suggested edits.
	Failed	Failed status indicates that the item does not meet the rules set by ClaimsManager and further edits are required.
	CMS Edits	This status indicates that the claim was flagged for CMS edits. **Note:** The CMS Edits status is deactivated by default. You must send a ToDo to CareTracker Support to request this feature.

Courtesy of Harris CareTracker PM and EMR

Figure 10-1 ClaimsManager Screening Status

Harris CareTracker PM automatically splits out the private payment amount owed, such as the patient's co-payment, for each procedure entered for the patient that requires a copayment. This only occurs if the amount of the patient's copayment is entered in the *Copay* field of the *Insurance* section in the *Demographics* application. The *Amt* field next to "Private Pay" displays the patient's copayment amount. If the patient's payment has not already been entered into Harris CareTracker PM, it can be entered now via the *Payments on Account* application fields that display in the bottom of the *Charge* screen. It is essential to enter the payment amount and the payment type.

EncoderPro

When all appropriate CPT® and ICD codes are entered, ***EncoderPro***, Harris CareTracker's partner for on-line code verification, can be run to verify the procedures, diagnoses, and modifiers entered for a patient. Running *EncoderPro* by clicking on the *EncoderPro.com* button (Figure 10-2) helps ensure that correct coding information is entered and claims are processed and paid promptly.

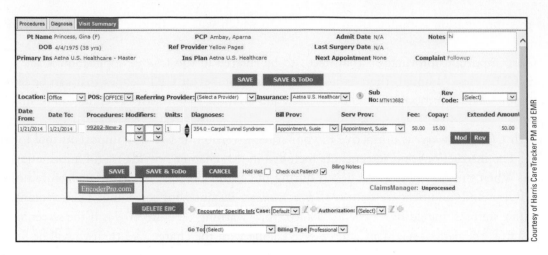

Figure 10-2 EncoderPro Button

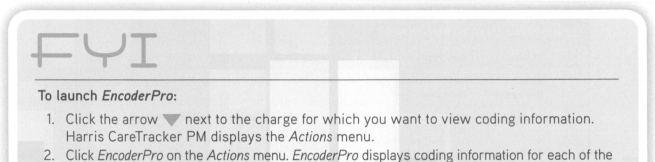

To launch *EncoderPro*:

1. Click the arrow ▼ next to the charge for which you want to view coding information. Harris CareTracker PM displays the *Actions* menu.
2. Click *EncoderPro* on the *Actions* menu. *EncoderPro* displays coding information for each of the codes included in the charge. This information can be used as a guide to correct the charge.
3. Review the coding information, and then close *EncoderPro*.

Claims Worklist Overview

Most claims are sent electronically in Harris CareTracker PM. Any claims identified with a problem that would prevent them from being paid will show up on a *Claims Worklist* to be resolved. The *Claims Worklist* identifies the following:

- Newly prepared claims that will be transmitted during your next claim run
- Claims that cannot be transmitted electronically due to a missing submitter number
- Claims that cannot be transmitted from Harris CareTracker PM because of missing information
- Claims that are not transmitted because of errors identified by *ClaimsManager*
- Claims that will not be accepted by a payer because of missing information
- Claims that you manually flagged as missing information or in review
- Claims that a payer does not have on file and claims with a denial status

Any claims flagged in any of the *Claims Worklist* columns, except *New/Prepared*, need to be followed up on, which typically requires you to add and/or edit information and rebill the claim. Harris CareTracker PM performs an electronic claim status check and, based on its status, moves the claim to one of the *Claims Worklist* categories. You can also manually flag a claim to move it to a *Claims Worklist* category.

Claims Worklist Categories. The *Claims Worklist* is grouped into four main categories: *New/Prepared, Claim Errors, Pending,* and *Other* (Figure 10-3). Claim categories are further subdivided as described in Table 10-1.

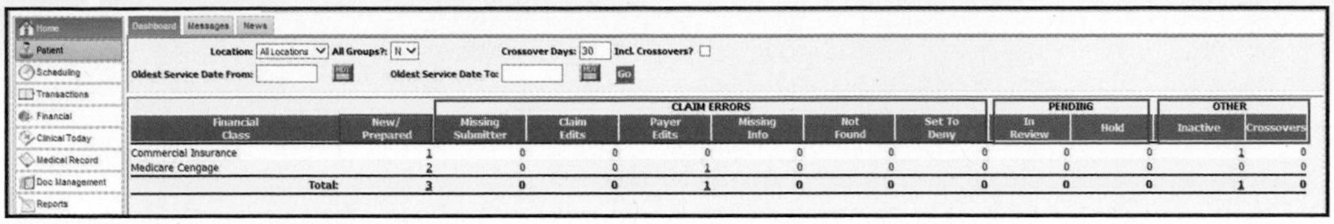

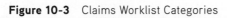

Figure 10-3 Claims Worklist Categories

TABLE 10-1 Claims Worklist Categories		
Category	**Column**	**Description**
New	New Prepared	Any claim listed in the *New/Prepared* column is a claim that will be transmitted during the next bill run. When a claim is edited and rebilled, it is added to this column. This column includes any claims that have been generated and that have been sent as well. Claims in the *New/Pending* column do not require follow-up.
Claim Errors	Missing Submitter	Claims will only appear in this column if there is a problem with the submitter numbers (as set up in the database). When a claim appears in this column, the enrollment specialist would be contacted to review/update. Claims in this column would either be rebilled when the enrollment is complete or dropped to paper.
	Claim Edits	Claims need to meet certain criteria to be transmitted from Harris CareTracker PM and EMR to a payer. When a claim does not meet these criteria (subscriber number, date of birth, and Harris CareTracker *ClaimsManager* database rules), the claim is placed in the *Claim Edits* column on the *Claims Worklist* screen. These claims have never been transmitted from Harris CareTracker PM. The required information needs to be added or edited to the claim and the claim needs to be rebilled in order for it to be removed from the *Claim Edits* column.
	Payer Edits	Claims in the *Payer Edits* column have been prepared by and transmitted from Harris CareTracker PM to a payer because they meet Harris CareTracker PM's claim criteria; however, the payer will not accept the claim because it is missing information the specific payer requires. These claims have not been reviewed by the payer because they cannot be accepted into its system electronically because the claims do not meet the payer's established claim criteria. These claims will appear on reports received back from insurance companies as rejected. Based on those reports, the status is automatically updated or you would be setting a claim with a status of *Payer Edit* manually. The required information needs to be added or edited to the claim and the claim needs to be rebilled in order for it to be removed from the *Payer Edits* column.
	Missing Info	When you manually flag a claim with having a status of *Missing Info*, the claim will appear in the *Missing Info* column. After reviewing a claim (an unpaid claim, and identifying information that the claim lacks), you can manually flag the claim as *Missing Info* and the claim will move to the *Missing Info* column. Claims remain in this column until the missing information is added or edited and the claim is rebilled. Claims are never automatically placed in this category. It must be a manual status change.
	Not Found	Claims are put into the *Not Found* category when you electronically check a claim's status and a claim is not on file with a payer. Harris CareTracker PM automatically flags the claim and moves it to this category. A claim will not be moved to the *Not Found Claims* category until seven days after the claim was originally transmitted, which allots time for transmission lag time and for the claim to be accepted into the payer's system. **Note:** When you electronically check a claim's status after the seven-day lag time and the payer does not have a claim accepted into its system, the claim will be moved to the *Not Found* category. When you call or check on claims with a payer not using the electronic claim status feature, you can manually flag a claim as *Not Found* and the claim will be moved to this category.

TABLE 10-1 *(Continued)*

Category	Column	Description
	Set to Deny	Claims are put into the *Claims Worklist* category of *Claim Status Denial* when you electronically check a claim's status and a payer flags a claim as set to deny. Harris CareTracker PM automatically flags the claim and moves it to this category. A claim will not be moved to the *Claim Status Denial* category until at least two weeks after the claim was originally transmitted, which allots time for transmission lag time, for the claim to be accepted into the payer's system, and for the payer to properly **adjudicate** the claim. Adjudication is the final determination of the issues involving settlement of an insurance claim, also known as a claim settlement. When you electronically check a claim's status after the two-week lag time, the payer has accepted into its system and has set the claim to deny, the claim will be moved to the *Claim Status Denial* category. The claim status window will show the details of each claim's denial. When you call or check on claims with a payer not using the electronic claim status feature, you can manually flag a claim as *Claim Status Denial*, and the claim will be moved to this category.
Pending	In Review	Claims are put into the *Claims Worklist* category of *In Review* when you electronically check a claim's status and the payer sends back a status of *In Review*. The claim is automatically moved to this category.
	Hold	A claim is only moved to the *Hold Claim* category if you manually flag the claim with a *Hold* status. For example, if there was an issue with a doctor's credentials, you would want to flag the claim with a *Hold* status to save it in the *Claims Worklist* screen until the issue was resolved and then you would rebill the claim. The status of claims saved in this category is not automatically checked by Harris CareTracker PM and EMR. However, you can do a manual recheck on the status of claims saved under this category if necessary.
Other	Inactive	A claim that has had no follow-up activity during the last 30 days is placed under this category.
	Crossover	Claims that are transferred from a patient's primary insurance to the supplementary insurance and are not paid within 30 days are placed under this category.

Courtesy of Harris CareTracker PM and EMR

Tip Box

The *form type* determines how the claim is produced, for example, on a paper 1500 form or in **American National Standards Institute (ANSI)** format to be sent electronically. ANSI (or CMS 1500) format can be changed to paper and Harris CareTracker PM ensures that the proper information is present on the claim form before releasing the claim to print. ANSI refers to form types that are claims electronically transmitted to a payer. If needed, a paper claim can be generated without Harris CareTracker PM verifying the accuracy of the information by clicking on the *Rebuild Paper Claim* button.

Claim Summary Fields and Features

Claim summary lines for each claim included in the *Claims Worklist* category you select for a particular financial class will display. Actions can be performed on multiple claims using this screen. Table 10-2 details claim summary lines.

TABLE 10-2	Claim Summary Lines
Field	**Description**
Back	Clicking on the *Back* button will bring you back to the *Unpaid/Inactive Claims* screen, where you can select an aged week of unpaid/inactive claims to work on for a particular financial class.
Select All	All claims included in the unpaid/inactive claims age for the financial class you chose to work on will be selected when the *Select All* button is clicked and a selected claim is indicated by a check mark in the *Select* column on the claim line. *Select All* is convenient to use if you need to perform an action on the selected batch of claims, such as electronically checking claim status, rebilling claims, or adding a note. When the *Select All* button is clicked, individual claims can be deselected by clicking on the check mark in the *Select* column.
Deselect All	Clicking on the *Deselect All* button will deselect any selected claim. A selected claim is indicated by a check mark in the *Select* column on a claim line. Deselecting a claim or all claims will remove the check mark.
Filing Limit	Claims approaching filing limit are highlighted red as a visual indication that these claims need to be handled in a timely manner. For most payers, a claim will turn red 25 to 30 days before its actual filing limit will be reached.
Inactive Limit	Claims that have not been worked in 30 days are considered inactive, and inactive claims are highlighted tan as a visual indication that these claims need to be worked.
Claim Summary Line	A claim summary line for each claim included in the unpaid/inactive claims age for the financial class you selected displays. The claim summary line shows the patient's name, Harris CareTracker PM and EMR ID number, the patient' date of birth, the insurance plan, the patient's subscriber number, the status of the claim, the claim's last activity date, the original claim date, the claim's age, the oldest service date, the provider, the original amount on the claim, the remaining open balance, the last transaction date, the description of the last transaction, the activity date, and the activity notes. More detailed claim summary information will display when an individual claim summary line is clicked.
Rebill	This *Rebill* button is used to rebill a batch of claims. Select the claims you need to rebill either by clicking on the *Select All* button or by clicking in the *Select* column for the appropriate claims and then click on the *Rebill* button. Rebilling claims changes their status to "New" and moves them to the *New/Pending* column on the *Claims Worklist* screen. Claims in the *New/Pending* column will be transmitted during your next bill run.

(Continues)

TABLE 10-2 *(Continued)*

Field	Description
Claim Status	Every evening, Harris CareTracker PM and EMR automatically checks the status of every claim on which there is an outstanding balance. A claim is checked for the first time after it has been flagged as TRANS OPEN for seven days. If the claim status continues to remain "In process," the second automated check is performed three days after the first check. Because a third check is not performed by Harris CareTracker PM and EMR, it is best practice to call the payer and follow up on the claim or manually recheck the claim status. There are particular statuses returned from a payer when a claim's status is checked: *In Process, Finalized, Set to Pay, Set to Deny, Pending In Review,* and *Not Found.* Each claim will be updated accordingly when the automated batch claim status check is complete. When a status of *Set to Deny, Pending in Review,* or *Not Found* is returned during an automated batch claim status check, the claim will be updated and flagged in the *Claims Worklist* link under the *Billing* section of the *Dashboard.* Harris CareTracker PM does not check any claims moved to the "Hold" category automatically. However, you can perform a manual claim status check if necessary.
Notes	Enter an activity note in regard to the selected claims in the *Notes* field and click on the *Save* button. The note will be saved in the *Activity Notes* section of each selected claim and adding a note restarts the claims aging used to determine inactive claims.
Status	The *Status* field can be used to manually change the status of the selected claims. "Select" defaults in the *Status* field; however, the selected claims' statuses can be changed by selecting the appropriate status from the *Status* field drop-down list of "Payer Edits," "Not Found," "Claim Status Denial," "Missing Info," or "In Review." Manually changing the claim's status will move the selected claims to the corresponding column on the *Claims Worklist* screen.
Save	Clicking on the *Save* button will save an activity note that has been entered in the *Notes* field and/or a claim status that has been selected from the *Status* list.

Courtesy of Harris CareTracker PM and EMR

Critical Thinking

Research claims filing limits for Medicare, Medicaid, Blue Cross/Blue Shield, and Aetna. Prepare a one-page paper on each insurer's claim filing limits. Contrast and compare and make best practice recommendations to the practice to process claims in a timely manner.

Claim Summary Screen. The *Claim Summary* screen (Figure 10-4) displays when an individual claim line is clicked. In this screen, actions can be performed on the selected claim only. The *Claim Summary* screen fields and descriptions are outlined in Table 10-3.

Work the Claims Worklist

Having identified a problem (or problems) that would prevent a claim from being paid, you will work the *Claims Worklist* to resolve the issue(s).

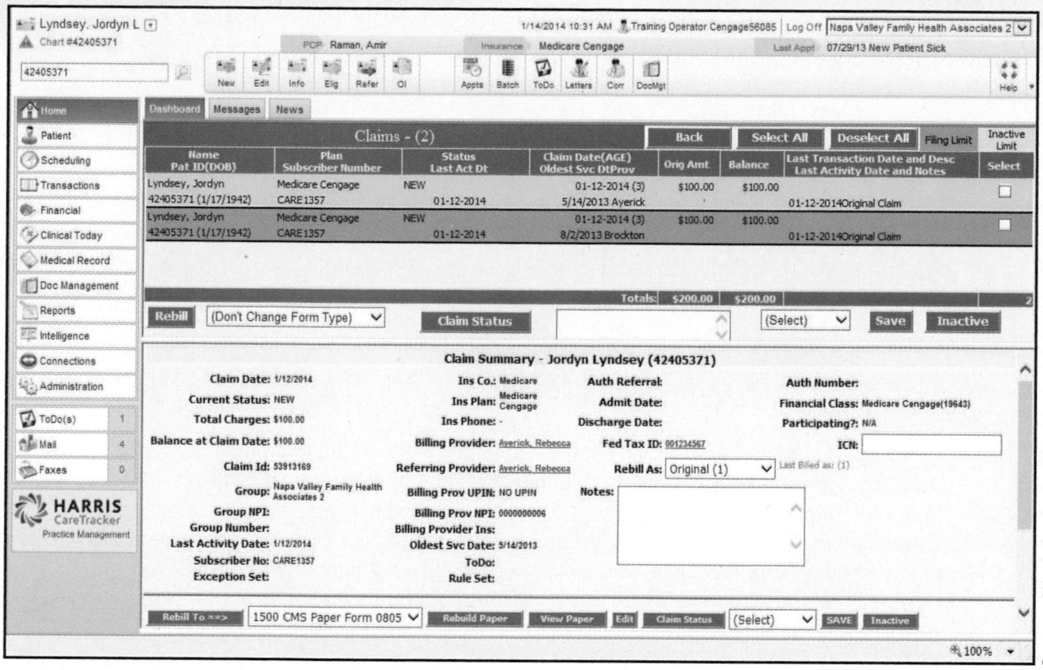

Figure 10-4   Claims Summary Screen

TABLE 10-3   Claims Summary Screen

Field	Description
Claim Information	The top part of the *Claim Summary* screen displays all of the information that was included on the claim; the status, balance, last activity date, subscriber number, insurance company, insurance plan, billing and servicing provider, billing provider UPIN and NPI, referring provider, admission date (if applicable) and authorization number (if applicable), provider's tax ID, provider's enrollment status in insurance, and the effective date of enrollment. These fields cannot be edited; however, the billing provider and the referring provider's insurance number details can be viewed by clicking on the respective provider's name. **Note:** A provider's participating status can be one of the following: • *N/A*—This indicates that the insurance carrier does not require specific enrollment/credentialing to participate. • *No*—This indicates that the provider does not participate with the insurance listed on the claim. • *Yes*—This indicates that the provider is enrolled with the insurance and displays the date of effective date.
Rebill As	The *Rebill As* field is used to flag an electronically resubmitted claim (ANSI 837 format) with a code that indicates the claim is a resubmission. Flagging a resubmitted claim prevents the claim from being denied as a duplicate. Code definitions: • *Insurance Default (I)*: Rebills each claim with the default code that was set for the insurance on that claim. • *Claim Default (C)*: Rebills the claim with its current status. • *Original (1)*: First generation of claim. **Note:** This code is not used for rebilling. • *Corrected (6)*: Adjustment of a prior claim. • *Replacement (7)*: Replacement of a prior claim. • *Void (8)*: Void/Cancel of a prior claim.

(Continues)

TABLE 10-3 *(Continued)*

Field	Description
Notes	An activity note can be added to the claim by entering the note in the *Notes* field and then clicking on the *Save* button. Adding a note restarts the claims aging used to determine inactive claims.
Rebill To==>	When the needed information has been added to or edited to the claim or the patient's demographic, the *Rebill To==>* button must be clicked to rebill the claim. When a claim is rebilled, it will be placed in the *New/Pending* column on the *Claims Worklist* screen and will be transmitted during your next bill run. Before clicking on the *Rebill To==>* button, verify the form type selected in the *Form Type* field. A form type must be changed before clicking on *Rebill To==>* button.
Form Type	ANSI form types are claims that are electronically transmitted to a payer, and paper form types are claims forms that are dropped to paper that must be printed from Harris CareTracker PM and then mailed to a payer. The default form type for the insurance plan the claim needs to be sent to is selected in the *Form Type* field. When a form type needs to be changed, select the appropriate form from the *Form Type* list and click on the *Rebill To==>* button. When ANSI format is changed to paper, Harris CareTracker PM ensures that the proper information is present on the claim form before releasing the claim to print.
Rebuild Paper Claim	The *Rebuild Paper* claim button can be used to print paper claims without Harris CareTracker PM verifying the accuracy of the information. The form type selected in the *Form Type* field must be a paper form. When the *Rebuild Paper* claim button is clicked, the claim displays in a window. Right-click on top of it and select *Print* from the gray pop-up menu. The claim will be removed from *Claims Worklist* when the *Rebuild Paper* claim button is clicked.
View Paper	The claim will display in a window when the *View Paper* claim button is clicked. Clicking on the *View Paper* button does not remove the claim from the *Claims Worklist* link.
Edit	Clicking on the *Edit* button on the *Claim Summary* screen displays the *Encounter* window from which you can add and/or edit claim information including the location, place of service, *Additional Claim Info*, referring provider, modifiers, and diagnoses. Dates of service, procedure codes, fees, the insurance company, and the amount of the claim may not be edited from this pop-up. **Note:** When the billing provider, dates of service, procedure codes, fee, units, servicing provider, or insurance needs to be changed, the charge will need to be reversed from Harris CareTracker PM via the *Edit* application in the *Transactions* module. The charge will then need to be put back into the system.
Claim Status	Every evening, Harris CareTracker PM will automatically check the status of every claim submitted on which there is an outstanding balance. A claim is checked for the first time after seven days and it is flagged as "TRANS OPEN" in the *Claim Status* box. If the claim status continues to remain "In process" the second automated check is performed three days after the first check and if the claim is not finalized it will be flagged as "Not Found". Because a third check is not performed by Harris CareTracker PM, it is best practice to call the payer and follow up on the claim or manually recheck the claim status. There are particular statuses returned from a payer when a claim's status is checked: "In Process," "Finalized," "Set to Pay," "Set to Deny," "Pending In Review," and "Not Found." Each claim will be updated accordingly when the automated batch claim status check is complete. When a status of "Set to Deny," "Pending in Review," or "Not Found" is returned during an automated batch claim status check, the claim will be updated and flagged in the *Claims Worklist* link under the *Billing* section of the *Dashboard*. The *Claim Status* button on the *Claim Summary* screen enables manual recheck of claims' status without having to wait for the automated process. **Note:** Harris CareTracker PM does not automatically check any claims moved to the "Hold" category. However, you can perform a manual claim status check if necessary.

TABLE 10-3 *(Continued)*

Field	Description
Status	The *Status* field can be used to manually change the status of the claim by selecting defaults in the *Status* field; however, the status can be changed by selecting the appropriate status from the *Status* list ("Payer Edits," "Not Found," "Claim Status Denial," "Missing Info," or "In Review"), and then clicking on the *Save* button. Manually changing the claim's status will move the claim to the corresponding column on the *Claims Worklist* screen.
Save	Clicking on the *Save* button will save an activity note that has been entered in the *Notes* field and/or a claim status that has been selected from the *Status* list.
Inactive	The *Inactive* button allows you to manually set an inactive date for one or more claims. When an inactive date is set, you can hover over the *Inactive* button to view the date. Additionally, Harris CareTracker PM adds an entry to the activity log below the *Claim Summary* each time an inactive date is set for a claim.
Status Column	The status column shows the claim's current status and all of the status steps the claim has gone through.
Activity Date	Activity date logs the date and time of all activity taken on the claim.
Activity Notes	Claim errors occur when a claim does not meet specific requirements set by Harris CareTracker PM and/or payers. Errors display under the *Activity Notes* section of the *Claim Summary* screen as a mnemonic code along with the error description. Error descriptions direct you as to what pieces of claim information needs to be fixed before the claim can be successfully transmitted to a payer. Example: "BPINNO - Billing Provider/Insurance Number is missing for this particular Billing Provider/Insurance combination" instead of "BPINNO" only.
Key	By clicking on the *Key* link, a list of all the possible system note codes and their corresponding messages will display. This key can be used to decipher a code that you do not understand.
Link	The *Acknowledgement* and the *Report* electronically received into Harris CareTracker PM from a payer that included the claim will be accessible from the *Claim Summary* screen. The *Acknowledgement* report can be viewed by clicking on the *ANSI 837* link and the *Report* can be viewed by clicking on the *Report* link. The *Report* shows all the claims that were transmitted in the same claim batch as the current claim's summary you are viewing.
Operator	This logs the operator who performed each action that has been taken on a claim.
Claim Batch ID	This shows the claim batch identification number.
Procedures	Each procedure line included on the claim will display in the lower part of the *Claim Summary* screen. Under each procedure line will be a record of all the financial transactions linked to each procedure.
Payment	The *Payments* screen displays when the *Payment* link is clicked from a financial transaction where a payment, adjustment, or transfer for the respective procedure line can be entered.
Separate Claim	When multiple procedure codes appear on one claim, those procedures can be separated to different claims by clicking on the *Separate Claim* link.

ACTIVITY 10-1: Work the Claims Worklist

1. Go to the *Home* module > *Dashboard* tab > *Billing* section > *Claims Worklist* link. There are three options: *Unbilled, Crossover,* and *Inactive* (Figure 10-5). Select *Unbilled.* This will take you to the *Claims Worklist* screen.

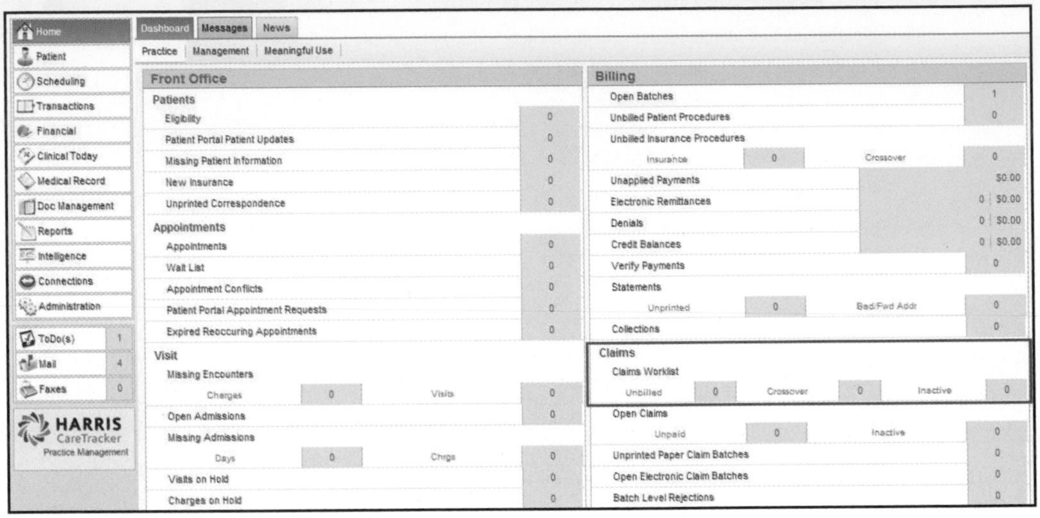

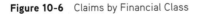

Figure 10-5 Claims Worklist Dashboard

Courtesy of Harris CareTracker PM and EMR

2. The *Location* list defaults to "All Locations." You have the option to select a specific location if needed. Leave as is.
3. The *All Groups* list defaults to "N" for No. Select "Y" for Yes if you want to include claims for all groups. Select "Y."
4. Select the *Incl. Crossovers* checkbox to include crossover claims and enter "180" in the *Crossover Days* field.
5. (Optional) Enter a date range in the *Oldest Service Date From/To* boxes to view claims from a specific time period.
6. Click *Go*. The application displays a list of all claims broken down by financial class (Figure 10-6).

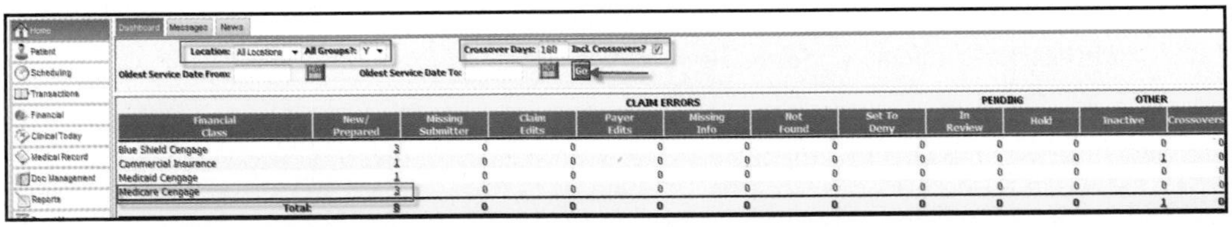

Figure 10-6 Claims by Financial Class

Courtesy of Harris CareTracker PM and EMR

7. Click on a number in the *New/Prepared* column for the corresponding financial class you need to work (select the column for "Medicare Cengage"). The *New/Prepared Claims* screen will display (Figure 10-7). **Note:** You can also click the *Total* at the bottom of the column. Harris CareTracker PM displays a claim line for all of the *Unbilled Claims* for the corresponding column and financial class.

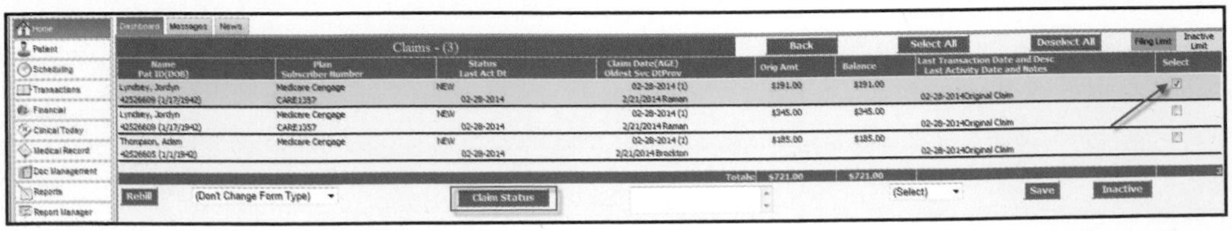

Figure 10-7 New/Prepared Claims Screen

Courtesy of Harris CareTracker PM and EMR

Tip Box

Click the column headings to re-sort the column data.

8. Select the checkbox in the *Select* column for each claim you want to work. Select the first claim for Jordyn Lyndsey and click the *Claim Status* button. (**Note:** You can select all of the claims by clicking *Select All*.) You will receive a pop-up (Figure 10-8) advising you of the claim's status (which displays "Processing...."). **DO NOT** click the *Close* button in the pop-up as this will remove the claim from the *Unbilled Claims* screen. Rather, click on the "X" in the upper right hand corner to close out of the window.

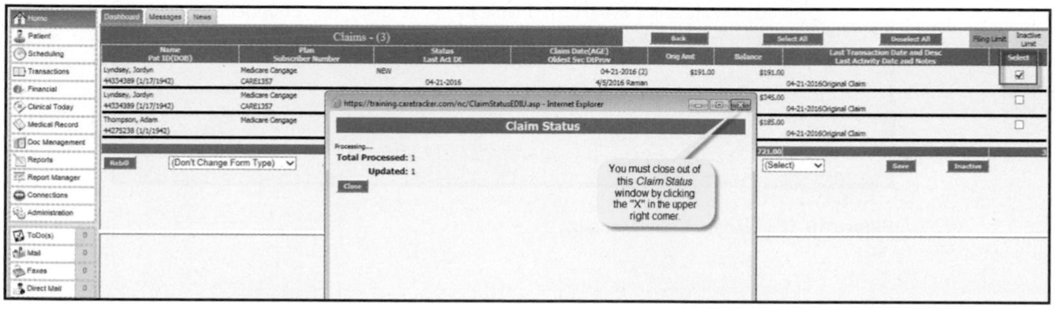

Figure 10-8 Claim Status Pop-Up

Courtesy of Harris CareTracker PM and EMR

9. To review, edit, check claim status, or rebill an individual claim, click in the claim summary line. The claim line now appears in yellow and the application displays the *Claim Summary* in the lower frame of the screen (see Figure 10-4). Look under the *Activity Notes* column to determine the inaccurate or missing claim information that, triggered by *ClaimsManager*, prevented the claim from being transmitted from Harris CareTracker PM, that prevented the claim from being accepted by a payer, or that caused the claim to be denied by the payer (Figure 10-9).

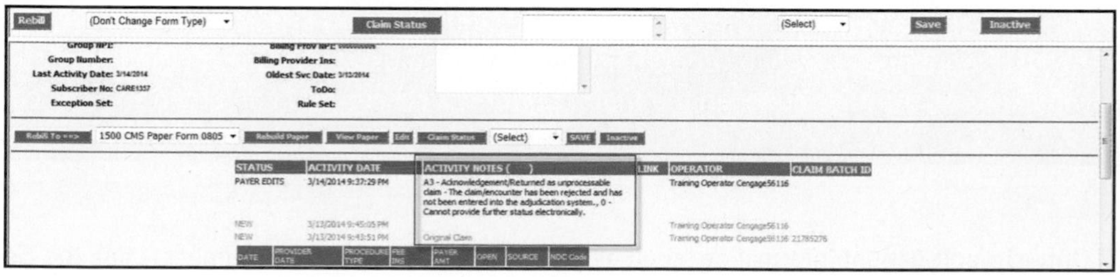

Figure 10-9 Activity Notes

Courtesy of Harris CareTracker PM and EMR

10. Perform the desired action on the claim(s):

a. To edit claim information, such as diagnosis code or referring provider, click *Edit* on the *Claim Summary* screen (Figure 10-10). The *Claim Transaction Summary* window displays the location, place of service, encounter specific claim information, referring provider, diagnosis code, and modifiers. Change the referring provider to "Dr. Raman," and then click *Save*. Once *Save* is clicked, you will briefly receive the "error" message noted in Figure 10-11. Click *OK*. Your *Claim Summary* will now reflect the change to Referring Provider.

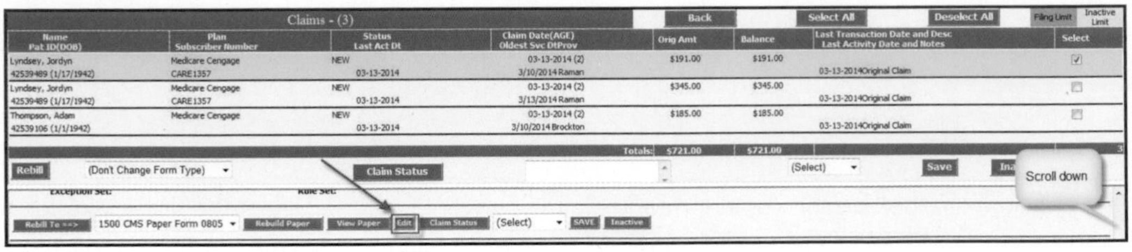

Courtesy of Harris CareTracker PM and EMR

Figure 10-10 Edit Claim Summary

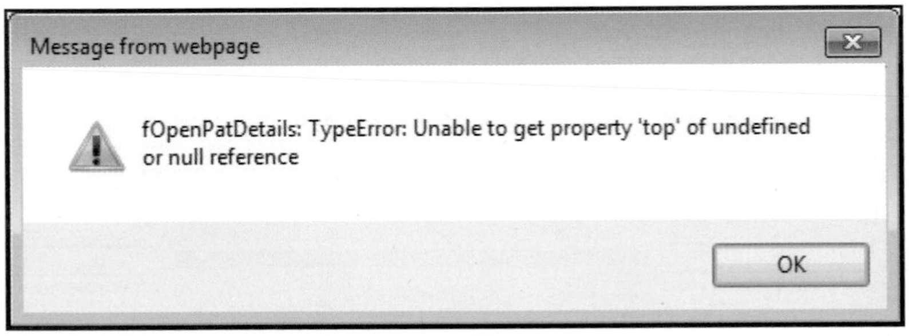

Courtesy of Harris CareTracker PM and EMR

Figure 10-11 Update Claim Message

PM SPOTLIGHT

In the medical setting the **National Drug Code (NDC)** number identifies a listed drug product that is assigned a unique 10-digit, 3-segment number. This number, known as the NDC, identifies the labeler, product, and trade package size. The first segment, the labeler code, is assigned by the Food and Drug Administration (FDA). A labeler is any firm that manufactures (including repackers or relabelers) or distributes (under its own name) the drug. The second segment, the product code, identifies a specific strength, dosage form, and formulation for a particular firm. The third segment, the package code, identifies package sizes and types. Both the product and package codes are assigned by the firm. The NDC will be in one of the following configurations and is required to be reported: 4-4-2, 5-3-2, or 5-4-1. The NDC enhances safety by documenting drugs and establishes a method to recall. **Note:** By clicking on the *Misc* button in the *Claim Summary* screen you can enter an NDC code.

b. (FYI Only) To edit patient information, such as date of birth or subscriber number, click the *Edit* button on the *Name Bar*. Harris CareTracker PM and EMR opens the patient's demographics in a new *Patient Edit* window.

c. (FYI Only) To inactivate a claim you would select the claim by placing a check mark in the *Select* column box. Click the *Inactive* button to inactivate a claim. A pop-up box appears. Enter the inactive date and then click *Accept* (Figure 10-12). Your screen will refresh and the *Inactive* date appears in the *Last Transaction Date and Desc* column (Figure 10-13).

CHAPTER 10   ClaimsManager and Collections   **543**

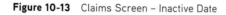

Figure 10-12   Enter Inactive Date

Figure 10-13   Claims Screen – Inactive Date

> ## Tip Box
>
> When the billing provider, dates of service, procedure codes, fee, units, servicing provider, or insurance need to be changed, the charge must be reversed from Harris CareTracker PM via the *Edit* application in the *Transactions* module. The charge will then be put back into the system.

   d. (FYI Only) Click the number link in the *Rule Set* field. The application displays descriptions of the rules for the insurance company where the claim is being submitted. Reviewing the rules can help you determine what claim information must be fixed.

   e. (FYI Only) In the *Claim Summary*, select a claim frequency code from the *Rebill As* field to indicate why the claim is being resubmitted (if applicable). Each code is described in Table 10-4.

> ## Tip Box
>
> When rebilling claims, the form type is not typically changed.

TABLE 10-4   Claims Frequency Codes

Code	Description
Insurance Default (I)	Rebills each claim with the default code that was set for the insurance on that claim.
Claim Default (C)	Rebills the claim with its current status.
Original (1)	First generation of claim. **Note:** This code is not used for rebilling.
Corrected (6)	Adjustment of a prior claim.
Replacement (7)	Replacement of a prior claim.
Void (8)	Void/Cancellation of a prior claim.

Courtesy of Harris CareTracker PM and EMR

11. Now select the same claim by clicking in the claim line (which will turn yellow) and checking the *Select* box. When all of the edits are complete, click *Rebill To*. Harris CareTracker PM places the claim in the *New/Pending* category of the *Claims Worklist* and the claim will be transmitted during the next claim run. Scroll down the screen and in the *Activity Notes* column, you will now see the activities completed (Figure 10-14).

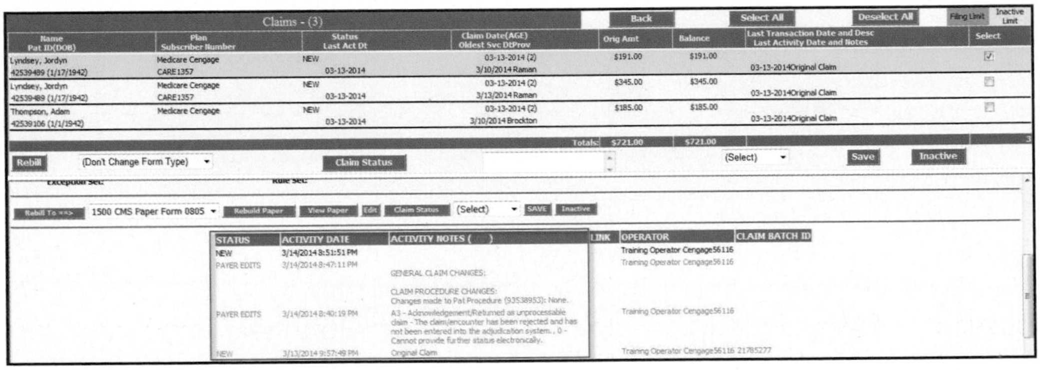

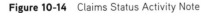

Figure 10-14   Claims Status Activity Note

Courtesy of Harris CareTracker PM and EMR

Print the Claim Status Activity screen, label it "Activity 10-1," and place it in your assignment folder.

Work Crossover Claims

A **crossover** claim is a claim that is automatically forwarded from Medicare to a secondary insurer after Medicare has paid its portion of a service.

ACTIVITY 10-2:   Search Crossover Claims

1. Go to the *Home* module > *Dashboard* tab > *Billing* section > *Claims Worklist* link. Select *Crossover* from the three options. Harris CareTracker PM opens the *Claims Worklist* application.

2. The *Location* list defaults to "All Locations." Leave as is.

3. The *All Groups* list defaults to "N" for No. Select "Y" for Yes to include claims for all groups.

4. Select the *Incl. Crossovers* checkbox. The *Crossover Days* field defaults to 30. **Note:** You can adjust the crossover days to 180 if claims are not displaying for you.

5. (Optional) Enter a date range in the *Oldest Service Date From/To* boxes.

6. Click *Go*. Harris CareTracker PM displays a list of all claims organized by financial class (Figure 10-15).

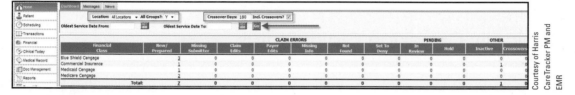

Figure 10-15   Crossover Claims

7. If there are crossover claims noted in the *Crossovers* column, click the number that corresponds to the financial class in which you want to work. Harris CareTracker PM displays a list of crossover claims (Figure 10-16). There are no *Crossover Claims* for you to work here; however, in a live environment you would do the following:

   a. In the *Bill?* column, select the checkbox next to each claim you want to bill to secondary insurance. Alternatively, click *Check All* to bill all claims as crossover claims.

   b. Click *Set to Bill*. All crossover claims are saved as Secondary 1500 Forms under the *Unprinted Paper Claims* link for printing in the next bill run.

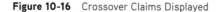

Figure 10-16   Crossover Claims Displayed

Print the **Crossovers search screen, label it "Activity 10-2," and place it in your assignment folder.**

WORK UNPAID CLAIMS

Learning Objective 2: Check status and work unpaid/inactive claims.

Unpaid claims are claims that have been submitted to an insurance company but have not been paid. **Inactive claims** are claims that are not only unpaid, but also have not had any follow-up activity on them for the last

30 days. *Unpaid* and *Inactive* claims are aged by week, broken down by financial class, and can be worked from the *Unpaid/Inactive* links in the *Claims* section of the *Practice Dashboard*. Inactive claims are highlighted in tan and claims that are nearing their filing limit are highlighted in red as a visual alert that these claims need to be worked immediately. From this list, you can drill down into each *Unpaid/Inactive* claim that requires follow-up. When an inactive claim has been worked it is removed from the inactive category; however, if there is no payment or additional activity on the claim for the next 30 days, it is recategorized as inactive.

The number of inactive claims should only be 5% to 10% of your unpaid claims. As best practice, you should focus your follow-up activities on the inactive claims category. This will significantly improve the efficiency of your claim follow-up activities and practice revenue cycle.

Harris CareTracker PM automatically checks the status of unpaid claims every evening with specific payers and will check the status of all claims with an outstanding balance. When a check is complete, the claim's status is updated, attached to the claims, and if necessary will also be flagged in *Claims Worklist* if a status of "Not Found," "Set to Deny," or "In Review" is returned.

Electronically Checking Claim Status

Claim status is automatically checked every evening for every claim that has an outstanding balance. Typically, a manual claim status check is not necessary. However, if you need to manually check claim status you do so individually or in a batch.

> ## PM SP⬤TLIGHT
>
> Harris CareTracker PM automatically performs a status check seven days after the claim is set to *Trans Open*. If the claim is not finalized, Harris CareTracker PM automatically performs another check three days later and then flags the claim as "Not Found."

Checking Individual Claim Status. Claim status for individual claims can be checked from any application in Harris CareTracker PM where the *Claim Summary* screen displays.

ACTIVITY 10-3: Individually Check Claim Status Electronically

1. Go to the *Home* module > *Dashboard* tab > *Billing* section > *Open Claims/Unpaid* link (Figure 10-17). Harris CareTracker PM displays the *Open Claims* application.

2. Select the desired filter options, as outlined:

   a. *Status*: NEW

   b. *Age By*: Oldest Service Date

   c. *Financial Class*: Leave as is

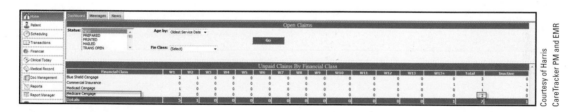

Figure 10-17   Unpaid Claims Link

3. Click *Go*. Harris CareTracker PM displays the *Unpaid/Inactive* claims, broken down by financial class and by week. The total inactive claims for a financial class displays in the *Inactive* column. Totals for all unpaid claims for a financial class displays in the *Total* column, and for each week the total number unpaid claims displays in the *Totals* row (Figure 10-18).

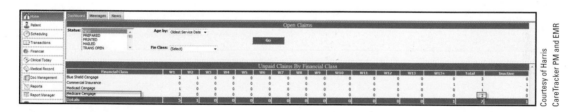

Figure 10-18   Open Claims

4. Determine the unpaid/inactive claims for which you would like to electronically check claim status. Select the *Financial Class* "Medicare Cengage" and click on the corresponding number in the *Total* column. Harris CareTracker PM displays a claim line for all corresponding *Unpaid/Inactive* claims with the patient's name, ID number, date of birth, subscriber number, the insurance plan for which the claim was transmitted, the claim status, last activity date on the claim, claim date, claim age, oldest service date on the claim, the provider on the claim, the original amount, balance remaining, and the last activity notes saved for the claim.

5. Place a check mark in the *Select* column, and then click on a claim summary line (select first claim). The line turns yellow and Harris CareTracker PM displays the *Claim Summary* in the lower frame of the screen.

6. Scroll down the screen and you will be able to view the claim history (Figure 10-19). Click *Claim Status*. When the *Claim Status* window has finished processing, close out of it by clicking the "X" in the upper right corner.

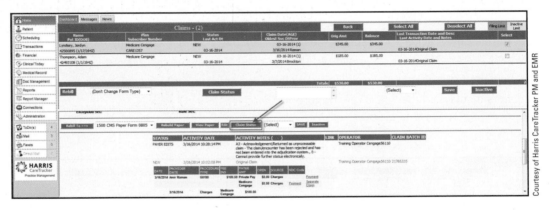

Figure 10-19 Claim History

7. Re-select the claim and click the *Claim Status* button above *Activity Notes* (Figure 10-20). Harris Care-Tracker PM displays the *Claim Status History* window (Figure 10-21), which includes all previous status checks that have occurred, including the date of the status check, the operator who performed the check, the claim status category, and the *Claim Status* code.

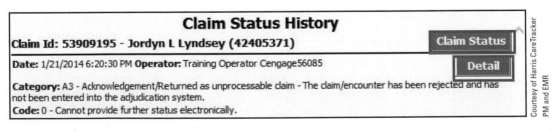

Figure 10-20 Select Claim Status Button

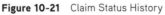

Figure 10-21 Claim Status History

8. Click on the *Claim Status* button on the top right corner of the *Claim Status History* window to perform another claim status check. When the claim status check is complete, the status of the current claim is automatically updated. Click on the "X" in the upper right corner of the *Claim Status* window to close it. Possible statuses are included in Table 10-5.

TABLE 10-5 Possible Claim Statuses	
In Process	When a claim status check is complete and the payer returns that it is "In Process," Harris CareTracker PM sets the claim status to "In Process." When a claim is set to "In Process" its status will not be checked during a batch electronic claim status check for the next seven days. However, you can manually recheck the individual claim's status, overriding the seven-day period.
Finalized	When a claim status check is complete and the payer returns that it is "Finalized," Harris CareTracker PM sets the claim status to "Finalized." A "Finalized"claim will have the details of the finalization listed under the *Activity Notes* section of the *Claims Summary* screen. After a claim has been set to "Finalized," no additional electronic claim status checks can be performed.
Set to Pay	When a claim status check is done and the payer returns that it is "Set to Pay," Harris CareTracker PM will set the claim status to "Set to Pay." "Set to Pay" claims are going to be paid by the respective payer. These claims will remain in *Unpaid/Inactive* claims until they are paid or adjusted off in full. After a claim has been set to "Set to Pay," no additional electronic claim status checks can be performed.
Set to Deny	This will send back as part of the claim status process. Any of these messages that constitute a claim status denial will set the claim's status to "Set to Deny." In addition to these claims being flagged in the *Unpaids/Inactive* link, they are flagged in the *Claims Worklist* link as well because they have been denied and will require follow-up. After a claim has been set to *Set to Deny*, no additional electronic claim status checks can be performed.
Pending in Review	There are also *Claim Status* messages that will come back from the payer that the claim is "In Review." Any of these statuses will set the claim to *In Review*. *In Review* claims should be followed up on until they have been adjudicated by a payer.
Not Found	Any payer that has electronic claim status where the claim is not on file after seven days of the original claim date will be set to "Not Found" status.

Courtesy of Harris CareTracker PM and EMR

Tip Box

When a claim's status has been returned, except for "Set to Pay," the claim will be moved to the corresponding column on the *Claims Worklist* screen.

9. To view the details of the check, click on the *Detail* button and the *Claim Status Detail* dialog box displays (Figure 10-22).

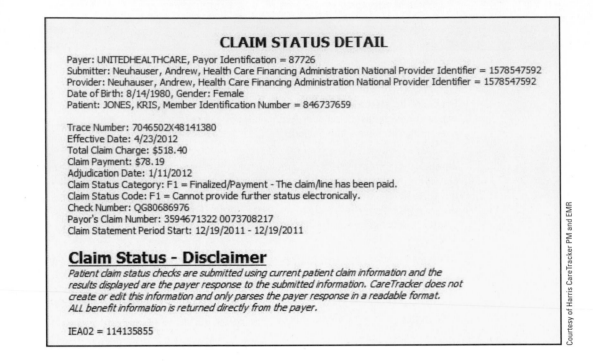

CLAIM STATUS DETAIL

Payer: UNITEDHEALTHCARE, Payor Identification = 87726
Submitter: Neuhauser, Andrew, Health Care Financing Administration National Provider Identifier = 1578547592
Provider: Neuhauser, Andrew, Health Care Financing Administration National Provider Identifier = 1578547592
Date of Birth: 8/14/1980, Gender: Female
Patient: JONES, KRIS, Member Identification Number = 846737659

Trace Number: 7046502X48141380
Effective Date: 4/23/2012
Total Claim Charge: $518.40
Claim Payment: $78.19
Adjudication Date: 1/11/2012
Claim Status Category: F1 = Finalized/Payment - The claim/line has been paid.
Claim Status Code: F1 = Cannot provide further status electronically.
Check Number: QG80686976
Payor's Claim Number: 3594671322 0073708217
Claim Statement Period Start: 12/19/2011 - 12/19/2011

Claim Status - Disclaimer

Patient claim status checks are submitted using current patient claim information and the
results displayed are the payer response to the submitted information. CareTracker does not
create or edit this information and only parses the payer response in a readable format.
ALL benefit information is returned directly from the payer.

IEA02 = 114135855

Courtesy of Harris CareTracker PM and EMR

Figure 10-22 Claim Status Detail

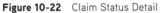 **Print the Claim Status Detail screen, label it "Activity 10-3," and place it in your assignment folder.**

10. Click "X" in the top right corner of the *Claim Status Detail* and *Claim Status History* windows to close out of them.

Working Unpaid/Inactive Claims

Now that you have checked the claim status, begin working the unpaid/inactive claims. The steps are similar to checking a claim status, but you are now working the claim.

ACTIVITY 10-4: Work Unpaid/Inactive Claims

1. Go to the *Home* module > *Dashboard* tab > *Billing* section > *Open Claims/Unpaid* link.

2. Harris CareTracker PM displays the *Open Claims* application. Enter the following:

   a. In the *Status* field, click on the status of the claims you want to view. Press the *[Ctrl]* key while clicking to select multiple statuses. Do not make a selection; leave as is.

   b. In the *Age by* drop-down list, select the age of claims to view. Select "Oldest Service Date."

   c. (Optional) From the *Fin Class* drop-down list, select the financial class containing the claims you want to view. Leave as "(Select)."

   d. Click *Go*. Harris CareTracker PM displays the unpaid/inactive claims by financial class and by week.

3. Locate the claims you want to work and click on the corresponding number in the chart. Harris CareTracker PM displays a claim line for each unpaid/inactive claim. Click the column headings to sort the columns. (**Note:** You cannot click on a zero total.) Select the number in the *Total* column for "Medicare Cengage."

4. When a number is clicked, a claim line for all corresponding *Unpaid/Inactive* claims displays with the patient's name, ID number, date of birth, subscriber number, the insurance plan for which the claim was transmitted, the claim status, last activity date on the claim, claim date, claim age, oldest service date on the claim, the provider on the claim, the original amount, balance remaining, and the last activity notes saved for the claim (Figure 10-23). Claims that have reached their *Filing Limit* will display in red.

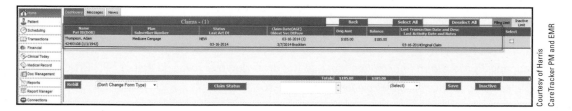

Figure 10-23   Unpaid/Inactive Claims

5. To work claims in a batch:

   a. (FYI Only) To work all claims, click *Select All* to select all of the claims, and then click on the *Claim Status* button.

   b. To review or work an individual claim, click on the claim summary line (select Adam Thompson's claim). Harris CareTracker PM displays the *Claim Summary* in the lower frame of the screen. You will need to scroll down on both the upper and lower screens to view all the claims and the *Claim Summary* information for the claim selected.

   c. To change the location, place of service, encounter specific claim information, referring provider, diagnosis code, and modifiers, scroll down and click *Edit* on the *Claim Summary* screen (Figure 10-24) (click *Edit* in Adam Thompson's claim). The *Claim Transaction Summary* window displays (Figure 10-25), where you can make changes. **Note:** Dates of service, procedure codes, fees, the insurance company, and the amount of the claim may not be edited from this window.

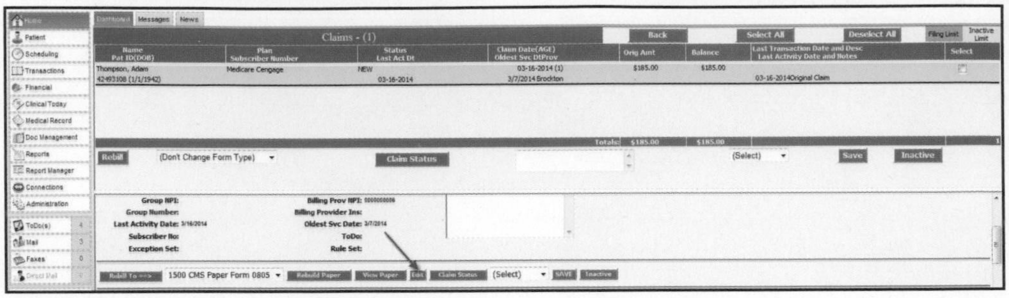

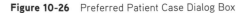

Figure 10-24   Edit Claim Summary

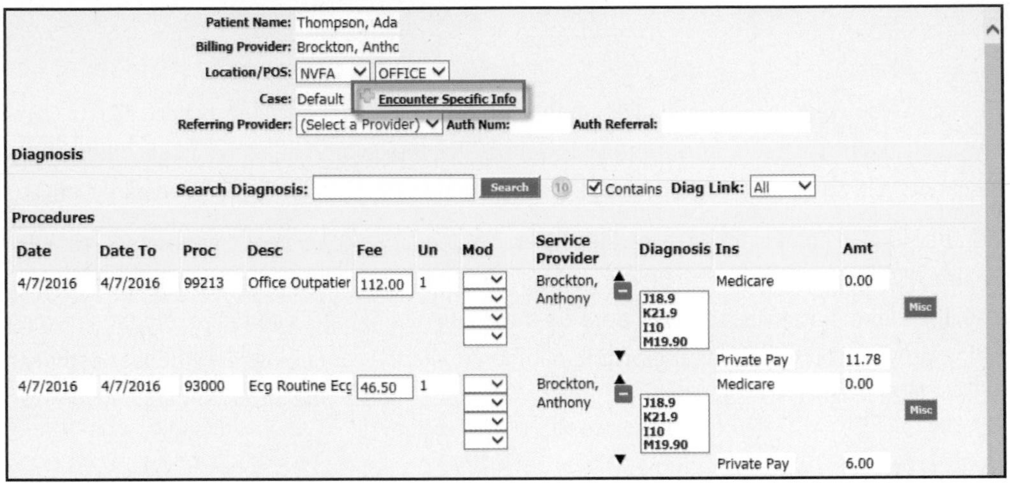

Figure 10-25   Encounters Window

d. Click on the [+] sign next to *Encounter Specific Info* and a pop-up *Preferred Patient Case* dialog box will appear. In the *Claim Information* tab, use the drop-down arrow and select "Dr. Brockton" as the *Supervising* and *Ordering Provider* (Figure 10-26).

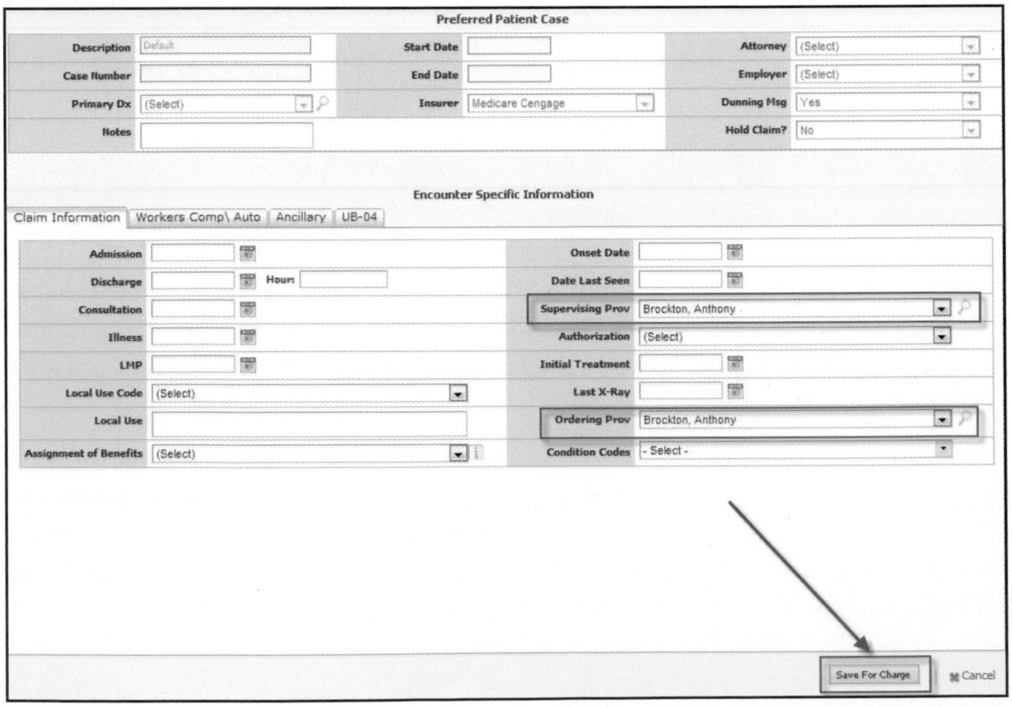

Figure 10-26   Preferred Patient Case Dialog Box

e. Click the *Save For Charge* button. The dialog box disappears and the screen returns to the *Encounters* dialog box.

f. Click the *Save* button at the bottom of the *Claim Transaction Summary* dialog box and it will close.

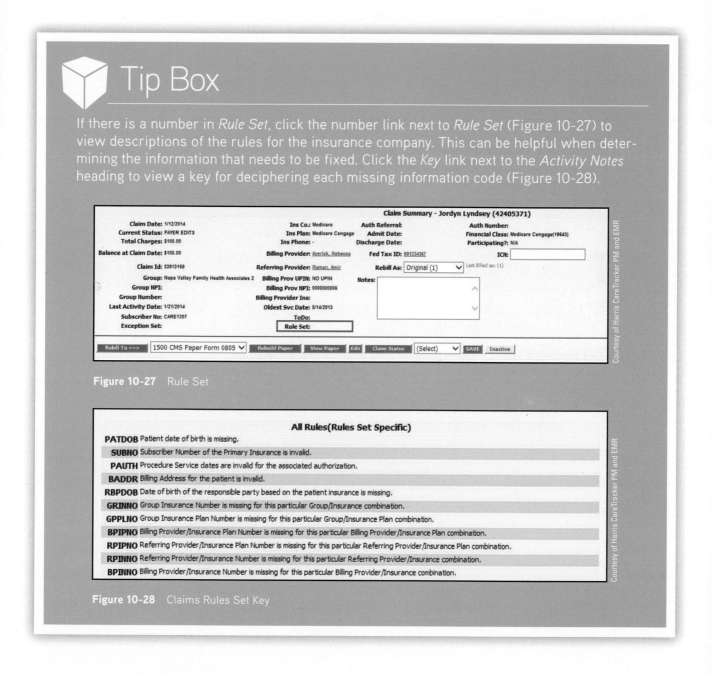

Tip Box

If there is a number in *Rule Set*, click the number link next to *Rule Set* (Figure 10-27) to view descriptions of the rules for the insurance company. This can be helpful when determining the information that needs to be fixed. Click the *Key* link next to the *Activity Notes* heading to view a key for deciphering each missing information code (Figure 10-28).

Figure 10-27   Rule Set

Figure 10-28   Claims Rules Set Key

6. (FYI Only) To edit patient demographic information, click the *Edit* button on the *Name Bar*. Harris CareTracker PM displays the patient's demographics in the *Patient Edit* window.

a. You would edit the information as needed, and then click *Save*.

7. After editing the claim or patient information, click *Rebill To*. Harris CareTracker PM will place the claim in the *New/Pending* category of the *Claims Worklist* screen and will transmit the claim during the next bill run (Figure 10-29).

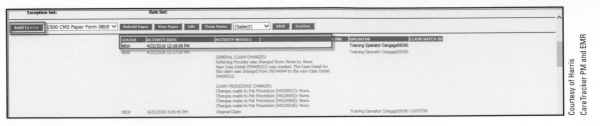

Figure 10-29 Last Transaction Update

Print the Unpaid/Inactive screen, label it "Activity 10-4," and place it in your assignment folder.

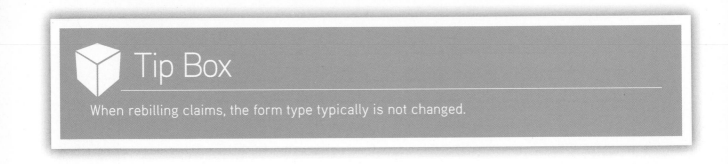

Tip Box

When rebilling claims, the form type typically is not changed.

GENERATE PATIENT STATEMENTS

Learning Objective 3: Generate patient statements.

Harris CareTracker PM automatically generates patient statements each week. Statements are sent to responsible parties who owe a private pay balance. Statements can also be sent for workers' compensation, nursing homes, and legal cases by setting up those organizations as an insurance company or an employer in Harris CareTracker PM.

Tip Box

A statement will not be generated for a patient if the patient has an unapplied balance saved on his or her account that is equal to or greater than the patient's current balance amount.

Patient statements will not be generated by Harris CareTracker PM until 5 p.m., regardless of when you submit the request.

ACTIVITY 10-5:   Generate Patient Statements

1. Before beginning this activity, post the following batches: "CrBalRefunds," "PostEOBs," and "LyndseySNF"

2. With patient Jordyn Lyndsey in context, go to the *Administration* module > *Practice* tab > *Daily Administration* section > *Financial* header > *Generate Statements* link (Figure 10-30). If a patient is in context, the application displays the option to generate statements for the parent company or the responsible party. You can generate statements for only the parent company when no patient is in context.

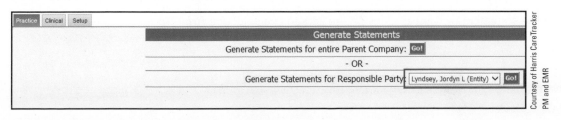

Figure 10-30   Generate Statements Link

3. In the *Generate Statements for Responsible Party* field, select the responsible party for whom you want to generate statements (patient "Jordyn Lyndsey") and then click *Go!* (Figure 10-31).

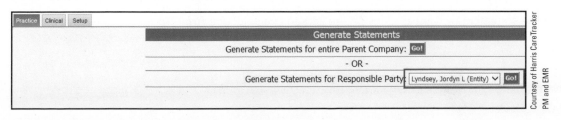

Figure 10-31   Generate Statements for Responsible Party - Jordyn Lyndsey

4. The application schedules the statements to be printed. Your screen will look like Figure 10-32. (FYI Only) In a live environment, patient statements will not be generated by Harris CareTracker PM until 5 p.m. (Figure 10-33) regardless of the time of day you request statements to be produced.

Courtesy of Harris CareTracker PM and EMR

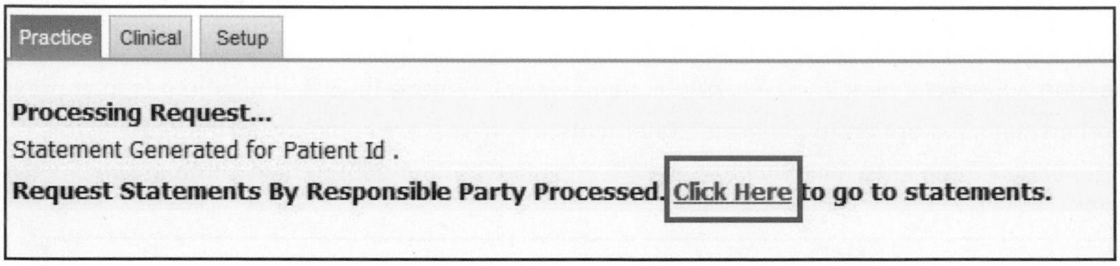

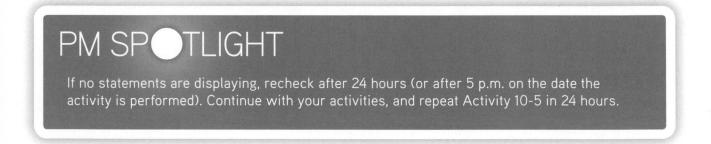

Figure 10-32 Statement Generated

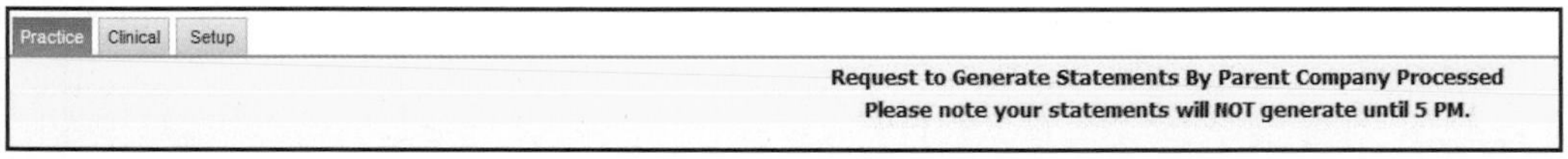

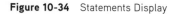

Figure 10-33 Statements Generate at 5 p.m.
Courtesy of Harris CareTracker PM and EMR

PM SPOTLIGHT

If no statements are displaying, recheck after 24 hours (or after 5 p.m. on the date the activity is performed). Continue with your activities, and repeat Activity 10-5 in 24 hours.

5. Click on the blue "Click Here" prompt (see Figure 10-32) to go to the statements. Your screen will now look like Figure 10-34. (**Note:** If no results are showing, change the *Date Range* to "All Dates.")

Courtesy of Harris CareTracker PM and EMR

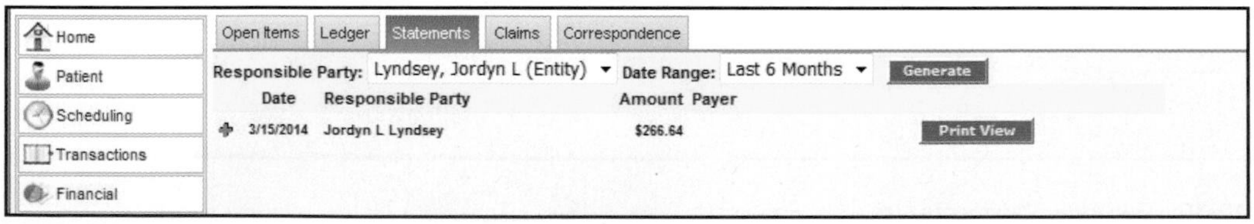

Figure 10-34 Statements Display

6. Click on the *Print View* button. The patient's statement will display in a new window (Figure 10-35).
7. Print the statement by right-clicking on the screen and selecting *Print* from the drop-down menu.

| Napa Valley Family Associates | ACCOUNT # | 38803-42539489 | STATEMENT DATE | 3/15/2014 |
| | LAST PAYMENT | $14.61 | STATEMENT TOTAL | $266.64 |

Statement - Page 1

DATE OF SERVICE	PATIENT	DESCRIPTION OF SERVICES	PROCEDURE CODE	SERVICING PROVIDER	AMOUNT	PATIENT AMT DUE
3/10/2014	Lyndsey, Jordyn L (42539489)	Office Outpatient New 30 Minutes	99203	Raman, Amir	-$86.55	$21.64
		Per Your Insurance Company, Your Copay Has Not Been Paid In Full. The Balance Is Your Responsibility. Thank You.				
		Transaction 03/10/2014, Adjustment - Contractual			-$82.81	
		Transaction 03/10/2014, Charges			$191.00	
3/13/2014	Lyndsey, Jordyn L (42539489)	Office Outpatient Visit 25 Minutes	99214	Raman, Amir	$245.00	$245.00
		See Billing Note				
		Transaction 03/13/2014, Non-Covered charge			$0.00	

MAKE CHECKS PAYABLE TO: Napa Valley Family Associates	**PLEASE PAY THIS AMOUNT**	$266.64

TO ENSURE PROPER CREDIT, PLEASE DETACH AND RETURN BOTTOM PORTION WITH YOUR PAYMENT

Napa Valley Family Associates
101 Vine Street
Napa, CA 94558

707- 555-1212 Ext:

	ACCOUNT #	38803-42539489	STATEMENT DATE	3/15/2014
	AMOUNT ENCLOSED $		STATEMENT TOTAL	$266.64

☐ CHECK BOX AND ENTER ADDRESS OR INSURANCE CORRECTIONS ON THE REVERSE SIDE

☐ IF PAYING BY CREDIT CARD, FILL OUT THE INFORMATION ON THE REVERSE SIDE

ADDRESSEE:
JORDYN L LYNDSEY
PO BOX 84557
FAIRFIELD, CA 94533

REMIT TO:
NAPA VALLEY FAMILY ASSOCIATES
101 VINE STREET
NAPA, CA 94558

IF ANY OF THE INFORMATION HAS BEEN CHANGED SINCE YOUR LAST STATEMENT, PLEASE INDICATE...

ABOUT YOU:	ABOUT YOUR INSURANCE:
YOUR NAME (Last, First, Middle Initial)	YOUR PRIMARY INSURANCE COMPANY'S NAME EFFECTIVE DATE
ADDRESS	PRIMARY INSURANCE COMPANY'S ADDRESS PHONE
CITY STATE ZIP	CITY STATE ZIP
TELEPHONE MARITAL STATUS ☐ Single ☐ Divorced	POLICYHOLDER'S ID NUMBER GROUP PLAN NUMBER
( ) ☐ Married ☐ Widowed	
EMPLOYER'S NAME TELEPHONE ( )	YOUR SECONDARY INSURANCE COMPANY'S NAME EFFECTIVE DATE
EMPLOYER'S ADDRESS CITY STATE ZIP	SECONDARY INSURANCE COMPANY'S ADDRESS PHONE
IF PAYING BY CREDIT CARD, FILL OUT BELOW	CITY STATE ZIP
☐ AMERICAN EXPRESS ☐ MASTERCARD ☐ VISA	POLICYHOLDER'S ID NUMBER GROUP PLAN NUMBER
CARD NUMBER	
CHARGE THIS AMOUNT EXPIRATION DATE	
SIGNATURE CARDHOLDER NAME	

Courtesy of Harris CareTracker PM and EMR

Figure 10-35   Patient Statement

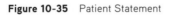
Print the patient statement, label it "Activity 10-5," and place it in your assignment folder.

When statements have been generated, you can use several locations in Harris CareTracker PM to print them either by batch or individually, as outlined in Table 10-6.

TABLE 10-6 Print Statements, Bulk and Individual

To Print Statements in Bulk	Go to the *Home* module > *Dashboard* tab > *Billing* section > *Statements/Unprinted Statements* link. Go to the *Reports* module > *Reports* tab > *Financial Reports* section > *All Statements* link.
To Print Individual Statements	Go to the *Financial* module > *Statements* tab. Go to the *Name Bar* > *Letters* button. (**Note:** This option is only applicable if your practice's statements are set up as a form letter.)

Courtesy of Harris CareTracker PM and EMR

Reprinting Statements

The *Statements* application in the *Financial* module (Figure 10-36) allows you to view and reprint statements that have been generated for the patient in context. A statement can be reprinted by clicking on the *Print View* button next to the appropriate statement line. When *Print View* is clicked, the patient's statement displays in a new window, and by right-clicking on top of it the statement can be printed.

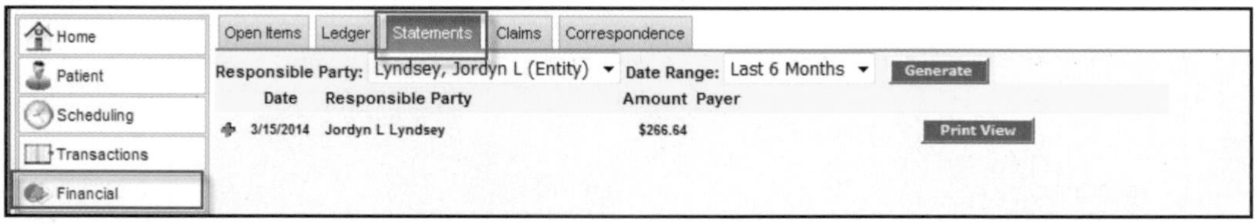

Figure 10-36 Statements Application in Financial Module
Courtesy of Harris CareTracker PM and EMR

ACTIVITY 10-6: View and Reprint a Patient Statement Using the Financial Module

1. Pull patient Jordyn Lyndsey into context.
2. Click the *Financial* module. Click *Go*. The *Open Items* for the patient display (Figure 10-37). (**Note:** You can also access the open items by clicking the *OI* icon on the *Name Bar*.)

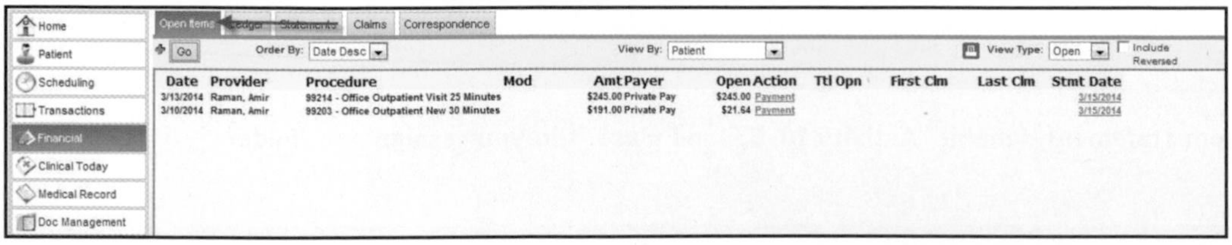

Figure 10-37 Financial Open Items

Courtesy of Harris CareTracker PM and EMR

3. Click the *Statements* tab. Harris CareTracker PM opens the *Statements* application (see Figure 10-36).

   a. The *Responsible Party* list defaults to the responsible party set in the patient's demographic. Leave as is. (**Note:** You can select a different responsible party or "(All)" responsible parties, if applicable.)

   b. The *Date Range* list defaults to "Last 6 Months." Use the drop-down next to *Date Range* and select "All Dates."

4. Click *Generate*. Harris CareTracker PM generates a list of the patient's statements and displays a processing message in the lower frame of the screen.

5. Select the *Click Here* link in blue. The application displays the list of statements.

Tip Box

Click on a statement line to view the statement details in the lower frame of the screen. Click the *plus sign* [+] next to a statement line to view the procedure details included in the statement. Click on a procedure line to view the complete procedure details (Figure 10-38).

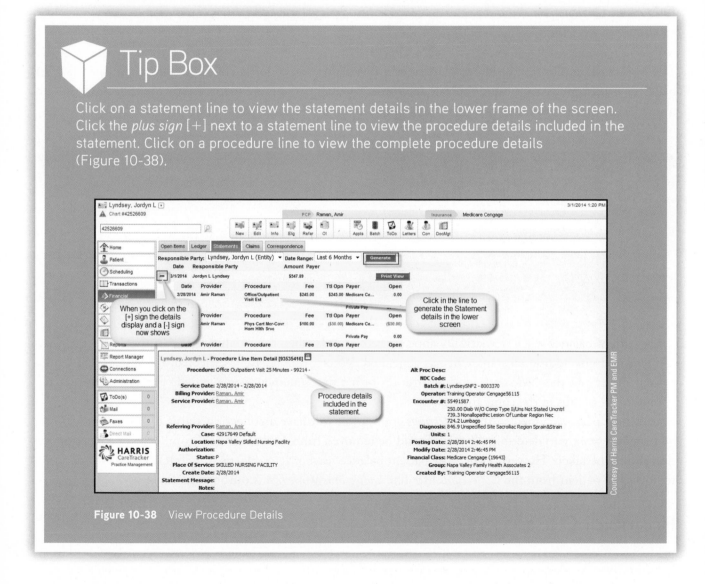

Figure 10-38   View Procedure Details

6. Click *Print View* next to the statement you want to print. Select the most recent statement. The application displays the statement in a new window. **Note:** It may take a few moments to display.

7. Right-click on the statement and then select *Print* from the shortcut menu.

Print the statement, label it "Activity 10-6," and place it in your assignment folder.

8. Close the statement window when the statement has printed.

PATIENT COLLECTIONS

Learning Objective 4: Describe and identify components of the patient collection process.

The *Collections* application in Harris CareTracker PM allows you to focus collection efforts on patients with balances at least 30 days overdue. You can determine whether patients are identified by the collections system immediately or after their balance is 30, 60, 90, or 120 days overdue.

Critical Thinking

Identify ways a medical practice can reduce the incidence of patient accounts going into collection status. How would a Practice Management/EMR program help facilitate this?

A patient balance will automatically appear in collections when the balance ages past the days set in *Days Overdue* and one additional statement has generated. When "Immediate" is selected, the system will send a patient directly to the *Collections* module after his or her first statement is generated. The collections setting applies to all groups in the company.

All new patients added to the *Collections* application will have a collection status of "New" and should be reviewed weekly to determine if they should be removed from *Collections* or if some type of collection action should be taken. However, when the patient balance reaches zero, Harris CareTracker PM automatically removes the patient from the *Collections* list. The *Collections Work List* is outlined in Table 10-7.

Financial Classes

While actively working on collecting **private pay** balances, you need to assign the private pay balances to a financial class. Private pay refers to patients without insurance or the balance due after insurance has adjusted the claim and paid any amount due under contract. In Harris CareTracker PM the financial class is linked to the insurance plan. While working collection balances, many practices prefer to move the private pay balances out of the *Patient* financial class and into another financial class to differentiate these monies. If you would like to move the patient's balance to a different financial class for reporting purposes, you will have several options. There are two financial classes that private pay balances can be transferred to: *collections pending* and *collections actual*, outlined in Table 10-7.

TABLE 10-7   Financial Classes (Collections Work List)

Name	Description
Collections Pending	Balances are typically first transferred to an insurance plan that is linked to the *Collections Pending* financial class to indicate that these are the patient balances that you are actively working. The *Collections Pending* financial class is linked to the "Collect Pend Statement" and "Collect Pend No Statement" insurance plans.
Collections Actual	Once you have exhausted your own collection activity on an account and you would like to transfer the patient's balance, you can either transfer the balance to the insurance plan "Collections Actual" or the specific collection agency your office works with. These balances would then be found in the *A/R* link on your *Dashboard* under the financial class "Collections Actual." All balance transfers can be done in bulk from the *Collections System*. In addition to transferring the patient's balance, the patient's collection status should also be changed to the corresponding status. The *Collections Actual* financial class is linking to the *Collections Actual* insurance plan and any collection agency insurance plans.

Courtesy of Harris CareTracker PM and EMR

Tip Box

To verify whether the patient qualifies for *Collections*, click the *Statements* tab in the *Financial* module. Click on the most recent statement and review the aging in the *Statement Detail* (Figure 10-39). If the aging has not met the *Days Overdue* setting, the patient will not appear in *Collections*.

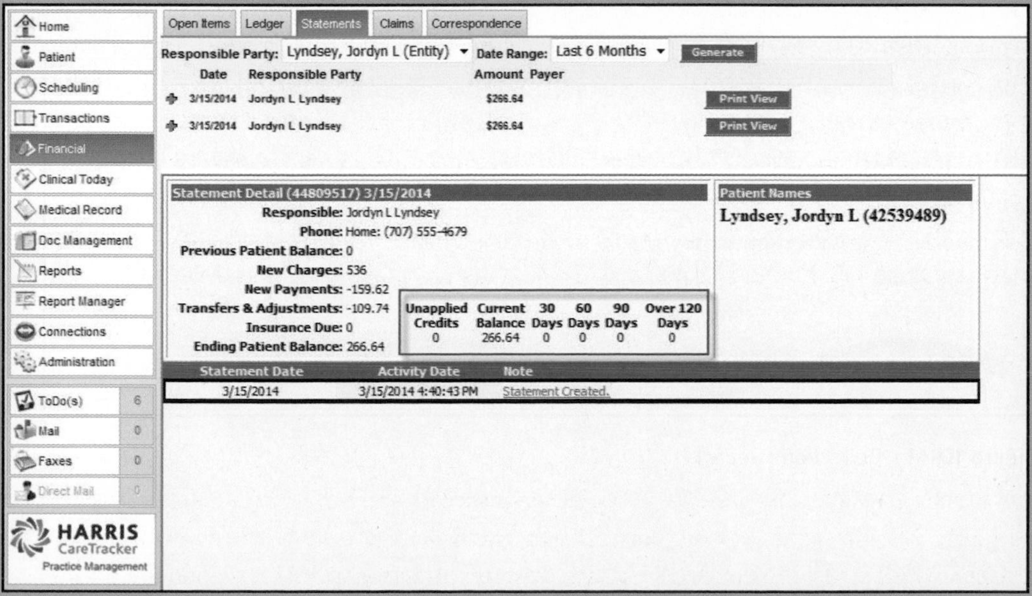

Figure 10-39   Statement Detail - Aging

In addition to managing the balance transfers, when you send a patient's balance to a collection agency, you should change his or her patient status to *Collections*. This can be done in the *Demographics* application by selecting "Collections" from the *Category* drop-down list (Figure 10-40). This status will always display next to the patient's name in Harris CareTracker PM (Figure 10-41) so all staff will know that this patient has been transferred to the collection agency. Table 10-8 describes the *Collections Reports* and *Last Activity Date* details.

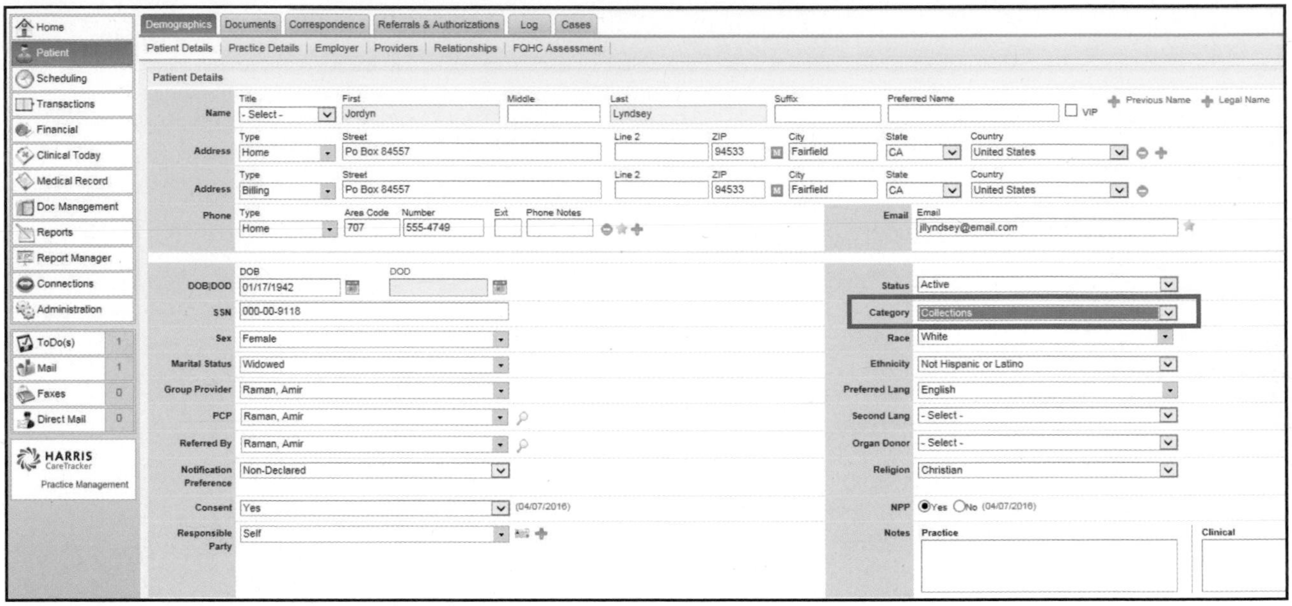

Courtesy of Harris CareTracker PM and EMR

Figure 10-40 Patient Category - Collections

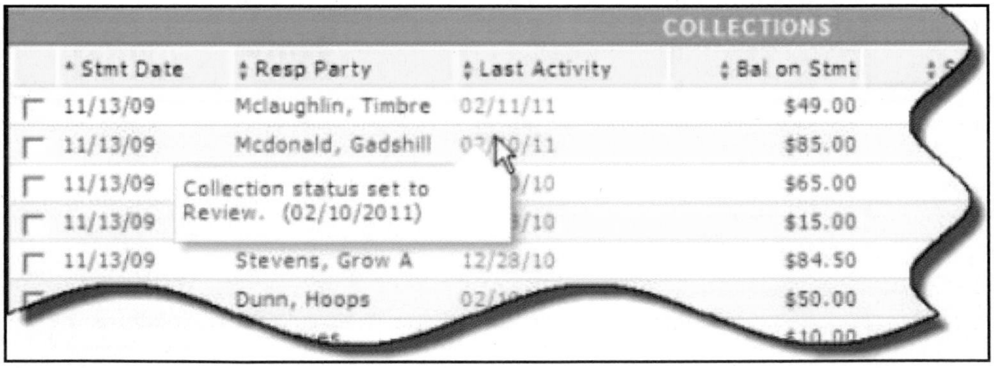

Courtesy of Harris CareTracker PM and EMR

Figure 10-41 Collections Report

TABLE 10-8	Collections
Collections Reports	There are *Collections* reports available in the *Reports* module > *Financial Reports* section > *Other Reports* link that can be used to identify balances to be transferred to your collection agency.
Last Activity Date	You can sort the collections list by last activity date by clicking the column heading. Harris CareTracker PM displays the last activity performed when the cursor is placed over the last activity date.

Courtesy of Harris CareTracker PM and EMR

COLLECTION STATUS

Learning Objective 5: Review collection status and transfer private pay balances.

The *Collections* application is accessed from the *Home* module > *Dashboard* tab > *Billing* section > *Collections* link (Figure 10-42). There are seven collection statuses in Harris CareTracker PM: New, Open Collections, Review, Collections Actual, Collections Pending, Collections Pending – NS, and Hold (Figure 10-43).

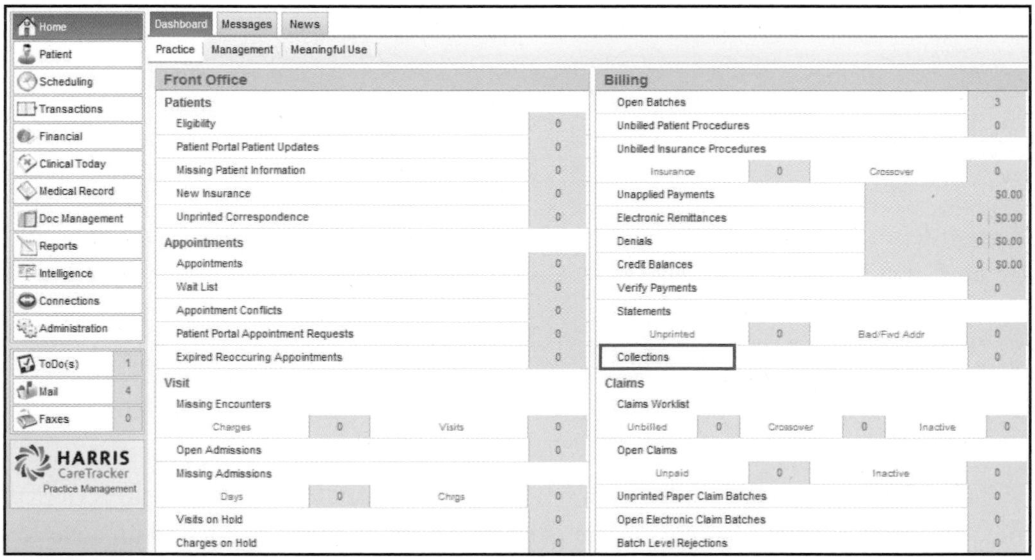

Figure 10-42   Collections Link

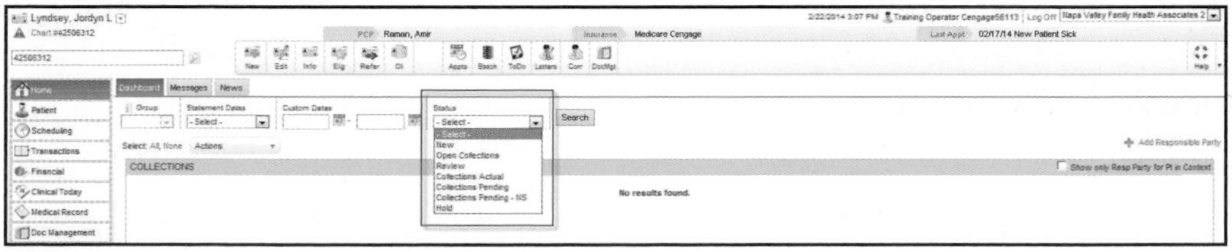

Courtesy of Harris CareTracker PM and EMR

Figure 10-43   Seven Collection Statuses

Courtesy of Harris CareTracker PM and EMR

New Status

After a patient has reached the set overdue period for your practice (i.e., immediate, 30, 60, 90, or 120 days overdue) they are automatically identified by the *Collections System* and assigned the status of "New." Patients and their balances with a status of "New" should be reviewed on a weekly basis to determine what action should be taken on the account and what collection status the patient should be assigned.

When a patient has been in the "New" status for more than six weeks, the system assumes that the item is not part of the collection process and is not included in the value displayed on the *Dashboard*. However, these collection items will continue to reside under the "New" status until the balance is paid off and removed from *Collections*.

Tip Box

If a patient in the "New" status is removed from *Collections* and he or she continues to have a patient balance that is 30, 60, 90, or 120 days overdue, the patient will be flagged again for the *Collections System* when a statement is generated and will be placed in the "New" status.

Open Collection Status

When a collection letter is sent to a patient, change his or her status to "Open Collections." A patient in "Open Collections" will continue to receive statements until his or her balance is transferred to "Collections Pending NS" or "Collections Actual."

Review Status

The "Review" status indicates that the physician or another office staff member should review the patient's account before any action is taken. Patients in the "Review" status should be reviewed on a weekly basis.

After "Review" patients have been reviewed, their status should be changed. Typically, the status would be changed to "Open" if an action is going to be taken (such as sending the patient a collection letter), or it should be changed to "Remove from Collections" if the patient needs to be removed from the *Collections System*.

Collections Actual Status

Any patient whose balance has been sent to a collection agency should be flagged with the "Collections Actual" status. These patients typically have been sent numerous collection letters but never made a payment or contacted the billing department/staff. When a patient is assigned the status of "Collections Actual," the patient's outstanding balance should be transferred to the "Collections Actual" insurance plan or to the actual collection agency your practice utilizes.

Collections Pending Status

The status "Collections Pending" identifies all patients with outstanding private pay balances transferred to the *Collect Pend Statement* insurance plan. Typically, patients are assigned to this status when you are still actively working on collecting owed money. Harris CareTracker PM continues to generate statements for patients in this status. When a patient is assigned the status of "Collections Pending," the patient's private pay outstanding balance should also be transferred to the *Collect Pend Statement* insurance plan.

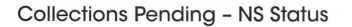

Tip Box

You must have a batch open to transfer any balances from private pay to *Collect Pend Statement*.

Collections Pending – NS Status

The status "Collections Pending – NS" is assigned to all patients whose outstanding private pay balances have been transferred to the *Collect Pend No Statement* insurance plan. Typically, patients are assigned to this status in the *Collections System* and their balances transferred to this insurance plan to identify patients who are pending collections but from whom you are still actively working on collecting owed money. Harris CareTracker PM does not generate statements for patients in this status.

Hold Status

The "Hold" status is assigned to patients who you want identified by the *Collections System* but for whom you do not want to take action. For example, a patient may make a small payment after receiving his or her first collection letter. Instead of sending the patient a second collection letter alerting the patient of the remaining overdue balance, you can flag the patient as "Hold" to see if he or she makes additional payments. Patients who have been assigned a status of "Hold" should be reviewed weekly to determine if additional collection activity is required on their account or if they should be removed from the *Collections System*.

Transfer Private Pay Balances

Transferring private pay balances coincides with changing a patient's collection status. For example, if you want to transfer a balance from the financial class "Private Pay" to the financial class "Collections Pending," you must change the patient's status from "Open Collections" to "Collections Pending." Both a status change and a balance transfer can happen at one time from the *Collections* application.

After private balances have been transferred to either the *Collections Actual* plan or a collection agency, some practices choose to adjust off these outstanding balances using the code "Adjustment-Collections." Adjusting off outstanding private pay balances must be performed from the *Open Items* application. You can use the list of patients with a status of "Collections Actual" in the *Collections System* as a work list to pull each patient into context and then click on the *OI* 🗋 icon on the *Name Bar* to complete the needed financial transaction.

Moving Patients to Collections

Harris CareTracker PM automatically moves patients into *Collections* when their overdue balance reaches the aging level assigned in the group settings and automatically removes patients from *Collections* when their overdue balance is paid. Operators can also move patients in and out of *Collections* manually. In *Open Items*, you can add a patient to *Collections* by clicking the *Add Responsible Party* link in the *Collections* work area or by transferring a balance to *Collections*.

Patients manually added to *Collections* are flagged with an asterisk (*) next to their name in the work area. Patients manually added to *Collections* must be removed from *Collections* manually as well. When manually adding a patient to *Collections*, Harris CareTracker PM pulls the patient into context and filters the *Collections* list to show the responsible party for that patient.

ACTIVITY 10-7: Transfer a Balance

1. Go to the *Home* module > *Dashboard* tab > *Billing* section > *Collections* link. Harris CareTracker PM displays a list of collection statuses and the number of patients in each status.

2. If there is no patient listed, click the *Add Responsible Party* link in the upper right corner of the screen. In the *Add Manual Collection* window click the *Search* icon and enter the name of the patient you are searching for (Jordyn Lyndsey). Click on the patient name in the *Results* window. The patient name now populates in the *Add Manual Collection* window. Click *Save*.

3. Click the *Edit* icon next to the balance you want to transfer to a new financial class. Harris CareTracker PM displays the *Edit* window (Figure 10-44).

   a. *Insurance*: Leave blank

   b. *Overdue*: Leave blank

   c. *Letter*: Leave blank

   d. *Change Status*: Select "Open Collections"

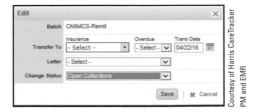

Figure 10-44 Edit Collections Dialog Box

4. Click *Save*. In the *Updates Processed* window that appears, click *Close*. Harris CareTracker PM updates the patient's status in the *Collections* application, transfers the outstanding balance to the selected financial class, and adds the selected "Transfer To" financial class to the patient's *Demographics* record.

Tip Box

To transfer multiple balances to a new financial class, select the checkbox next to each balance you want to transfer and then click *Actions > Edit* (Figure 10-45).

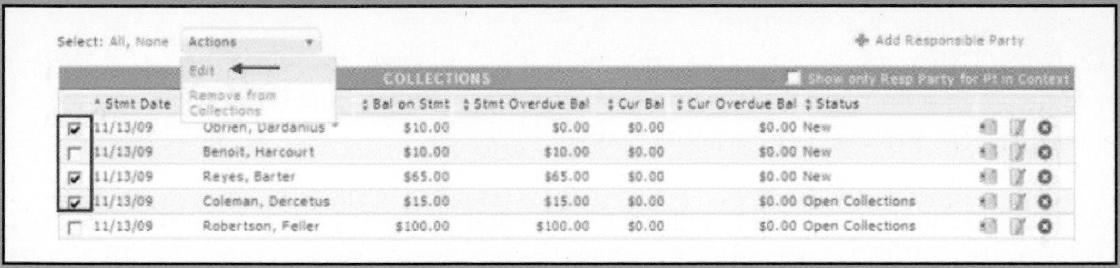

Figure 10-45   Select Multiple Patients for Collections

Tip Box

You can add the *Collections Pending Statement, Collections Pending No Statement, Collections Actual* financial classes, or your collection agency name to the *Insurance Plans* "quick pick" list in the *Quick Picks* application in the *Administration* module.

Print the Balance Transfer screen, label it "Activity 10-7," and place it in your assignment folder.

COLLECTION ACTIONS

Learning Objective 6: Perform collection actions.

There are four collection actions in Harris CareTracker PM: *Transfer, Remove from Collections, Group Collections,* and *Global Collection Letters.*

Transfer is used when a patient's private pay balance needs to be transferred to a different insurance plan/financial class. Possible insurance plans you would be transferring to a private pay balance are:

a. Collect Pend Statement
b. Collect Pend No Statement
c. Collections Actual
d. Your practice's collection agency

FYI

To remove a balance from *Collections*:

1. Go to the *Home* module > *Dashboard* tab > *Billing* section > *Collections* link. Harris Care-Tracker PM displays a list of collection statuses and the number of patients in each status.
2. To remove an individual balance:
   a. Click the *Delete* icon next to the statement line you want to delete. Harris CareTracker PM displays a confirmation dialog box. Click *OK*. Harris CareTracker PM removes the balance from the *Collections* application.
3. To remove multiple balances:
   a. Select the checkbox next to each statement line you want to remove from *Collections* (Figure 10-46).
   b. Click *Actions* > *Remove from Collections* at the top of the page. The application displays a confirmation dialog box.
   c. Click *OK*. Harris CareTracker PM removes the balance from the *Collections* application.

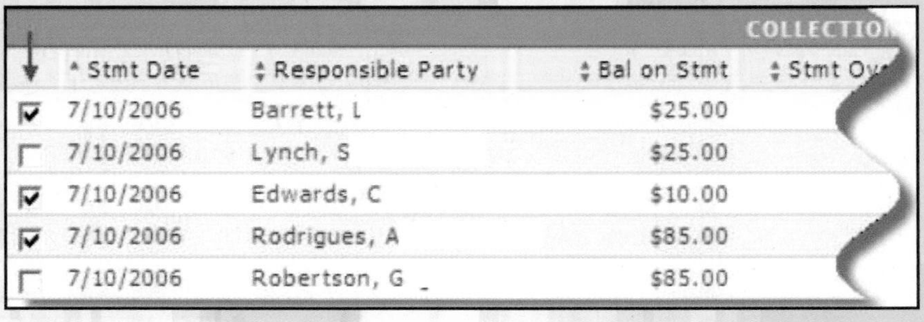

	▲ Stmt Date	⇕ Responsible Party	⇕ Bal on Stmt	⇕ Stmt Ov
☑	7/10/2006	Barrett, L	$25.00	
☐	7/10/2006	Lynch, S	$25.00	
☑	7/10/2006	Edwards, C	$10.00	
☑	7/10/2006	Rodrigues, A	$85.00	
☐	7/10/2006	Robertson, G _	$85.00	

Figure 10-46 Remove Multiple Collections

Each insurance plan is linked to a financial class. There are two collection financial classes: *Collections Actual* and *Collections Pending*. After the private pay balance is transferred to the appropriate insurance plan, the money will automatically be moved to the appropriate financial class. A bulk transfer to one insurance plan can be done for multiple patients at one time from the *Collections* application.

The *Remove from Collections* action removes the patient from the *Collections System*. The patient will be put back into the *Collections System* if any portion of his or her private pay balance ages beyond the number of days set in the group's collections flag, when statements are generated again for the patient.

Tip Box

A patient is automatically removed from *Collections* when his or her private pay or collection balances are paid in full or adjusted off, regardless of the patient's collection status.

Group Collection Letters, which are specific to your practice, are built in the *Letter Editor* application in the *Administration* module. After creating a custom collection letter, you must add the letter to your *Form Letters Quick Picks* via the *Quick Picks* application in the *Administration* module. This will allow you to select the letter in the *Collections* module.

The *Global Collection Letters* application contains the following letters, which are available to all users in Harris CareTracker PM.

- "Collections 1": Explains that the account is overdue and lists the overdue balance (Figure 10-47).

IF PAYING BY CREDIT CARD FILL OUT BELOW

CareTracker Support
70 LITTLE ROYAL DRIVE
xxxxxxxxxxxxxx
Providence, RI 02940

(401) 274-0103
support@lighthousemd.com

CHECK CARD USING FOR PAYMENT

MASTERCARD AMERICAN EXPRESS DISCOVER

CARD NUMBER		AMOUNT
SIGNATURE		EXP. DATE
DATE February 5, 2008	AMOUNT DUE $.00	ACCT# 9163-2877327
	SHOW AMOUNT PAID HERE $	

ADDRESSEE:

Derek Brown
1oo Broad St
Apt4
Providence, RI 02906

REMIT TO:

CareTracker Support
70 LITTLE ROYAL DRIVE
xxxxxxxxxxxxxx
Providence, RI 02940

Please check box if address is incorrect or insurance information has changed, and indicate change(s) on reverse side.

PLEASE DETACH AND RETURN TOP PORTION WITH YOUR PAYMENT

To: Derek Brown

From: CareTracker Support - Collections Division

RE: Overdue balance

Please be advised this letter serves as an official notice to the overdue balance of $35.00 on your account.

If you do not send payment in full or contact this office within 10 working days, we will be left with no choice but to continue with our collection policy. Our collection policy may include sending your balance to a collection agency or pursuing legal action. Should this be necessary, it may have a negative impact on your credit history.

If you feel you have received this letter in error or if you have any questions regarding your balance, please call our office immediately. Your anticipated cooperation in this matter is appreciated.

Sincerely,

Billing Office
CareTracker Support

Courtesy of Harris CareTracker PM and EMR

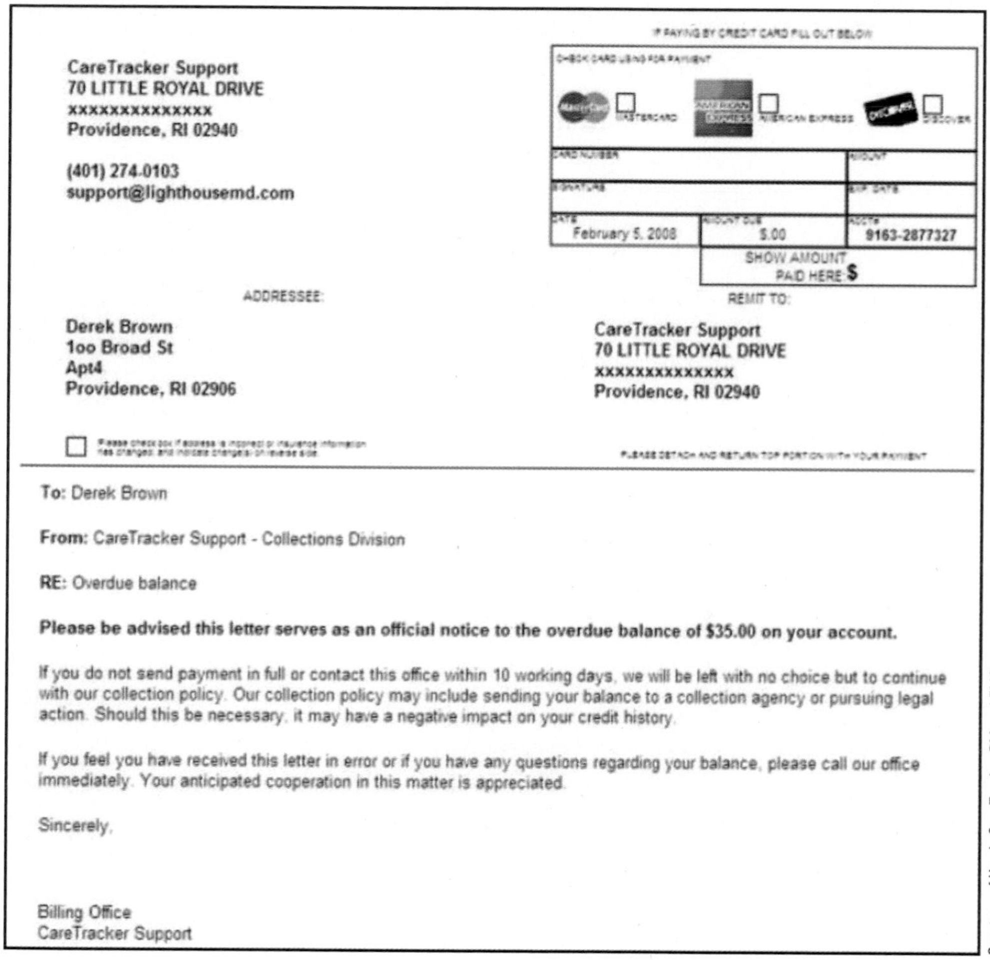

Figure 10-47 Collections 1 Letter

- "Past Due": Explains that the overdue balance or a portion of the balance is more than 60 days past due (Figure 10-48).
- "Delinquent": Explains that the overdue balance or a portion of the balance is more than 90 days past due (Figure 10-49).
- "Final Notice": Tells the patient that her overdue balance or a portion of her balance is more than 120 days past due. This is the final written notice the patient will receive, and, if payment is not received, the account will be sent to *Collections* (Figure 10-50).
- "75 Collection": States that if the overdue balance is not paid in full, the billing office will continue with its collection policy, which may include using a collection agency (Figure 10-51).

PAST DUE

Dear Sarah Seri

Our records show that a portion of your account balance is now more than 60 days past due.

Please remit payment immediately.

If you made a payment on this account within the last 10 days, please accept our apology and disregard this notice. If you have any questions, comments or if you need to make special arrangements for payment of this balance, please feel free to contact me at (508)777-0202.

Thank you,

Account Manager

Mayflower Cardiology Inc. 2 Mayflower Way Plymouth, MA 02360	Date: June 23, 2006	Account Number: 3670824
	Total Patient Amount Overdue: $20.00	Show Amount Paid Here: $

Figure 10-48 Past Due Letter

DELINQUENT

Dear Sarah Seri

Our records indicate that a portion of your account balance is now more than 90 days past due.

Please remit payment immediately.

If you made a payment on this account within the last 10 days, please accept our apology and disregard this notice. If you have any questions or comments, or if you need to make special arrangements for payment of this balance, please feel free to contact me at (508)777-0202.

Thank you,

Account Manager

Mayflower Cardiology Inc. 2 Mayflower Way Plymouth, MA 02360	Date: June 23, 2006	Account Number: 3670824
	Total Patient Amount Overdue: $20.00	Show Amount Paid Here: $

Figure 10-49 Delinquent Letter

FINAL NOTICE

Dear Sarah Seri

Our records indicate that a portion of your account balance is more than 120 days past due.

Please remit payment immediately.

This is your final written notice of payment due. Despite the difficulty we have in taking this kind of action our policy dictates that unless payment is received within 10 days of the postmark of this letter, this account may be turned over to a Collection Agency.

If you have made a payment on this account within the last 10 days, please accept our apology and disregard this notice. If you have any questions or comments, or if you need to make special arrangements for payment of this balance, please feel free to contact me at (508)777-0202.

Thank you,

Account Manager

Mayflower Cardiology Inc.	Date:	Account Number:
2 Mayflower Way	June 23, 2006	3670824
		Show Amount

Figure 10-50   Final Notice Letter

Mayflower Cardiology Inc.
2 Mayflower Way
Plymouth, MA 02360
(508)777-0202

June 23, 2006   **Account Number:** 3670824
                                                                          Overdue Balance: $20.00
                                                                          Balance Due: $20.00

Sarah Seri
5 Cook St.
Portsmouth, RI 02871

To: Sarah Seri
From: Mayflower Cardiology Inc. - Collections Division

Please be advised this letter serves as an official notice to the overdue balance on your account.

If you do not send payment in full or contact this office within 10 working days, we will be left with no choice but to continue with our collection policy. Our collection policy may include sending your balance to a collection agency or pursuing legal action. Should this be necessary, it may have a negative impact on your credit history.

If you feel you have received this letter in error or if you have any questions regarding your balance, please call our office immediately. Your anticipated cooperation in this matter is appreciated.

Sincerely,

Figure 10-51   75 Collections Letter

- "Collection Payment Plan": Informs the patient that she can set up a weekly or monthly payment plan to pay off the overdue balance. On a "Collection Payment Plan" letter, the patient can also indicate if she has insurance that covered the services for which she has an overdue balance. When a patient indicates that he or she has insurance to cover the services, the patient must also complete the insurance section on the back of a statement (Figure 10-52).

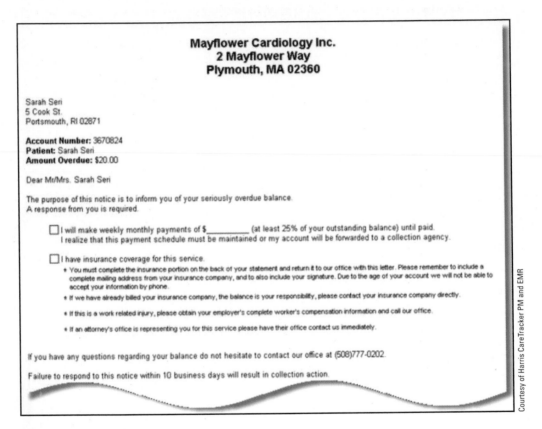

Figure 10-52 Collection Payment Plan Letter

You can also create custom collection letters in the *Letter Editor* application in the *Administration* module.

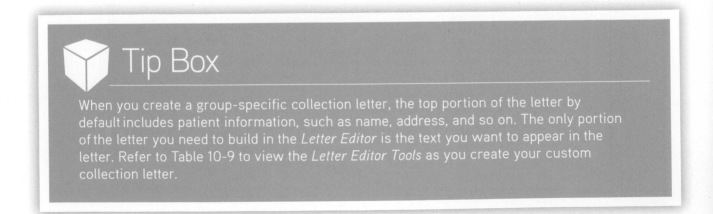

Tip Box

When you create a group-specific collection letter, the top portion of the letter by default includes patient information, such as name, address, and so on. The only portion of the letter you need to build in the *Letter Editor* is the text you want to appear in the letter. Refer to Table 10-9 to view the *Letter Editor Tools* as you create your custom collection letter.

COLLECTION LETTERS

Learning Objective 7: Create collection letters.

Group-specific collection letters are built in the *Practice Letter Editor* in the *Administration* module. After creating a custom collection letter, you must add the letter to your *Form Letters Quick Picks* via the *Quick Picks* application in the *Administration* module. This will allow you to access the letter in the *Collections* module.

ACTIVITY 10-8: Create a Custom Collection Letter

1. Go to the *Administration* module > *Practice* tab > *Forms and Letters* section > *Practice Letter Editor* link (Figure 10-53).

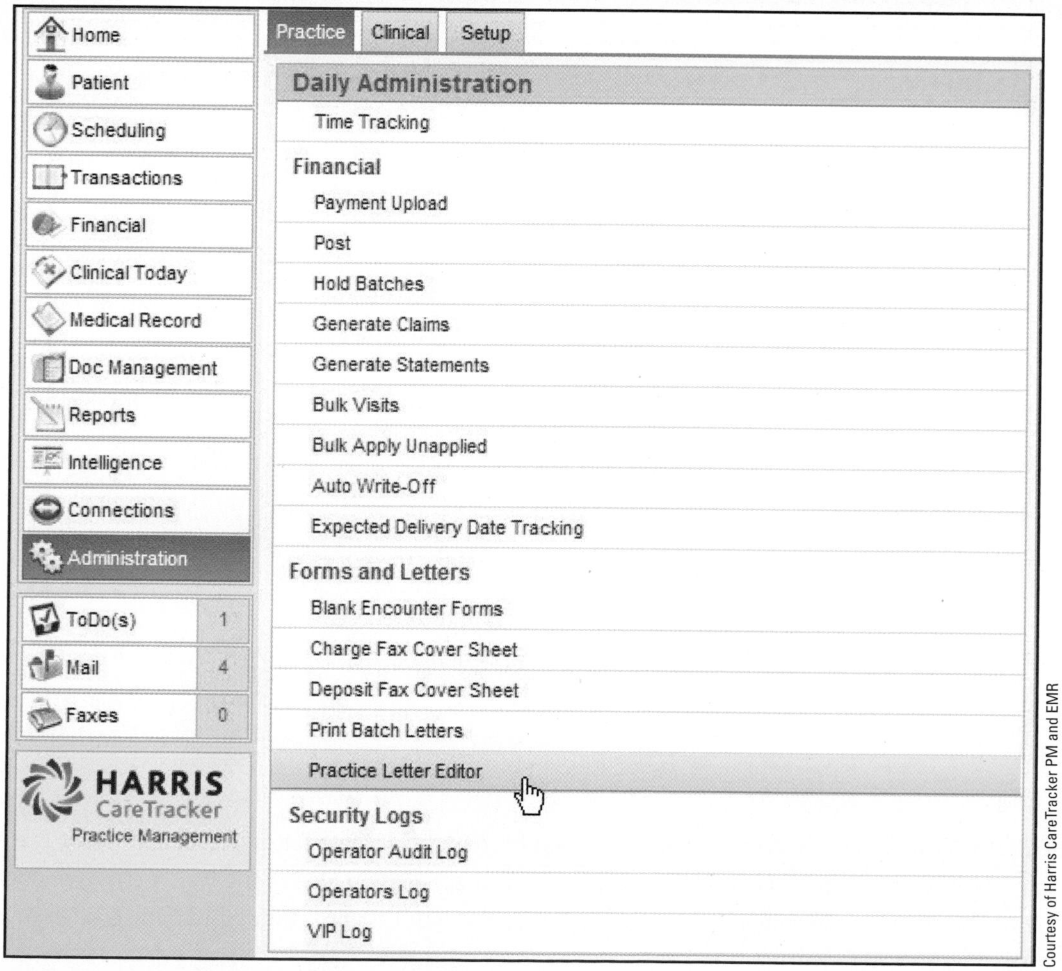

Figure 10-53 Practice Letter Editor Link

2. From the *Letters* drop-down list, select "Create New Letter" (Figure 10-54). The application displays the *New Letter* window (Figure 10-55).

3. Enter a descriptive name for the form letter in the *Letter Name* field. Enter "Late Cancel Fee Letter."

Courtesy of Harris CareTracker PM and EMR

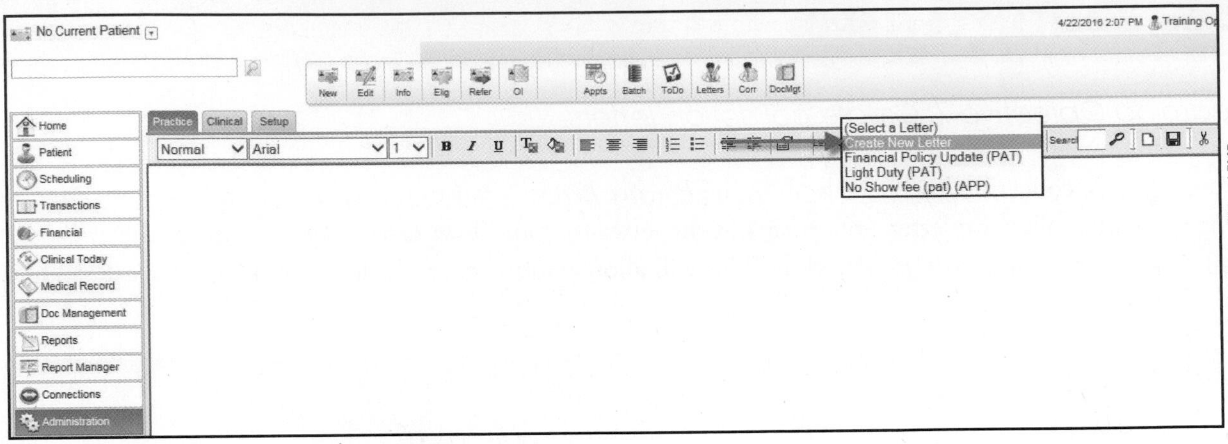

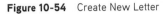

Figure 10-54 Create New Letter

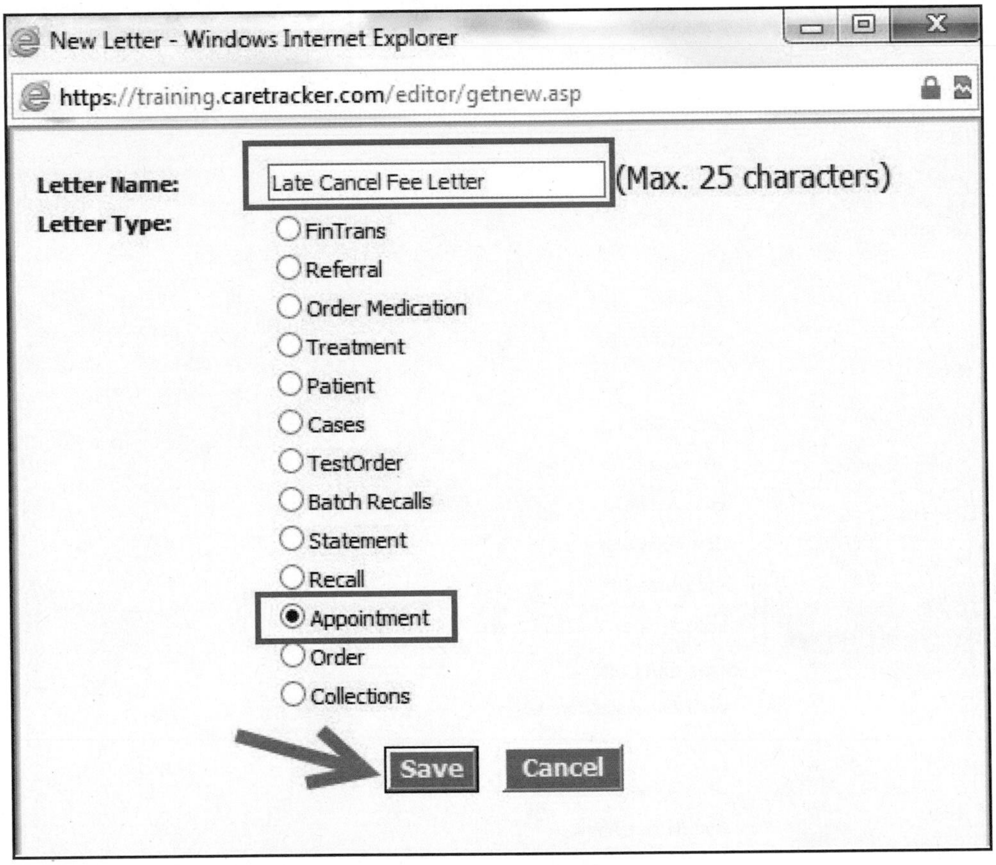

Courtesy of Harris CareTracker PM and EMR

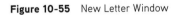

Figure 10-55 New Letter Window

4. In the *Letter Type* field, select the radio button next to the type of form letter you are creating (select "Appointment"), and then click *Save* (Figure 10-55). The application closes the *New Letter* window and pulls the new letter name and type into the *Letters* field (Figure 10-56). **Note:** It may take a few moments for the screen to refresh.

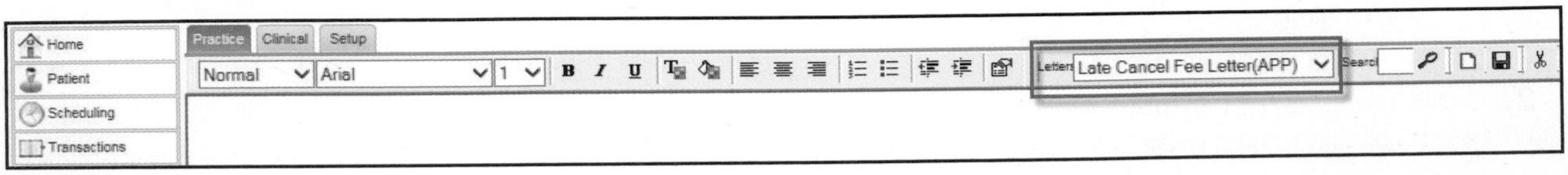

Figure 10-56 Letters Field
Courtesy of Harris CareTracker PM and EMR

5. Enter the text from Figure 10-57 to appear in the form letter and insert data fields where necessary using the *Select Field* {··} icon. Select data fields from the drop-down list in the *Select Field* list (Figure 10-58) to complete your letter. (For example, for the first line of the letter, select "Current Date - Long" from the *Special Fields* section in the *Select Field* list.) Be sure to format the letter as you would like it to appear.

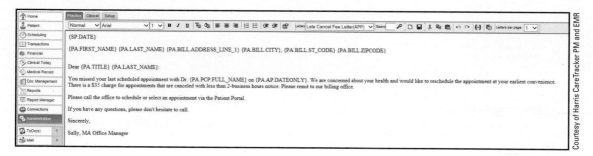

Figure 10-57 Late Cancel Fee Letter

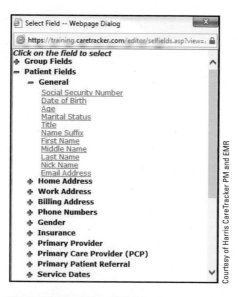

Figure 10-58 Select Field List

Tip Box

The *Letter Editor* is preset to double space when you hit the [Enter] key to enter a new line of text. For single spacing hold the [Shift] key down as you press the [Enter] key.

6. Click the *Save File* 🖫 icon when you are finished with your form letter. (As a best practice, you should click *Save* periodically while building your letter.)

Print the screen that displays the Custom Collection Letter, label it "Activity 10-8," and place it in your assignment folder.

Critical Thinking

Using your experience as a medical assistant, create several custom letters, and cite their purpose. Submit the letters to your instructor for discussion. Add them to your *Quick Picks* (Activity 10-9) upon completion.

1. Custom Collection letter
2. Custom Missed Appointment letter
3. Custom Annual Physical Exam reminder letter

TABLE 10-9 Letter Editor Tools

Tool	Icon	Description
Style	Normal	When you create a new letter, the text style defaults to "Normal" and the text displays as normal. There are also various Heading styles of different sizes that will present the selected text in a bigger, bolder format. A Heading format is typically how company names are displayed in headers of form letters. Other selections in the Style list are "Address" and "Formatted," and these will also change the formatting of the text accordingly.
Font & Font Size	Arial 1	Arial is the default font in *Letter Editor*. Tahoma, Courier New, Times New Roman, and Wingdings are the other available fonts for building a letter. These fonts appear in *Letter Editor* as they would in a Microsoft® Word document.
		Unlike in Microsoft® Word, the font sizes in *Letter Editor* only range from 1 to 7, with 1 being the smallest font and 7 being the largest.
		Note: You must have the small "IDAutomationHC39S" font installed on your computer to utilize the barcode font in the *Letter Editor*.
Bold, Italics, & Underline	**B** *I* U	**B:** Selected text will be **bolded** when this button is clicked.
		I: Selected text will be *italicized* when this button is clicked.
		U: Selected text will be underlined when this button is clicked.
Text Color	T	Allows you to change the color of the selected text.
Background Color		Allows you to highlight text with a background color.
Text Justification	≡ ≡ ≡	Used to justify the text to the left, center, or right.
Numbering	≔	Adds numbering to a list. Number 1 will be assigned to the first line, and when you hit [Enter], 2 will automatically be put on the second line, etc.
Bulleted	≔	Adds bullets to a nonsequential list.
Indenting	⇥ ⇤	Used to adjust the indentation of text in a paragraph. The left arrow decreases the indent. The right arrow increases the indent.

TABLE 10-9   (Continued)

Tool	Icon	Description
Edit Description/ Status		Used to edit the description and status of a form letter already saved in Harris CareTracker PM and EMR. The status indicates whether a form letter is active or inactive. Before clicking on this icon, select the name of the letter you would like to edit or make inactive in the *Letters* field.
Selecting a Letter	Letters: (Select a Letter) ⌄	Form letters already created for your practice will be listed in the *Letters* list. To edit a letter, select the letter from the list, and then edit the letter accordingly. To create a new form letter, select "Create New Letter" from the *Letters* list and begin building your letter.
Search	Search: ___ 🔍	Used to search all global form letters saved in Harris CareTracker PM and EMR. Enter the name of the letter you would like to search for and then click on the magnifying glass.
New File		Creates a new form letter.
Save		Saves a new form letter or saves edits made to an existing form letter.
Cut		Selected text will be deleted from your form letter when this button is clicked.
Copy/Paste		Clicking on the first icon copies selected text. Then by clicking on the clipboard icon, you can paste the copied text into the current or another form letter. **Note:** You cannot copy fields from one letter type and paste them into another letter type. The letter types must be the same. For example, you cannot copy fields from an *Appointment* letter and paste them into a *Recall* letter.
Undo & Redo	↺ ↻	Clicking on the Undo button will undo the last action performed while creating your form letter. Clicking on the Redo button will redo the last action you selected to undo while creating your form letter.
Select Field	{··}	Inserts a data field into the form letter. When your form letter is generated, the data fields pull in the respective data from Harris CareTracker PM and EMR. There are three types of data fields you can insert into a form letter: "Group," "Patient," or "Special." Within each of these categories are specific data fields that you can insert. To insert a field: 1. Place your cursor in the location where you want the data field to appear in the letter and then click the *Select Field* button. Harris CareTracker PM displays the *Select Field* dialog box. 2. Click the plus signs [+] to expand each category. 3. Click on the underlined link to insert the field in the letter. Harris CareTracker PM and EMR adds the data field to the letter in brackets. When a letter is generated for a patient, the patient-specific information will be pulled into the field from the patient's record.
Toggle HTML		Clicking on this button will allow you to toggle between the HTML code for the letter and the text format.
Numbers of Letters	Letters per page: 1 ⌄	When you create a form letter, Harris CareTracker PM and EMR defaults to generate and print one letter per 8½ × 11 inch page. However, you have the option of modifying the system so that more than one letter will be printed on one page.

Adding a Form Letter to Quick Picks

After creating a new form letter, you must add it to your *Quick Picks* to make it available for use in Harris CareTracker PM and EMR.

ACTIVITY 10-9: Add a Form Letter to Quick Picks

1. Go to the *Administration* module 〉 *Setup* tab 〉 *Financial* section 〉 *Quick Picks* link.

2. From the *Screen Type* drop-down list, select "Form Letters" (Figure 10-59).

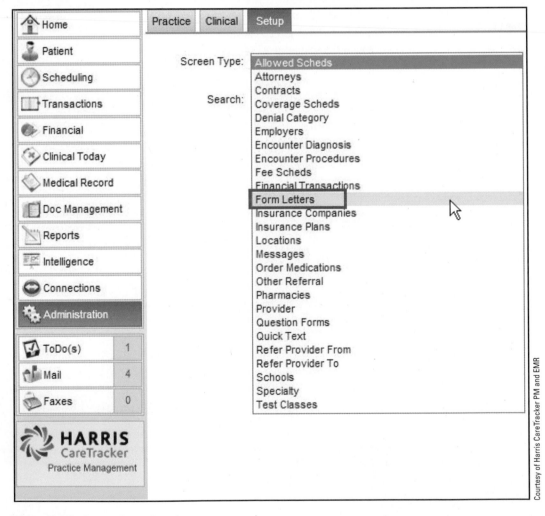

Figure 10-59 Screen Type - Form Letters

3. Enter the name of the new form letter you created in Activity 10-8 in the *Search* field (enter "Late") and then click the *Search* 🔍 icon. The application displays a pop-up of all of the letters that match the search criteria (Figure 10-60).

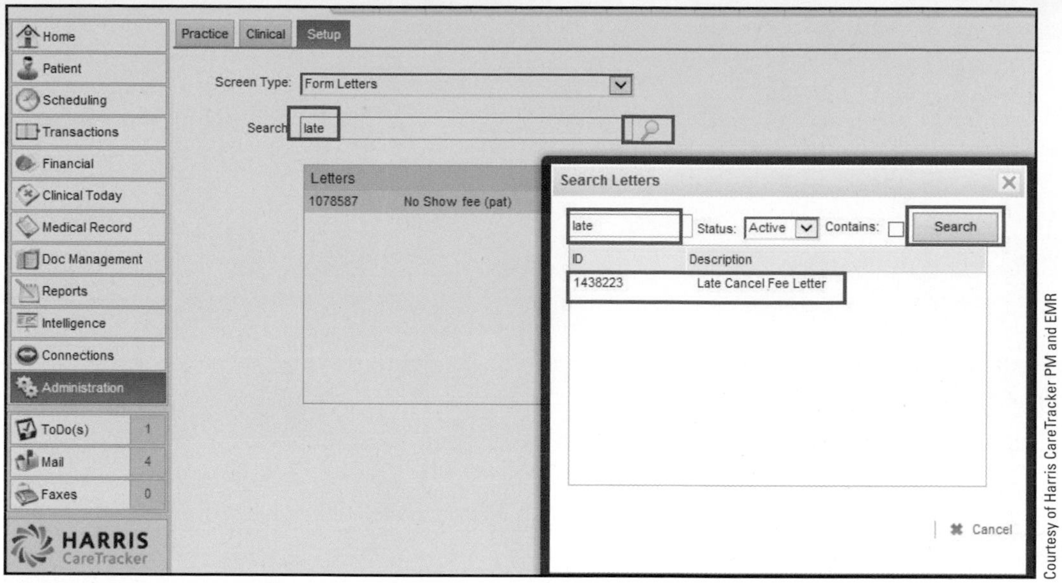

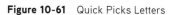

Figure 10-60   Search Letters Window

4. Click on the form letter you want to add to your *Quick Pick* list (select "Late Cancel Fee Letter"). You will receive a pop-up *Success* box stating "Quick Pick information has been updated." Click *Close* on the *Success* box (Figure 10-61).

5. The application adds the letter to the *Quick Pick* list where it will be available to generate for patients (Figure 10-61).

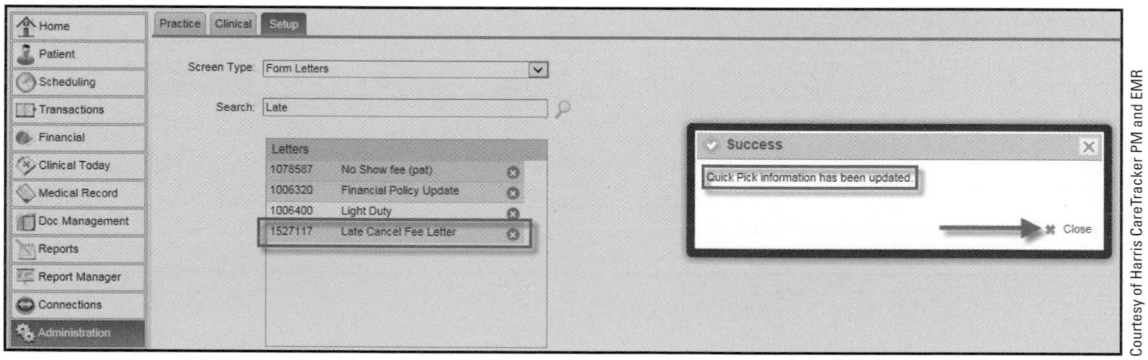

Figure 10-61   Quick Picks Letters

Print the Quick Pick list screen, label it "Activity 10-9," and place it in your assignment folder.

GENERATE COLLECTION LETTERS

Learning Objective 8: Generate collection letters.

To generate collection letters, use one of two options: Harris CareTracker PM and EMR's global collection letters, or build a custom collection letter specific to your practice. After collection letters have been generated they must be printed from the *Print Batch Letters* application in the *Administration* module. Generated collection letters are saved in the patients' record in the *Correspondence* application of the *Financial* module.

Tip Box

You can click the column headings in the work area to sort the *Collections* list by statement date, responsible party, statement balance, overdue balance, current balance, and status.

ACTIVITY 10-10: Generate Collection Letters

1. Go to the *Home* module > *Dashboard* tab > *Billing* section > *Collections* link. Harris CareTracker PM displays a list of collection statements.
2. To search *Collections*, select an option from one or more of the following search fields and then click *Search* (Figures 10-62 and 10-63).
    - *Group* – This field is only available when statements for the company are set up by group.
    - *Statement Dates* – This allows you to view a week's worth of statements.
    - *Custom Dates* – Enter a custom date range in the fields provided.
    - *Status* – Select the status of the collection statements you want to view.

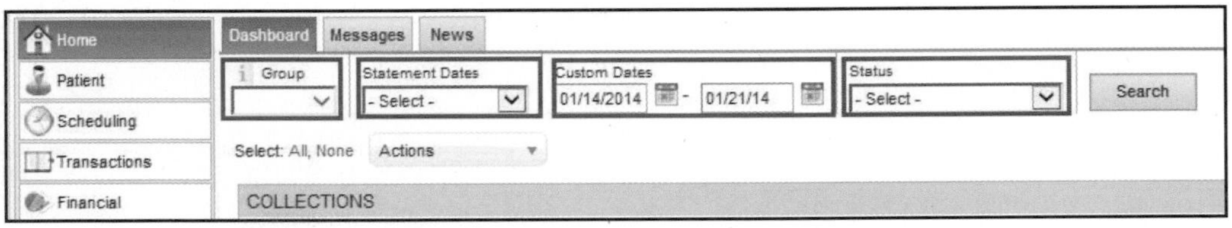

Courtesy of Harris CareTracker PM and EMR

Figure 10-62 Search Collections Fields

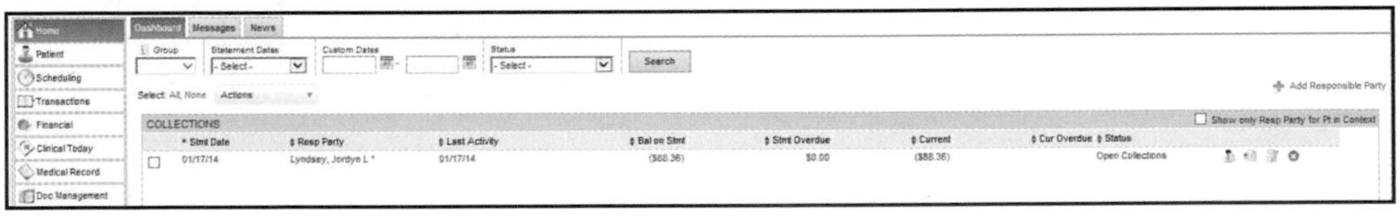

Figure 10-63 Search Collections Results

Courtesy of Harris CareTracker PM and EMR

3. Use the filters at the top of the page to view statements by *Group, Status,* or date range. For this activity, in the drop-down list in the *Status* field, leave as (-Select-).
4. Double-click the name "Jordyn Lyndsey" in the line of the *Responsible Party* column to view the *Statement Details* (Figure 10-64). It is helpful to review this information when determining a status change and/or deciding what action to take on a patient's balance. Close the *Statement Details* dialog box.
5. Click the *Edit* icon next to the statement line for which you want to generate a collection letter (Jordyn Lyndsey). Harris CareTracker PM displays the *Edit* box.
6. From the *Letter* list, select the letter you want to generate. Select "Past Due 60 1st."
7. If needed, select a new status from the *Change Status* list. (Leave blank.)

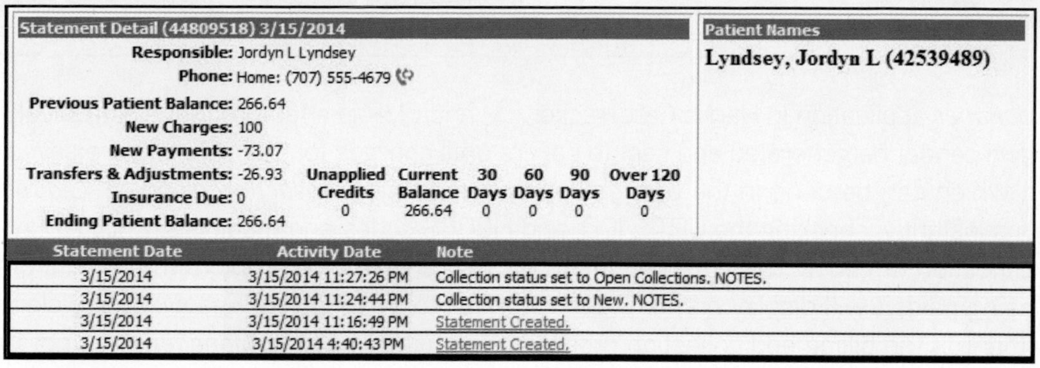

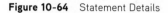

Statement Detail (44809518) 3/15/2014
Responsible: Jordyn L Lyndsey
Phone: Home: (707) 555-4679
Previous Patient Balance: 266.64
New Charges: 100
New Payments: -73.07
Transfers & Adjustments: -26.93
Insurance Due: 0
Ending Patient Balance: 266.64
Unapplied Credits 0
Current Balance 266.64
30 Days 0
60 Days 0
90 Days 0
Over 120 Days 0
Patient Names
Lyndsey, Jordyn L (42539489)
Statement Date
Activity Date
Note
3/15/2014 3/15/2014 11:27:26 PM Collection status set to Open Collections. NOTES.
3/15/2014 3/15/2014 11:24:44 PM Collection status set to New. NOTES.
3/15/2014 3/15/2014 11:16:49 PM Statement Created.
3/15/2014 3/15/2014 4:40:43 PM Statement Created.

Figure 10-64 Statement Details

Tip Box

To generate letters for multiple patients, select the checkbox next to each patient for whom you want to generate a letter and then click *Actions > Edit*.

Print the Edit window, label it "Activity 10-10," and place it in your assignment folder.

8. Click *Save* and then close out of the *Updates Processed* window. Generated collection letters can be printed from the *Print Batch Letters* application in the *Administration* module (Figure 10-65). You will receive an error message because you are not able to print batch letters in your student version of Harris CareTracker.

Batch Letters
Printed Batch Letters application
Status:
Notes:
Save
Print Letters
Print Labels

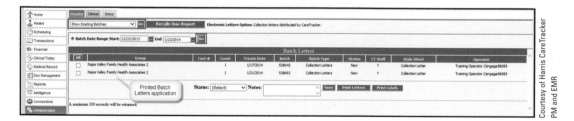

Figure 10-65 Print Batch Letters Application

Tip Box

If you do not print the collection letters, Harris CareTracker PM and EMR will automatically print the letters to send out to the patient the next day.

SUMMARY

The *ClaimsManager* application in Harris CareTracker PM and EMR is a feature that electronically screens a claim. A claim cannot be generated and sent to payers until charges for patient visits are saved in Harris CareTracker, which can be done in the *Charge* application of the *Transactions* module. *ClaimsManager* screens claims instantly, checking the CPT®, ICD, and HCPCS codes and modifiers. *EncoderPro* provides an online verification of codes. If *ClaimsManager* identifies an error or problem that would prevent the claim from being paid, it will display on the *Claims Worklist* to be resolved. Resolving any claim issue is a critical element of the billing and collection process. Although the *ClaimsManager* does not function in your student environment, it is important that you understand how it works.

Collections are the final step of the Harris CareTracker PM administrative and billing tasks. *Billing* and *Collections* are vital to the financial health of a medical practice. Harris CareTracker PM streamlines the billing and collection processes by provided global templates, the ability to create custom letters, and automatically generate statements. Patient information is pulled in to the collection letter template, eliminating the need to create and enter individual information and letters, improving accuracy and efficiency.

As with the entire text, the information learned and activities completed in this chapter will prepare you to successfully pass an EHR certification exam, a valued quality desired by medical practices. The comprehensive case studies in Chapter 11: Applied Learning Activities will provide you with more valuable "hands-on" experience with Harris CareTracker PM and EMR, allowing you to master the use of an integrated Practice Management and Electronic Medical Records application.

Check Your Knowledge

Select the best response.

_____ 1. The *Charge* application is where you enter the appropriate CPT® and ICD codes. What is the limit of CPT® codes? ICD codes? Modifiers?

    a. CPT® codes – 4; ICD codes – 4; Modifiers – 4
    b. CPT® codes – no limit; ICD codes – 4; Modifiers – 4
    c. CPT® codes – 4; ICD codes – no limit; Modifiers – 4
    d. CPT® codes – no limit; ICD codes – no limit; Modifiers – 4

_____ 2. Harris CareTracker PM automatically splits out the private payment amount owed, such as the patient's copayment, for each procedure entered for the patient that requires a copayment. This only occurs if the amount of the patient's copayment is entered where?

    a. In the *Billing* tab
    b. In the *ClaimsManager* field
    c. In the *Copay* field of the *Insurances* section in the *Demographics* application
    d. In the *Transactions* module

_____ 3. In which claims list category would you find claims that are transferred from a patient's primary insurance to the supplemental insurance and are not paid within 30 days?

    a. PENDING, In Review   c. OTHER, Set to Deny
    b. CLAIM ERRORS, Payer Edits   d. OTHER, Crossover

_____ 4. When the billing provider, dates of service, procedure codes, fee, units, servicing provider, or insurance need to be changed, the charge must be reversed from Harris CareTracker PM and EMR via the _____ application in the _____ module. The charge will then be put back into the system.

    a. *Edit; Transactions*   c. *Financial; Batch*
    b. *Edit; Patient*   d. *Batch; Edit*

_____ 5. A patient is automatically removed from *Collections* when the patient's private pay or collection balances are _____, regardless of his or her collection status.

    a. transferred   c. adjusted off
    b. paid in full   d. Both b and c

_____ 6. Of the four collection actions in Harris CareTracker PM, which is used when a patient's *Private Pay* balance needs to be assigned to a different insurance plan/financial class?

    a. Transfer   c. Group collections letter
    b. Remove from *Collections*   d. Global collections letter

_____ 7. Which *Global Collection* letter would be sent when an account balance is more than 60 days past due?

    a. Collection 1   c. Delinquent

    b. Past due   d. Final notice

_____ 8. After collection letters have been generated, they must be printed from the _____ application in the _____ module.

    a. *Batch Letters; Transactions*   c. *Print; Transactions*

    b. *Print; Patient*   d. *Batch Letter; Administration*

_____ 9. To generate letters for multiple patients, select the checkbox next to each patient for whom you want to generate a letter, and then click:

    a. *Collections > Billing*   c. *Actions > Edit*

    b. *Billing > Transfer*   d. *Edit > Multiple*

_____ 10. When a patient has reached the set overdue period for your company, the patient is automatically identified by the *Collections System* and assigned the status of:

    a. Collections actual   c. Collections pending

    b. New   d. Review

_____ 11. Patients manually added to *Collections* are flagged with [a(n)] _____ next to their name in the work area.

    a. asterisk (*)   c. exclamation point (!)

    b. plus sign [+] vs. (+)   d. brackets ([ ])

_____ 12. What type of *Global Collection* letter to a patient states that if the overdue balance is not paid in full, the billing office will continue with its collection policy, which may include a collection agency?

    a. Final notice   c. 75 Collection

    b. Collection payment plan   d. Collection 1

_____ 13. Which is not a letter editor tool?

    a. Search   c. Background color

    b. Copy/paste   d. Print

_____ 14. Name the two financial classes that private pay balances can be transferred to.

    a. Collections pending and collections actual

    b. Collections actual and financial

    c. Collections pending and status

    d. Collections and pending insurance

mini-case studies

Note: Case studies must be completed in every chapter since future chapter activities build upon them.

Complete all case studies for the following patients (**Note:** Prior to completing case studies, post any open batches):

a. Jane Morgan
b. Adam Thompson
c. Ellen Ristino
d. Barbara Watson

Case Study 10-1

1. Prior to beginning Case Study 10-1, create a new batch and name it "Ch10MCS".

2. Repeat Activity 10-5 and generate statements for all patients.

 Print the Generated Statements, label them "Case Study 10-1a through 10-1d," and place them in your assignment folder.

Case Study 10-2

Repeat Activity 10-7 and transfer any remaining balance for all patients.

 Once all balances have been transferred, print the screen showing all Transferred Balances, label it "Case Study 10-2," and place it in your assignment folder.

Case Study 10-3

Repeat Activity 10-10 and generate collection letters for all patients.

 Print the Edit screens showing the Collection Letters generated for each patient, label them "Case Study 10-3a through 10-3d" and place them in your assignment folder.

Case Study 10-4

1. Run a journal for your batch. Review and make any corrections if necessary.
2. Post the batch.

 Print the screens of the Journal and Open Batch, label them "Case Study 10-4a" and "Case Study 10-4b," and place them in your assignment folder.

Resources

The Harris CareTracker PM and EMR Help homepage represents a wealth of information for the electronic health record (https://training.caretracker.com/help/CareTracker_Help.htm).

American Medical Association

National Healthcare Association. (n.d.). *Certified Electronic Health Records Specialist (CEHRS™)*. Retrieved from http://www.nhanow.com/health-record.aspx.

Chapter 11
Applied Learning for the Paperless Medical Office

Learning Objectives

This module is designed to apply the skills you have learned to several patient case studies without the step-by-step instruction given in the previous chapters.

CASE STUDY 11-1: JULIA HERNANDEZ

Julia Hernandez calls the office this morning to schedule a new patient visit and would like to select Dr. Rebecca Ayerick as her primary care provider. (**Note:** Use the first date available that corresponds with Napa Valley Family Health Associates open office hours for Dr. Rebecca Ayerick.)

Step 1: Register a New Patient and Schedule an Appointment

Schedule a new patient CPE appointment for Julia Hernandez with Dr. Ayerick on the first available date. You will need to create a mini-registration to add the patient to the database before scheduling the appointment for her.

1. First search your database to see if Julia had ever been registered as a patient with the practice, using two patient identifiers: last name and date of birth. Upon confirming she is not already registered, create a new patient registration for Julia, starting with the following information (you will complete the full registration process when she arrives for her first appointment):
   - *Name:* Julia Hernandez
   - *Address:* 5224 Sunset Landing, Vacaville, CA 95688
   - *Home Phone:* (707) 468-4457
   - *Date of Birth:* 06/24/1987
   - *Social Security Number:* 123-45-2137
   - *Sex:* Female

2. Schedule an appointment for Julia with Dr. Ayerick, using the first available morning appointment slot.
   - *Appointment Type:* New Patient CPE
   - *Chief Complaint:* New Patient
   - *Location:* NVFA

While still on the phone with Julia, refer her to the Napa Valley Family Health Associates website to download the patient registration forms to complete and bring to her first appointment, along with photo ID and her insurance card(s). Advise Julia to arrive 15 minutes before her scheduled appointment to complete the registration process.

Step 2: Enter Payment, Check In Patient, and Complete Patient Registration

When you arrive at the office on the day of Julia's appointment, log in to Harris CareTracker and create a new batch titled "HernandezCopay". When Julia arrives for her appointment, review her patient registration forms for completeness. You see from her insurance card that she has a $25.00 copay.

1. Accept and enter Julia's cash payment for her copay and print a receipt for her.
2. Check Julia in for her visit with Dr. Ayerick.
3. While Julia is waiting to see Dr. Ayerick, record her complete patient registration information (see Source Document 11-1 in Appendix A).

Print the patient receipt and patient Demographics screen. Label them "Case Study 11-1a and 11-1b".

Step 3: Patient Work-Up

To begin EMR activities, review your *Batch* to set up operator preferences for clinical workflows.

When you have completed Step 3: Patient Work-Up, print the patient's Chart Summary and label it "Case Study 11-1c".

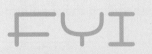

Background Information about Julia Hernandez
Julia Hernandez is a new patient here for a complete physical exam. Her company just started a new health and wellness program, which offers insurance premium discounts to employees who have one physical per year, as well as other preventive profiles and procedures. Julia does not have any current health concerns other than acid reflux. She is committed to a healthy lifestyle. Julia currently has an OB-GYN and is deferring a breast or genitourinary exam today.

1. *Transfer* Julia to Exam Room #1.
2. Referring to Table 11-1, enter Julia's medical information into her patient record.

TABLE 11-1	Medical Information for Julia Hernandez
Medication	Ortho Novum 1/35 (SIG: Take 1 tablet daily according to packet instructions.)
Allergies	Sulfa 10 (*Reaction:* Hives and Rash; *Start Date*: 06/15/2008; *Alert Status*: Popup Alert)
Immunizations	Skip this section. Julia does not have her immunization record with her and does not remember the dates of her immunizations. She states that her last tetanus shot was well over 10 years ago, so Dr. Ayerick will likely order a tetanus shot today. Julia signed a consent form for her medical records to be sent to Dr. Ayerick, but until her records arrive you will not be able to enter any information into this section.

3. Now enter the patient's medical history. Refer to Tables 11-2 and 11-3 for Julia's history information.

TABLE 11-2	Patient History for Julia Hernandez	
Section	**Item**	**Entry**
General Medical History	*Fracture*	Spiral fracture of left tibia at age 14. Treatment: Leg cast for 10 weeks. No complications.
	GERD	Acid reflux problems at least 3–4 days/week. OTC meds give little relief.
		All other sections are negative.
Hospitalizations		None
Other Medical History		None
Tobacco Assessment	*Smoking Status*	Never smoker
Social History	*Alcohol Use*	Occasional
	Caffeine Use	2 servings per day
	Drug Use	"N"
	Sun Protection (SPF 30)	"Y"
	Tattoos	"Y"
	Sexually Active	"Y"
	Race	Hispanic
	Native Language	Spanish
	Physical and Domestic Abuse	"N"
	Educational Level	Technical/vocational school
	Marital Status	Single
	Exercise Habits	strenuous > 3x/wk
	Seatbelts	"Y"
	Body Piercings	"Y"
	Birth Control Method	Oral contraceptive
	Religion	Roman Catholic
	Occupation	Server

(Continues)

TABLE 11-2 *(Continued)*

Section	Item	Entry
Depression Screening	*Little interest or pleasure in doing things*	At no time
	Feeling down, depressed, or hopeless	At no time
	Date of last depression screening	Leave blank
OB/GYN History	*LMP*	Enter a date that is two weeks ago from today's date
	Frequency of menstrual cycle	28 days
	History of abnormal Pap smears	"N"
	Sexually active	"Y"
	Ectopic pregnancy	"N"
	Birth Control	Oral contraceptive
		Leave remaining boxes in this section blank.
Pregnancy Summary	*Gravida*	0
		Leave all other boxes blank in this section.
Surgical/Procedural		Click on the box that states *"No prior surgical history."*
Preventive Care	*Flu Vaccine*	November 13 of last year
	Pap Smear	May 2 of last year
		Leave all other boxes blank.
Self-Management Goal		1. Increase workout schedule to 7 days/week.
		2. Get caught up on all preventive testing and procedures.

TABLE 11-3 General Family History for Julia Hernandez

Disease	Comment
Cardiovascular disease	Maternal grandmother died of a heart attack at age 65.
COPD	Paternal grandfather died from complications of COPD at age 72.
Hypertension	*Mother:* Controlled with medication
Osteoporosis	*Mother:* Controlled with medication
All other diseases should be marked "N."	

4. Next, take Julia's vital signs and record them in her chart. Refer to Table 11-4 for Julia's vital sign information.

TABLE 11-4 Vital Signs for Julia Hernandez

Height	5' 4"	**Blood Pressure**	94/66	**Respiratory Rate**	12
Weight	115	**Pulse Rate**	66 bpm	**Pain Level**	0/10
LMP	14 days ago from today's date	**Temperature**	97.8°F	**Chief Complaint**	New Patient – CPE. Patient here for a complete physical.

5. Because Julia is now ready to see Dr. Ayerick, create a *Progress Note* for her. Select a template of "IM OV Option 4 (v4) w/A&P." Refer to Table 11-5 while completing the progress note.

TABLE 11-5   Progress Note for Julia Hernandez

Tab	Item	Entry
ROS	*Gastrointestinal*	Click "N" on all the selections in this grouping.
	Other gastrointestinal symptoms	GERD
		Select "No symptoms" in all other sections.
PE		Click on "Y" for *patient deferred full body exam*.
	General	Select "awake," "well developed," and "well nourished."
	Head	Enter "Normocephalic" in the *Other head findings* box
	Eyes	Click "Y" for "PERRL" and "EOMI."
	Other eye findings	Fundi normal, vision grossly intact.
	Other ENT findings	External auditory canals and tympanic membranes clear. No nasal drainage, oral cavity and pharynx normal. No oral lesions or drainage. Teeth and gingiva in very good condition.
	Neck	Click "Y" beside "supple," click "N" beside "tenderness," "thyroid enlargement," and "carotid bruit."
	Lymphatics	Click "No" for "cervical adenopathy" and "tenderness."
	Chest	Click the box next to "Negative chest exam."
	Lungs	Click on "N" for "wheezing," "rhonchi," and "diminished breath sounds."
	Other lung findings box	Clear to auscultation
	Heart	Click on the "Y" beside "S1" and "S2." Click on the "N" beside "S3," "S4," and "irregular heart rhythm."
	Other heart findings box	No bruits, extremities are warm and well perfused, capillary refill is less than 2 seconds.
	Abdomen	Click on "Y" beside "soft"; click on "N" beside "rebound," "mass," "tenderness," "distention," and "muscle guarding."
	Other abdomen findings	Positive bowel sounds
	Musculoskeletal	Click on the "Y" beside "normal movement of all extremities"; click on the "N" beside "muscle tenderness," "joint tenderness," and "edema."
	Back	Negative back exam
	Neurologic	Click on the "Y" beside "cranial nerves II–XII intact"; click on the "N" beside "sensation," "motor," "gait and stance," and "reflexes."
	Other neurologic findings	Strength and sensation symmetric and intact throughout, reflexes good
	Mental Status Exam	Click on the "N" beside "affect," "attitude," and "mood."
	Skin	Click on the "Y" beside "warm," "dry," and "normal turgor."
Assess	*Today's Selected Diagnosis*	Normal routine history and physical examination (Z00.00)
Plan	*Additional Plan Details*	1. Basic metabolic panel in Blood
		2. Rx for PriLOSEC oral capsules, delayed release, 20 mg, Sig 1 cap daily. # 30, 0 refills
		3. Tetanus toxoid, absorbed (VIS form)
		4. Provide the patient with patient information sheets for "What is GERD?" and "MEDICATION: PRILOSEC."
		5. Set up a referral for the patient to see Dr. David Wong, gastroenterologist in San Ramon.
		6. Patient should follow up in one year for her next physical exam.

Step 4: Complete the Visit

Julia's visit is now over with Dr. Ayerick. It is your responsibility to complete orders as indicated in the *Plan* section of the progress note.

1. Enter the new lab order.

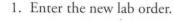 **Print the lab order and label it "Case Study 11-1d".**

2. Create and print the new prescription.

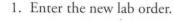 **Label the prescription "Case Study 11-1e".**

3. Add a new immunization: "Tetanus Toxoid Absorbed." Refer to Table 11-6 for additional immunization information.
4. Provide Julia with a copy of the Patient Information sheets ordered in the *Plan* section of the progress note.

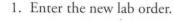 **Print the Patient Information sheets and label them "Case Study 11-1f-1 and 11-1f-2".**

5. Create an outgoing referral to the gastroenterologist noted in the *Plan* section of the progress note: Dr. David Wong in San Ramon.

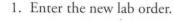 **Print the outgoing referral and label it "Case Study 11-1g".**

TABLE 11-6 Immunization for Julia Hernandez			
Manufacturer	Abbott Laboratories	Dose Route	IM
Lot Number	25698GBC	Amount	0.5 mL
Expiration Date	November 1 of next year	Series	1
Administration Date	Date of Julia Hernandez's appointment	Site	Left Deltoid
Administration Time	30 minutes following the start of the appointment	VIS Date	10/01/Last year
Administered By	You	Date VIS Given to Patient	Date of appointment
Ordering Provider	Dr. Ayerick	Adverse Reaction	Patient tolerated well

Step 5: Capture the Visit and Sign the Note

Having completed all the orders as indicated in the progress note, now capture the *Visit* and sign the progress note.

1. Capture the *Visit* by entering:
   a. *CPT® code(s):* 99203; 90718; and 90471

   Source: Current Procedural Terminology © 2013 American Medical Association.

   b. *ICD-10 code(s):* Z00.00 and K21.9
2. Sign the progress note.

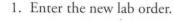 **Print the signed progress note and label it "Case Study 11-1h".**

3. Before Julia leaves the office, add a *Recall* for her annual physical, scheduled one year from the date of this visit. Her recall appointment will be for an "Established Patient CPE."

Step 6: Other Clinical Documentation

The *Results* of Julia's lab order have been received.

1. Manually enter the lab order results. Refer to Table 11-7 to enter results. All results are normal and final. (**Hint:** You will need to add the selected electrolytes to the results page. Click on the [+] sign next to "Basic Metabolic Panel in Blood." In the search window, search for each electrolyte separately. To add each one you will select the name of the electrolyte followed by "[Moles/volume] in Blood.")
2. Enter a *ToDo* to call the patient with the lab results.

Print a screenshot of the Manual Lab Results and label it "Case Study 11-1i".

TABLE 11-7	Results for Julia Hernandez Lab Order					
Test Name	**Result**	**Normal Range**	**Test Name**	**Result**	**Normal Range**
Glucose	86	74–100 mg/dL	Electrolytes		
			Sodium	141	134–144 mmol/L
			Potassium	4.3	3.5–5.3 mmol/L
			Chloride	104	98–107 mmol/L
			Carbon dioxide	23.5	22–30 mmol/L
Creatinine	0.7	0.1–1.2 mg/dL	Urea Nitrogen	16	6–22 mg/dL
Calcium	9.2	8.7–9.7 mg/dL			

Step 7: Verify Charges

Verify charges for Julia's *Visit*.

1. Using the batch you created at the beginning of this case study, run a journal and verify charges.

Step 8: Process Remittance (EOB) and Transfer to Private Pay

1. Create a new batch to record Julia's EOB titled "HernandezEOB".
2. Refer to Julia's EOB (Source Document 11-2 in Appendix A) and process the remittance. (**Hint:** Be sure to build all claims first.)
3. Run a journal to verify charges.

Print the journal and label it "Case Study 11-1j".

Step 9: Work Claims and Generate Patient Statement

1. Work the *Claims Worklist*.
2. Post all open batches.
3. Generate a statement for Julia.

Print the statement and label it Case Study 11-1k".

CASE STUDY 11-2: DELORES SIMPSON

Delores Simpson is an established patient of the practice who calls the office this morning to schedule an appointment with Dr. Raman, her primary care provider. She tells you she has not been feeling well and complains of chest discomfort. She has taken her blood pressure at home several times this morning and says it is normal. Just to be on the safe side, you encourage the patient to call the EMS so that she can be evaluated. The patient refuses to call and insists on coming into the office. Due to her age and the severity of her complaint, you message Dr. Raman and he replies to have her come in to the office this morning. If there are no appointments open, double-book the first available appointment for her to be seen. Delores has not been in to see Dr. Raman since the office converted to electronic records, but she is registered in the database.

Step 1: Search the Database and Schedule an Appointment

1. Search the database, confirming the patient's DOB, current address, phone number, and insurance.
2. Schedule an appointment for Delores with Dr. Raman, using the first available morning slot, or by double-booking the 11:00 a.m. slot.
   - *Appointment Type:* Follow Up
   - *Complaint:* Chest pain (resolved, normal BP readings)
   - *Location:* NVFA

Step 2: Check In Patient

1. When Delores arrives for her appointment, view her *At-A-Glance* patient information to confirm that she is still insured with Medicare and has no copay.
2. Check Delores in for her visit with Dr. Raman.

Step 3: Patient Work-Up

To begin EMR activities, create a new *Batch* titled "SimpsonEncounter" and edit your operator preferences for clinical workflows with Dr. Raman as the provider.

When you have completed Step 3: Patient Work-Up, print the patient's Chart Summary and label it "Case Study 11-2a".

FYI

Background Information about Delores Simpson
Delores is a kind, older patient who rarely complains. This morning she has been experiencing some chest discomfort. Upon her arrival, you immediately escort Delores to the cardiac bay. This room has equipment that can be used during a cardiac event. Normally, you would update the patient's medical history information, but the provider tells you just to get the patient's medication and allergy information to expedite the process.

1. *Transfer* Delores to the cardiac bay.
2. Referring to Table 11-8, enter Delores's medical information into her patient record.

3. Take Delores's vital signs and record them in her patient chart. Refer to Table 11-9 for Delores's vital sign information.
4. Because Delores is now ready to see Dr. Raman, create a *Progress Note* for her. Use progress note template "Cardio OV Option 3 (v4)." Refer to Table 11-10 while completing the progress note.

TABLE 11-8	Medical Information for Delores Simpson
Medications	Levothyroxine, 100 mcg tab, 1 per day
	Lisinopril, 20 mg tab, 1 per day
Allergies	Codeine (*Reaction*: Hives and Rash; *Start Date*: 02/15/1999; *Alert Status*: Popup Alert)

Copyright © 2015 Cengage Learning®.

TABLE 11-9	Vital Signs for Delores Simpson
Height	5' 2"
Weight	143
Blood Pressure	122/68
Pulse Rate	68 bpm
Temperature	97.4°F
Respiratory Rate	14

Copyright © 2015 Cengage Learning®.

TABLE 11-10 Progress Note for Delores Simpson		
Tab	**Item**	**Entry**
CC/ HPI	*Reason for Visit*	Chest pain
	HPI	Patient complains of early morning chest pain that lasted approximately 15 minutes and then subsided. No current pain. Patient described the pain as midsternal "tight, squeezing pressure radiating slightly to the left side of sternum." Pain rating at its worst around a "6." Patient denies any radiation of pain to other parts of the body, shortness of breath, or diaphoresis. There was no change in pain intensity upon movement. Patient took her blood pressure at least three times during the event but stated that each time her blood pressure was normal ("Around 110/68"). Patient denies any gastrointestinal or neurologic symptoms. Patient states that she has been under a great deal of stress lately because her daughter just moved to Boston. She feels that the pain may be related to stress. Patient does not recall any history of chest pain prior to this morning's event.
ROS		Select "N" for all categories in the *Cardiovascular ROS* sections. Do not mark any of the boxes in the *Review of Systems* section.
	Other Review of Systems box	Denies fatigue, fever, weight changes or pain (other than the chest discomfort she experienced this morning). *HEENT*: Denies headache, dizziness, or voice changes. *CHEST*: As stated in the HPI, patient denies any current chest pain or shortness of breath. *CV*: Refer to HPI. *GI*: Patient denies any nausea or vomiting, abdominal pain, or reflux. Has had some constipation lately but nothing out of the "ordinary." *GU*: Denies any frequency, dysuria, or changes in voiding habits. *MUSC*: Denies any muscular or joint pain or any joint swelling. *NEURO*: Denies vertigo, headache, ataxia, or syncope. *PV*: No changes in temperature or any swelling in extremities. *PSYCH*: As stated in the HPI, patient feels anxious over daughter moving to Boston. Feels like she will never see her daughter now that she is so far away.

(Continues)

TABLE 11-10 *(Continued)*

Tab	Item	Entry
PE		Select "N" for all applicable categories in the *Cardio PE* section. Click in the box beside *regular rate and rhythm*.
		Do not click on any of the responses in the *Physical Examination* box.
	Other Physical Findings box	*General*: Patient appears alert and well.
		HEENT: Head, normocephalic, no pharyngeal exudate or erythema, uvula midline.
		NECK: Supple, no palpable masses or nodules, thyroid normal in size, trachea midline.
		CHEST: Thorax without distortion. Respiration regular and unlabored, no cough. Lung fields normal. Negative rales or rhonchi. Breath sounds clear.
		ABDOMEN: Round and soft. No tenderness, rash, or palpable mass. Nail beds pink with less than 2 sec capillary refill. Pedal pulse 2+l.
		NEURO: Patient alert and oriented. No speech problems. Patient able to move all extremities and appears coherent. Other than being a little anxious regarding daughter's move, patient appears in good overall spirits.
A&P	*Today's Selected Diagnosis*	Chest pain (R07.9)
	Assessment Notes	R/O angina pectoris and MI. Chest discomfort may be related to the stress of her daughter's move.
	Other Plan Items box	1. 12-Lead EKG
		2. Patient information sheet "Your Body's Response to Anxiety"
		3. F/U in one week
		4. Refill for levothyroxine tabs, 100 mcg, Sig 1 tab daily, # 30, 3 refills

Step 4: Complete the Visit

Delores's visit is now over with Dr. Raman. It is your responsibility to complete orders as indicated in the *A&P* section of the progress note.

1. Create and print the new prescription.

 Label the printed prescription "Case Study 11-2b".

2. In the *Procedures* tab within the progress note, type the following: "Performed 12-Lead EKG per Dr. Raman."
3. Provide Delores with a copy of the Patient Information sheet(s) ordered in the *Plan* section of the progress note.

 Print the Patient Information sheet and label it "Case Study 11-2c".

Step 5: Capture the Visit and Sign the Note

Having completed all of the orders as indicated in the *Progress Note*, now capture the *Visit* and sign the progress note.

1. Capture the *Visit* by entering:
   a. *CPT® code(s):* 99213 and 93000

   Source: Current Procedural Terminology © 2013 American Medical Association.

   b. *ICD-10 code(s):* R07.9

2. Sign the progress note.

Print the signed progress note and label it "Case Study 11-2d".

3. Before Delores leaves schedule her follow-up appointment noted in the *Plan* section of the progress note.

Step 6: Verify Charges

Verify charges for Delores's *Visit*.

1. Using the batch you created at the beginning of this case study, run a journal and verify charges.

Print the journal and label it "Case Study 11-2e".

Step 7: Process Remittance (EOB) and Transfer to Private Pay

1. Create a new batch to record Delores's EOB titled "SimpsonEOB".
2. Refer to Delores's EOB (Source Document 11-3 in Appendix A) and process the remittance. (**Hint:** Be sure to build all claims first.)
3. Run a journal to verify charges.

Print the journal and label it "Case Study 11-2f".

Step 8: Work Claims and Generate Patient Statement

1. Work the *Claims Worklist*.
2. Post all open batches.
3. Generate a statement for Delores.

Print the statement and label it "Case Study 11-2g".

CASE STUDY 11-3: ADAM ZOTTO

Adam Zotto is an established patient who calls the office this morning to schedule an appointment with Dr. Ayerick, his primary care provider. He says he wants to see Dr. Ayerick regarding his diabetes management. Adam has not been in to see Dr. Ayerick since the office converted to electronic records, but he is registered in the database. Search the database confirming his DOB, current address, phone number, and insurance, and then schedule the appointment for him.

Step 1: Search the Database and Schedule an Appointment

1. Search the database confirming the patient's DOB, current address, phone number, and insurance.
2. Schedule an appointment for Adam with Dr. Ayerick, using the first available morning slot.
   - *Appointment Type:* Follow Up
   - *Complaint:* Follow-up; Diabetes management
   - *Location:* NVFA

Step 2: Enter Payment and Check In Patient

When Adam arrives for his appointment, view his *At-A-Glance* patient information and confirm that he is still insured with Senior Gap and has a $10.00 copay. Before accepting Adam's payment, create a new batch titled "ZottoCopay".

  1. Accept and enter Adam's cash payment for his copay and print a receipt for him.

Label the printed receipt "Case Study 11-3a".

  2. Check Adam in for his visit with Dr. Ayerick.

Step 3: Patient Work-Up

To begin EMR activities, edit your *Batch* operator preferences for clinical workflows with Dr. Ayerick as the provider.

When you have completed Step 3: Patient Work-Up, print the patient's Chart Summary and label it "Case Study 11-3b".

FYI

Background Information about Adam Zotto

Adam was diagnosed with type 2 diabetes mellitus approximately 20 years ago—around the same time he was diagnosed with hypertension. He has been very compliant over the years and remains on an oral hypoglycemic. He is here for a routine follow-up appointment exam. He recently discovered at a church health fair that his cholesterol is elevated and wants to discuss the findings with the doctor.

  1. *Transfer* Adam to Exam Room #1.
  2. Referring to Table 11-11, enter Adam's medical information into his patient record.

TABLE 11-11 Medical Information for Adam Zotto	
Medications	Glyburide: one 5 mg tablet twice a day
	Metoprolol tartrate: one 50 mg tablet daily
	Aspirin chewable: one 81 mg tablet daily
Allergies	None
Immunizations	Tetanus Toxoid Absorbed, 07/02/last year
	Influenza, seasonal injectable, 10/04/two years ago

Copyright © 2015 Cengage Learning®.

  3. Now enter the patient's medical history. Refer to Tables 11-12 and 11-13 for Adam's history information.

	TABLE 11-12	Patient History for Adam Zotto

Section	Item	Entry
General Medical History	DM Type 2	Diagnosed in June of 1995. Controlled with diet and Micronase. Well controlled.
	Gastric Ulcer	April of 2008. Controlled with medication. Last EGD in April of 2012. Ulcer resolved. Medication discontinued.
	Hypertension	Diagnosed in March of 1995. Well controlled with metoprolol.
	Osteoarthritis	Diagnosed in May of 2004. Hands, hips, and knees affected.
		All other sections are negative.
Hospitalizations		Right TKA in August of 2009. No complications.
		Left TKA in July of 2011. No complications.
Other Medical History		None
Tobacco Assessment	Smoking Status	Former smoker
	# Pack Years	20
Social History	Alcohol Use	Occasional
	Caffeine Use	3 servings per day
	Drug Use	"N"
	Sun Protection (SPF 15)	"Y"
	Tattoos	"Y"
	Sexually Active	"N"
	Race	Caucasian
	Physical Abuse	"N"
	Domestic Violence	"N"
	Educational Level	Grades 9-12
	Marital Status	Single
	Exercise Habits	Moderate < 3 x/wk
	Seatbelts	"Y"
	Body Piercings	"Y"
	Religion	Christian
	Occupation	Retired
Depression Screening	Select Patient Refused.	
	Date of last depression screening	Leave blank.
OB/GYN History		Skip
Pregnancy Summary		Skip
Surgical/Procedural	Other Surgical History	Right TKA in August of 2009. No complications.
		Left TKA in July of 2011. No complications.
Preventive Care	A1c %	10/12 of the previous year
	Blood Glucose	02/05 of last year
	Colonoscopy	02/15/2005
	Dilated Eye Exam	04/15 of last year
	PSA	04/22 of last year

(Continues)

TABLE 11-12 *(Continued)*

Section	Item	Entry
Preventive Care	*Td*	Check immunization table
	Zoster Vaccine	09/02/2006
	Leave all other boxes blank.	
Self-Management Goal		1. Get caught up on all preventive testing and procedures.
		2. Get a gym membership at the "Y."

TABLE 11-13   General Family History for Adam Zotto

Disease	Comment
Cardiovascular Disease	Father died of a heart attack at age 65.
CHF	Mother died at age 69 of congestive heart failure.
Diabetes	Mother, type 2; Age of onset, 42
Hypertension	Both mother and father
Kidney Disease	Mother
Osteoarthritis	Both mother and father
Leave all other sections blank.	

4. Next, take Adam's *Vital Signs* and record them in his chart. Refer to Table 11-14 for Adam's *Vital Sign* information.

TABLE 11-14   Vital Signs for Adam Zotto

Height	5′ 11½″	Pulse Rate	78 bpm
Weight	205	Temperature	98.4°F
Blood Pressure	130/84	Respiratory Rate	16

5. Because Adam is now ready to see Dr. Ayerick, create a *Progress Note* for him. Select a template of "IM OV Option 4 (v4) w/A&P." Refer to Table 11-15 while completing the progress note.

TABLE 11-15   Progress Note for Adam Zotto

Section	Item	Entry
CC/HPI	*CC*	Follow-up visit
	Other Complaints	Wants cholesterol checked. Had blood test (finger stick) at a church health fair. Result was elevated. Does not recall reading.
	HPI	Pt. here for a F/U exam for diabetes and hypertension. Pt. states he checks his blood sugar in the morning when he first gets up and 2 hours after each meal. "Readings have stayed below 130 mg/dL." Last A1c was in October of last year, result 6.4. Pt. also states that home blood pressure readings have been running between 110 and 130 on the systolic side and between 64 and 80 on the diastolic side. Pt. has some tingling in his toes but not often. Regularly sees an ophthalmologist for eye care. Overall, pt. states that he feels very good!

TABLE 11-15   *(Continued)*

Section	Item	Entry
ROS	*Constitutional*	No constitutional symptoms
	Eyes	No eye symptoms
	Cardiovascular	"Y" for "cold hands or feet" and "N" for all other symptoms in this category
	Genitourinary	No GU symptoms
	Neurological	"Y" for "tingling" (Both feet mainly when in a sitting position); "N" for all other symptoms in this category.
		Leave other sections blank.
PE	*General*	Select "awake," "alert," and "General appearance normal."
	Head/Other head findings	Normocephalic
	Eyes	"Y" for "PERRL" and "EOMI"
	Heart	"N" for "bradycardia," "tachycardia," "irregular heart rhythm," "murmurs," "rubs," and "gallop"; "Y" for "S1" and "S2" and "N" for "S3" and "S4"
	Genitourinary	Negative genitourinary exam
	Neurologic	"A" for "sensation"
	Other neurologic findings	Some lower extremity numbness. Microfilament test shows two regions without sensation bilaterally. Bottoms of feet appear slightly calloused and dry. Skin is intact. Cranial nerves II–XII grossly intact. Cerebellar function intact demonstrated through RAM
	Skin	"Y" for "warm," "dry," and "normal turgor"
	Other skin findings	Feet slightly cooler than the rest of the body
Assess	*Today's Selected Diagnosis*	1. Diabetes mellitus type 2, uncomplicated (E11.9) 2. Diabetic peripheral neuropathy (E11.42) 3. Hypertension (I10)
Plan	*Additional Plan Details*	1. Hemoglobin A1c/Hemoglobin total in Blood 2. Lipid panel with direct LDL in Serum or Plasma 3. Have patient follow up with podiatrist 4. Rx: Glyburide: One 5 mg tablet twice a day, 60 tabs, 3 refills 5. Rx: Metoprolol tartrate: One 50 mg tablet daily, 30 tabs, 3 refills 6. Patient information sheet: What is Peripheral Neuropathy? 7. 3-month follow-up appointment 8. Referral to podiatrist: Dr. Katrina Di Pasqua, DPM in Napa, CA

Step 4: Complete the Visit

Adam's visit is now over with Dr. Ayerick. It is your responsibility to complete orders as indicated in the *Plan* section of the progress note.

1. Enter the new lab orders.

Print the lab orders and label them "Case Study 11-3c".

2. Create and print the new prescriptions.

Label the printed prescriptions "Case Study 11-3d-1 and 11-3d-2".

3. Provide Adam with a copy of the Patient Information sheet(s) ordered in the *Plan* section of the progress note.

Print the Patient Information Sheet and label it "Case Study 11-3e".

4. Create an outgoing referral to Dr. Katrina Di Pasqua, DPM.

Print the referral and label it "Case Study 11-3f".

Step 5: Capture the Visit and Sign the Note

Having completed all the orders as indicated in the *Progress Note*, now capture the *Visit* and sign the progress note.

1. Capture the *Visit* by entering:
   a. *CPT® code(s):* 99213

   Source: Current Procedural Terminology © 2013 American Medical Association.

   b. *ICD-10 code(s):* E11.9, E11.42, and I10
2. Sign the progress note.

Print the signed progress note and label it "Case Study 11-3g".

3. Before Adam leaves the office, add a *Recall* for his CPE one year from today's date.

Step 6: Other Clinical Documentation

The *Results* of Adam's lab order have been received.

1. Manually enter the lab order results. Refer to Table 11-16 to enter results. All results are final.

Print a screenshot of the Manual Lab Results and label it "Case Study 11-3h".

2. Enter a *ToDo* to call the patient with the lab results.

TABLE 11-16	Lab Results for Adam Zotto	
Test Name	**Result**	**Normal Value**
Hemoglobin A1c/Hemoglobin, total in Blood	6.8%	Less than 7%
Lipid Panel with Direct LDL in Serum or Plasma		
Cholesterol in LDL/Cholesterol in HDL [Mass Ratio]	Leave blank	Leave blank
Cholesterol in VLDL in Serum or Plasma	32 mg/dL	5–40 mg/dL
Cholesterol in LDL in Serum or Plasma	104 mg/dL	Less than 100 mg/dL
Cholesterol in HDL in Serum or Plasma	44 mg/dL	Greater than 40 mg/dL
Cholesterol in Serum or Plasma	232	Less than 200
Triglyceride in Serum or Plasma	160 mg/dL	Less than 150 mg/dL
Cholesterol Total/Cholesterol in HDL [Mass Ratio]	Leave blank	Leave blank

Step 7: Verify Charges

Verify charges for Adam's *Visit*.

1. Using the batch you created at the beginning of this case study, run a journal and verify charges.

Print the journal and label it "Case Study 11-3i".

Step 8: Process Remittance (EOB) and Transfer to Private Pay

1. Create a new batch to record Adam's EOB titled "ZottoEOB".
2. Refer to Adam's EOB (Source Document 11-4 in Appendix A) and process the remittance. (**Hint:** Be sure to build all claims first.)
3. Run a journal to verify charges.

Print the journal and label it "Case Study 11-3j".

Step 9: Work Claims and Generate Patient Statement

1. Work the *Claims Worklist*.
2. Post all open batches.
3. Adam does not have an outstanding balance, so you do not need to generate a patient statement.

CASE STUDY 11-4: BARBARA WATSON

Barbara is an established patient who was last seen in the office for a fever. Her history has been previously entered in Harris CareTracker EMR during that visit (see Case Study 6-3). She calls the office this morning to schedule a visit with Dr. Raman, her primary care provider. She is concerned about the flu that is going around and currently has cold symptoms.

Step 1: Search the Database and Schedule an Appointment

1. Search the database confirming the patient's DOB, current address, phone number, and insurance.
2. Schedule an appointment for Barbara with Dr. Raman, using the first available morning slot.
   - *Appointment Type:* Follow Up
   - *Complaint:* Follow-up; Fever and flu symptoms
   - *Location:* NVFA

Step 2: Enter Payment and Check In Patient

When Barbara arrives for her appointment, view her *At-A-Glance* patient information and confirm that she is still insured with Blue Cross Blue Shield and has a $20.00 copay. Before accepting Barbara's payment, create a new batch titled "WatsonCopay".

1. Accept and enter Barbara's cash payment for her copay and print a receipt for her.

Print the receipt and label it "Case Study 11-4a".

2. Check Barbara in for her visit with Dr. Raman.

Step 3: Patient Work-Up

To begin EMR activities, edit your *Batch* operator preferences for clinical workflows with Dr. Raman as the provider.

When you have completed Step 3: Patient Work-Up, print the patient's Chart Summary and label it "Case Study 11-4b".

FYI

Background Information about Barbara Watson

Barbara is a fit older adult who recently retired. She has a history of osteoporosis but no other significant health problems. She likes to travel and is planning to fly out tomorrow morning to visit her friend in Texas. She is concerned that her symptoms will worsen because of the pressurized cabin on the plane. Barbara wants something that will help relieve her symptoms before tomorrow.

1. *Transfer* Barbara to Exam Room 2.
2. Review the patient's medical history with her. (Barbara tells you that there have been no changes since the last visit.)
3. Next, take Barbara's vital signs and record them in her chart. Refer to Table 11-17 for Barbara's vital sign information.
4. Because Barbara is now ready to see Dr. Raman, create a *Progress Note* for her. Select a template of "IM OV Option 4 (v4) w/A&P." Refer to Table 11-18 while completing the progress note.

TABLE 11-17 Vital Signs for Barbara Watson			
Height	5' 10"	**Temperature**	98.8°F
Weight	131	**Respiratory Rate**	16
Blood Pressure	130/86	**Pulse Oximetry**	95%
Pulse Rate	78 bpm	**Pain Level**	6/10

TABLE 11-18	Progress Note for Barbara Watson	
Section	**Item**	**Entry**
CC/HPI	*CC/Other Complaints*	Stuffy nose, sore throat, sinus headache, and frequent sneezing for the past week. Intermittent dry cough.
	HPI	Nasal congestion, rhinorrhea, and sinus congestion that began approximately one week ago. Reports frontal head pain (6/10) and facial pressure around cheekbones and eyes. Moderate amount of clear to green drainage from nose with intermittent congestion. Denies fever. Patient reports that she has a sore throat upon awakening in the mornings but it usually subsides by midday. No history of seasonal allergies.
ROS	*Constitutional*	"N" for "fever" and "Y" for "chills" and "headache"
	Eyes	"N" for "double vision," "blurred vision," and "photophobia"
	Other eye symptoms	Watery eyes
	ENT	"Y" for "nasal congestion," "nasal discharge," and "sore throat." "N" for "earache," "tinnitus," and "dysphagia"
	Other ENT symptoms	Intermittent bilateral ear pressure but no pain
	Neck	No neck symptoms
	Respiratory	"Y" for "cough" and "N" for all other symptoms
		Leave all other sections blank.
PE	*General*	Select "awake" and "alert."
	Other general findings	Denies significant changes in weight, fatigue, or appetite
	Head/Other head findings	Normocephalic with the exception of mild pressure reported upon palpation of forehead region
	Eyes	"Y" for "PERRL" and "EOMI"
	Ears	"N" for all symptoms associated with the ear
	Nose	"Y" for "rhinorrhea," "coryza," and "sinus tenderness"
	Pharynx	"N" for "oropharyngeal hemorrhage" and "Y" for "oropharyngeal exudate" and "pharyngeal inflammation"
	Other ENT findings	Ears: Bilateral canals patent without erythema, exudate, or edema. Bilateral tympanic membranes intact, pearly gray with sharp cone of light. Nose: Bilateral nares congested with rhinorrhea, mild erythema of nasal mucosa. Throat: Posterior oropharynx has a moderate discharge (clear to white). No ulcerations. Uvula midline.
	Neck	"Y" for "supple" and "N" for all other symptoms in this category
	Lymphatics	Negative lymph node exam
	Chest	Negative lung exam
	Lungs/Other lung findings	Lungs clear upon auscultation
	Heart	"Y" for "S1" and "S2". "N" for all other symptoms
Assess	*Today's Selected Diagnosis*	1. Acute URI (J06.9) 2. Acute Sinusitis (J01.90) 3. Acute pharyngitis (R/O Strep) (J02.9)
Plan	*Additional Plan Details*	1. Rapid Streptococcus Group Identification (Kit) 2. Rx: Zithromax Oral Packet, 1 GM, Take as directed, # 1 Packet, No refills 3. Patient Information Sheet: Acute Sinusitis 4. Obtain an OTC decongestant to help with congestion.

Step 4: Complete the Visit

Barbara's visit is now over with Dr. Raman. It is your responsibility to complete the orders as indicated in the *Plan* section of the progress note.

1. Enter the results for the *Rapid Streptococcus Group Identification* test in the *Tests* tab of the patient's progress note. The result is negative.
2. Create and print the new prescription.

Label the printed prescription "Case Study 11-4c".

3. Provide Barbara with a copy of the Patient Information sheet(s) ordered in the *Plan* section of the progress note.

Print the Patient Information sheet and label it "Case Study 11-4d".

Step 5: Capture the Visit and Sign the Note

Having completed all the orders as indicated in the *Progress Note*, now capture the *Visit* and sign the progress note.

1. Capture the *Visit* by entering:
   a. *CPT® code(s):* 99213 and 87430 (enter $30.00 as the *Fee* for 87430 in the *Missing Encounters/ Visits* screen for Barbara Watson [see Tip Box on pages 501–502] because it is not listed on the NVFHA encounter form)

   Source: Current Procedural Terminology © 2013 American Medical Association.

   b. *ICD-10 code(s):* J06.9, J01.90, and J02.9
2. Sign the progress note.

Print the signed progress note and label it "Case Study 11-4e".

Step 6: Verify Charges

Verify charges for Barbara's *Visit*.

1. Using the batch you created at the beginning of this case study, run a journal and verify charges.

Print the journal and label it "Case Study 11-4f".

Step 7: Process Remittance (EOB) and Transfer to Private Pay

1. Create a new batch to record Barbara's EOB titled "WatsonEOB".
2. Refer to Barbara's EOB (Source Document 11-5 in Appendix A) and process the remittance. (**Hint:** Be sure to build all claims first.)
3. Run a journal to verify charges.

Print the journal and label it "Case Study 11-4g".

Step 8: Work Claims and Generate Patient Statement

1. Work the *Claims Worklist*.
2. Post all open batches.
3. Generate a statement for Barbara.

Print the statement and label it "Case Study 11-4h".

CASE STUDY 11-5: CRAIG X. SMITH

Craig is an established patient who was last seen in the office for wheezing. His history has been previously entered in Harris CareTracker EMR during that visit (Case Study 6-4). He is returning today for a recheck from his prior visit.

Step 1: Search the Database and Schedule an Appointment

1. Search the database confirming patient's DOB, current address, phone number, and insurance.
2. Schedule an appointment for Craig with Dr. Raman, using the first available morning slot.
   - *Appointment Type:* Follow Up
   - *Location:* NVFA

Step 2: Enter Payment and Check In Patient

1. When Craig arrives for his appointment, view his *At-A-Glance* patient information and confirm that he is still insured with Medicaid and has no copay.
2. Check Craig in for his visit with Dr. Raman.

Step 3: Patient Work-Up

To begin EMR activities, create a new *Batch* titled "SmithEncounter" and edit your operator preferences for clinical workflows with Dr. Raman as the provider.

When you have completed Step 3: Patient Work-Up, print the patient's Chart Summary and label it "Case Study 11-5a".

FYI

Background Information about Craig X. Smith
Craig was seen two weeks ago for a fever and wheezing. His mother was unable to keep his follow-up appointment last week so she is following up today. Craig's symptoms have completely resolved. Fever has subsided and wheezing is gone.

1. *Transfer* Craig to Exam Room #1.
2. Now review the patient's medical history with his mother. Mom reports that there is no change since the last visit.

3. Next, take Craig's vital signs and record them in his chart. Refer to Table 11-19 for Craig's vital sign information.

4. Because Craig is now ready to see Dr. Raman, create a *Progress Note* for him. Select a template of "Pediatric OV Option 1 (v1)." Refer to Table 11-20 while completing the progress note.

TABLE 11-19 Vital Signs for Craig X. Smith

Category	Entry
Height	N/A
Weight	26 lb 8 oz
Body Mass Index	Automatically populates after entering height and weight
LMP	N/A
Blood Pressure	94/60
Pulse Rate	96 bpm
Temperature	98.6°F
Respiratory Rate	20
Pulse Oximetry	98%
Pain Level	N/A
Head Circumference	N/A
Length	32.9"

Copyright © 2015 Cengage Learning®.

TABLE 11-20 Progress Note for Craig X. Smith

Section of OV Tab	Entry
CC	Follow-up from last visit.
History of Present Illness	Patient's mother states that patient is doing much better. His symptoms have completely subsided and he is once again a happy little boy.
Past Medical/Social/Family History	No changes since last visit.
Review of Systems	*General:* No acute distress at this time. *Ears, Nose, and Throat:* Symptoms have dissipated from previous exam. *Respiratory:* No wheezing or coughing at this time.
Physical Examination	*General:* Awake, well developed. *Ears, Nose, and Throat:* Normal oropharyngeal discharge, ears and nose clear. *Respiratory:* All lung fields clear, SaO_2 reading is 98% today. *Cardiovascular:* Normal rate and peripheral pulses are normal.
Tests	Leave blank.
Procedure Note	Leave blank.
Assessment	No active problems today.
Plan	1. Mother to call if symptoms return.

Copyright © 2015 Cengage Learning®.

Step 4: Capture the Visit and Sign the Note

Having completed all the orders as indicated in the *Progress Note*, now capture the *Visit* and sign the progress note.

1. Capture the *Visit* by entering:
   a. *CPT® code(s):* 99392

   Source: Current Procedural Terminology © 2013 American Medical Association.

   b. *ICD-10 code(s):* R06.2 (**Note:** Although the symptoms have resolved, Craig is still being seen for a follow-up of this diagnosis.)
2. Sign the progress note.

 Print the signed progress note and label it "Case Study 11-5b".

Step 5: Verify Charges

Verify charges for Craig's *Visit*.

1. Using the batch you created at the beginning of this case study, run a journal and verify charges.

Print the journal and label it "Case Study 11-5c".

Step 6: Process Remittance (EOB) and Transfer to Private Pay

1. Create a new batch to record Craig's EOB.
2. Refer to Craig's EOB (Source Document 11-6 in Appendix A) and process the remittance. (**Hint:** Be sure to build all claims first.)
3. Run a journal to verify charges.

Print the journal and label it "Case Study 11-5d".

Step 7: Work Claims and Generate Patient Statement

1. Work the *Claims Worklist*.
2. Post all open batches.
3. Craig does not have an outstanding balance, so you do not need to generate a patient statement.

CASE STUDY 11-6: TRANSFER TO COLLECTIONS

It has now been more than 60 days since you generated statements for Julia, Delores, and Barbara. Their final payments have not been received. Create a new batch for collections activities titled "Ch11Collections".

1. Manually transfer their accounts to *Collections*.
2. Generate a collection letter appropriate to the office policy for accounts older than 60 days.

Print a screenshot of the Collections screen listing these outstanding accounts and label it "Case Study 11-6".

3. Run a journal and post the batch.

CASE STUDY 11-7: OPERATOR ACTIVITY LOG

Having completed the activities in this textbook and applied learning case studies, run an activity log to review the entries (refer to Activity 2-5).

CASE STUDY 11-8: VIEW THE VIP LOG

Having completed the activities in this textbook and applied learning case studies, view the VIP log entries (refer to Activity 2-5 FYI box).

CASE STUDY 11-9: CLOSE THE FISCAL PERIODS AND FISCAL YEARS

Having completed the activities in this textbook and the applied learning case studies, close any open fiscal periods and fiscal years (following the instructions in Activities 2-6 and 2-7, only this time closing the periods and years).

WARNING!! Once a fiscal period or fiscal year is closed, it cannot be reopened. Be sure you have completed all activities and assignments in this text prior to closing. (**Note:** You may want to wait until the end of the semester so that you can review your assignments with your instructor or make any necessary changes to the activities.)

1. Access *Open Fiscal Period(s)/Open Fiscal Year*(s). Write down a list of all open periods.
2. Review *Open Batches* and run a *Journal* for any open batches.
3. Review your *Open Batches, Journal,* and *Open Fiscal Period(s)/Open Fiscal Year(s)* with your instructor.
4. Upon confirmation that all activities have been completed as assigned and that any open batches have been posted, close all the fiscal period(s) and fiscal year(s).

Appendix A

Source Documents

Source Document 3-1

Patient Registration Form

NVFHA

Patient's Last Name	First (legal name)	First (Preferred name)	Middle Name
SMITH	JAMES	JIM	M

Address (Number, Street, Apt #)	City	State	Zip Code
2455 E. Front, Apt. 205	Napa	CA	94558

Mail will be sent to the address listed above, unless patient indicates a different address (leave blank if same as above)

Send mail to Address (Number, Street, Apt #)	City	State	Zip Code

Phone Options	Phone Number	Okay to leave detailed message	Call this number (circle one)
Home	(707) 221 - 4040	Yes _×_ No _____	(1st) 2nd 3rd choice
Cell	( ) -	Yes _____ No _____	1st 2nd 3rd choice
Work	(877) 833 - 7777	Yes _____ No _×_	1st (2nd) 3rd choice

Would you like to communicate by Email Yes _×_ No __	Email Address	Jmsmith@email.com

Date of Birth	Gender	Social Security Number
2/23/1965	Female ____ Male _×_	000-00-9009

Marital Status (**circle one**)	What is your preferred language / secondary language
(Single)/ Married / Divorced / Widow /Partner	English

Race (circle one)

African American-Black / Asian / Bi-Multi-racial / Pacific Islander-Hawaiian / (Caucasian–White) / Native American Eskimo Aleut / Decline to state / Other

Ethnicity (circle one)

Hispanic-Latino / Non-Hispanic-Latino / Other

Religion	Organ Donor	Yes _____	No _____

Are you new to our practice	Who referred you to our practice	Who is your Primary Care Physician
Yes _×_ No _____	David Dodgin	Rebecca Ayerick

Additional Notes	No call after 8 pm

Emergency Contact

Emergency Contact's Name	Relationship to patient	Phone
Joan Smith	Mother	(510) 478 - 5151

On-Line Patient Portal Communication via Email

On-Line communication is used for non-urgent message/requests only. NVFHA uses secure technology to protect the privacy and confidentiality of your personal information. Only you, your physician, and authorized staff can read your message.

What is your preferred method of communication	Phone _×_ Letter _____ Patient Portal _____

Insurance Information

Subscriber (Insurance Holder) Name	Date of Birth	Relationship to patient	Subscriber Phone Numeber
James M. Smith	2/23/1965	Self	(707) 221 - 4040

Health Plan Information	Primary Health Plan	Secondary Health Plan
Health Plan Name	Blue Shield Cengage	
Health Plan Address	PO Box 32245, Los Angeles, CA, 90002	
Group Number	BCBS987	
Subscriber Number	BCBS987	

Elig Date From	1/1/2010	Copay	$ 25.00

Patient Employer Information

Employer Name & Address (Number, Street, Apt #, City, State, Zip Code)	Employer Phone Number
River Rock Casino, 3250 Highway 128, Geyersville, CA 95441	(877) 833 - 7777

Occupation	IT Support	Start Date	8/25/2009

Assignment of Benefits • Financial Agreement

I hereby give lifetime authorization for payment of insurance benefits to be made directly to **Napa Valley Family Health Assoc.**, and any assisting physicians, for services rendered. I understand that I am financially resposible for all charges whether or not they are covered by insurance. In the event of default, I agree to pay all costs of collection, and reasonable attorney's fees. I hereby authorize this healthcare provider to release all information necessary to secure the the payment of benefits.

I further agree that a photocopy of this agreement shall be as vaild as the original.

Date: __XX/XX/20XX__   Your Signature: _____ *James M. Smith* _____

Method of Payment: ■ Cash   ■ Check   ■ Credit Card

Source Document 3-2

NOTICE OF PRIVACY PRACTICES (NOPP)

ACKNOWLEDGEMENT OF RECEIPT

Patient Name: James M. Smith
_____
(Please Print)

By signing this form, you acknowledge receipt of the Notice of Privacy Practices of NAPA VALLEY FAMILY HEALTH ASSOCIATES. Our Notice of Privacy Practices provides information about how we may use and disclose your protected health information (PHI). We encourage you to read it in full.

Our Notice of Privacy Practices is subjected to change. If we change our notice, we will provide you with the revised notice or you may obtain a copy of the revised notice by accessing our web-site at http://www.nvfha.org or contacting our organizations' customer service department at (707) 555-1212.

If you have any questions about our Notice of Privacy Practices, please contact the Privacy Officials at the medical practice you visit or the Quality Improvement Department at (707) 555-1212.

. . . .

I acknowledge receipt of the Notice of Privacy Practices of NAPA VALLEY FAMILY HEALTH ASSOCIATES.

By: _James M. Smith_____   Date: __XX/XX/20XX_____
       (Patient/Legal Representative's Signature)

Name: __James M. Smith_____
                    (Please Print)

If legal representative give relationship: _____

Inability to Obtain Signature	Date: _____
Why: _____	
_____	
Provider Representative: _____ (Print)	Provider Rep Signature: _____

Source Document 3-3

Patient Registration Form

NVFHA

Patient's Last Name	First (legal name)	First (Preferred name)	Middle Name
Perrisi	Rachelle		M

Address (Number, Street, Apt #)	City	State	Zip Code
254 Chardonnay	Sonoma	CA	95476

Mail will be sent to the address listed above, unless patient indicates a different address (leave blank if same as above)

Send mail to Address (Number, Street, Apt #)	City	State	Zip Code

Phone Options	Phone Number	Okay to leave detailed message	Call this number (circle one)
Home	(707) 833 - 0087	Yes __X__ No _____	(1st) 2nd 3rd choice
Cell	( ) -	Yes ____ No _____	1st 2nd 3rd choice
Work	(707) 299 - 4900	Yes ____ No __X__	1st (2nd) 3rd choice

Would you like to communicate by Email Yes _X_ No __   Email Address   rmperrisi@email.com

Date of Birth	Gender	Social Security Number
11/17/1986	Female __X__ Male ____	000-00-9109

Marital Status (*circle one*)	What is your preferred language / secondary language
Single / Married /(Divorced)/ Widow /Partner	English/Farsi

Race (*circle one*)	Ethnicity (*circle one*)
African American-Black / Asian / Bi-Multi-racial / Pacific Islander-Hawaiian / Caucasian–White / Native American Eskimo Aleut /(Decline to state)/ Other	Hispanic-Latino / Non-Hispanic-Latino / Other

Religion		Organ Donor	Yes _____	No __X__

Are you new to our practice	Who referred you to our practice	Who is your Primary Care Physician
Yes __X__ No _____	Richard Shinaman	Anthony Brockton

Additional Notes

Emergency Contact

Emergency Contact's Name	Relationship to patient	Phone
Amir Perrisi	Brother	(707) 555 - 2334

On-Line Patient Portal Communication via Email

On-Line communication is used for non-urgent message/requests only. NVFHA uses secure technology to protect the privacy and confidentiality of your personal information. Only you, your physician, and authorized staff can read your message.

What is your preferred method of communication	Phone __X__ Letter _____ Patient Portal _____

Insurance Information

Subscriber (Insurance Holder) Name	Date of Birth	Relationship to patient	Subscriber Phone Numeber
Self	/ /		( )

Health Plan Information	Primary Health Plan	Secondary Health Plan
Health Plan Name	Blue Shield Cengage	
Health Plan Address	PO Box 32245, Los Angeles, CA, 90002	
Group Number	BCBS987	
Subscriber Number	BCBS987	

Elig Date From	7/1/2009		Copay	$ 0

Patient Employer Information

Employer Name & Address (Number, Street, Apt #, City, State, Zip Code)	Employer Phone Number
The Cameros Inn, 4048 Sanoma Highway, Napa, CA 94559	(707) 299 - 4900

Occupation	Manager	Start Date	7/1/2009

Assignment of Benefits • Financial Agreement

I hereby give lifetime authorization for payment of insurance benefits to be made directly to **Napa Valley Family Health Assoc.,** and any assisting physicians, for services rendered. I understand that I am financially resposible for all charges whether or not they are covered by insurance. In the event of default, I agree to pay all costs of collection, and reasonable attorney's fees. I hereby authorize this healthcare provider to release all information necessary to secure the the payment of benefits.

I further agree that a photocopy of this agreement shall be as vaild as the original.

Date: __XX/XX/20XX__   Your Signature: ___rachelle M. perrisi_____

Method of Payment: ■ Cash   ■ Check   ■ Credit Card

Source Document 3-4

Patient Registration Form

NVFHA

Patient's Last Name	First (legal name)	First (Preferred name)	Middle Name
Lyndsey	Jordyn		L

Address (Number, Street, Apt #)		City	State	Zip Code
Po Box 84557		Fairfield	CA	94533

Mail will be sent to the address listed above, unless patient indicates a different address (leave blank if same as above)

Send mail to Address (Number, Street, Apt #)		City	State	Zip Code

Phone Options	Phone Number	Okay to leave detailed message	Call this number (circle one)
Home	(707) 555 - 4749	Yes __X__ No _____	(1st) 2nd 3rd choice
Cell	( ) -	Yes ____ No _____	1st 2nd 3rd choice
Work	( ) -	Yes ____ No _____	1st 2nd 3rd choice

Would you like to communicate by Email	Yes _X_ No __	Email Address	jllyndsey@email.com

Date of Birth	Gender	Social Security Number
1/17/1942	Female _X_ Male ___	000-00-9118

Marital Status (*circle one*)	What is your preferred language / secondary language
Single / Married / Divorced /(Widow)/Partner	English

Race (*circle one*)		Ethnicity (*circle one*)
African American (Black)/ Asian / Bi-Multi-racial / Pacific Islander-Hawaiian / Caucasian–White / Native American Eskimo Aleut / Decline to state / Other		Hispanic-Latino / (Non-Hispanic-Latino)/ Other

Religion	Baptist	Organ Donor	Yes ___X___ No _____

Are you new to our practice	Who referred you to our practice	Who is your Primary Care Physician
Yes __X__ No _____	Amir Raman	Amir Raman

Additional Notes

Emergency Contact

Emergency Contact's Name	Relationship to patient	Phone
Janet Jones	Daughter	(510) 555 - 2246

On-Line Patient Portal Communication via Email

On-Line communication is used for non-urgent message/requests only. NVFHA uses secure technology to protect the privacy and confidentiality of your personal information. Only you, your physician, and authorized staff can read your message.

What is your preferred method of communication	Phone _X_ Letter _____ Patient Portal _____

Insurance Information

Subscriber (Insurance Holder) Name	Date of Birth	Relationship to patient	Subscriber Phone Numeber
Self	/ /		( )

Health Plan Information	Primary Health Plan	Secondary Health Plan
Health Plan Name	Medicare Cengage	
Health Plan Address	PO Box 234434, San Francisco, CA, 94134	
Group Number	CARE 1357	
Subscriber Number	CARE 1357	

Elig Date From	1/17/2007	Copay	N/A

Patient Employer Information

Employer Name & Address (Number, Street, Apt #, City, State, Zip Code)	Employer Phone Number
N/A	( )
Occupation	Start Date

Assignment of Benefits • Financial Agreement

I hereby give lifetime authorization for payment of insurance benefits to be made directly to **Napa Valley Family Health Assoc.,** and any assisting physicians, for services rendered. I understand that I am financially resposible for all charges whether or not they are covered by insurance. In the event of default, I agree to pay all costs of collection, and reasonable attorney's fees. I hereby authorize this healthcare provider to release all information necessary to secure the payment of benefits.

I further agree that a photocopy of this agreement shall be as vaild as the original.

Date: **XX/XX/20XX**   Your Signature: *Jordyn Lyndsey*

Method of Payment: ■ Cash ■ Check ■ Credit Card

Source Document 3-5

Patient Registration Form

NVFHA

Patient's Last Name	First (legal name)	First (Preferred name)	Middle Name
Riley	Justin		I

Address (Number, Street, Apt #)	City	State	Zip Code
308 Foxwood	Napa	CA	94559

Mail will be sent to the address listed above, unless patient indicates a different address (leave blank if same as above)

Send mail to Address (Number, Street, Apt #)	City	State	Zip Code

Phone Options	Phone Number	Okay to leave detailed message	Call this number (circle one)
Home	(707) 255 - 6555	Yes ____ No __X__	(1st) 2nd 3rd choice
Cell	( ) -	Yes ____ No ____	1st 2nd 3rd choice
Work	( ) -	Yes ____ No ____	1st 2nd 3rd choice

Would you like to communicate by Email	Yes __ No _X_	Email Address

Date of Birth	Gender	Social Security Number
8/31/2006	Female ____ Male _X_	000-00-9120

Marital Status (*circle one*)	What is your preferred language / secondary language
(Single) Married / Divorced / Widow /Partner	

Race (*circle one*) | **Ethnicity (*circle one*)**

African American-Black / Asian / Bi-Multi-racial / Pacific Islander-Hawaiian / Caucasian–White / Native American Eskimo Aleut / (Decline to state) / Other

Hispanic-Latino / Non-Hispanic-Latino / Other

Religion		Organ Donor	Yes _____	No _____

Are you new to our practice	Who referred you to our practice	Who is your Primary Care Physician
Yes _X_ No ____	Emily Riley	Anthony Brockton

Additional Notes

Emergency Contact

Emergency Contact's Name	Relationship to patient	Phone
Jeff Riley	Grandfather	(510) 555 - 2246

On-Line Patient Portal Communication via Email

On-Line communication is used for non-urgent message/requests only. NVFHA uses secure technology to protect the privacy and confidentiality of your personal information. Only you, your physician, and authorized staff can read your message.

What is your preferred method of communication	Phone _X_ Letter _____ Patient Portal _____

Insurance Information

Subscriber (Insurance Holder) Name	Date of Birth	Relationship to patient	Subscriber Phone Numeber
Emily D. Riley	11/1/1966	Mother	(707) 255 - 6555

Health Plan Information	Primary Health Plan	Secondary Health Plan
Health Plan Name	Century Medical PPO	
Health Plan Address	PO Box 87542, San Jose, CA, 95101	
Group Number		
Subscriber Number	CMED 2478	

Elig Date From		Copay	$ 35.00

Patient Employer Information

Employer Name & Address (Number, Street, Apt #, City, State, Zip Code)	Employer Phone Number
Emily Riley - Silverado Resort and Spa, 1600 Atlas Peak Road, Napa, CA 94558	(707) 257 - 0200
Occupation	Start Date

Assignment of Benefits • Financial Agreement

I hereby give lifetime authorization for payment of insurance benefits to be made directly to **Napa Valley Family Health Assoc.,** and any assisting physicians, for services rendered. I understand that I am financially resposible for all charges whether or not they are covered by insurance. In the event of default, I agree to pay all costs of collection, and reasonable attorney's fees. I hereby authorize this healthcare provider to release all information necessary to secure the the payment of benefits.

I further agree that a photocopy of this agreement shall be as vaild as the original.

Date: __XX/XX/20XX__   Your Signature: __Emily Riley__

Method of Payment: ■ Cash   ■ Check   ■ Credit Card

Source Document 3-6

Patient Registration Form

NVFHA

Patient's Last Name	First (legal name)	First (Preferred name)	Middle Name
Ramirez	Sonia		S

Address (Number, Street, Apt #)	City	State	Zip Code
989 Riverwood	Rio Vista	CA	94571

Mail will be sent to the address listed above, unless patient indicates a different address (leave blank if same as above)

Send mail to Address (Number, Street, Apt #)	City	State	Zip Code

Phone Options	Phone Number	Okay to leave detailed message	Call this number (circle one)
Home	(707) 555 - 8441	Yes __X__ No _____	(1st) 2nd 3rd choice
Cell	( ) -	Yes ____ No _____	1st 2nd 3rd choice
Work	(707) 253 - 5000	Yes ____ No __X__	1st (2nd) 3rd choice

Would you like to communicate by Email   Yes _X_ No __   Email Address   ssramirez@email.com

Date of Birth	Gender	Social Security Number
7/16/1986	Female _X_ Male ____	000-00-9125

Marital Status (***circle one***)	What is your preferred language / secondary language
Single / (Married) / Divorced / Widow / Partner	Spanish/English

Race (*circle one*)

African American-Black / Asian / Bi-Multi-racial / Pacific Islander-Hawaiian /
Caucasian–White / Native American Eskimo Aleut / (Decline to state) / Other

Ethnicity (*circle one*)

(Hispanic-Latino) /
Non-Hispanic-Latino / Other

Religion	Roman Catholic	Organ Donor	Yes ___X___ No _____

Are you new to our practice	Who referred you to our practice	Who is your Primary Care Physician
Yes __X__ No _____	Rebecca Ayerick	Rebecca Ayerick

Additional Notes

Emergency Contact

Emergency Contact's Name	Relationship to patient	Phone
Guadalupe Monroy	Mother	(704) 555 - 5580

On-Line Patient Portal Communication via Email

On-Line communication is used for non-urgent message/requests only. NVFHA uses secure technology to protect the privacy and confidentiality of your personal information. Only you, your physician, and authorized staff can read your message.

What is your preferred method of communication   Phone _X_   Letter _____   Patient Portal _____

Insurance Information

Subscriber (Insurance Holder) Name	Date of Birth	Relationship to patient	Subscriber Phone Numeber
Hector Ramirez	4/14/1980	Husband	(707) 555 - 8441

Health Plan Information	Primary Health Plan	Secondary Health Plan
Health Plan Name	Century Medical PPO	
Health Plan Address	PO Box 87542, San Jose, CA, 95101	
Group Number	CMED 2478	
Subscriber Number	CMED 2478	

Elig Date From	1/1/2011	Copay	$ 25.00

Patient Employer Information

Employer Name & Address (Number, Street, Apt #, City, State, Zip Code)	Employer Phone Number
The Carneros Inn, 4048 Sonoma Hloy, Napa, CA94559	(707) 253 - 5000
Occupation Admin	Start Date

Assignment of Benefits • Financial Agreement

I hereby give lifetime authorization for payment of insurance benefits to be made directly to <u>Napa Valley Family Health Assoc.,</u> and any assisting physicians, for services rendered. I understand that I am financially resposible for all charges whether or not they are covered by insurance. In the event of default, I agree to pay all costs of collection, and reasonable attorney's fees. I hereby authorize this healthcare provider to release all information necessary to secure the the payment of benefits.

I further agree that a photocopy of this agreement shall be as vaild as the original.

Date: __XX/XX/20XX__   Your Signature: *Sonia Ramirez* _____

Method of Payment: ■ Cash   ■ Check   ■ Credit Card

Case Study 6-2 Information Packet

PATIENT'S NAME: Adam Thompson

DATE OF BIRTH: 01/01/1942

PROVIDER: Dr. Anthony Brockton

MEDICATIONS

Mr. Thompson is currently taking all of the medications listed in the following table. Leave the Rx *Start Date* and *End Date* boxes blank, as well as the *Original Date*.

Medication	Strength	Directions
Norvasc Oral	5mg	Sig 1 tab per day
Isopto® Carpine Ophthalmic Solution	2%	Sig 2 drops in each eye twice a day
Prevacid Solutab Oral Tablets Dispersib	15 mg/bid	Sig 1 tab twice a day

ALLERGIES

Confirm No Known Allergies

IMMUNIZATIONS

Category	Entry
Immunization	Influenza, seasonal, injectable
Admin Date	09/15/Last Year
Administration Notes	Administration Location: Walgreens on South Central Blvd.

Note: Leave all other sections blank.

VITAL SIGNS

Category	Entry
Height	6 ft 2 in
Weight	195 Pounds
Body Mass Index	Automatically populates after entering height and weight
LMP	N/A
Blood Pressure	168/78
Pulse Rate	95 bpm
Temperature	101° F
Respiratory Rate	26

Pulse Oximetry	94%
Pain Level	N/A
Head Circumference	N/A
Length	N/A
Chief Complaint	Cough x 2 weeks

HISTORY

Patient History

First, using the patient history information listed in Source Document 6-1A (found on page 627), enter Mr. Thompson's information in the *History* module of his medical record. Then, for any "Yes" responses entered in the *General Medical History* section, you will need to add additional information to each corresponding *Finding Details* box. The following table provides you with the detailed information that Mr. Thompson gave when questioning him regarding the "Yes" responses. (**Hint:** The *Patient History* tab should be highlighted at the top of the *History* window when entering the information from Source Document 6-1A.)

Disease	Entry in Finding Details Box
Cardiovascular Disease	The patient has a past medical history of a Cardiac pacemaker placed in 2011 for a third-degree complete heart block. He reports no problems with his pacer.
Gastric Ulcer	Positive for H Pylori. Treated with ATBs. No further issues.
GERD	10-Year History of GERD. Treatment PPIs. Well controlled.
Hypertension	15-Year History of Hypertension. Treated with Norvasc. Patient states it is usually well controlled.
Osteoarthritis	Mild osteoarthritis of head and neck. Reports occasional Tylenol or Advil use, less than once per week.

Sensitive Information

Using the information listed in Source Document 6-1B (found on page 629), enter Mr. Thompson's sensitive information in the *History* module of his medical record. (**Hint:** The *Sensitive Info* tab should be highlighted at the top of the *History* window when entering the information from Source Document 6-1B.)

Family History Information

First, using the information listed in Source Document 6-1C (found on page 629), enter Mr. Thompson's family history information in the *History* module of his medical record. Then, for any "Yes" responses entered in the *General Family History* section, you will need to add additional information to each corresponding *Finding Details* box. The following table provides you with the detailed information that Mr. Thompson gave when questioning him regarding the "Yes" responses. (**Hint:** The *Family History* tab should be highlighted at the top of the *History* window when entering the information from Source Document 6-1C.)

Disease	Entry in Finding Details Box
Asthma	Mother and brother
Cardiovascular Disease	Father and brother
COPD	Mother
Diabetes	Aunt and maternal grandfather
Hypertension	Mother, father, brother, and sister
Stroke	Father died of stroke at age 78
Cancer	Mother; Comment: Mother died of lung cancer at the age of 66.

PROGRESS NOTE

Template: IM OV Option 4 (v4) w/A&P (**Note:** If the template you need is not listed on the *Template* drop-down, click on the *Search* icon to the left of the *Save* button. In the pop-up window, enter "IM OV Option 4 (v4)" in the *Template* field and click the *Search* button. Click the [+] sign to the left of *Internal Medicine* and select "IM OV Option 4 (v4) w/A&P". This will add the template to your progress note.)

Using the information in the following table, complete the progress note for your provider.

Tab	Entry
CC/HPI	*Chief Complaint:* Select "Cough".
	History of Present Illness: Here today for cough that started ten days ago. It is now worse. He reports he has shortness of breath with moving around the house. The shortness of breath is a new symptom as of a few days ago. He thinks he might have a fever because he has been chilling and shivering.
History	*Reviewed:* Select Medication List Reviewed, Allergy List Reviewed, Past Medical History Reviewed, Social History Reviewed, Family History Reviewed.
ROS	*Constitutional:* "Y" for fever, chills; "N" for headache.
	Other constitutional symptoms: He reports he is feeling "poorly."
	Eyes: No eye symptoms
	ENMT: "Y" for nasal congestion and nasal discharge
	Respiratory: "Y" for shortness of breath, difficulty breathing, and coughing up sputum
	Cardiovascular: No cardiovascular symptoms
	Gastrointestinal: No GI Symptoms
	Genitourinary: No GU Symptoms
PE	*General:* Well developed and well nourished
	HEENT/ENT/Ears: "N" for all responses
	HEENT/ENT/Nose: "Y" for rhinorrhea
	HEENT/ENT/Pharynx: "Y" for oropharyngeal exudate
	Other ENT Findings: Rhinorrhea (yellow discharge), No tonsils present
	Lymphatics: "N" for cervical adenopathy
	Chest: "N" for chest wall tenderness
	Heart: "Y" for S1, S2 and tachycardia
	Other Heart Findings: Mild tachycardia, Regular rhythms, S1, S2.
	Other Abdomen Findings: Normal gastrointestinal exam
Assessment	*Diagnosis:* Bilateral Pneumonia (J18.9)
Plan	*Additional Plan Details:* 1. CXR 2. CBC with diff, lytes 3. EKG 4. Ibuprofen 800 mg oral now and instruct for every six hours while awake 5. Return visit in one day 6. Seek treatment in the ED if symptoms worsen 7. Zithromax Z-Pack one as directed

Directions:

The source documents below represent what each section of the patient *History* module will look like on the printed patient history report forms. These source documents will look different from your *History* screen as you are entering information. Your goal is to make certain that anything that is highlighted in these documents is entered into the correct section of the *History* screen. Leave everything else blank. (**Hint:** For those sections where you must enter a "yes" or "no," a check mark indicates "yes" and an X indicates "no.")

Adam Thompson DOB: 1/1/1942

Source Document 6-1A: Patient History

Reviewed

✔ Medication List Reviewed		✔ Past Medical History Reviewed	
✔ Allergy List Reviewed		✔ Social History Reviewed	
☐ Problem List Reviewed		✔ Family History Reviewed	
☐ Denies significant past history.		☐ No recent change in medical history.	

GENERAL MEDICAL HISTORY

☐ Alcoholism	☐ Depression	☐ Kidney Infections
☐ Allergies/Hayfever	☐ DM Type 1	☐ Kidney stone
☐ Anemia	☐ DM Type 2	☐ Migraine
☐ Anxiety	☐ Epilepsy	☐ Multiple Sclerosis
☐ Asthma	☐ Fracture	☐ Obesity
☐ Atrial Fibrillation	✔ Gastric ulcer	☐ Old MI
☐ Blood Transfusions	☐ Gastrointestinal Disease	✔ Osteoarthritis
☐ CAD	✔ GERD	☐ Osteoporosis
☐ Cancer	☐ Gestational Diabetes	☐ Pneumonia
☐ Cardiac Pacer	☐ Glaucoma	☐ Progressive Neurological Disorder
✔ Cardiovascular Disease	☐ Heart Murmur	☐ Pulmonary Disease
☐ CHF	☐ Hepatitis	☐ Rheumatic Fever
☐ Cirrhosis	☐ High Cholesterol	☐ Rheumatoid Arthritis
☐ Colitis	☐ Hyperlipidemia	☐ STD
☐ COPD	✔ Hypertension	☐ Terminal Illness
☐ CRF	☐ Hyperthyroidism	☐ Thyroid Disease
☐ Crohn's disease	☐ Hypothyroidism	☐ TIA
☐ CVA	☐ Joint Pain	☐ Tuberculosis

HOSPITALIZATIONS Cardiac Pacemaker Placement 02/15/2011. Overnight stay at Napa Valley Medical Center. No complications

OTHER MEDICAL HISTORY

Tobacco Assessment

This section supports Stage 1 Meaningful Use
Smoking Status   Former smoker

☐ Tobacco User

pack-years **20**

Date quit smoking **03/14/1990**

☐ Counseling on tobacco cessation
☐ Rx therapy for tobacco cessation
☐ Discussed Smoking/Tobacco Use Cessation Strategies

Social History

Alcohol Use Occasional	Educational level
Caffeine Use 2 servings per Day	Marital Status
☒ Drug Use	Exercise Habits
☒ sun protection	✔ seatbelts
☒ Tattoos	☐ Body piercings
☒ sexually active	birth control method
Race	Birth Control Device insertion date
Native language	Birth Control Device removal date
☐ physical abuse	Religion
☐ domestic violence	Occupation
Other Social History	

Depression Screening

☐ Patient Refused
Little interest or pleasure in doing things
Feeling down, depressed, or hopeless

Date of Last Depression Screening/PHQ-2
PHQ-2 Score **PHQ2 Score: incomplete**

OB/GYN HISTORY

LMP
Frequency of menstrual cycle
☐ Menopause has occurred
☐ History of abnormal pap smears
☐ Sexually Active

☐ ectopic pregnancy
PREGNANCY SUMMARY
Gravida
Term
Preterm
AB
Live children
OTHER OB-GYN HISTORY

Menarche Age
Days menstrual cycle

Birth Control
Birth Control Device insertion date
Birth Control Device removal date

Miscarriage
Elective Abortion
C-Section:

SURGICAL / PROCEDURAL

☐ No prior surgical history
☐ Appendectomy
☐ Breast Lumpectomy
☐ Cataract Surgery
☐ Colectomy
☐ Cone Biopsy
☐ D&C
OTHER SURGICAL
HISTORY

☐ Endometrial Ablation
☐ Gall Bladder
☐ Heart Surgery
☐ Hemorrhoids
☐ Hernia
☐ Hysterectomy

Cardiac Pacemaker in 2011

☐ Laparoscopy
Mastectomy
☐ Myomectomy
☐ Oophorectomy
☐ Tonsil/Adenoidectomy
☐ Tubal Ligation

PREVENTIVE CARE

A1c %
Air Contrast Barium Enema
Ankle Brachial Index
Blood Glucose
Bone Density
Chest X-Ray
Chlamydia Screening
Colonoscopy   10/01/2008
Dilated Eye Exam
DTaP Vaccine (90700)
Echocardiogram
Electrocardiogram
Flexible Sigmoidoscopy
Flu vaccine   09/15/2013
Foot Exam Date
HIV Test Date:

Self-Management Goal

HPV Test
HPV Vaccine
Last Complete Physical Exam
Lipids
Mammography
Pap Smear
Pneumovax
PSA
Pulmonary Function Tests
Routine Eye Exam
Stool Occult Blood   05/10/2010
Stress Test   10/10/2013
Td
Tdap Vaccine, Adult
Tuberculin PPD
Varicella
Zoster Vaccine (90736)   03/22/2007

Adam Thompson DOB: 1/1/1942

Source Document 6-1B: Sensitive Information

STD

☒ Vaginosis	☒ Gonorrhea
☒ Trichomonas	☒ Chlamydia
☒ Genital Warts	☒ Syphillis
☒ PID	☒ HPV
STD Info	

SUBSTANCE ABUSE

☒ History of Substance Abuse
Abused Substances

MENTAL HEALTH

☒ Seeing mental health provider
Mental Health Provider Name
Mental Health Condition(s)

HIV Status

HIV Status
HIV Test Date
HIV Notes

Medicare High Risk Criteria

Age when became sexually active
☐ More than 5 sexual partners in lifetime
☐ DES history in mother
Pap Smear
☐ History of abnormal pap smears

Courtesy of Harris CareTracker PM and EMR

Adam Thompson DOB: 1/1/1942

Source Document 6-1C: Family History

GENERAL FAMILY HISTORY

☐ Adopted	☐ Denial of any knowledge of significant family history	
☐ Unknown Paternal Hx	☐ Unknown Maternal Hx	
☐ Alcoholism	☐ Congenital Anomaly	☑ Hypertension
☐ Anemia	☑ COPD	☐ Hypothyroidism
☐ Anxiety	☐ Crohn's Disease	☐ Kidney Disease
☑ Asthma	☐ Depression	☐ Liver Disease
☐ Birth Defects	☑ Diabetes	☐ Multiple Births
☐ CAD	☐ Epilepsy	☐ Osteoarthritis
☑ Cardiovascular Disease	☐ GERD	☐ Osteoporosis
☐ CHF	☐ Hypercholesterolemia	☐ Pulmonary Disease
Cancer lung	☐ Hyperlipidemia	☑ Stroke
Other conditions		

Courtesy of Harris CareTracker PM and EMR

Case Study 6-3 Information Packet

PATIENT'S NAME: Barbara Watson

DATE OF BIRTH: 02/18/1951

PROVIDER: Dr. Amir Raman

MEDICATIONS:

Ms. Watson is currently taking the medication listed in the following table. Leave the Rx *Start Date* and *End Date* boxes blank, as well as the *Original Date*.

Medication	Strength	Directions	Override Reason
Boniva Oral Tablet	150 mg	Take 1 tab every month	Benefit outweighs risk

ALLERGIES

Confirm No Known Allergies

IMMUNIZATIONS

Skip this section

VITAL SIGNS

Category	Entry
Height	5 ft 10 in
Weight	135 Pounds
Body Mass Index	Automatically populates after entering height and weight
LMP	N/A
Blood Pressure	122/78
Pulse Rate	66 bpm
Temperature	98.2° F
Respiratory Rate	16
Pulse Oximetry	98%
Pain Level	0/10
Head Circumference	N/A
Length	N/A

HISTORY

Patient History

First, using the patient history information listed in Source Document 6-2A (found on page 632), enter Ms. Watson's information in the *History* module of her medical record. Then, for any "Yes" responses, you will need to add additional information to each corresponding *Finding Details* box. The following table provides you with the detailed information that Ms. Watson gave when questioning her regarding the "Yes" responses. (**Hint:** The *Patient History* tab should be highlighted at the top of the *History* window when entering the information from Source Document 6-2A.)

Section	Entry in Finding Details Box
General Medical History *Osteoporosis*	Diagnosed in 2010; Taking Boniva (Once/Month)
OB-GYN History *Menopause has occurred*	Full menopause at the age of 46

Sensitive Information

Using the information listed in Source Document 6-2B (found on page 634), enter Ms. Watson's sensitive information in the *History* module of her medical record. (**Hint:** The *Sensitive Info* tab should be highlighted at the top of the *History* window when entering the information from Source Document 6-2B.)

PROGRESS NOTE

Template: IM OV Option 4 (v4) w/A&P

Using the information in the following table, complete the progress note for your provider.

Tab	Entry
CC/HPI	CC: Fever x two days
	History of Present Illness: Patient states that she ran a fever the last two days that ranged between 100.0° F–101.0° F. She denies any other symptoms and states that this morning her fever was gone.
History	*Reviewed*: Select Medication List Reviewed, Allergy List Reviewed, Past Medical History Reviewed, Social History Reviewed.
ROS	*Constitutional*: "Y" for fever; "N" for chills and headache.
	Other constitutional symptoms: Had fever for two days but the fever is gone today.
	Eyes: No eye symptoms
	ENMT: No ENT symptoms
	Neck: No neck symptoms
	Respiratory: No respiratory symptoms
	Cardiovascular: No cardiovascular symptoms
	Gastrointestinal: No GI Symptoms
	Genitourinary: No GU Symptoms
PE	*General*: Awake; alert; oriented to time, place, and person; general appearance normal; well developed and well nourished
	HEENT/Head: Other head findings; normal head exam
	HEENT/ENT/: Other ENT Findings; normal ENT Findings exam
	Neck: Other neck findings; normal neck exam
	Lymphatics: Other lymph node findings; normal lymph node exam
	Chest: Other lung findings; normal lung exam
	Heart: Other heart findings; normal heart exam
	Other Abdomen Findings: normal abdominal exam
Assessment	Diagnosis: Fever, unspecified (R50.9)
Plan	*Additional Plan Details*:
	1. Patient appears to be healthy overall.
	2. Instructed patient to call back if symptoms return

Directions:

The source documents below represent what each section of the patient *History* module will look like on the printed patient history report forms. These source documents will look different from your *History* screen as you are entering information. Your goal is to make certain that anything that is highlighted in these documents is entered into the correct section of the *History* screen. Leave everything else blank. **Hint:** For those sections where you must enter a "yes" or "no," a check mark indicates "yes" and an X indicates "no."

Barbara Watson DOB: 2/18/1951

Source Document 6-2A: Patient History

Reviewed

✔	Medication List Reviewed	✔	Past Medical History Reviewed
✔	Allergy List Reviewed	✔	Social History Reviewed
☐	Problem List Reviewed	☐	Family History Reviewed
☐	Denies significant past history.	☐	No recent change in medical history.

GENERAL MEDICAL HISTORY

☐ Alcoholism	☐ Depression	☐ Kidney Infections
☐ Allergies/Hayfever	☐ DM Type 1	☐ Kidney stone
☐ Anemia	☐ DM Type 2	☐ Migraine
☐ Anxiety	☐ Epilepsy	☐ Multiple Sclerosis
☐ Asthma	☐ Fracture	☐ Obesity
☐ Atrial Fibrillation	☐ Gastric ulcer	☐ Old MI
☐ Blood Transfusions	☐ Gastrointestinal Disease	☐ Osteoarthritis
☐ CAD	☐ GERD	✔ Osteoporosis
☐ Cancer	☐ Gestational Diabetes	☐ Pneumonia
☐ Cardiac Pacer	☐ Glaucoma	☐ Progressive Neurological Disorder
☐ Cardiovascular Disease	☐ Heart Murmur	☐ Pulmonary Disease
☐ CHF	☐ Hepatitis	☐ Rheumatic Fever
☐ Cirrhosis	☐ High Cholesterol	☐ Rheumatoid Arthritis
☐ Colitis	☐ Hyperlipidemia	☐ STD
☐ COPD	☐ Hypertension	☐ Terminal Illness
☐ CRF	☐ Hyperthyroidism	☐ Thyroid Disease
☐ Crohn's disease	☐ Hypothyroidism	☐ TIA
☐ CVA	☐ Joint Pain	☐ Tuberculosis

HOSPITALIZATIONS None

OTHER MEDICAL HISTORY None

Tobacco Assessment

This section supports Stage 1 Meaningful Use

Smoking Status Never smoker

pack-years

☐ Counseling on tobacco cessation
☐ Rx therapy for tobacco cessation
☐ Discussed Smoking/Tobacco Use Cessation Strategies

☐ Tobacco User

Date quit smoking

Social History

Alcohol Use Non-Drinker
Caffeine Use 1 serving per day
☒ Drug Use
☒ sun protection
☒ Tattoos
☒ sexually active
Race African American
Native language
☒ physical abuse
☒ domestic violence
Other Social History

Educational level
Marital Status Divorced
Exercise Habits   moderate >3 x/wk
✔ seatbelts
☐ Body piercings
birth control method
Birth Control Device insertion date
Birth Control Device removal date
Religion Jehovah's Witness
Occupation

Depression Screening

☐ Patient Refused
Little interest or pleasure in doing things
Feeling down, depressed, or hopeless

Date of Last Depression Screening/PHQ-2
PHQ-2 Score **PHQ2 Score: incomplete**

OB/GYN HISTORY

LMP   Menarche Age **12**

Frequency of menstrual cycle   Days menstrual cycle

[✔] Menopause has occurred

[ ] History of abnormal pap smears

[✗] Sexually Active   Birth Control

                                                            Birth Control Device insertion date
[ ] ectopic pregnancy   Birth Control Device removal date

PREGNANCY SUMMARY

Gravida 0

Term

Preterm   Miscarriage

AB   Elective Abortion

Live children   C-Section:

OTHER OB-GYN HISTORY ···

SURGICAL / PROCEDURAL

[ ] No prior surgical history

[ ] Appendectomy   [ ] Endometrial Ablation   [ ] Laparoscopy

[ ] Breast Lumpectomy   [ ] Gall Bladder   Mastectomy

[ ] Cataract Surgery   [ ] Heart Surgery   [ ] Myomectomy

[ ] Colectomy   [ ] Hemorrhoids   [ ] Oophorectomy

[ ] Cone Biopsy   [ ] Hernia   [✔] Tonsil/Adenoidectomy

[ ] D&C   [ ] Hysterectomy   [ ] Tubal Ligation

OTHER SURGICAL
HISTORY ···

PREVENTIVE CARE

A1c %	HPV Test
Air Contrast Barium Enema	HPV Vaccine
Ankle Brachial Index	Last Complete Physical Exam
Blood Glucose	Lipids
Bone Density 06/04/2013	Mammography 06/04/2013
Chest X-Ray	Pap Smear 02/05/2013
Chlamydia Screening	Pneumovax
Colonoscopy 10/13/2011	PSA
Dilated Eye Exam 05/27/2013	Pulmonary Function Tests
DTaP Vaccine (90700)	Routine Eye Exam
Echocardiogram	Stool Occult Blood
Electrocardiogram	Stress Test
Flexible Sigmoidoscopy	Td
Flu vaccine	Tdap Vaccine, Adult
Foot Exam Date	Tuberculin PPD
HIV Test Date:	Varicella
	Zoster Vaccine (90736)
Self-Management Goal	

Barbara Watson DOB: 2/18/1951

Source Document 6-2B: Sensitive Information

STD

☒ Vaginosis		☒ Gonorrhea	
☒ Trichomonas		☒ Chlamydia	
☒ Genital Warts		☒ Syphillis	
☒ PID		☒ HPV	

STD Info

SUBSTANCE ABUSE

☒ History of Substance Abuse

Abused Substances

MENTAL HEALTH

☒ Seeing mental health provider

Mental Health Provider Name

Mental Health Condition(s)

HIV Status

HIV Status   Negative

HIV Test Date

HIV Notes

Medicare High Risk Criteria

Age when became sexually active
☐ More than 5 sexual partners in lifetime
☐ DES history in mother
Pap Smear
☐ History of abnormal pap smears

Case Study 6-4 Information Packet

PATIENT'S NAME: Craig X. Smith

DATE OF BIRTH: 01/06/2012

PROVIDER: Dr. Amir Raman

ALLERGIES:

Confirm No Known Allergies

VITAL SIGNS:

Category	Entry
Height	NA
Weight	26 lbs 6 oz
Body Mass Index	Automatically populates after entering height and weight
LMP	N/A
Blood Pressure	92/62
Pulse Rate	110 bpm
Temperature	100.6° F
Respiratory Rate	40
Pulse Oximetry	93%
Pain Level	N/A
Head Circumference	N/A
Length	32.8"

PROGRESS NOTE:

Template: Pediatric OV Option 1 (v1) (**Note:** If the template you need is not listed on the *Template* drop-down, click on the *Search* icon to the left of the *Save* button. In the pop-up window, enter "Pediatric OV Option 1" in the *Template* field and click the *Search* button. Click the [+] sign to the left of *Pediatrics* and select "Pediatric OV Option 1 (v1)". This will add the template to your progress note.)

Using the information in the following table, complete the progress note for your provider.

OV Tab Field	Entry
Chief Complaint	Wheezing x 3 days
History of Present Illness	Patient's mother states that he has had a cold for the past 3 days. She noticed he was "breathing funny" this morning and coughing a lot. She states that his temperature at home was 102 degrees F and she gave him Tylenol an hour before the visit.
Past Medical/Social/ Family History	Other past medical history includes 36-week gestation, mother had elevated blood pressure, no preeclampsia. C-section (failure to progress). Apgars 8 at one minute, 9 at 5 minutes. Infant went home with mom at time of her discharge.

Review of Systems	*General*: fever, loss of appetite
	Ears, nose and throat: nasal congestion clear in appearance
	Respiratory: coughing up thick yellow mucus at times
	Otherwise normal review of systems
Physical Examination	*General*: Awake, well developed
	Ears, Nose, and Throat: oropharyngeal exudate; yellow discharge in oropharynx
	Respiratory: Wheezing over all lung fields, mild intercostal retractions, no grunting or nasal flaring. RR is increased, mild respiratory distress. SaO_2 initial reading was 93%, now reading 96-98% with activity during exam.
	Cardiovascular: Mild tachycardia at 100's, regular rate, peripheral pulses normal
	Genitourinary: Mother reports normally wet diapers last night and today
	Skin: Warm and dry to touch
Tests	Leave Blank
Procedure Note	Leave Blank
Assessment	1. Wheezing (R06.2)
	2. Mild respiratory distress (J98.9)
Plan	1. Isoetharine HCL, Inhalation A (STAT)
	2. Albuterol Sulfate Inhalation Nebulization Solution (2.5 mg/mL) 0.083%, sig 1 ampoule every 6 hours (q6h) as needed, Rx quantity 8, Refills: None
	3. Recheck in 24 hours
	4. Chest X-ray PA & Lat

Case Study 6-5 Information Packet

PATIENT'S NAME: Ellen Ristino

DATE OF BIRTH: 11/01/1956

PROVIDER: Dr. Anthony Brockton

MEDICATIONS

Mrs. Ristino is currently taking the medications listed in the following table. Leave the Rx *Start Date* and *End Date* boxes blank, as well as the *Original Date*.

Medication	Strength	Directions	Override Reason
Lipitor	20 mg	Sig 1 tab per day	Benefit outweighs risk

ALLERGIES

Allergy Source	Reaction	Reported Start Date	Reported End Date
Peanuts	Anaphylaxis	10/30/2008	N/A

IMMUNIZATIONS

Leave the Immunization section blank

VITAL SIGNS

Category	Entry
Height	5 ft 9 in
Weight	165 Pounds
Body Mass Index	Automatically populates after entering height and weight
LMP	N/A
Blood Pressure	130/75
Pulse Rate	84 bpm
Temperature	100.8° F
Respiratory Rate	16
Pulse Oximetry	96%
Pain Level	N/A
Head Circumference	N/A
Length	N/A
Chief Complaint	Nasal congestion and sore throat

HISTORY

Patient History

First, using the patient history information listed in Source Document 6-3A (found on page 640), enter Mrs. Ristino's information in the *History* module of her medical record. Then, for any "Yes" responses entered, you will need to add additional information to each corresponding *Finding Details* box. The following table provides you with the detailed information that Mrs. Ristino gave when questioning her regarding the "Yes" responses. (**Hint:** The *Patient History* tab should be highlighted at the top of the *History* window when entering the information from Source Document 6-3A.)

Section	Entry in Finding Details Box
General Medical Information	
High Cholesterol	The patient has a medical history of high cholesterol lasting 5 years. States she has been on high cholesterol meds for the past 5 years.
Osteoarthritis	Patient states she has mild arthritis which does not affect her in her daily life.
Social History	
Sun Protection	*Type*: Sunglasses, sunscreen, and hats SPF: 30
OB-GYN	
Menopause has occurred	Patient states full menopause occurred at age 52
Surgical Procedure	
Appendectomy	Emergency appendectomy at age 22. No complications.
Breast Lumpectomy	*Location*: Left August 2011: History of microcalcifications. Biopsy negative for cancer.

Sensitive Information

Leave this section blank

Family History Information

First, using the information listed in Source Document 6-3B (found on page 641), enter Mrs. Ristino's family history information in the *History* module of her medical record. Then, for any "Yes" responses entered in the *General Family History* section, you will need to add additional information to each corresponding *Finding Details* box. The following table provides you with the detailed information that Mrs. Ristino gave when questioning her regarding the "Yes" responses. (**Hint:** The *Family History* tab should be highlighted at the top of the *History* window when entering the information from Source Document 6-3B.)

Disease	Entry in Finding Details Box
Cardiovascular Disease	Father and aunt
COPD	Father and brother
Hypertension	Mother, father, aunt, and brother

PROGRESS NOTE

Template: IM OV Option 4 (v4) w/A&P (**Note:** If the template you need is not listed on the *Template* drop-down, click on the *Search* icon to the left of the *Save* button. In the pop-up window, enter "IM OV Option 4 (v4)" in the *Template* field and click the *Search* button. Click the [+] sign to the left of *Internal Medicine* and select "IM OV Option 4 (v4) w/A&P". This will add the template to your progress note.)

Using the information in the following table, complete the progress note for your provider.

Tab	Entry
CC/HPI	*Chief Complaint:* Select "Sore Throat" *History of Present Illness:* Complaining of sore throat which started two days ago and now is worse. Denies difficulty with swallowing, only pain. Nose is stuffy and generally "does not feel good."
History	*Reviewed:* Select Medication List Reviewed, Allergy List Reviewed, Past Medical History Reviewed, Social History Reviewed, Family History Reviewed.
ROS	*Constitutional:* "Y" for fever; "N" for chills; "N" for headache. *Eyes:* No eye symptoms *ENMT:* "Y" for nasal congestion, nasal discharge and sore throat; "N" for earache, tinnitus and dysphagia. *Respiratory:* "Y" for cough and coughing up sputum; "N" for the remainder of categories under this heading. *Cardiovascular:* No cardiovascular symptoms
PE	*General:* Well developed and well nourished *HEENT/ENT/Ears:* "Y" Serous exudate of TM and retraction of TM; "N" for all other responses in the ear category *HEENT/ENT/Nose:* "Y" for rhinorrhea *HEENT/ENT/Pharynx:* "Y" for oropharyngeal exudate and pharyngeal inflammation; "N" for oropharyngeal hemorrhage *Lymphatics:* "Y" for cervical adenopathy; "N" for axillary adenopathy and tenderness *Lungs:* "Y" for rhonchi; "N" for all other categories in this section *Heart:* Negative heart exam
Assessment	*Diagnosis:* Select "Acute Upper Respiratory Infection (J06.9)" and "Acute Pharyngitis (J02.9)"
Plan	*Additional Plan Details:* 1. Rapid Strep test 2. CBC with diff 3. Mono spot with EBV titer if negative 4. Ibuprofen 800 mg every 6 hours 5. Increase fluids 6. Return in 5 days if symptoms do not improve 7. Schedule routine preventative care visit for follow-up 8. Call patient with lab results

Directions:
The source documents below represent what each section of the patient *History* module will look like on the printed patient history report forms. These source documents will look different from your *History* screen as you are entering information. Your goal is to make certain that anything that is highlighted in these documents is entered into the correct section of the *History* screen. Leave everything else blank. (**Hint:** For those sections where you must enter a "yes" or "no," a check mark indicates "yes" and an X indicates "no.")

Ellen Ristino DOB: 11/1/1956

Source Document 6-3A: Patient History

Reviewed

☑ Medication List Reviewed	☑ Past Medical History Reviewed
☑ Allergy List Reviewed	☑ Social History Reviewed
☐ Problem List Reviewed	☑ Family History Reviewed
☐ Denies significant past history.	☐ No recent change in medical history.

GENERAL MEDICAL HISTORY

☐ Alcoholism	☐ Depression	☐ Kidney Infections
☐ Allergies/Hayfever	☐ DM Type 1	☐ Kidney stone
☐ Anemia	☐ DM Type 2	☐ Migraine
☐ Anxiety	☐ Epilepsy	☐ Multiple Sclerosis
☐ Asthma	☐ Fracture	☐ Obesity
☐ Atrial Fibrillation	☐ Gastric ulcer	☐ Old MI
☐ Blood Transfusions	☐ Gastrointestinal Disease	☑ Osteoarthritis
☐ CAD	☐ GERD	☐ Osteoporosis
☐ Cancer	☐ Gestational Diabetes	☐ Pneumonia
☐ Cardiac Pacer	☐ Glaucoma	☐ Progressive Neurological Disorder
☐ Cardiovascular Disease	☐ Heart Murmur	☐ Pulmonary Disease
☐ CHF	☐ Hepatitis	☐ Rheumatic Fever
☐ Cirrhosis	☑ High Cholesterol	☐ Rheumatoid Arthritis
☐ Colitis	☐ Hyperlipidemia	☐ STD
☐ COPD	☐ Hypertension	☐ Terminal Illness
☐ CRF	☐ Hyperthyroidism	☐ Thyroid Disease
☐ Crohn's disease	☐ Hypothyroidism	☐ TIA
☐ CVA	☐ Joint Pain	☐ Tuberculosis

HOSPITALIZATIONS
OTHER MEDICAL
HISTORY

Tobacco Assessment

This section supports Stage 1 Meaningful Use
Smoking Status   Former smoker

pack-years **28**

☐ Counseling on tobacco cessation
☐ Rx therapy for tobacco cessation
☐ Discussed Smoking/Tobacco Use Cessation Strategies

☐ Tobacco User
Date quit smoking **10/01/2005**

Social History

Alcohol Use Occasional	Educational level Junior College
Caffeine Use 2 servings per Day	Marital Status Married
☒ Drug Use	Exercise Habits moderate <3 x/wk
☑ sun protection	☑ seatbelts
☒ Tattoos	☒ Body piercings
☑ sexually active	birth control method
Race Caucasian	Birth Control Device insertion date
Native language	Birth Control Device removal date
☒ physical abuse	Religion None
☒ domestic violence	Occupation **Registration Supervisor**
Other Social History	

Depression Screening

☐ Patient Refused
Little interest or pleasure in doing things
Feeling down, depressed, or hopeless

Date of Last Depression Screening/PHQ-2
PHQ-2 Score **PHQ2 Score: incomplete**

OB/GYN HISTORY

LMP

Frequency of menstrual cycle

☑ Menopause has occurred

☐ History of abnormal pap smears

☑ Sexually Active

☐ ectopic pregnancy

PREGNANCY SUMMARY

Gravida 4

Term 3

Preterm 1

AB 0

Live children 4

OTHER OB-GYN HISTORY Tubal ligation at age 32

Menarche Age **14**

Days menstrual cycle

Birth Control

Birth Control Device insertion date

Birth Control Device removal date

Miscarriage 0

Elective Abortion 0

C-Section: 0

SURGICAL / PROCEDURAL

☐ No prior surgical history

☑ Appendectomy

☑   Breast Lumpectomy

Location:

left

☐ Cataract Surgery

☐ Colectomy

☐ Cone Biopsy

☐ D&C

OTHER SURGICAL

HISTORY

☐ Endometrial Ablation

☐ Gall Bladder

☐ Heart Surgery

☐ Hemorrhoids

☐ Hernia

☐ Hysterectomy

☐ Laparoscopy

Mastectomy

☐ Myomectomy

☐ Oophorectomy

☐ Tonsil/Adenoidectomy

☐ Tubal Ligation

PREVENTIVE CARE

A1c %

Air Contrast Barium Enema

Ankle Brachial Index

Blood Glucose

Bone Density 11/07/2012

Chest X-Ray

Chlamydia Screening

Colonoscopy 11/10/2010

Dilated Eye Exam

DTaP Vaccine (90700)

Echocardiogram

Electrocardiogram

Flexible Sigmoidoscopy

Flu vaccine

Foot Exam Date

HIV Test Date:

Self-Management Goal

1. Healthier diet
2. Increase exercise
3. Lose 20 pounds

HPV Test

HPV Vaccine

Last Complete Physical Exam

Lipids

Mammography 05/16/2012

Pap Smear 05/18/2012

Pneumovax

PSA

Pulmonary Function Tests

Routine Eye Exam

Stool Occult Blood

Stress Test

Td 04/09/2013

Tdap Vaccine, Adult

Tuberculin PPD 04/09/2013

Varicella

Zoster Vaccine (90736)

Courtesy of Harris CareTracker PM and EMR

Ellen Ristino DOB: 11/1/1956

Source Document 6-3B: Family History

GENERAL FAMILY HISTORY

☐ Adopted

☐ Unknown Paternal Hx

☐ Alcoholism

☐ Anemia

☐ Anxiety

☐ Asthma

☐ Birth Defects

☐ CAD

☑ Cardiovascular Disease

☐ CHF

Cancer

Other

conditions

☐ Denial of any knowledge of significant family history

☐ Unknown Maternal Hx

☐ Congenital Anomaly

☑ COPD

☐ Crohn's Disease

☐ Depression

☐ Diabetes

☐ Epilepsy

☐ GERD

☐ Hypercholesterolemia

☐ Hyperlipidemia

☑ Hypertension

☐ Hypothyroidism

☐ Kidney Disease

☐ Liver Disease

☐ Multiple Births

☐ Osteoarthritis

☐ Osteoporosis

☐ Pulmonary Disease

☐ Stroke

Courtesy of Harris CareTracker PM and EMR

Case Study 6-6 Information Packet

PATIENT'S NAME: Jordyn Lyndsey

DATE OF BIRTH: 01/14/1942

PROVIDER: Dr. Amir Raman

MEDICATIONS

Mrs. Lyndsey is currently taking the medications listed in the following table. Leave the Rx *Start Date* and *End Date* boxes blank, as well as the *Original Date*.

Medication	Strength	Directions	Override Reason
Januvia Oral Tablets	50 mg	Sig 1 tab per day	N/A
Metoprolol Tartrate Oral Tablets	50 mg	Sig 1 tab per day	Benefit outweighs risk

ALLERGIES

Confirm No Known Allergies

IMMUNIZATIONS

Leave the Immunization section blank

VITAL SIGNS

Category	Entry
Height	5 ft 7 in
Weight	132 Pounds
Body Mass Index	Automatically populates after entering height and weight
LMP	N/A
Blood Pressure	148/92
Pulse Rate	92 bpm
Temperature	98.4° F
Respiratory Rate	18
Pulse Oximetry	98%
Pain Level	9/10
Head Circumference	N/A
Length	N/A

HISTORY

Patient History

First, using the patient history information listed in Source Document 6-4A (found on page 645), enter Mrs. Lyndsey's information in the *History* module of her medical record. Then, for any "Yes" responses entered, you will need to add additional information to each corresponding *Finding Details* box. The following table provides you with the detailed information that Mrs. Lyndsey gave when questioning her regarding the "Yes" responses. (**Hint:** The *Patient History* tab should be highlighted at the top of the *History* window when entering the information from Source Document 6-4A.)

Section	Entry in Finding Details Box
General Medical Information	
DM Type 2	Control Status: Diet controlled; medication controlled
	Comment: Fifteen-year history of diabetes type II.
Hypertension	Twenty-year history. Usually well controlled. Patient thinks today's reading is related to her pain level.
OB-GYN	
Menopause has occurred	Full menopause occurred at the age of 55. No hormonal therapy.
Surgical Procedure	
Appendectomy	May of 1986; No complications
Cataract Surgery	Right IOL in 10/2010
	Left IOL in 04/14/11
	No complications

Sensitive Information

Using the information listed in Source Document 6-4B (found on page 647), enter Mrs. Lyndsey's sensitive information in the *History* module of her medical record. (**Hint:** The *Sensitive Info* tab should be highlighted at the top of the *History* window when entering the information from Source Document 6-4B.)

Family History Information

First, using the information listed in Source Document 6-4C (found on page 647), enter Mrs. Lyndsey's family history information in the *History* module of her medical record. Then, for any "Yes" responses entered in the *General Family History* section, you will need to add additional information to each corresponding *Finding Details* box. The following table provides you with the detailed information that Mrs. Lyndsey gave when questioning her regarding the "Yes" responses. (**Hint:** The *Family History* tab should be highlighted at the top of the *History* window when entering the information from Source Document 6-4C.)

Disease	Entry in Finding Details Box
Diabetes	Mother, sister, and brother. *Comments*: All family members mentioned were diagnosed with Type 2 Diabetes Mellitus.
GERD	Sister. *Comments*: Had surgery to repair hiatal hernia. GERD is much better now.
Hyperlipidemia	Sister and brother. *Comments*: Both siblings are on medications to lower their cholesterol.
Hypertension	Mother, father, brother, sister, maternal grandmother, and paternal grandfather. *Comments*: Several family members have been diagnosed with hypertension. All family members still living with hypertension are on some form of antihypertensive medication.
Kidney Disease	Mother. *Comments*: Mother had kidney disease secondary to diabetes. Was on dialysis for the last several years of her life.

PROGRESS NOTE

Template: IM OV Option 4 (v4) w/A&P

Using the information in the following table, complete the progress note for your provider.

Tab	Entry
CC/HPI	*Chief Complaint*: Back pain. *Other Complaints:* Patient continues to have intense lower back pain following an injury to her back six weeks ago. *HPI*: Patient picked up a large box approximately six weeks ago and immediately felt a burning sensation in her lower back. Pain started at a 5/10 and subsided to a 2/10 the following day. Pain has been steadily increasing and is now a 9/10. Patient describes pain as tight and continuous. Activity makes pain worse; sitting still in an upright position makes it feel slightly better. Patient has been taking Tylenol and using a heating pad since onset (little relief). Patient denies any numbness, tingling, or pain that radiates down either leg or previous low back pain or trauma.
History	*Reviewed*: Select Medication List Reviewed, Allergy List Reviewed, Past Medical History Reviewed, Social History Reviewed, Family History Reviewed.
ROS	*Constitutional*: "N" for fever, chills, and headache. *Other constitutional symptoms*: Patient in quite a bit of distress due to severe back pain *Eyes*: No eye symptoms *ENMT*: No ENT symptoms *Neck*: No neck symptoms *Cardiovascular*: No cardiovascular symptoms *Genitourinary*: No GU symptoms *Musculoskeletal*: "Y" for back pain *Other musculoskeletal symptoms*: Lower back pain after lifting a heavy box 6 weeks ago. Pain is intensifying.
PE	*General*: Alert; oriented to time, place, and person; General appearance normal. *HEENT/Other head findings:* Normal head exam *Other eye findings:* Normal eye exam *Neck/Other neck findings:* Normal neck exam *Heart/Other heart findings:* Normal heart exam *Abdomen/Other abdomen findings:* Normal abdominal exam *Musculoskeletal/Other musculoskeletal findings:* Moderate tenderness around L5 and sacroiliac junction. Normal range of motion for waist flexion/extension and lateral flexion. Increased tenderness upon flexion of waist. *Neurologic/Other neurological findings:* Lower extremity strength 4/5 and slightly asymmetric. Lower extremity reflexes +3/4 at patella and Achilles, gait is normal, Negative straight leg test.
Assessment	*Assessment*: 1. Low back pain (M54.5) 2. Somatic Dysfunction -Lumbar, Pelvis (M99.03 and M99.05) 3. Hypertension (I10) 4. Type II Diabetes Mellitus (E11.9)
Plan	*Additional Plan Details*: Plan 1. LS MRI 2. Referral to Orthopedist 3. Oxycodone-Acetaminophen 10-325 mg tabs

Directions:
The source documents below represent what each section of the patient *History* module will look like on the printed patient history report forms. These source documents will look different from your *History* screen as you are entering information. Your goal is to make certain that anything that is highlighted in these documents is entered into the correct section of the *History* screen. Leave everything else blank. (**Hint:** For those sections where you must enter a "yes" or "no," a check mark indicates "yes" and an X indicates "no.")

Jordyn L. Lyndsey DOB: 1/17/1942

Source Document 6-4A: Patient History

Reviewed

✓ Medication List Reviewed	✓ Past Medical History Reviewed
✓ Allergy List Reviewed	✓ Social History Reviewed
☐ Problem List Reviewed	✓ Family History Reviewed
☐ Denies significant past history.	☐ No recent change in medical history.

GENERAL MEDICAL HISTORY

☐ Alcoholism	☐ Depression	☐ Kidney Infections
☐ Allergies/Hayfever	☐ DM Type 1	☐ Kidney stone
☐ Anemia	✓ DM Type 2	☐ Migraine
☐ Anxiety	☐ Epilepsy	☐ Multiple Sclerosis
☐ Asthma	☐ Fracture	☐ Obesity
☐ Atrial Fibrillation	☐ Gastric ulcer	☐ Old MI
☐ Blood Transfusions	☐ Gastrointestinal Disease	☐ Osteoarthritis
☐ CAD	☐ GERD	☐ Osteoporosis
☐ Cancer	☐ Gestational Diabetes	☐ Pneumonia
☐ Cardiac Pacer	☐ Glaucoma	☐ Progressive Neurological Disorder
☐ Cardiovascular Disease	☐ Heart Murmur	☐ Pulmonary Disease
☐ CHF	☐ Hepatitis	☐ Rheumatic Fever
☐ Cirrhosis	☐ High Cholesterol	☐ Rheumatoid Arthritis
☐ Colitis	☐ Hyperlipidemia	☐ STD
☐ COPD	✓ Hypertension	☐ Terminal Illness
☐ CRF	☐ Hyperthyroidism	☐ Thyroid Disease
☐ Crohn's disease	☐ Hypothyroidism	☐ TIA
☐ CVA	☐ Joint Pain	☐ Tuberculosis

HOSPITALIZATIONS 1962-C-Section (No complications)
1986-Appendectomy (No complications)

OTHER MEDICAL HISTORY

Tobacco Assessment

This section supports Stage 1 Meaningful Use
Smoking Status   Current Everyday Smoker

\# pack-years **25**

☐ Counseling on tobacco cessation
☐ Rx therapy for tobacco cessation
☐ Discussed Smoking/Tobacco Use Cessation Strategies

☒ Tobacco User
Date quit smoking

Social History

Alcohol Use Occasional	Educational level
Caffeine Use 2 servings per Day	Marital Status Widow
☒ Drug Use	Exercise Habits moderate >3 x/wk
☒ sun protection	✓ seatbelts
☒ Tattoos	☐ Body piercings
☒ sexually active	birth control method
Race African American	Birth Control Device insertion date
Native language	Birth Control Device removal date
☒ physical abuse	Religion
☒ domestic violence	Occupation **Retired**
Other Social History	

Depression Screening

☐ Patient Refused
Little interest or pleasure in doing things   At no time
Feeling down, depressed, or hopeless   Occasionally

Date of Last Depression Screening/PHQ-2
PHQ-2 Score **PHQ2 Score: 1**

OB/GYN HISTORY

LMP	Menarche Age **13**
Frequency of menstrual cycle	Days menstrual cycle
☑ Menopause has occurred	
☒ History of abnormal pap smears	
☒ Sexually Active	Birth Control
	Birth Control Device insertion date
	Birth Control Device removal date
☐ ectopic pregnancy	

PREGNANCY SUMMARY

Gravida 1	
Term 1	
Preterm	Miscarriage
AB	Elective Abortion
Live children 1	C-Section: 1

OTHER OB-GYN HISTORY

SURGICAL / PROCEDURAL

☐ No prior surgical history

☑ Appendectomy	☐ Endometrial Ablation	☐ Laparoscopy
☐ Breast Lumpectomy	☐ Gall Bladder	Mastectomy
☑ Cataract Surgery	☐ Heart Surgery	☐ Myomectomy

Location:
Right

Location:
Left

☐ Colectomy	☐ Hemorrhoids	☐ Oophorectomy
☐ Cone Biopsy	☐ Hernia	☐ Tonsil/Adenoidectomy
☐ D&C	☐ Hysterectomy	☐ Tubal Ligation

OTHER SURGICAL
HISTORY

PREVENTIVE CARE

A1c % 05/01/2013	HPV Test
Air Contrast Barium Enema	HPV Vaccine
Ankle Brachial Index	Last Complete Physical Exam
Blood Glucose	Lipids
Bone Density	Mammography 01/03/2013
Chest X-Ray	Pap Smear
Chlamydia Screening	Pneumovax
Colonoscopy 10/15/2009	PSA
Dilated Eye Exam 04/16/2013	Pulmonary Function Tests
DTaP Vaccine (90700)	Routine Eye Exam
Echocardiogram	Stool Occult Blood
Electrocardiogram	Stress Test
Flexible Sigmoidoscopy	Td
Flu vaccine 10/09/2012	Tdap Vaccine, Adult
Foot Exam Date	Tuberculin PPD
HIV Test Date:	Varicella
	Zoster Vaccine (90736)
Self-Management Goal	

Jordyn L. Lyndsey DOB: 1/17/1942

Source Document 6-4B: Sensitive Information

STD

[X] Vaginosis		[X] Gonorrhea	
[X] Trichomonas		[X] Chlamydia	
[X] Genital Warts		[X] Syphillis	
[X] PID		[X] HPV	

STD Info

SUBSTANCE ABUSE

[X] History of Substance Abuse

Abused Substances

MENTAL HEALTH

[X] Seeing mental health provider

Mental Health Provider Name

Mental Health Condition(s)

HIV Status

HIV Status

HIV Test Date

HIV Notes

Has never had an HIV test.

Medicare High Risk Criteria

Age when became sexually active **18**

[X] More than 5 sexual partners in lifetime

[✔] DES history in mother .

Pap Smear

[X] History of abnormal pap smears

Jordyn L. Lyndsey DOB: 1/17/1942

Source Document 6-4C: Family History

GENERAL FAMILY HISTORY

[ ] Adopted	[ ] Denial of any knowledge of significant family history	
[ ] Unknown Paternal Hx	[ ] Unknown Maternal Hx	
[ ] Alcoholism	[ ] Congenital Anomaly	[✔] Hypertension
[ ] Anemia	[ ] COPD	[ ] Hypothyroidism
[ ] Anxiety	[ ] Crohn's Disease	[✔] Kidney Disease
[ ] Asthma	[ ] Depression	[ ] Liver Disease
[ ] Birth Defects	[✔] Diabetes	[ ] Multiple Births
[ ] CAD	[ ] Epilepsy	[ ] Osteoarthritis
[ ] Cardiovascular Disease	[✔] GERD	[ ] Osteoporosis
[ ] CHF	[ ] Hypercholesterolemia	[ ] Pulmonary Disease
Cancer	[✔] Hyperlipidemia	[ ] Stroke
Other conditions	....	

Activity 8-5 Information Packet: 9-Month Exam

PATIENT'S NAME: Spencer Douglas

DATE OF BIRTH: 01/10/2013 (**Note:** Since patient Spencer Douglas's date of birth is fixed in the database, his age may show as older than 9 months when you are completing this activity. However, he was 9 months old at the time of his September 2013 appointment.)

PROVIDER: Dr. Anthony Brockton

PROGRESS NOTE

Template: Pediatric: 9 month well-child visit (You will need to search for this template)

Tab	Entry
Interval History	*Accompanied by:* Mother *Concerns and Questions:* Mother has no questions or concerns at this time. *Interval History:* Pt. is here a bit early for son's 9-month visit. Family will be out of the country for the next two months so she wanted to bring Spencer in before leaving for their trip.
ROS	**Nutrition** Select "Y" for *breast fed* *Times per day:* 3 *Minutes per side:* 10 Check the following boxes: *Drinks from cup, source of water, solid foods, juice* Add comment to the *solid foods* note box: "Eats approximately 3 jars of baby food/day. Solid foods include cereal with applesauce, peas, squash, and bananas." **Elimination** *Wet diapers per day:* 6 *Bowel movements per day:* 1 **Sleep** Select "Y" for *sleeping through the night* **Development** *Gross Motor:* Select "Y" for *sits well*, and *crawls*; Select "N" for *pulls to feel with support* *Fine motor:* Select "Y" for *Feeds self, bangs objects together*, and *pincer grasp* *Communication:* Select "Y" for *Responds to name, waves bye-bye*, and *imitates sound* *Social:* Select "Y" for *Peekaboo, Patty-cake*, and *Stranger anxiety*
PE	**Vital Signs** *Weight:* 22 lbs 05 oz *Height:* 2 ft 6 in *Temperature:* 98.3 F *Heart Rate:* 104 bpm *Respiration Rate:* 22 **Physical Examination** Select "N" for normal for all categories except female genitalia (leave that blank)
Anticipatory Guidance	*Nutrition:* Select "avoid choke foods" *Injury Prevention:* Select "crib safety," "choking hazards," "First Aid, CPR," and "sun exposure"
Assess & Plan	Click on the box beside "established patient birth to 1 year (99391)" Click on the box beside "DTap-HepB-IPV (90723)" *Plan:* Click on the drop-down box beside *Follow-up/Next Visit* and select "1 Year"

Activity 8-5 Information Packet: 12-Month Exam

PATIENT'S NAME: Spencer Douglas

DATE OF BIRTH: 01/10/2013 (**Note:** Since patient Spencer Douglas's date of birth is fixed in the database, his age may show as older than 12 months when you are completing this activity. However, he was 12 months old at the time of his December 2013 appointment.)

PROVIDER: Dr. Anthony Brockton

PROGRESS NOTE

Template: Pediatric: 12 month well-child visit (You will need to search for this template.)

Tab	Entry
Interval History	*Accompanied by:* Father *Concerns and Questions:* Father has no questions or concerns at this time.
ROS	**Nutrition** Select "N" for *breast fed.* Add comment to the *breast fed* note box: "Mom stopped breast feeding last month. Patient has adjusted well according to dad." Select "Y" for the following: *Drinks from cup, table foods, finger foods* **Elimination** *Wet diapers per day:* 6 *Bowel movements per day:* 2 **Sleep** Select "Y" for *sleeping through the night* **Development** *Gross Motor:* Select "Y" for *walks without assistance*, and *stands well alone* *Fine motor:* Select "Y" for *has a pincer grasp, bangs objects together, scribbles spontaneously* *Communication:* Select "Y" for *says mama/dada specifically, imitates simple daily tasks, language at 12 months* *Social:* Select "Y" for *plays pat-a-cake, waves bye-bye*
PE	**Vital Signs** *Weight:* 21 lbs *Height:* 2 ft 9 in *Temperature:* 98.2 F *Heart Rate:* 100 bpm *Respiration Rate:* 22 **Physical Examination** Select "N" for normal for all categories except female genitalia (leave that blank)
Anticipatory Guidance	*Nutrition:* Select "whole milk," "healthy food choices," and "nutritious snacks, limit sweets" *Social competence:* Select "toilet training" *Injury Prevention:* Select "electrical outlets"
Assess & Plan	Click on the box beside "established patient birth to 1 year (99391)" *Immunizations:* Select "DTAP/HIB/IPV (90698)," "Polio Virus Vaccine (90713)," and "Measles, Mumps, Rubella Vaccine (90707)." Click on the drop-down box beside *Follow-up/Next Visit* and select "1 Month." *Plan:* Enter "Will bring patient back in for a weight check in 30 days."

Source Document 8-1

Patient Name	DOB	Age	Gender		
Morgan, Jane W	**1/22/1955**	**58**	**F**	Report Status:	**Final**
Ordering Provider				Reported:	**11/11/2013 10:07:05 PM**
Amir Raman DO				Accession:	
				Collected:	**7/30/2013**

A	Test	Results	Abnormal Results	Units	Reference Range
URINALYSIS DIPSTICK PANEL IN URINE BY AUTOMATED TEST STRIP					
A	**Clarity of Urine**		**Cloudy**		**Clear**
N	Ketones [Mass/volume] in Urine by Automated test strip	Negative			Negative
A	**Nitrite [Presence] in Urine by Automated test strip**		**Positive**		**Negative**
A	**Hemoglobin [Mass/volume] in Urine by Automated test strip**		**Trace**		**None**
N	pH of Urine by Automated test strip	7.5			5.0-9.0
A	**Protein [Mass/volume] in Urine by Automated test strip**		**Trace**		**Negative**
N	Urobilinogen [Mass/volume] in Urine by Automated test strip	Normal			Normal
N	Specific gravity of Urine by Automated test strip	1.030			< 1.030
N	Bilirubin [Mass/volume] in Urine by Automated test strip	Negative			Negative
N	Glucose [Mass/volume] in Urine by Automated test strip	Negative		mg/dL	Negative
N	Color of Urine	Dark Yellow			Yellow
URINALYSIS MICROSCOPIC PANEL [#/VOLUME] IN URINE BY AUTOMATED COUNT					
A	**Leukocyte clumps [#/volume] in Urine by Automated count**		**Present**		**Absent**
A	**Mucus [#/volume] in Urine by Automated count**		**Present**		**Absent**
N	Spermatozoa [#/volume] in Urine by Automated count	None			Absemt
A	**Bacteria [#/volume] in Urine by Automated count**		**Moderate**		**None-Few**
N	Crystals [#/volume] in Urine by Automated count	Absent			Absent
N	Casts [#/volume] in Urine by Automated count	None		#/LPF	None

Patient Name	DOB	Age	Gender			
Morgan, Jane W	**1/22/1955**	**58**	**F**	Report Status:	**Final**	
Ordering Provider				Reported:	**11/11/2013 10:07:05 PM**	
Amir Raman DO				Accession:		
				Collected:	**7/30/2013**	

A	Test	Results	Abnormal Results	Units	Reference Range
N	Hyaline casts [#/volume] in Urine by Automated count	1		#/LPF	0-3
A	**Epithelial cells.non-squamous [#/volume] in Urine by Automated count**		**2 (Renal)**	**#/LPF**	**Absent**
N	Epithelial cells.squamous [#/volume] in Urine by Automated count	Few			None-Few
A	**Leukocytes [#/volume] in Urine by Automated count**		**18-20**	**#/HPF**	**<5/HPF**
A	**Erythrocytes [#/volume] in Urine by Automated count**		**8-9**	**#/HPF**	**<5/HPF**

© Cengage Learning 2015

Source Document 8-2

Patient Name	DOB	Age	Gender	
Thompson, Adam	**1/1/1942**	**71**	**M**	Report Status: **Final**
Ordering Provider				Reported: **11/10/2013 7:17:14 PM**
Anthony Brockton MD				Accession:
				Collected: **8/12/2013**

A	Test	Results	Abnormal Results	Units	Reference Range
CBC W AUTO DIFFERENTIAL PANEL IN BLOOD					
N	Granulocytes %				
N	Erythrocyte distribution width				
N	Neutrophils.band form #				
N	Platelet distribution width				
N	Platelet mean volume				
N	Neutrophils.band form %				
N	Lymphocytes Variant %				
N	Lymphocytes Variant #				
N	Hematocrit %	41.2		%	39.0-50.0
N	Leukocytes other #				
N	Auto Differential panel in Blood				
N	Other cells %				
N	Complete blood count (hemogram) panel in Blood by Automated count				
N	Other cells #				
N	Monocytes %	12.9		%	0.0-13.0
N	Leukocytes #	5.2		Thous/cu. mm	3.9-11.1
N	Basophils #				
H	**Basophils %**		**3.0**	**%**	**0.0-2.0**
N	Eosinophils #				
N	Eosinophils %	0.6		%	0.0-8.0
N	Hemoglobin	14.5		g/dL	13.2-16.9
N	Lymphocytes #				
N	Lymphocytes %	46.1		%	15.0-48.0
N	Monocytes #				
N	Neutrophils #				
N	Neutrophils %	40.1		%	38.0-80.0
N	Platelets #	172		Thous/cu. mm	140-390
H	**Erythrocyte mean corpuscular hemoglobin**		**41.4**	**pg**	**27.0-34.0 pg**
N	Erythrocyte mean corpuscular hemoglobin concentration	35.3		%	32.0-35.5 g/dL
H	**Erythrocyte mean corpuscular volume**		**117**	**fL**	**78.0-100.0 fL**

Patient Name	DOB	Age	Gender		
Thompson, Adam	**1/1/1942**	**71**	**M**	Report Status:	**Final**
Ordering Provider				Reported:	**11/10/2013 7:17:14 PM**
Anthony Brockton MD				Accession:	
				Collected:	**8/12/2013**

A	Test	Results	Abnormal Results	Units	Reference Range
N	Erythrocyte distribution width %				
L	**Erythrocytes #**		**3.51**	**Mil/cu.mm**	**4.2-5.7 Mil/cu.mm**

ELECTROLYTES 1998 PANEL IN SERUM OR PLASMA

A	Test	Results	Abnormal Results	Units	Reference Range
N	Carbon dioxide, total [Moles/volume] in Serum or Plasma	31		mEq/L	22-32
N	Chloride [Moles/volume] in Serum or Plasma	122		mEq/L	118-132
N	Potassium [Moles/volume] in Serum or Plasma	4.2		mEq/L	3.5-5.0
N	Sodium [Moles/volume] in Serum or Plasma	140		mEq/L	135-145
H	**Anion gap in Serum or Plasma**		**18**	**mEq/L**	**7-16**

© Cengage Learning 2015

Source Document 8-3

Patient Name	DOB	Age	Gender		
Ristino, Ellen	11/1/1956	57	F	Report Status:	**Final**
Ordering Provider				Reported:	**11/11/2013 8:12:58 AM**
Anthony Brockton MD				Accession:	
				Collected:	**7/29/2013**

A	Test	Results	Abnormal Results	Units	Reference Range
		FASTING			
HETEROPHILE AB [TITER] IN SERUM BY AGGLUTINATION					
N	Heterophile Ab [Titer] in Serum by Agglutination	Negative			Negative
CBC W AUTO DIFFERENTIAL PANEL IN BLOOD					
N	Granulocytes %				
N	Erythrocyte distribution width				
N	Neutrophils.band form #				
N	Platelet distribution width				
N	Platelet mean volume				
N	Neutrophils.band form %				
N	Lymphocytes Variant %				
N	Lymphocytes Variant #				
N	Hematocrit %	42		%	39.0-50.0
N	Leukocytes other #				
N	Auto Differential panel in Blood				
N	Other cells %				
N	Complete blood count (hemogram) panel in Blood by Automated count				
N	Other cells #				
N	Monocytes %	3		%	0.0-13.0
N	Leukocytes #	4.2		Thous/cu. mm	3.9-11.1
N	Basophils #				
N	Basophils %	0		%	0.0-2.0
N	Eosinophils #				
N	Eosinophils %	1		%	0.0-8.0
N	Hemoglobin	14		g/dL	13.2-16.9
N	Lymphocytes #				
H	**Lymphocytes %**		**52**	**%**	**15.0-48.0**
N	Monocytes #				
N	Neutrophils #				
N	Neutrophils %	44		%	38.0-80.0
N	Platelets #	320		Thous/cu. mm	140-390

Patient Name	DOB	Age	Gender		
Ristino, Ellen	**11/1/1956**	**57**	**F**	Report Status:	**Final**
Ordering Provider				Reported:	**11/11/2013 8:12:58 AM**
Anthony Brockton MD				Accession:	
				Collected:	**7/29/2013**

A	Test	Results	Abnormal Results	Units	Reference Range
N	Erythrocyte mean corpuscular hemoglobin	31.8		pg	27.0-34.0
N	Erythrocyte mean corpuscular hemoglobin concentration	33.3		%	32.0-35.5
N	Erythrocyte mean corpuscular volume	95.5		fl	78.0-100.0
N	Erythrocyte distribution width %				
N	Erythrocytes #	4.4		Mil/cu.mm	4.2-5.7

© Cengage Learning 2015

Source Document 9-1: Explanation of Benefits

MEDICARE CENGAGE

Medicare Cengage
P.O. Box 234434
San Francisco, CA 94137

AMIR RAMAN, D.O.
Napa Valley Family Health Associates (NVFHA)
101 Vine Street
Napa, CA 94558

Date: MM/DD/YYYY (Appt. date used in Activity 4-1)
Payment Number: 12808957
Payment Amount: $ 145.01

Account Number	Patient Name				Subscriber Number		Claim Number			
Dates of Service	Description of Service	Amount Charged	Not Covered	Prov Adj Discount	Amount Allowed	Deduct/ Coins/ Copay	Paid to Provider	Adj Reason Code	Rmk Code	Patient Resp
CARE1357	Lyndsey, Jordyn									
(Appt. date used in Activity 4-1)	99203	$191.00	$0.00	$82.81	$108.19	$21.64	$86.55	45*		$21.64

Account Number	Patient Name				Subscriber Number		Claim Number			
Dates of Service	Description of Service	Amount Charged	Not Covered	Prov Adj Discount	Amount Allowed	Deduct/ Coins/ Copay	Paid to Provider	Adj Reason Code	Rmk Code	Patient Resp
CARE1357	Lyndsey, Jordyn									
(Appt. date used in Activity 9-3)	99214	$245.00	$245.00		$0.00	$245.00	$0.00	20*		$245.00
(Appt. date used in Activity 9-3)	G0180	$100.00		$26.93	$73.07	$14.61	$58.46			$14.61

Amount Allowed (45*) = Charges exceed your contracted/legislated fee arrangement
Amount Allowed (20*) = Not a covered code

© Cengage Learning 2015

Source Document 9-2:   Explanation of Benefits

BLUE SHIELD CENGAGE

Blue Shield Cengage
P.O. Box 32245
Los Angeles, CA 90002

AMIR RAMAN, M.D.
Napa Valley Family Health Associates (NVFHA)
101 Vine Street
Napa, CA 94558

Date: MM/DD/YYYY (Appt. date used in Activity 4-1)
Payment Number: 5564856
Payment Amount: $0.00

Account Number	Patient Name				Subscriber Number		Claim Number			
Dates of Service	Description of Service	Amount Charged	Not Covered	Prov Adj Discount	Amount Allowed	Deduct/ Coins/ Copay	Paid to Provider	Adj Reason Code	Rmk Code	Patient Resp
BCBS97	**Morgan, Jane**									
(Appt. date used in Activity 4-1)	99213	$112.00	$0.00	$36.00	$76.00	$76.00	$0.00	22*		$76.00
(Appt. date used in Activity 4-1)	90746	$100.00		$23.00	$77.00	$77.00	$0.00	22*		$77.00

Amount Allowed (45*) = Charges exceed your contracted/legislated fee arrangement
Amount Allowed (20*) = Not a covered code
Amount Allowed (22*) = Patient has not yet met annual policy deductible ($6,000.00). All balances are patient's responsibility.
Amount Allowed (25*) = Requires Modifier 25 to be paid as a separate service

© Cengage Learning 2015

Source Document 9-3:   Explanation of Benefits

MEDICARE CENGAGE

Medicare Cengage
P.O. Box 234434
San Francisco, CA 94137

Date: MM/DD/YYYY (Appt. date used in Activity 4-1)
Payment Number: 11235784
Payment Amount: $81.12

ANTHONY BROCKTON, M.D.
Napa Valley Family Health Associates (NVFHA)
101 Vine Street
Napa, CA 94558

© Cengage Learning 2015

Account Number	Patient Name				Subscriber Number		Claim Number			
Dates of Service	Description of Service	Amount Charged	Not Covered	Prov Adj Discount	Amount Allowed	Deduct/ Coins/ Copay	Paid to Provider	Adj Reason Code	Rmk Code	Patient Resp
CARE1357	Thompson, Adam									
(Appt. date from Activity 4-1)	94760	$13.00	$0.00	$10.36	$2.64	$0.53	$2.11	45*		$0.53
(Appt. date from Activity 4-1)	99213	$112.00	$0.00	$53.11	$58.89	$11.78	$47.11	45*		$11.78
(Appt. date from Activity 4-1)	71020	$13.50	$0.00	$3.50	$10.00	$2.00	$8.00	45*		$2.00
(Appt. date from Activity 4-1)	93000	$46.50	$0.00	$16.50	$30.00	$6.00	$24.00	45*		$6.00

Amount Allowed (45*) = Charges exceed your contracted/legislated fee arrangement
Amount Allowed (20*) = Not a covered code

Source Document 9-4:   Explanation of Benefits

BLUE SHIELD CENGAGE

Blue Shield Cengage
P.O. Box 32245
Los Angeles, CA 90002

ANTHONY BROCKTON, M.D.
Napa Valley Family Health Associates (NVFHA)
101 Vine Street
Napa, CA 94558

Date: MM/DD/YYYY (Appt. date used in Activity 4-1)
Payment Number: 5564854
Payment Amount: $81.64

Account Number	Patient Name				Subscriber Number			Claim Number			
Dates of Service	Description of Service	Amount Charged	Not Covered	Prov Adj Discount	Amount Allowed	Deduct/ Coins/ Copay	Paid to Provider	Adj Reason Code	Rmk Code	Patient Resp
BCBS97	**Ristino, Ellen**									
(Appt. date used in Activity 4-1)	99213	$112.00	$0.00	$36.00	$76.00	$15.20	$60.80	45*		$15.20
(Appt. date used in Activity 4-1)	86308	$45.00			$16.55	$3.31	$13.24	45*		$3.31
(Appt. date used in Activity 4-1)	3210F	$24.00			$9.50	$1.90	$7.60	45*		$1.90
(Appt. date used in Activity 4-1)	36415	$15.00	$15.00		$0.00			25*		$15.00
(Appt. date used in Activity 4-1)	94760	$13.00	$13.00		$0.00			20*		$13.00

Amount Allowed (45*) = Charges exceed your contracted/legislated fee arrangement
Amount Allowed (20*) = Not a covered code
Amount Allowed (25*) = requires Modifier 25 to be paid as a separate service

Source Document 9-5:   Explanation of Benefits

MEDICAID CENGAGE

Medicaid Cengage
P.O. Box 221352
Fresno, CA 93701

AMIR RAMAN, D.O.
Napa Valley Family Health Associates (NVFHA)
101 Vine Street
Napa, CA 94558

Date: MM/DD/YYYY (Appt. date used in Activity 4-1)
Payment Number: 5644425
Payment Amount: $46.00

Account Number	Patient Name				Subscriber Number			Claim Number			
Dates of Service	Description of Service	Amount Charged	Not Covered	Prov Adj Discount	Amount Allowed	Deduct/ Coins/ Copay	Paid to Provider	Adj Reason Code	Rmk Code	Patient Resp
CAID8002	**Smith, Craig X.**									
(Appt. date used in Activity 4-1)	99213	$112.00	$79.00	$79.00	$33.00	$0.00	$33.00	45*		$0.00
(Appt. date used in Activity 4-1)	J7650	$25.00	$18.00	$18.00	$7.00	$0.00	$7.00	45*		$0.00
(Appt. date used in Activity 4-1)	71020	$13.50	$7.50	$7.50	$6.00	$0.00	$6.00	45*		$0.00

Amount Allowed (45*) = Charges exceed your contracted/legislated fee arrangement
Amount Allowed (20*) = Not a covered code

© Cengage Learning 2015

Source Document 9-6:   Explanation of Benefits

BLUE SHIELD CENGAGE

Blue Shield Cengage
P.O. Box 32245
Los Angeles, CA 90002

AMIR RAMAN, M.D.
Napa Valley Family Health Associates (NVFHA)
101 Vine Street
Napa, CA 94558

Date: MM/DD/YYYY (Appt. date used in Activity 4-2)
Payment Number: 5564855
Payment Amount: $0.00

Account Number	Patient Name					Subscriber Number			Claim Number			
Dates of Service	Description of Service	Amount Charged	Not Covered	Prov Adj Discount	Amount Allowed	Deduct/ Coins/ Copay	Paid to Provider	Adj Reason Code	Rmk Code	Patient Resp
BCBS97	**Watson, Barbara**									
(Appt. date used in Activity 4-2)	99213	$112.00	$0.00	$36.00	$76.00	$76.00	$0.00	22*		$76.00
(Appt. date used in Activity 4-2)	94760	$13.00		$11.00	$2.00	$2.00	$0.00	22*		$2.00

Amount Allowed (45*) = Charges exceed your contracted/legislated fee arrangement
Amount Allowed (20*) = Not a covered code
Amount Allowed (22*) = Patient has not yet met annual policy deductible ($5,000.00). All balances are patient's responsibility.
Amount Allowed (25*) = requires Modifier 25 to be paid as a separate service

© Cengage Learning 2015

Source Document 11-1

Patient Registration Form

NVFHA

Patient's Last Name	First (legal name)	First (Preferred name)	Middle Name
HERNANDEZ	JULIA		

Address (Number, Street, Apt #)	City	State	Zip Code
5224 Sunset Landing	Vacaville	CA	95688 - 5688

Mail will be sent to the address listed above, unless patient indicates a different address (leave blank if same as above)

Send mail to Address (Number, Street, Apt #)	City	State	Zip Code

Phone Options	Phone Number	Okay to leave detailed message	Call this number (circle one)
Home	(707) 468 - 4457	Yes _X_ No _____	(1st) 2nd 3rd choice
Cell	( ) -	Yes ____ No _____	1st 2nd 3rd choice
Work	(877) 883 - 7777	Yes ____ No _X_	1st (2nd) 3rd choice

Would you like to communicate by Email Yes _X_ No __	Email Address Jhernandez@email.com

Date of Birth	Gender	Last 4 digits Social Security Number
06/24/1987	Female _X_ Male ___	2137

Marital Status (circle one)	What is your preferred language / secondary language
(Single) / Married / Divorced / Widow / Partner	Spanish/English

Race (circle one)	Ethnicity (circle one)
African American-Black / Asian / Bi-Multi-racial / Pacific Islander-Hawaiian / Caucasian–White / Native American Eskimo Aleut / Decline to state / Other	(Hispanic-Latino) Non-Hispanic-Latino / Other

Religion	Roman Catholic	Organ Donor	Yes _X_ No _____

Are you new to our practice	Who referred you to our practice	Who is your Primary Care Physician
Yes _X_ No _____	Rebecca Ayerick	Rebecca Ayerick

Additional Notes

Emergency Contact

Emergency Contact's Name	Relationship to patient	Phone
Cynthia Hernandez	SISTER	(707) 555 - 0454

On-Line Patient Portal Communication via Email

On-Line communication is used for non-urgent message/requests only. NVFHA uses secure technology to protect the privacy and confidentiality of your personal information. Only you, your physician, and authorized staff can read your message.

What is your preferred method of communication	Phone _X_ Letter _____ Patient Portal _____

Insurance Information

Subscriber (Insurance Holder) Name	Date of Birth	Relationship to patient	Subscriber Phone Numeber
Self	/ /		( )

Health Plan Information	Primary Health Plan	Secondary Health Plan
Health Plan Name	Blue Shield Cengage	
Health Plan Address	PO Box 32245, Los Angeles, CA, 90002	
Group Number	BCBS 987	
Subscriber Number	BCBS 987	

Elig Date From	2/21/2011	Copay	$ 25.00

Patient Employer Information

Employer Name & Address (Number, Street, Apt #, City, State, Zip Code)	Employer Phone Number
River Rock Casino, 3250 Highway 128, Goyersville, CA, 95441	(877) 883 - 7777

Occupation	Server		Start Date	2/21/2011

Assignment of Benefits • Financial Agreement

I hereby give lifetime authorization for payment of insurance benefits to be made directly to **Napa Valley Family Health Assoc.**, and any assisting physicians, for services rendered. I understand that I am financially resposible for all charges whether or not they are covered by insurance. In the event of default, I agree to pay all costs of collection, and reasonable attorney's fees. I hereby authorize this healthcare provider to release all information necessary to secure the the payment of benefits.

I further agree that a photocopy of this agreement shall be as vaild as the original.

Date: **XX/XX/20XX** _____   Your Signature: *Julia hernandez* _____

Method of Payment: ■ Cash   ■ Check   ■ Credit Card

Source Document 11-2:   Explanation of Benefits

BLUE SHIELD CENGAGE

Blue Shield Cengage
P.O. Box 32245
Los Angeles, CA 90002

REBECCA AYERICK, M.D.
Napa Valley Family Health Associates (NVFHA)
101 Vine Street
Napa, CA 94558

Date: MM/DD/YYYY (per Case Study 11-1)
Payment Number: 556774
Payment Amount: $176.80

Account Number	Patient Name				Subscriber Number		Claim Number			
Dates of Service	Description of Service	Amount Charged	Not Covered	Prov Adj Discount	Amount Allowed	Deduct/ Coins/ Copay	Paid to Provider	Adj Reason Code	Rmk Code	Patient Resp
42507342	Hernandez, Julia									
(Appt. date used in Case Study 11-1)	99203	$191.00			$191.00	$38.20	$152.80			$38.20
(Appt. date used in Case Study 11-1)	90718	$15.00			$15.00	$3.00	$12.00			$3.00
(Appt. date used in Case Study 11-1)	90471	$15.00			$15.00	$3.00	$12.00			$3.00

Amount Allowed (45*) = Charges exceed your contracted/legislated fee arrangement
Amount Allowed (20*) = Not a covered code
Amount Allowed (25*) = requires Modifier 25 to be paid as a separate service

© Cengage Learning 2015

Source Document 11-3: Explanation of Benefits

MEDICARE CENGAGE

Medicare Cengage
P.O. Box 234434
San Francisco, CA 94137

AMIR RAMAN, D.O.
Napa Valley Family Health Associates (NVFHA)
101 Vine Street
Napa, CA 94558

Date: MM/DD/YYYY (Appt. date used in Case Study 11-2)
Payment Number: 1280977
Payment Amount: $126.80

Account Number	Patient Name					Subscriber Number		Claim Number			
Dates of Service	Description of Service	Amount Charged	Not Covered	Prov Adj Discount	Amount Allowed	Deduct/ Coins/ Copay	Paid to Provider	Adj Reason Code	Rmk Code	Patient Resp
42399647	Simpson, Delores									
(Appt. date used in Case Study 11-2)	99213	$112.00	$0.00		$112.00	$22.40	$89.60			$21.64

Account Number	Patient Name					Subscriber Number		Claim Number			
Dates of Service	Description of Service	Amount Charged	Not Covered	Prov Adj Discount	Amount Allowed	Deduct/ Coins/ Copay	Paid to Provider	Adj Reason Code	Rmk Code	Patient Resp
CARE1357	Simpson, Delores									
(Appt. date used in Case Study 11-2)	93000	$46.50	$0.00		$46.50	$9.30	$37.20			$9.30

Amount Allowed (45*) = Charges exceed your contracted/legislated fee arrangement
Amount Allowed (20*) = Not a covered code

Source Document 11-4:   Explanation of Benefits

SENIOR GAP - CENGAGE

Senior Gap
P.O. Box 87956
Oakland, CA 94601

REBECCA AYERICK, M.D.
Napa Valley Family Health Associates (NVFHA)
101 Vine Street
Napa, CA 94558

Date: MM/DD/YYYY (Appt. date used in Case Study 11-3)
Payment Number: 4566751
Payment Amount: $102.00

© Cengage Learning 2015

Account Number	Patient Name				Subscriber Number		Claim Number			
Dates of Service	Description of Service	Amount Charged	Not Covered	Prov Adj Discount	Amount Allowed	Deduct/ Coins/ Copay	Paid to Provider	Adj Reason Code	Rmk Code	Patient Resp
42399658	Zotto, Adam									
(Appt. date used in Case Study 11-3)	99213	$112.00	$0.00		$112.00	$10.00	$102.00	CP*		$10.00

Amount Allowed (45*) = Charges exceed your contracted/legislated fee arrangement
Amount Allowed (20*) = Not a covered code
Amount Allowed (25*) = requires Modifier 25 to be paid as a separate service
Adj Reason Code (CP*) = patient's copay

Source Document 11-5: Explanation of Benefits

BLUE SHIELD CENGAGE

Blue Shield Cengage
P.O. Box 32245
Los Angeles, CA 90002

AMIR RAMAN, D.O.
Napa Valley Family Health Associates (NVFHA)
101 Vine Street
Napa, CA 94558

Date: MM/DD/YYYY (Appt. date used in Case Study 11-4)
Payment Number: 556776
Payment Amount: $93.60

Account Number	Patient Name				Subscriber Number			Claim Number			
Dates of Service	Description of Service	Amount Charged	Not Covered	Prov Adj Discount	Amount Allowed	Deduct/ Coins/ Copay	Paid to Provider	Adj Reason Code	Rmk Code	Patient Resp
42399626	Watson, Barbara									
(Appt. date used in Case Study 11-4)	99213	$112.00			$112.00	$20.00	$69.60	CP*		$42.40
(Appt. date used in Case Study 11-4)	87430	$30.00			$30.00	$6.00	$24.00			$6.00

Amount Allowed (45*) = Charges exceed your contracted/legislated fee arrangement
Amount Allowed (20*) = Not a covered code
Amount Allowed (25*) = requires Modifier 25 to be paid as a separate service
Adj Reason Code (CP*) = copay amount

© Cengage Learning 2015

Source Document 11-6:   Explanation of Benefits

MEDICAID CENGAGE

Medicaid Cengage
P.O. Box 221352
Fresno, CA 93701

AMIR RAMAN, D.O.
Napa Valley Family Health Associates (NVFHA)
101 Vine Street
Napa, CA 94558

Date: MM/DD/YYYY (Appt. date used in Case Study 11-5)
Payment Number: 2321442
Payment Amount: $30.00

Account Number	Patient Name				Subscriber Number			Claim Number		
Dates of Service	Description of Service	Amount Charged	Not Covered	Prov Adj Discount	Amount Allowed	Deduct/ Coins/ Copay	Paid to Provider	Adj Reason Code	Rmk Code	Patient Resp
42399649	**SMITH, CRAIG X.**									
(Appt. date used in Case Study 11-5)	99392	$195.00	$0.00	$165.00	$30.00	$0.00	$30.00	45*		$0.00

Amount Allowed (45*) = Charges exceed your contracted/legislated fee arrangement
Amount Allowed (20*) = Not a covered code
Amount Allowed (25*) = requires Modifier 25 to be paid as a separate service

Appendix B

Workflow Assessment Guide and Checklist

HealthInsight

Workflow Assessment Guide

Before you start the analysis, note the names of the various clinic roles (e.g., front desk, medical records, medical assistant, operator, etc.). As you move through the guide, note who does what on each step.

This tool is meant to guide your workflow analysis. It includes processes that are common to most primary care offices, but it may not include all the processes of a particular office. So, before the analysis ends make sure to ask if any processes were missed. Then write down those steps.

As you proceed through the guide, think about hand-offs (of the chart, super-bill, etc.). Where do things end up--in bins, on desks, in drawers, etc.?

If you ask a clinic to fill out a guide (not recommended), make sure they note: (1) roles, (2) who does what, (3) missing processes, (4) and hand-offs.

Clinic name: _____

Individuals interviewed: _____

_____

Assessors: _____

Assessment date: _____

Pre Visit

Do you make reminders?
  ❑ Calls
  ❑ Letters/cards
  ❑ Does your system generate reminders?
  ❑ Do you send forms to the patient to complete before their visit?

What do you do to prepare for the next day's appointments (ask same-day appts. And walk-in patients)?
  ❑ Add forms to chart
  ❑ Print and add superbill/encounter form

When the chart is pulled does someone check for outstanding labs, missing consults, etc.? What is done if something is missing?

Patient Visit
What do you do about no-shows?

What do you do with the chart with a no-show (policy vs. what really happens)?

What is your check-in process once the patient arrives?
- ☐ Information verification (how)
- ☐ Co-pay
- ☐ Papers the patient must sign
- ☐ Do you add forms to the chart before putting it up for the MA?

What do you do with papers the patient brings in/forms the patient signs?

How do you let the MA know the patient is ready to be seen?

Patient Visit: Nurse

Nurse begins visit (include where these items are done):
- ☐ Weight
- ☐ Vitals
- ☐ Review medications
- ☐ Chief complaint
- ☐ Ask about preventive/screening services due (e.g., mammogram, immunizations, lab tests)
- ☐ Other (e.g., foot exam, UA, strep screen, procedure set up)

What else does the MA document?

How does the MA notify the provider that the patient is ready and which is the next room?
- ☐ Chart in door
- ☐ Walkie-talkie
- ☐ Whiteboard
- ☐ Other:

Is there any communication between the MA and the MD other than that the patient is ready to be seen?
- ☐ Face-to-face
- ☐ Walkie-talkie
- ☐ Sticky note on the chart
- ☐ Whiteboard
- ☐ Other:

What type of information is communicated?
- ☐ Chief complaint
- ☐ Medications
- ☐ Preventive/screening services due
- ☐ Other:

Are there variations between MAs and between MA/provider teams?

Patient Visit: Provider Exam

Does the provider review the patient's chart prior to entering the room?

What is the process for reviewing the:
- ❑ Problem list
- ❑ Medication list
- ❑ Lab tests
- ❑ Preventive/screening services that are due

What does provider do if she needs something or needs the MA during visit (e.g., lab, equipment, exam assistance)?

What is the process when a patient has to leave the room for lab, x-ray, etc. and then comes back?

How are prescriptions written?
- ❑ Prescription pads in room
- ❑ Prescription pads carried by doctor
- ❑ Computer/printer (with an option to select drug and dosage from a list)
- ❑ Computer directly to pharmacy

Does the provider have a method to check for interactions/contraindications for medications?

What else does the provider document?

Does MA put anything else in the chart after the patient leaves?

Patient Visit Concludes

When is the visit documentation completed?
- ❑ As the visit concludes – yes on most
- ❑ Immediately after the visit in the nursing station
- ❑ Between visits, when the MD has time
- ❑ At the end of the day
- ❑ Days/weeks later
- ❑ Usually within _____hours/days

How is the plan of care documented?

Does the patient receive documentation of the plan?

Is there variability between providers in the time it takes to complete the chart?

What happens to the chart?
- ❑   Goes with patient to check out
- ❑   Goes to the doctors office
- ❑   Sits in the work area for MD to work on as he has time
- ❑   Other

Super-bill/Encounter form

   Who documents on the super-bill?
   Where does it go at the end of the visit?
   How does it get there?
   What are the steps until a bill is dropped?

Coders

   Do they have the information they need?
   How do they get their questions answered?

Patient Visit: Check-out Process

Who checks the patient out?

When are follow-up appointments made?

How is payment handled?
- ❑   Co-pay (before or after visit)
- ❑   Billing (e.g., for self-payers)

Who completes the super bill/encounter form?
Where does it go after the visit?

Care Management

Do you track any clinical indicators for patients with a specific disease or condition?
- ☐ Diabetes
- ☐ Heart disease
- ☐ Hypertension
- ☐ Mammography/Pap tests
- ☐ Other:

How do you identify the indicators?

How do you handle patients needing tests, monitoring, teaching, etc?

Patient Visit: Labs

Do you have an in-house lab? (describe the process): **no**

Outside lab (describe the process):
- ☐ Hospital
- ☐ Quest
- ☐ Labcorps
- ☐ Other:

How are lab results returned to the clinic, reviewed, and communicated to the patient?

What happens if patient can't be reached?

How do you know that labs were ordered, done, results returned, reviewed by provider, and given to patient?

Patient Visit: Referrals

Describe the ways patients obtain referrals (e.g., MA makes call, provider fills out form, etc.)?

How do you know the patient actually completes the referral?

Prescription Refills (phone, fax, pharmacy calls)

Describe process when a patient calls in for a refill:

Describe process when a patient asks for a refill during an office visit:

What happens when the pharmacy calls about a refill?

Phone Calls (other than for prescription refills)

What types of phone calls do you get most often:

Describe process for taking messages:

Describe process for returning patient phone calls:

Arkansas Foundation for Medical Care

Work Flow Assessment Checklist

Scheduling

How are appointments made?
  Phone in advance

  Phone for same day appointment

  Previous visit

Does anything happen between the time an appointment is made and the patient arrives?
  Cancellation

  Rescheduling

Do you do reminders?
  Calls

  Letters/cards

  Does your system generate reminders?

  Do you send forms to the patient to complete before their visit?

What do you do to prepare for the next day's appointments?
  What about work-ins?

  Do you get walk-in patients?

Who pulls the chart?
  Regular appointments

  Same day appointments/nurse visits

  Phone calls

When the chart is pulled do you check for outstanding labs, missing consults, etc.?
  What do you do if something is missing?

(By alerting pt./MD of missing information upstream, time and unnecessary visits can be saved)

Originated: April 2005
Revised: June 2005

Where do you put the next day's charts?

What do you do if you can't find them?

Scheduling - continued

Is there anything else?

Add additional questions here:

Patient Arrives (or not)

What do you do about no-shows?

Is there a standard process?

What do you do with the chart?

Policy vs. what really happens

What is your check-in process?

Information verification (how)

Papers the patient must sign

What is done with signed forms?

Do you add forms to the chart before putting it up for the MA?
(Can we get copies of the forms you use routinely?)

What do you do with papers the patient brings in, e.g., driver license, PE, etc.?

What forms (e.g., DOT, etc.) do you have on hand?

Are any electronic? Which?

Would you like to have forms electronically?

How do you let the MA know the patient is ready to be seen (patient and paperwork are ready)?

Do you do things differently for any of the MAs?

Is there anything else?

Add additional questions here:

Patient Visit: MA

MA picks up the chart and calls patient back	
MA begins visit	
Weight	Where is this done?
Vitals	Where is this done?
Review medications	
Other (e.g., foot exam, UA, strep screen, procedure set up)	
What does the MA document?	

How does the MA notify the MD the patient is ready and which is the next room?
   Chart in door
   Walkie-talkie
   Whiteboard	

Is there any communication between the MA and the MD other than that the patient is ready to be seen?
   Face-to-face
   Walkie-talkie
   Sticky note on the chart
   Whiteboard
What type of information is communicated?
	Are there variations between MAs, between MA & provider?

Is there anything else?	

Add additional questions here:

Exam

MD does exam

What does MD do if he needs something or needs the MA during visit?

    Lab

    Equipment

    Assistance with exam

Does the MA keep the MD on schedule? How?

What is the process when a patient has to leave the room for lab, x-ray, etc. and then comes back?

Visit documentation
    MD
    MA

Does MA put anything else in the chart after the patient leaves?

Is there anything else?

Add additional questions here:

End of visit

When is the visit documentation completed?

    As the visit concludes

    Immediately after the visit in the nursing station

    Between visits, when the MD has time

    At the end of the day

    Days/weeks later

    Usually within _____ hours/days

Originated: April 2005
Revised: June 2005

Is there variability between providers in the time it takes to complete the chart?

End of visit – cont.

What happens to the chart?

Goes with patient to check out

Goes to the doctors office

Sits in the work area for MD to work on as he has time

Other

Superbill

Who documents on the superbill?

Where does it go at the end of the visit?

How does it get there?

What are the steps until a bill is dropped?

Coders

Do they have the information they need?

How do they get their questions answered?

Data entry

Billers

Is there anything else?

Add additional questions he

Prescriptions

Does the MD ask if refills are needed?

If Rx needs to be written, do they have Rx pad, or do they have to leave the room?

How are they handled?

Written and given to patient

Fax

Other

Is there anything else?

Originated: April 2005
Revised: June 2005

Add additional questions here:

Lab

In house (describe the process)

Outside (describe the process)

    Hospital

    LabCorp

    Quest

How are lab results returned to the clinic?

    Who gets them?

    What do they do with them?

    When are they matched with the chart?

    Who matches them?

    Are results prioritized by type of test, or for abnormal results?

Do all results go to the doctor?

    How?

    What does the doctor do with them?

    How does the MD notify MA what needs to be done about the results and how does the MA get the information?

    How long does it take?

    Do results get to the patient?

    How?

        Letter

        Phone call

        What happens if patient can't be reached?

    Who?

    When?

    All results or only abnormal?

    What is documented?

How do you know that labs were ordered, done, results returned, seen by MD, and given to patient?

How is the loop closed?

Originated: April 2005
Revised: June 2005

Lab – cont.

Is there anything else?

Add additional questions here:

Referrals

What are your most common referral types?
Outside your practice
Internally within your practice

What are the ways the patients gets the referral?

How do you know the patient actually completes the referral?

How do you receive results of the referral, and what do you do with them?

How is the patient notified?

How do results get into the chart?

Is there anything else?

Add additional questions here:

Originated: April 2005
Revised: June 2005

Check out process

How does the patient check out?

Who checks out the patient?

Are follow up appointments made?

How is payment handled?
    Co-pay
    Billing

Who completes the super bill/encounter form?

Where does it go after the visit?

Is there anything else?

Add additional questions here:

Originated: April 2005
Revised: June 2005

Source: Arkansas Foundation for Medical Care

Glossary

A

abstract. to abstract data means to condense a record. In the context of medical records, entering data from the patient's paper chart into an EHR is abstracting. For example, the patient's problem list, current medications, allergies, personal history, and family history are entered into the electronic chart as a baseline of medical history (Ch. 1).

accession. a unique identifier (usually a number) (Ch. 7).

accounts receivable (A/R). arise when a company provides goods or services on credit; money that is owed to your group broken out by financial class (e.g., Private Pay, Medicare, Blue Shield, Commercial, etc.) and also by age (e.g., current to 30 days old, 31 to 60 days old, etc.) (Ch. 2 and 10).

addendum. text that is added to a progress note after it is signed (Ch. 8).

adjudicate. final determination of the issues involving settlement of an insurance claim; also known as a claim; settlement (Ch. 7 and 10).

advance beneficiary notice (ABN). a written notice (the standard government form CMS-R-131) that a patient receives from physicians, providers, or suppliers before they furnish a service or item to the patient, notifying him or her that Medicare will probably deny payment for that specific service or item; the reason the physician, provider, or supplier expects Medicare to deny payment; and that the patient will be personally and fully responsible for payment if Medicare denies payment. ABNs alert beneficiaries that Medicare might not reimburse for certain services even though physicians have ordered them; ABNs ask for patients' consent regarding financial liability when Medicare denies coverage; ABNs notify patients with Medicare insurance that either a service or services rendered will be the patients' financial responsibility to the physician/facility (lab) for payment (Ch. 7).

advance directive. legal documents, such as a living will, durable power of attorney, and health care proxy, that allow people to convey their decisions about end-of-life care ahead of time (Ch. 6).

aging. the classification of accounts by the time elapsed after the date of billing or the due date (Ch. 10).

American National Standards Institute (ANSI). form types that are claims electronically transmitted to a payer (Ch. 10).

American Recovery and Reinvestment Act (ARRA). also known as the "stimulus bill" signed into law by President Obama on February 17, 2009, which authorized the HHS to establish programs to improve health care quality through the promotion of HIT.

anthropometric. refers to a measurement or description of the physical dimensions and properties of the body, especially on a comparative basis; typically used on upper and lower limbs, neck, and trunk (Ch. 6).

Ask at Order Entry (AOE). represents questions you must provide to the lab when sending an order electronically or submitting a printed order (Ch. 7).

attestation period. the date that begins the 90-day reporting period of meeting the core and menu measures for meaningful use (Ch. 5).

B

batch. establishes defaults and assigns a name to a batch (group) of financial transactions you will be entering into Harris CareTracker PM and EMR. A new batch must be created to enter financial transactions (Ch. 3, 4, and 9).

C

cache. a space in your computer's hard drive and random access memory (RAM) where your browser saves copies of recently visited web pages (Ch. 2).

carve-out. when charges are entered for the patient, Harris CareTracker PM and EMR will automatically calculate and "carve out" the copayment amount for private pay (the amount for which the patient is responsible) (Ch. 3).

Certification Commission for Health Information Technology (CCHIT®). an organization appointed by the Department of Health and Human Services (HHS) to certify electronic medical record software (Ch. 5). An independent, not-for-profit group that certifies electronic health records (EHR) and networks for health information exchange (HIE) in the United States (Ch. 1).

chief complaint. in the patient's own words, the reasons for being seen for the visit (Ch. 4).

classification systems. organize related terms into categories for easy retrieval; used for billing and reimbursement, statistical reporting, and administrative functions (Ch. 1).

clearinghouse. a private or public company that processes health information and executes electronic transactions. It provides connectivity and often serves as a "middleman" between physicians and billing entities, payers, and other health care partners for transmission and translation of claims information (primarily electronic) into the specific format required by payers (American Medical Association) (Ch. 1, 2, and 9).

clinical templates. progress notes made within the EHR; allows documentation into EHR; must be interoperable (Ch. 1).

clinical vocabularies. a standardized system of medical terminology; set of common definitions for medical terms (Ch. 1).

compendium. a summary or abstract containing the essential information in a concise but brief form (Ch. 7).

Computer Physician Order Entry (CPOE). an application used by physicians and other health care providers to enter patient care information (Ch. 1).

context. a patient is "in context" when his or her information appears in the *Name* list and *ID* box. Pulling a patient into context populates the *Name Bar* with the patient's name and Harris CareTracker PM and EMR *ID* number, allowing you to perform patient-specific tasks. When a patient is in context, many transactions can take place in the patient's account, including editing the demographic record, rescheduling an appointment, and viewing any open balances (Ch. 3).

contraindication. a symptom or condition that makes a particular treatment or procedure inadvisable (Ch. 6 and 7).

copayment. a predetermined (flat) fee that an individual pays for health care services, in addition to what the insurance covers. For example, some HMOs require a $10 "copayment" for each office visit, regardless of the type or level of services provided during the visit. Copayments are not usually specified by percentages (Ch. 4).

covered entity. covered entities can include health plans, health care clearinghouses, and health care providers (Ch. 1).

crossover. a claim that is automatically forwarded from Medicare to Medicaid (or any other insurer) after Medicare has paid its portion of a service (Ch. 10).

crosswalk. (sometimes referred to as a "link") refers to a relationship between a medical procedure (CPT®/HCPCS code) and a diagnosis (ICD-9 code) (Ch. 9).

Current Procedural Terminology (CPT®). a nationally recognizable five-digit numeric coding system maintained by the American Medical Association (AMA) that is used to represent a service provided by health care providers in an outpatient setting (Ch. 1).

D

demographics. basic patient identifying information; defining or descriptive information on the patient (e.g., name, address, phone number(s), gender, insurance information, DOB (age), ethnicity, etc.) and defined as relating to the dynamic balance of a population, especially with regard to density and capacity for expansion or decline (Ch. 3).

designated record sets (DRS). any item, collection, or grouping of information that includes protected health information and is maintained by a covered entity (Ch. 1).

dispensable (drug). capable of being dispensed, administered, or distributed (Ch. 7).

E

edit. modifying the content of the input by inserting, deleting, or moving characters, numbers, or data (Ch. 3).

electronic health record (EHR). refers to the interoperability of electronic medical records or the ability to share medical records with other health care facilities (Ch. 1).

electronic medical record (EMR). patient records in a digital format (Ch. 1).

electronic protected health information (ePHI). protected health information that is created, received, maintained, or transmitted in electronic form (Ch. 1).

eligibility. (checks) determining whether a person is entitled to receive insurance benefits for health care services (Ch. 3).

EncoderPro. Harris CareTracker's partner for online code verification. It can be run to verify all the procedures, diagnoses, and modifiers entered for a patient. Running *EncoderPro* helps to ensure that correct coding information is entered and that claims are processed and paid quickly (Ch. 1 and 10).

encounter. an interaction with a patient on a specific date and time. Encounter types include visits, phone calls, referrals, results of a test, and more (Ch. 5 and 6).

encryption. refers to the conversion of letter or numbers to code or symbols so that its contents cannot be viewed or understood (Ch. 3).

event type. an action that is triggered by a macro such as a *ToDo*, fax, or mail message (Ch. 2).

explanation of benefits (EOB). detail of the amount of claim to the insurance company (or Medicare), any discounts for contracted rates, the percentage paid by the insurance or Medicare, denial reasons (codes), and balance due from the patient; sometimes accompanied by a benefits check (Ch. 3 and 9).

explosion codes. In Harris CareTracker PM and EMR, explosion codes can be built to include multiple CPT codes, which eliminates the need to enter each procedure individually. Creating one explosion code for this procedure reduces the amount of time it takes to enter the charge into the system. Valid modifiers for each procedure code can also be linked to them. Explosion codes are practice-specific and you can determine the descriptive name of the code set along with the CPT codes it will include (Ch. 9).

F

family history. displays part of a patient's medical history in which questions are asked in an attempt to find out whether the patient has hereditary tendencies toward particular diseases. Family history is to be present in all members' charts, including children (Ch. 6).

fee schedule. determines the amount charged for each CPT® code entered into Harris CareTracker PM and EMR (Ch. 2).

flowsheet template. a profile with selected items. Data in a patient medical record can be pulled into a flow sheet, eliminating the need for double entry. It accommodates multidisciplinary documentation requirements and is linked to progress notes, vital signs, and the results applications (Ch. 6).

formulary. defined by the Centers for Medicare & Medicaid Services as a list of prescription drugs covered by a prescription drug plan or another insurance plan offering prescription drug benefits (also called a drug list) (Ch. 7).

G

group number. typically identifies the employer (insurance) related (Ch. 3).

growth chart. provides a graphical method to compare a child's achieved growth with that of children of the same age and sex from a suitable reference population (Ch. 6).

H

Health Information Technology for Economic and Clinical Health (HITECH) Act. created as part of the ARRA ("Stimulus Bill"), that was signed into law on February 17, 2009 to promote the adoption and meaningful use of health information technology.

Health Insurance Portability and Accountability Act (HIPAA). passed in 1996, providing new directives for protecting patient information and providing security measures as well as specific instruction for electronically transmitting patient data where required (Ch. 1).

Health Level 7 (HL7). one of the world's leading developers of health care standards for exchanging information between medical applications, to devise a common industry standard for EHR functionality that will guide the efforts of software developers; a messaging standard used to transfer data between applications (Ch. 1).

Healthcare Common Procedure Coding System (HCPCS). (called level II) managed by CMS and classifies medical equipment, injectable drugs, transportation services, and other services not classified in CPT® (Ch. 9).

history of present illness (HPI). the patient's account of related symptoms for today's visit. The HPI is generated with the use of problem-focused templates, voice dictation, or handwriting and voice recognition (Ch. 4).

hybrid conversion. using a combination of paper and electronic data (Ch. 1).

I

inactive claims. claims that are not only unpaid, but also have not had any follow-up activity on them for the last 30 days (Ch. 10).

International Classification of Diseases (ICD). the internationally recognizable three- to five-digit code set representing medical conditions or signs and symptoms (standardized categorization of diseases); diagnosis codes used in a health care setting; standards developed by the World Health Organization (WHO) (Ch. 1).

iterations. the act of repeating (Ch. 6).

K

Knowledge Base. a repository of constantly updated product troubleshooting tips and procedures (Ch. 2).

L

Logical Observation Identifiers Names and Codes (LOINC®). a universal code system for identifying laboratory and clinical observations. LOINC® enables the exchange and aggregation of electronic health data from many independent systems and includes standardized terms for all kinds of observations and measurements (Ch. 1).

lot. a collection of primary containers or units of the same size, type, and style manufactured or packed under similar conditions and handled as a single unit of trade (Ch. 5).

M

macros. a grouping of one or more templates (Ch. 2).

meaningful use. the set of standards defined by the Centers for Medicare and Medicaid Services (CMS) incentive programs that governs the use of electronic health records and allows eligible providers and hospitals to earn incentive payments by meeting specific criteria; a term used by the CMS to ensure that electronic medical records are being used in a meaningful way or to their fullest potential. Medicare and Medicaid payments are affected by meaningful use (Ch. 1 and 5).

member number. a number that is typically assigned to individual family members on the insurance policy (Ch. 3).

minimum necessary. must provide only PHI in the minimum necessary amount to accomplish the purpose for which use or disclosure is sought (Ch. 1).

mnemonics. assisting memory (Ch. 9).

modifier. a two-character code added to a CPT® or HCPCS code that is used to help in the reimbursement process. For example, a modifier is used to explain that a procedure not normally covered when billed on the same day as another is actually a separate and significant process, or that it is a rural health procedure that gets higher reimbursement. Up to four modifiers can be attached to each CPT®, although in most cases only one or two are used (Ch. 1 and 9).

multi-resource appointment. an appointment that requires two or more resources. For example, if a patient is to be seen by a provider, but also needs an ultrasound at the same visit, the *Advanced* application allows you to book one appointment for both resources (Ch. 4).

N

National Drug Code (NDC). a code that identifies all medications recognized by the Food and Drug Administration (FDA) by vendor (manufacturer), product, and package size; number identifies a listed drug product that is assigned a unique 10-digit, 3-segment number (Ch. 1 and 10).

nomenclature. a system of terms used in a particular science (Ch. 1).

nonparticipating payer. a payer who chooses not to enter into a participating agreement to provide electronic eligibility checks for free (Ch. 3).

nonverbal communication. includes body language, gestures, eye contact, and expressions to communicate a message (Ch. 4).

notice of privacy practices (NPP). a document that describes medical practices policies and procedures regarding the use and disclosure of PHI (Ch. 1 and 3).

O

open encounter. documentation of a patient visit that took place that was never completed (Ch. 6).

open order. test or X-ray that the provider has ordered for a patient but the practice has not received the results of that test or X-ray (Ch. 2 and 6).

order. consists of a list of tests to perform on one or more patient specimens, for example, blood or urine (Ch. 7).

order set. a grouping of treatment options for a specific diagnosis or condition; predefined groupings of standard orders for a condition, disease, or procedure (Ch. 1).

override. used to either restrict an operator's access to certain applications and functionality, or it can be used to grant an operator additional privileges that may not be included in the operator's role (Ch. 2).

P

patient history. part of the medical record where you enter the patient's personal medical history, past medical history, and family medical history (Ch. 6).

practice management. referring to the "front office" of a medical practice, including functions such as the patient's record, financial, demographic, and nonmedical information (Ch. 3).

primary. first in order (Ch. 3).

private pay. refers to patients without insurance, or the balance due after insurance has adjusted the claim and paid any amount due under contract (Ch. 10).

progress note. the heart of the patient record, written by the clinician or provider, that describes the details of a patient's encounter and is sometimes referred to as a chart note. It serves as a chronological listing of the patient's overall health status. Data pertaining to the findings from the visit are entered into a progress note (Ch. 6 and 8).

protected health information (PHI). individually identifiable health information, held or maintained by a covered entity or its business associates acting for the covered entity that is transmitted or maintained in any form or medium (including the individually identifiable health information of non-U.S. citizens). This includes identifiable demographic and other information relating to the past, present, or future physical or mental health or condition of an individual, or the provision or payment of health care to an individual that is created or received by a health care provider, health plan, employer, or health care clearinghouse. For purposes of the Privacy Rule, genetic information is considered to be health information (HHS/NIH) (Ch. 1 and 3).

providers. people or organizations that furnish, bill, or are paid for health care in the normal course of business (Ch. 1).

R

Real Time Adjudication (RTA). refers to the immediate and complete adjudication of a health care claim upon receipt by the payer from a provider (Ch. 7).

recall. reminders to patients that an appointment needs to be booked. Rather than scheduling a future appointment, a recall (reminder) date is set for the appointment (Ch. 2 and 4).

receipt. receipts in Harris CareTracker PM and EMR identify a patient's previous balance, the activity of charges and payments for that date of service, and the new patient balance (Ch. 4).

resource. can be people, places, or things. Providers are always considered a resource, but an exam room or a piece of equipment can also be considered a resource. Something that requires a schedule is considered a resource because it has specific availability with days and times it can provide certain services. If the resource does not need a set schedule then it is not considered a "resource" in Harris CareTracker PM and EMR (Ch. 2 and 4).

responsible party. the individual who is responsible for any private pay balances; the remaining amount, if any, after insurance has paid its portion (Ch. 3).

revenue codes. practice-specific codes that give you an alternative way of reporting financial data in Harris CareTracker PM and EMR. Revenue codes can either be linked to specific CPT® codes on your fee schedule (e.g., "New Patient Office Visits"), or can be selected during the visit or charge entry to represent a specific servicing provider, billing provider, and location combination (e.g., "Evening Clinic") (Ch. 2).

roles. determine which Harris CareTracker PM and EMR modules and applications an operator can access (Ch. 2).

routed (drug). refers to the way that a drug is introduced into the body, such as oral, enteral, mucosal, parenteral, or percutaneous (Ch. 7).

Rx Norm. a standardized nomenclature for clinical drugs and drug delivery devices produced by the National Library of Medicine (NLM). The Rx Norm code supports interoperability between EHR systems (Ch. 7).

S

scope of practice. there is no single definition of a medical assistant and his or her scope of practice. All medical assistants must work under the direction of a physician or licensed health care professional. The employer is ultimately responsible and accountable for actions of the medical assistant. A medical assistant is not allowed to independently assess or triage patients, make medical evaluations, independently refill prescriptions, or give out drug samples without the approval of the physician (Ch. 1).

scrub. to verify technical and coding accuracy before claims are filed by identifying potential problems that will cause claim rejection or reduction in payment. The claim scrubber provides a comprehensive set of coding and technical edits. Each individual edit may be enabled or disabled completely for a specific claim type or for an individual payer (Ch. 1 and 9).

secondary. second in order (Ch. 3).

sensitive information. information regarding the patient's STD and HIV history as well as alcohol and drug history (Ch. 6).

sequelae. an after-effect of disease, condition, or injury; a secondary result (Ch. 1).

SIG. an abbreviation for *signa* in Latin (meaning "label" or "sign"). SIG codes are specific dosage instructions that are given when prescribing medications (Ch. 6 and 7).

stat. refers to "immediately" or "without delay" (Ch. 7).

subscriber. an individual who is a member of a benefits plan. For example, in the case of family coverage, one adult is ordinarily the subscriber. A spouse and children would ordinarily be dependents (Ch. 3).

subscriber number. refers to the insurance policy number (Ch. 3).

Surescripts®. the largest network of its kind and provides electronic connectivity between pharmacies (Ch. 6).

sustainability. the responsible use of resources (Ch. 1).

Systemized Nomenclature of Medicine, Clinical Terms (SNOMED-CT®). a comprehensive clinical terminology covering diseases, clinical findings, and procedures that allows for a consistent way of indexing, storing, retrieving, and aggregating clinical data across specialties and sites of care (Ch. 1).

T

"Tall Man" lettering. medication names that have mixed case lettering in the description name, for example, NEXium. This is to comply with the patient safety initiative endorsed by the Food and Drug Administration (FDA) and Institute for Safe Medication Practices (ISMP), which helps reduce errors between medication names that either look or sound alike (Ch. 7).

task classes. determine what types of appointments can be seen at what times; are the building blocks for a resource's schedule (Ch. 2).

TeleVox®. an automated appointment reminder and confirmation system that can be used to notify patients of upcoming appointments (Ch. 4).

template. a preformatted body of text; assigned to a specific group and a single macro (Ch. 2).

tertiary. third in order (Ch. 3).

titer. (having labs drawn) determines how much antibody is present in the patient's blood to fight a specific antigen (disease-causing agent) (Ch. 8).

ToDos. Harris CareTracker's internal messaging system (Ch. 6).

total conversion. when all paper records are converted to electronic records at once (Ch. 1).

transfer. the status of a patient when he or she has been taken to an exam room (Ch. 6).

treatment, payment, and operations (TPO). conditions under which protected health information can be released without consent from the patient (Ch. 1).

U

Unified Medical Language System (UMLS®). another clinical standard, which is a set of files and software that brings together many health and biomedical vocabularies and standards to enable interoperability between computer systems; that is, a thesaurus database of medical terminology (Ch. 1).

unknown status. results when the patient's primary insurance is a non-participating (non-par) payer (Ch. 3).

unpaid claims. claims that have been submitted to an insurance company but have not been paid (Ch. 10).

unsigned note. a progress note that was never signed (Ch. 6).

V

variance. difference between the allowed and payment amounts; the difference between the actual amount of money you received from the insurance company and the negotiated rate the insurance is responsible for paying (Ch. 9).

verbal communication. the use of language or the actual words spoken (Ch. 4).

W

workflow. how tasks are performed throughout the office (usually in a specific order); for example, the patient is checked in, insurance cards are scanned, the patient is taken to the exam room, vital signs are taken/recorded, and so on (Ch. 1 and 3).

Index

The letter *t* following a page number denotes a table; the letter *f* following a page number denotes a figure.

A

abstraction, of data, 7
AC (prescription abbreviation), 33*t*
access, to health information, 4
accession identifiers, 319
accounts receivable (A/R), 61*t*, 530
acronyms, 33, 33*t*–35*t*
action terms, in medical terminology, 40*t*
activation
    appointment recall, 195
    correspondence, 363–364
    patient address, 123
    of *TeleVox*® app, 198
activity logs, 81, 353–354, 354*t*
acute care, 33*t*
addendum, 410–411
addresses, 123–124, 137
adjudication, 381, 534*t*
adjustments, 64*t*, 489
Administration app, *Setup* tab, 86–99
Administration module, 14–15, 65
administrators, 128
Admissions app, 61*t*
advance beneficiary notices (ABNs), 323
advance directives, 285*t*
Advanced app, 159*t*, 192–193
Affordable Care Act (ACA), 6–7, 31
aging, of accounts, 530, 561
alerts
    duplicate charge, 470
    for missing documentation, 118, 121, 146
    purpose of, 115*f*, 118
    during registration, 146*f*
    types of, 236, 240*t*
    viewing, 240–241

Allergies app, 36*t*, 280–283
allergy information
    adding, 280–283
    viewing, 239–240
ambulatory care, 30, 33*t*
American Association of Professional Coders (AAPC), 18
American Medical Association (AMA), 23
American National Standards Institute (ANSI), 534
American Recovery and Reinvestment Act (2009), 6, 226
anthropometric variables, 298
appointment calendars, 188–191
appointment history, 158, 195–196
appointment types
    customization of, 161
    scheduling by, 92–93
    selection of, 164
appointments
    booking, 159–170
        directly, 163–165
        using Find, 166–168
        using Force, 169–170
    cancelling
        in *Advanced* application, 193
        with conflicts, 178–180
        upcoming, 175–178
    cancel/reschedule reasons for, 93–94
    conflicting, 178–180
    double-booking, 169–170
    existing, 163
    for family members, 191–192
    in front office management, 12
    monthly total of, 187
    multi-resource, 193
    non-patient, 180–182
    patient requests for, 61*t*
    recall, 193–195
    recurring, 61*t*
    reminders for, 63*t*, 193–201
    rescheduling, 171–175
        in *Advanced* application, 193
        conflicts, 178–180

        directly, 171–173
        using Find, 173–175
    viewing
        daily, 60*t*, 265–266
        by patient, 158
        for VIP patients, 185
        wait lists for, 60*t*, 183–187
Appointments app, 265
Ask at Order Entry (AOE), 320
Assessment and Plan (A&P) tab, 316
attachments
    handling, 244*t*, 285*t*
    insurance card, 146–147
    mail message, 443
    untranscribed voice, 63*t*
    viewing, 363
attestation period, 227, 230
audio files, transcription of, 63*t*
authorizations, 34*t*, 35*t*, 366–369, 375, 473

B

Back tab, 58
bank deposits, 64*t*, 523–524
Bar Chart format, 158, 191
Batch application, 203, 264
Batch Deposits, 64*t*, 523–524
Batch Level Rejections, 63*t*
batches
    clinical, 203, 204*f*
    creating, 208–211, 457–461
    definition of, 456
    eligibility check, 151–152
    financial, 203, 204*f*
    open, 61*t*
    paper claim, 481–487
    posting, 216–221, 477–478
    settings for, 204–206
    totals only view of, 217
    types of fields available for, 207*t*–208*t*
billing, for medical services
    batch creation for, 457–461
    certification requirements, 455
    completing a visit for, 376–391

Billing feature, 12–13, 59, 61*t*–63*t*, 456
billing statements. *See* statements
Book app, 158*t*, 159–187
Brandt, Jon S., 7
"break the glass" privileges.
    See overrides
Bulk Charges app, 61*t*, 513
Bush, George W., 6

C

cache
    clearing your, 47–48
    definition of, 46
calculators, dosing, 336
Calendar format, 158*t*, 188–191
cancellations, 93, 94
care management registries, 233–235
carve-out payments, 143
CCHIT® (Certification Commission for Health Information Technology), 2, 226
CDC (Centers for Disease Control and Prevention), 346
Centers for Disease Control and Prevention (CDC), 346
Centers for Medicare and Medicaid Services (CMS), 3, 59, 245
certification
    benefits of, 8, 9
    requirements
        appointment scheduling, 158
        billing, 455
        claims and collections, 529
        clinical documentation management, 397
        demographics and registration, 113
        electronic health record specialists, 2
        electronic medical records, 45, 225
        patient visit documentation, 315
        work-ups, 263

Certification Commission for Health Information Technology (CCHIT®), 2, 226
Certified Electronic Health Record Specialist (CEHRS™)
    clinical duties and definitions, 36
    employment opportunities, 29–30
    exam, 7–10, 36
    responsibilities, 8, 29
charges
    batch creation for, 457–461
    capturing, 382
    duplicate, 470
    editing, 471–475
    entering, 461–467
    for hospital visits, 473
    reversing, 471–475
Charges app, 64*t*, 513, 530–531
Charges on Hold app, 61*t*
chart numbers, 125, 133–134, 138
Chart Summary, 245–246
Chart Viewer, 243*t*, 429
charts
    accessing, 123
    printing, 245*t*
    updating
        allergy information, 280–283
        immunization, 283–284
        medications, 275–278
    viewing, 243*t*
check in, patient, 201–203, 266
Chief Complaint Maintenance app, 94–96
chief complaint (CC)
    adding, 95–96
    definition of, 36
    documenting, 291
    recording, 161, 164
claim numbers, search by, 134
claim statuses
    checking, 546–550
    possible, 549*t*
claims
    batch level rejection of, 63*t*
    editing, 470
    frequency codes, 544*t*
    inactive, 62*t*, 534*t*, 545–554
    open, 62*t*
    paper
        generating, 483
        printing, 481–483, 486
    processing, 532
    resolving, 536–544
    scrubbing, 3, 456
    settlement, 381
    submitting
        electronically, 478–481
        paper, 481–487
    unbilled, 19, 61*t*
    unpaid, 545–554
claims summary
    lines, 535–536
    screen, 537*f*, 537*t*–539*t*
ClaimsManager app
    claim scrubbing in, 456
    functions and purpose of, 530
    screening statuses, 469*f*
ClaimsManager Edit, 382
ClaimsWorklist app
    definition of, 62*t*
    functions and purpose of, 532–539
    working in, 540–544

classification systems, definition of, 15
clearinghouses, 4, 62, 478
Clinical Alerts, 240*t*
clinical batches, 203, 204*f*
Clinical Letter Editor, 357
clinical letters, 357–359
Clinical module
    application summaries, 59, 63*t*
    Daily Administration, 82–84
    Import/export, 86, 398, 448–449
    System Administration, 84–86
    toolbar, 243–245
Clinical Notes, 127, 240*t*
clinical templates, 33*t*
Clinical Today module
    Appointments app in, 265–267
    function and purpose of, 264, 265
    log in to, 206
    Tasks app in, 267–271
    viewing prescriptions in, 272–274
Clinical Toolbar, 243–245
clinical vocabularies, 34*t*
code set standards, 15
coding systems, 16–25
collection letters
    creating, 573–575
    form letters for, 569–572
    generating, 579–581
    global, 569–572
    group, 569
collection reports, 561*f*, 563*t*
collection statuses, 563–565
Collections Actual, 568
Collections app
    accessing, 563
    available actions in, 567–568
    financial classes, 561–562
    functions and purpose of, 62*t*, 560
Collections Pending, 565, 567, 568
Collum, T. H., 30
combining forms, in medical terminology, 39*t*
communication skills, 159
compendium, 325, 326
Computer Physician Order Entry (CPOE), 36–37
consent fields, 136*f*, 139
contact information, for operators, 75
Contents tab, 52
context, patient in, 116, 145
Contracts & Fees feature, 86–87
contraindications, 278
conversion, medical record, 7, 34*t*, 35
copayments, 215, 489, 522*t*
correspondence
    active/inactive, 363–364
    adding, 360–362
    attachments to, 363
    collection letters, 569–577
    printing
        attachments, 363
        log, 364–366
    recall, 443–444
    viewing, 363
Correspondence app, 357–366
    accessing, 359
    columns overview for, 357–366
Correspondence Log, 364–366
co-signatures, 387, 388*t*, 389, 390*t*
covered entities, 4, 17
CPOE (Computer Physician Order Entry), 36–37

CPT® codes, 23–24, 378, 468
credit balances, 62, 490, 497, 509–513, 521*t*
Credit Balances app, 62
credit cards, processing, 215
crossover claims, 534*t*, 544–545
crosswalk codes, 468
Current Procedural Terminology. *See* CPT® codes
Custom Order Questions, 325
Custom Resources, 96–97, 250–251
customization
    of appointment types, 161
    of education materials, 356
    of letter templates, 357
    of orders, 320, 325
CVX, 33

D

Daily Administration
    in *Clinical* module, 82–84
    in *Practice* module, 66–71
daily schedule management, 187–201
Dashboard, 58–65
    on *Home* module, 58
    Management, 58*f*, 59, 64*t*
    Meaningful Use, 58*f*, 59*f*, 65, 229–232
    Practice, 58*f*, 59, 60*t*–63*t*
Date Book format, 188
date of birth (DOB), 125, 138
deactivation
    appointment recall, 195
    correspondence, 363–364
    employment information, 129
    insurance information, 143–144
    patient address, 123
    phone number, 124–125
demographic reports, 148–149
demographics
    access restrictions to, 69
    claims billing and, 12–13
    definition of, 114, 118–119
Demographics app, 115*f*, 118–129, 146, 147, 149
denials
    adjusting balance after, 508–509
    entering, 504–505, 521*t*
    processing, 490
    transferring, to private pay, 507
    viewing, 503–504
Denials app, 62, 502–509
designated record sets, 34
diagnoses, searching for, 323
diagnosis and assessment, 36*t*
diagnosis codes
    explosion codes for, 468
    mapping, 21*f*, 465–466
    modifiers, 467, 468*f*
    searching for, 464
    systems for, 16–25
diagnostic orders, 316–317
DICOM (Digital Imaging and Communication in Medicine), 34*t*
Digital Imaging and Communication in Medicine (DICOM), 34*t*
directional terms, in medical terminology, 40*t*
disclosures, 360–361
Disease Management registries, 302*t*, 305

Document Management Upload app, 244*t*
documentation
    alerts for missing, 121, 146
    support, 51, 56–57
    uploading, 146–147, 245*t*
dosing calculators, 336
dropdowns. *See* Quick Picks lists
drug interactions, screening for, 245*t*
drug lists. *See* formularies
Drug Type list, 334, 335

E

E&M Evaluator, 245*t*
education materials, 354–356
EHR Incentive Programs, 6–7, 59, 65, 227, 229
electronic health networks, 26
electronic health record specialists
    duties of, 10
    employment opportunities, 29–30
    responsibilities of, 29
electronic health record systems, 9–10, 27*t*–28*t*
electronic health records (EHRs)
    acronyms and terminology associated with, 33*t*–35*t*
    advantages, 28–29
    components, 237–246
    conversion to, 7
    definition of, 2
    disadvantages, 30–31
    in electronic health networks, 26
    in hospitals, 30
    incentives for implementing, 6–7
    as legal records, 4
electronic medical records (EMRs). *See also Medical Record* module
    advantages, 28–29
    certification requirements, 225
    core functions, 27
    creating new patient, 119–120
    definition of, 2, 26
    and meaningful use, 226–229
    minimum requirements for, 118
    retrieving and updating, 274–275
Electronic Medication Administration Records (eMars), 34*t*, 36–37
electronic protected health information (ePHI), 34
Electronic Remittances app, 61*t*, 488–499
eligibility checks, 114, 151–153
eligibility field, 143
email messages, 105, 138
eMars. *See* Electronic Medication Administration Records
employer information, 145
employment information, 129–130
EncoderPro®, 16, 41, 469, 531–532
encounters
    creating, 239–240
    definition of, 239, 267
    for drop-in patients, 292
    forms for, 88
    in ICD-10 codes, 21
    and letters, 359
    missing, 61
    open
        definition of, 268
        resolving, 385–387

encounters (*continued*)
   in *Tasks* app, 269
   viewing, 383–384
   types of, 382
   viewing, 239–240
Encounters app, 387
encryption, 122, 125
entities. *See* covered entities
e-prescribing, 28
etiquette, 159–160, 311
event types, 100
explanation of benefits (EOB)
   definition of, 134, 456
   manually entering, 489
   printing, 499–502
explosion codes, 468

F

Family app, 158t, 191–192
family history, 36t, 284, 285t
family members
   editing and deleting, 192
   linking, 191–192
Favorite Labs app, 82–84, 251–254
Favorites tab
   adding tests to, 325
   education materials on, 354, 355
   for medications, 334–336
faxes, 99, 108–110, 345
fee schedules, 87
Financial apps
   in *Management* dashboard, 59, 64t
   in *Setup* module, 88–92
   in *System Administration*, 71–74
financial batches, 61t, 203, 204f
financial classes, 560–561, 568
fiscal periods, 71–74, 209
flash notes, 127, 138
flowsheets, 296–298
foreign addresses, 13, 124
form letters, 578–579
form types, for claims, 534
formularies
   definition of, 337
   tiered, 339
Forward tab, 58
front office management, 12, 59,
   60t–61t, 114. *See also* practice
   management

G

gender, 125, 126f, 138
general authorizations, 34t
generic drugs. *See* medications
Global Collection Letters, 569–572
Glossary tab, 57
Group Collection Letters, 569
group number, 142
Group Operators, 81
group providers, 139
growth charts, 298–301

H

Harris CareTracker Physician EMR, 3, 46
Harris CareTracker PM and EMR
   administration features and
      functions in, 65–71

background of, 2
care management registries,
   233–235
Help system for, 51–58
logging in to, 46–51
maintenance functions in, 251–262
navigation in, 58–65, 235–245
tools for assistance with meaningful
   use, 229–233
Harris CareTracker Practice
   Management (PM), 2–3, 46
Hash Cpt box, 210
Health Care Financing Administration
   (HFCA), 484–486
health information exchange (HIE), 2
Health Information Technology for
   Economic and Clinical
   (HITECH) Act, 226
health information technology (HIT), 34t
Health Insurance Portability and
   Accountability Act (HIPAA),
   5–6, 17
Health Level 7 (HL7), 9
Health Maintenance registries, 302t, 305
health plans, definition of, 34t
Health Tracker. See Patient Portal
Healthcare Common Procedural Coding
   System (HCPCS), 15, 23,
   24–25, 467, 468
Help system, 51–58
   Back tab, 58
   Contents tab, 52
   conventions used, 52
   Forward tab, 58
   Glossary tab, 57
   navigation methods in, 51–52
   Print tab, 57
   recorded training sessions, 53–54
   Search tab, 52–53
   Support tab, 56–57
   toolbar, 52, 52f
HFCA (Health Care Financing
   Administration), 484–486
HHS. *See* U.S. Department of Health
   and Human Services
History app, 159t, 195–196
   accessing, 284–291
   functions and purpose of, 284
   information found in, 285t
history of present illness (HPI), 36, 161
History tab
   appointment management in, 171,
      175, 177
   functions and purpose of, 159,
      195–196
HITECH (Health Information
   Technology for Economic and
   Clinical) Act, 226
Hold status
   charges on, 61t
   claims, 534t, 536t
   visits on, 61t, 382
Home module, 58–59
hospital admissions, 61t, 473
HPI (History of Present Illness), 36t, 161
HS (prescription abbreviation), 34t
hybrid conversion, of paper records, 7

I

ICD. *See* International Classification of
   Diseases
identification (ID) numbers

assignment of, 145
search by, 132–133
identifiers
   order, 319
   patient, 120, 130
idle time, Optum™ PM, 78
Immunization Export app, 86, 448–449
immunization lots
   adding, 255–257, 349–350
   managing, 244, 254–258
   modifying, 257–258
   reports for, 448–451
immunization records
   adding, 347–352
   printing, 352–353
   updating, 283–284
   where to manage, 244
Immunization Writer app, 347
Immunizations Activity Log, 353–354,
   354t
Immunizations app
   accessing, 346–347
   columns overview for, 347t
   functions and purpose of, 244,
      283, 352
Import/export
   applications on *Practice* tab, 67f
   clinical, 86, 398
In Network labs, 251
inactive claims, 62t, 534t, 545–554
incentive programs, 6–7, 59, 65,
   226–227, 229
incremental conversion, 34t
Institute of Electric and Electronics
   Engineering (IEEE), 33
Institute of Medicine (IOM), 27
insurance cards, 146–147
insurance information
   adding multiple, 143
   adding new, 129, 139–143
   deactivation, 143–144
   eligibility checks of, 151–153
   entering, 12–13
insurance payments
   pending, 88
   processing, 497–513
   verification, 517–523
Interactions Screening box, 278, 279f,
   343, 344t
International Classification of Diseases,
   17–23, 34t
   mapping system, 21f, 465–466
   9th edition, 17, 17t–18t, 20t,
      22t–23t
   10th edition, 18–20, 20t, 22t–23t
Internet Explorer, cache clearing in, 47
iterations, of vital data, 294

J

journals, 215, 216–220, 475–476

K

Knowledge Base, 56, 66
Krames StayWell, 354

L

lab orders. *See* orders

lab results
   browsing, 416
   codes for, 417
   color-coding of, 415
   electronic, 414, 415
   graphing, 423–424
   manually entering, 416–419
   printing, 424–426
   in *Results* app, 63
   unmatched, 415
   viewing, 414, 420
labs
   adding, 82–84, 251–254
   removing, 254
   searching for, 322
Letter Editor app, 569, 572, 576t–577t
letters. *See also specific types of letters, e.g.
      collection letters*
   creating, 357–359
   form, 578–579
Letters app, 357–359
locations, adding, 89–90
Locations app, 88
Logical Observation Identifiers Names
   and Codes (LOINIC®), 15
logos, company, 357
logs
   audit
      operator, 66–68
      user access, 64t
lot, definition of, 244
lot numbers. *See* immunization lots

M

macros and templates, 100
Mail app, 99, 103–106, 432
Main menu, 58
Manage Immunization Lots app, 254
Management dashboard, 58f, 59, 64t
marital status, 138
meaningful use, 6, 226–229
Meaningful Use dashboard, 65, 229–232
   screenshots, 230f, 231f, 233f
   tab, 58f, 59f, 232f
Medicaid, 6, 31, 227
medical history, 66t, 241, 284–291.
      See also Patient Medical History
Medical Record module
   advantages of, 235
   components, 235, 236t
   navigation, 235–246
Medicare, 6, 24, 31, 226–227, 245,
   290, 323
medications
   adding to Favorites list, 334–338
   interaction screening of, 343
   lists of, 36t
   mixed case lettering for, 343
   reconciliation, 35t
   updating, 275–278
   viewing active, 239–240
Medications app
   columns overview for, 331t
   functions in, 339, 345
   lists in, 330
   status categories in, 275t–276t
member number, 142
Menachemi, N., 30
Message Center, 99–110, 427–428, 433
messages
   accessing, 436
   addressing, 105

with attachments, 443
creating, 102–106, 432–436
deleting, 442
forwarding, 441–442
moving, 438–440
recording, 427–432
reply to, 440
ToDos, 100–103
viewing, 437–438
when to use, 432
Messages app, 58, 427–428
mini-menus
accessing, 185
check-in, 202–203
scheduling, 185–187
minimum necessary rule, 6
Missing Encounters app, 61
mnemonics, claims editing, 470
modifiers, for codes, 24, 467, 468*f*
Month app, 158*t*, 187–191
multi-resource appointments, 193
MVX, 35*t*
MyFax®, 345

N

Name Bar, 114–116
accessing *Chart Summary* through, 246
table of applications, 115*f*
names, of patients
entering, 122
search by, 130–132
National Center for Health Statistics (NCHS), 18
National Council for Prescription Drug Program (NCPDP), 35*t*
National Drug Code (NDC), 15, 376, 378, 542
National Health Information Network, 35*t*
National Healthcareer Association (NHA), 7–9
National Immunization Program (NIP), 35*t*
News app, 58, 59*f*
NIP (National Immunization Program), 35*t*
nomenclature, 15
nonparticipating payers, 151, 152
nonverbal communication skills, 159
notes
in cancelled appointments, 177
editing, 387–389
field, 126–127
flash, 127, 138
signing, 389–391
unsigned, 270, 386, 387
use of symbols in, 164
notice of privacy practices (NPP), 35, 121, 139, 140

O

Obama, Barack, 6, 31
Office of the National Coordinator-HIT (ONCHIT), 35*t*
ONCHIT (Office of the National Coordinator-HIT), 35*t*
online help, 51
Open Encounters app
accessing, 382–383

columns overview for, 384*t*
functionality of, 63
resolving visits in, 385–387
Open Items app, 489–490
Open Orders app, 319, 327*t*, 329
open orders, definition of, 63, 268
Open/Close Period, 71–74
Operator Activity Log, 81
Operator Audit Log, 66–68
Operator Settings app, 75
operators
adding, 77–80
monitoring, 68, 81
overriding roles of, 79, 80*f*
and roles, 77
setting preferences for, 204–206, 457
storing contact information for, 75
Operators & Roles app, 76–81
Operators Log, 68, 69*f*
Order Actions, 327*t*
Order Set app, 244*t*
order sets, 37
order types, 319*t*, 321, 325
orders
actions for, 327*t*
adding, 319–329
definition of, 319
identifiers for, 319
multiple, 327
open, 63, 268
printing, 329
requisitioning diagnostic, 316–317
searching for, 325
Orders app
accessing, 316–318
advanced features, 329
columns overview for, 319*t*
functions and purpose of, 242*t*, 244*t*
overrides
for accessing patient information, 69, 128
adding, 79–80
purpose of, 77

P

paper versus paperless records, 4
paperless records. *See* electronic health records
passwords
changing, 50–51, 75–76
formats of, 49, 78
override, 80*f*
preassigned, 46
requirements for, 15
past medical history, 36*t*, 285*t*
Patient Alerts, 120–122, 146*f*, 201
Patient Care Management Alerts, 240*t*
Patient Care Management app
accessing, 235, 302–303
columns overview for, 302*t*–303*t*
functions and purpose of, 302
sections within, 302*t*
updating in, 303–305
Patient Detail Bar
components, 236*t*–237*t*
location of, 236
purpose of, 236*t*
viewing, 237–239
Patient Education, 354–356
Patient Education app, 244*t*

patient history, 285*t*
patient identifiers, 120, 130
patient information
editing, 114, 146, 150
encryption of, 122
finding, 114–116, 117*ff*
viewing summary, 237–239
Patient Medical History
accessing, 246
functions of, 242*t*
purpose of, 236*t*, 241
Patient Portal, 61, 86–87, 103, 272–273
Patient Registration module, 114
demographics, 114–129
insurance information, 129–130
new patient registration, 122–128
patients
checking in, 201–203
pulling, into context, 116
searching for, 116
tracking, 202, 265–267
transferring, 266–267
payment history, 522*t*
payments
accepting, 211–215
accessing, 212
carve-out, 143
credit card, 215
entering, 212–215
insurance, 88, 497–513, 517–523
monthly total of, 64*t*
posting, 461–462, 489–494
unapplied, 61*t*, 513–515
unmatched, 498–499
with variances, 517–523
Payments on Account, 211
PDF Documents, 56
Pending Insurance, 88
personal health records (PHRs), 33*t*, 34*t*, 35*t*, 116, 117*t*
pharmacies, 330, 333, 334, 340–342
phone calls
etiquette during, 159–160
reminder, 196–197
phone numbers, 124–125, 137–138
photos, of patients, 123,
plan and treatment, 36*t*
PO (prescription abbreviation), 35*t*
positional terms, in medical terminology, 40*t*
Practice dashboard, 58*f*, 59, 60*t*–63*t*
practice management, 12–15, 66–71, 114
Practice module
Daily Administration, 66–71
on *Home* module, 58*f*
System Administration, 71–81
preferences, setting operator, 204–206, 457
prefixes, medical, 38*t*
prescriptions
abbreviations used with, 33*t*, 34*t*, 35*t*
creating, 332–333
electronic submission of, 345–346
faxing, 345
new, 274
printing, 339–340
viewing, 272–274
Prescriptions app, 63*t*
primary care providers (PCPs), 138, 140*f*
primary insurance, 143, 151
Print tab, 57
privacy, 31, 121
private pay balances, 531, 560, 565–567
progress notes, 306–311

addendums to, 410–411
and chief complaint, 161, 164
definition of, 36*t*, 398
deleting, 408–409
editing, 406–408
filtering, 389, 404–406
printing, 413
signing, 389–391, 411–412
templates, 306–307
unsigned, 270
unsigning, 412–413
viewing, 398–399
Progress Notes app, 398–404
columns overview for, 400*t*–401*t*
templates, 306–307
and website links, 356
protected health information (PHI), 4, 5, 121
Provider Portal, 103, 105
providers
definition of, 35
eligible Medicare, 227
group and primary care, 138
multiple, 167
searching for, 322

Q

queues, 99, 107–108
Quick Picks lists
adding
form letters, 578–579
items, 90–92
providers, 371–372
removing items from, 93

R

radiology orders. *See* orders
Real Time Adjudication (RTA), 381
recalls
adding, 444–446
appointment, 193–195
correspondence for, 443–444
overdue, 63*t*, 443
updating, 447
using TeleVox, 196
Recalls app, 158*t*, 193–195, 244*t*, 443–447
Recalls/Letter Due app, 443
receipts, printing, 215–216
Recorded Training feature, 53–56
reference tools, quick, 51
Referral app, 245*t*
referrals
incoming, 371–375
outgoing, 367–370
referred by field, 139
Referrals and Authorizations app, 364–375
registration
new patient, 122–127
VIP, 69, 127–128
registries
care management, 233–235
Disease Management and Health Maintenance, 302*t*, 305
relationship field and responsible party, 129
Release Notes, 57
release of information (ROI), 121
reminders. *See* recalls
remittances, electronic, 61*t*, 488–499

Remove from Collections, 568
renewals, prescription, 272–274
reports
    collection, 561*f*, 563*t*
    immunization lot number,
        448–451
    patient demographic, 148–149
    referrals and authorizations, 375
reschedules. *See* appointments
resources
    adding custom, 96–97, 250–251
    definition of, 96
    scheduling, 158
responsible party, 129, 139
Results app, 414–426
    columns overview for, 420*t*–421*t*
    customized views in, 421–422
    filtering by patient name in,
        422–423
    graph view in, 423–424
    and *Orders* app, 316
    printing options in, 424–426
revenue codes, 87, 88
Review of Systems (ROS), 36*t*
Rights of Individuals, 35, 121
roles, operator, 77–81
Room Maintenance
    adding, 98–99, 247–249
    editing, 249–250
ROS (Review of Systems), 36*t*
routed drugs, 335
Rowley, Robert, 30
RX New app, 274
Rx Norm, 332
RX Renewal app, 272–274
Rx Writer, 243*t*, 332–334, 336,
        340–341, 343

S

Safari, cache clearing in, 48
Scheduling app
    appointment types in, 92–93
    building schedules in, 92–99
    cancel/reschedule reasons in, 93–94
    chief complaint maintenance in,
        94–96
    custom resources in, 96–97
    room maintenance in, 98–99
Scheduling module, 158, 158*t*–159*t*
scope of practice, of medical assistants, 5
Screen feature, 245*t*
screening statuses, *ClaimsManager*, 531
scrubbing, a claim, 3, 456
Search tab, 52–53

secondary insurance, 143, 148
sensitive information, 285*t*
sequelae, 21
Setup module, 86–92
SIGs, 279, 334
Snipit Training feature, 55–56
social history, 36*t*, 284, 285*t*
social security numbers
    encryption of, 125, 126*f*
    entering, 138
    search by, 134–135
specialists orders. *See* orders
specific authorizations, 35*t*
Staff Measures app, 59, 64*t*
standards
    for classification, 15
    clinical, 33*t*
    definition of, 35*t*
stat, definition of, 319
statements
    generating, 554–557
    printing, 516–517, 558
    reprinting, 558–560
Statements app, 62
subscriber number, 142
subscribers
    adding new, 140–143
    definition of, 140
suffixes, medical, 38*t*–39*t*
Support tab, 56–57
Surescripts®, 272, 332
sustainability and electronic medical
        records, 4
symbols, use of, in notes and complaints,
        164
System Administration
    in *Clinical* tab, 84–86
    in *Practice* tab, 71–81
system readiness requirements, 46–47
Systemized Nomenclature of
        Medicine Clinical Terms
        (SNOMED-CT®), 15

T

Tab key, 119, 136
"Tall Man" lettering, 343
task classes, for appointments, 93
task sheets, 13*f*, 32*f*
Tasks app, 267–271
telephone calls. *See* phone calls
TeleVox® app, 158*t*, 159, 159*t*, 196–201
templates
    clinical, 33
    flowsheet, 296

letter, 357
    mail message, 104
    Message Center, 100, 427–428, 433
    progress note, 306–307
    removing selected, 96
terminology
    associated with electronic health
        records, 33*t*–35*t*
    medical, 37–40
        action, 40*t*
        combining forms, 39*t*
        common, 33–35
        directional, 40*t*
        positional, 40*t*
        prefixes, 38*t*
        suffixes, 38*t*–39*t*
tertiary insurance, 143
test frequency, 324
tests. *See* orders
titers, 448
ToDo app, 100–103
ToDos, 244*t*, 427–431
    creating, 100–101, 428–430
    definition and function of, 99
    filtering, 108
    for sending referrals, 375
    Support Center, 102
total conversion, of paper records, 7, 35
TPO (treatment, payment, and
        operations), 35*t*
tracking logs, viewing, 202
training sessions
    recorded, 53–56
    Snipit, 55–56
transactions. *See* financial batches;
        payments
Transactions module, 88, 489–490
transcription, of voice attachments, 63*t*
Transcription Import, 86
Transfer action, 567
transfers
    credit balance, 521*t*
    patient, 266–267
    private pay, 565–567
treatment, payment, and operations
        (TPO), 35*t*

U

Unapplied payments app, 61*t*, 513–515
Unbilled Procedures, 61*t*
Unified Medical Language System®
        (UMLS®), 15
unknown status, of insurance, 152
unpaid claims, 545–546, 550–554

unposted charges, 471–475
Unprinted statements app, 516
unsigned notes
    definition of, 270
    filtering for, 389
Unsigned Notes app, 386–389
    accessing, 387
    columns overview for, 388*t*
Untranscribed Voice Attachments, 63*t*
U.S. Department of Health and Human
        Services, 2, 9, 27, 31
User Access Audit, 64*t*
usernames
    case sensitivity in, 49
    and passwords, 15
    preassigned, 46

V

variances, 517–520
verbal communication skills, 159
Verify Payments app, 62, 517–523
View feature, 245*t*
VIP flag, 127–128, 139
VIP Patient Log, 69–71, 128
Visit Summary app,
        84–86, 316
visits
    capturing, 377–381
    completing, 316
    editing, 377, 380
Visits app, 245*t*, 316, 376–382
Visits By Day, 64*t*
Visits on Hold app, 61*t*, 382
vital signs
    definition of, 36*t*
    flowsheets for viewing, 296–298
    recording, 291–295
Vital Signs app
    filtering vital data in, 295
    functions and purpose of, 291

W

Wait List app, 60, 183–187
webinars, 51, 53
words, medical, analysis of, 37–38
workflow
    administrative, 10–11, 114
    clinical, 31–33
    definition of, 10
    in front office management, 114
    under ICD-10, 19